CLINICS IN DEVELOPMENTAL MEDICINE NO. 99/100

ORTHOPAEDIC MANAGEMENT IN CEREBRAL PALSY

Clinics in Developmental Medicine No. 99/100

ORTHOPAEDIC MANAGEMENT IN CEREBRAL PALSY

EUGENE E. BLECK, MD
Stanford University School of Medicine,
Stanford, California

1987
Mac Keith Press
OXFORD: Blackwell Scientific Publications Ltd.
PHILADELPHIA: J. B. Lippincott Co.

© 1987 Mac Keith Press
5a Netherhall Gardens, London NW3 5RN

First published 1987

British Library Cataloguing in Publication Data

Bleck, Eugene E.
  Orthopaedic management in cerebral palsy—
  (Clinics in Developmental Medicine No. 99/100)
  1. Cerebral palsy
  I. Title
  616.8'36   RC388

ISBN (UK) 0-632-01523-3
     (USA) 0-397-48004-0

Printed in Great Britain at The Lavenham Press Ltd., Lavenham, Suffolk
Mac Keith Press is supported by **The Spastics Society, London, England**

CONTENTS

FOREWORD

This book has two origins: Dr Samilson's 1975 monograph *Orthopaedic Aspects of Cerebral Palsy**, and Professor Bleck's own original volume, published by W. B. Saunders in 1979. The Samilson volume sought to bring together all that was then known about the subject, by collecting the work of experts from all over the world. By the time Professor Bleck came to write his volume, centres such as his own had developed and accumulated enough experience for one principal to write a comprehensive account of the orthopaedic management of cerebral palsy. Now, seven years after the first edition came out, considerably more experience and data have accumulated: particularly in relation to the management of hip and spinal problems in cerebral palsy.

The book aims to give a general account, so that it will be as useful to the paediatrician and therapist wanting to understand the orthopaedist as it will be to the orthopaedic surgeon who has decided to become involved in the care of people with cerebral palsy. It does not always provide the latter with technical details of how to perform the surgery, but it does provide him with the right approach and philosophy with which to select the appropriate procedure.

This is because the book is about management rather than surgery. The dramatic intervention of surgery forms only one part of the orthopaedist's involvement with the child with cerebral palsy. Too often in the past, the orthopaedist has intervened dramatically without trying to understand either the underlying neurology of the child's motor disorder, or the way in which the physical and social environment can modify the disorder. The thoughtful chapter on 'Goals, Treatment and Management' (Chapter 6) emphasises the integrated approach to the motor disorder in cerebral palsy. We thank him for sharing his experience with us.

MARTIN C. O. BAX

**Clinics in Developmental Medicine Nos. 52/53.* London: S.I.M.P. with Heinemann; Philadelphia: J. B. Lippincott.

PREFACE

When the first edition of this book* went out of print, many of my orthopaedic colleagues around the world asked me if there would be a new edition. The result is this new monograph on the same subject. Many colleagues told me that they liked the first edition because it was concise and well illustrated. In this new volume I have again tried to be as concise as possible without omitting important details, particularly in surgical procedures. I have drawn attention to the pitfalls of surgery, in the hope that the unintended results of instant and dramatic change in form and function due to the intervention will not be disappointing too often.

This is not a comprehensive work on all aspects of cerebral palsy. The associated defects and developmental problems (*e.g.* convulsive disorders, communication and education) are touched on, to give orthopaedic surgeons a perspective on the complexity of the condition and enable them to be conversant about it with their colleagues in pediatrics, general practice, neurology, and physical medicine and rehabilitation. In case more information on a particular defect in function is wanted, I have included a list of suggestions for further reading.

When indicated, I have added new sections and new information. In descriptions of operative procedures I have attempted to reference new procedures reported in the literature. The procedures I recommend have been tested with my own experience, although I am sure that other surgeons have their own preferences.

The format remains essentially the same, because of my opinion that the patient should be treated comprehensively rather than as isolated anatomical parts. Accordingly, the major sections are on spastic hemiplegia, spastic diplegia and total body involvement, with the operative procedures most commonly needed to correct the structural deformity in each of these three categories of geographical involvement. However, procedures described in one section will apply in another section when a particular deformity occurs. For example, the management of spastic equinus is in the chapter on hemiplegia, but would equally apply to equinus in diplegia.

The surgical treatment of paralytic scoliosis has changed so dramatically in the past six years that an entire chapter is devoted to it. I have updated the chapter dealing with neurobiology and its importance in the use of physical therapy. A separate chapter is devoted to physical therapy because physicians are usually asked to approve of a particular therapy program, or to certify it (in the United States a prescription is required). Consequently, a critique of current methods seems important if the physician's advice or authority to approve is requested. It would be most unwise for the physician to take responsibility for recommending the management of a child with cerebral palsy, and be detached from the physical and occupational therapists and their methods.

*Published by W. B. Saunders Company, 1979.

Some chapters such as those on the family and counseling might seem to have more to do with philosophy than science. So be it. No apology needs to be made for an apparent lack of science. Medicine, after all, fulfils a social need: it is an applied science and an art. To rise above the mere technocrat, the physician needs a philosophical base from which to work in this difficult, often frustrating, and sometimes depressing field.

I would like to acknowledge here the painstaking task of translating the entire first edition of my book into Chinese by Dr Cheng Chao-peng, Fourth Municipal Hospital, Zhengzhou, Henan, People's Republic of China. Despite my fairly intense efforts to find a publisher, I have failed to find any (including international agencies) to undertake the publication in Chinese. Perhaps with the growing awareness of China's importance in the world, this might be accomplished eventually.

Dr Sue Jenkins, Dr Martin Bax and Mr Edward Fenton of the Mac Keith Press deserve my thanks for all of their careful editing and many useful suggestions.

As in the first edition, I must thank the people of France: specifically Mme John Pila of Lyon who allowed us to use her villa in the 'presqu'Île Giens', Dr and Mrs Eric Bérard and their children who were our constant source of guidance in the ways of French living, and the people of the village of Giens-Hyêres, for allowing us to live so well while writing. To them I say: 'Je vous prie de croire dans mes sentiments très amicaux'.

EUGENE E. BLECK

1
INTRODUCTION

Definitions

Cerebral Palsy. Despite attempts to label the syndrome differently (*e.g.* static encephalopathy, permanent brain damage, or infirme moteur cérébrale), the term 'cerebral palsy' appears to have been adopted and understood worldwide (Stanley and Alberman 1984).

Many definitions have been offered over the years. The original descriptions by Little, Osler, and Freud left no doubt that it was not a disease but a collection of motor disorders due to lesions of the brain that originated at the time of birth or early childhood. Perhaps the most suitable description is Ingram's (1955):

> Cerebral palsy is used as an inclusive term to describe a group of non-progressive disorders occurring in young children in which disease of the brain causes impairment of motor function. The impairment of motor function may be the result of paresis, involuntary movement or inco-ordination, but motor disorders which are transient or are the result of progressive disease of the brain or attributable to abnormalities of the spinal cord are excluded.

Tone. This term has come into common usage in the United States, particularly with physical therapists. People speak of 'hypertonicity' and 'tone'-inhibiting plasters rather than spasticity or spastic paralysis. Muscle tone is defined as: 'The state of partial contraction in which the muscles maintain their posture without fully relaxing. It is due to low-frequency asynchronous impulses from the anterior horn cells which produces a tetanus' (Butterworths 1978). Muscles have visco-elastic properties, that create resistance and tension (McMahon 1984), as well as contractile ability initiated by nerve impulses. The definition of tone given here resembles what one would expect in what we call dystonic posturing. Muscles at rest, *e.g.* during sleep, show no electrical activity when examined with electromyography.

Reflexes. A reflex is a simple motor action, stereotyped and repeatable; it is elicited by a sensory stimulus, the strength of the motor action being graded with the intensity of the stimulus (Shepherd 1983). In 1950 Konrad Lorenz suggested that many of the individual motor actions and motor responses of animals could be described as *fixed action patterns*. The characteristics of these are a complex motor act, involving a specific temporal sequence of component acts; it is generated internally, or elicited by a sensory stimulus. The stimulus acts as trigger, and should cause release of the motor act (Shepherd 1983).

A *myostatic reflex* is when the muscle that was stretched contracts and the reflex feeds back to the stretched muscle via the neural circuit through the spinal cord. It is also called a *stretch reflex* because it is elicited by stretch (Shepherd 1983).

1

The nature of spastic paralysis is usually described as a condition of increased sensitivity of the muscle to stretch, resulting in contraction from the recruitment of all the fibers within the muscle. The continuous contraction of a spastic muscle when it responds to passive or active stretch (*e.g.* during walking) can be called a 'myostatic reflex'—*i.e.* the contraction of the muscle feeds back to cause more contraction.

In contrast to spastic paralysis, muscle in athetosis (when examined with electromyograms) demonstrated tonic patterns of electrical activity on both voluntary and involuntary movements. Hallett (1983) found that in ballistic movement patterns, there was excessive firing of both agonist and antagonist muscle groups. Classification based upon electromyographic analysis has been tried, but is unsuccessful in refining what we can observe by clinical examination.

Infantile reflexes and automisms can be considered as 'fixed action patterns'. They are a complex motor act elicited by a sensory stimulus. Examples are the Babinski sign, the Moro reflex, and the tonic neck reflexes (Baird and Gordon 1983).

Classification
The original classification by Freud (1892) was based upon a presumed pathological lesion in the brain, and was used for many years (Ingram 1984). Some of these classifications are complex. Some were introduced after the long hiatus between Little's and Freud's descriptions, during which time cerebral palsy was relegated to the 'wastebasket' of diseases which did not fit into the paradigms of the 19th century (Accardo 1982). The classifications now used date from developments after World War II, when the interest in cerebral palsy was rekindled because of the success of the poliomyelitis vaccine.

To be valid, a classification has 'to be repeatable in relation to the same subject, both by the same and different observers'. It also needs to be sensitive, *i.e.* efficient in labeling cases which may or may not fall into a class according to an established reference. This ability to classify correctly cases which are not 'genuine' is called 'specificity' (Alberman 1984*a*).

I prefer the term *spastic diplegia* to paraplegia. The mental picture we have of a spastic diplegic child is one who has obvious spasticity in the lower limbs, and none in the upper limbs except for fine motor co-ordination defects. Most were born prematurely with a birthweight less than 2500g, and their prognosis for life function is generally good.

Paraplegia means that there is absolutely no involvement in the upper limbs, and no associated defects. The importance of precision in describing a patient as paraplegic is that if the child is a genuine paraplegic, the diagnosis may not be cerebral, and a spinal-cord lesion or hereditary spastic paraplegia should be considered.

Total body involved has become increasingly accepted as a term appropriate to those who have obvious involvement of all four limbs, together with abnormal posturing and movement of the trunk, head and neck. Most of those called 'quadriplegic' fit this term better. Isolated spastic paralysis of four limbs without truncal involvement must be rare.

2

Triplegia exists if we are describing definite and gross spastic paralysis in three limbs. In this text the surgical treatment applicable would be that done in hemiplegia (upper limb) and diplegia.

Because this monograph is concerned mainly with the orthopaedic management of the spastic type of cerebral palsy, the classification submitted attempts to be precise in describing the movement disorder. Frequently dystonia is confused with spasticity. Dystonic postures are not amenable to orthopaedic surgery. The *tension athetosis* described by Phelps does seem different from spasticity. These patients are usually total body involved, and overzealous release of presumed spastic muscles can result in the opposite deformity, *e.g.* total hip flexor 'release' can become a postoperative extension contracture of the hip.

Athetoid patients sometimes do develop structural changes such as scoliosis and degenerative arthritis of the spine or hips. Their orthopaedic problems can be surgically treated as in normal patients. Limb surgery is rarely required, because contractures are uncommon.

Classification of severity
Attempts have recently been made to refine the terminology used to describe severity, and base it on a set of standards of functional ability (Jarvis and Hey 1984). The evolving consensus is that the severity of the motor disability ought to be analyzed from the standpoint of function. Terver and colleagues (1981) devised a set of scorable functional abilities in both independence and efficiency in a prospective study of goal-setting for 71 total body involved children. The details of these assessments of function are presented in Chapter 6.

It is harder to quantify the severity of the spasticity, athetosis, dysequilbrium, or ataxia itself. An attempt was made by Jarvis and Hey (1984), who used three tests: (i) grip strength with a hand-held dynamometer, (ii) manual dexterity utilizing the Purdue pegboard test, and (iii) the lower-limb running, speed and agility subtest of Bruininks and Oseretsky. Again the results are preliminary because of lack of normal controls, and the relatively small number of cerebral-palsied children tested. Their data did suggest a correlation with the over-all score of the functional assessment.

Quantification of the motor disorder by instrumentation is an attractive and fascinating option. Cinematography has been used for years, but again the assessment of severity was a perception of the viewer. Electromyography seems limited in quantifying the degree of spasticity in the muscles tested; one should be cautious in placing too much emphasis on the peaks and volume of electrical discharges recorded graphically. As pointed out by Murray (1976), the volume and strength of the electrical discharges is dependent upon the density of motor endplates in the muscle. For example, the obicularis oris muscles are packed with motor endplates and will have stronger and denser muscle firing, while the peroneus longus (with more sparsely distributed motor units) will have less proportionate firing, especially with fine wire or needle electrodes.

The optical recording of movement of the lower limbs and trunk in ambulatory patients appears to be the best way to measure abnormal movement compared to

3

normal standards. The cadence, velocity, and step length in gait are easy to measure (Chapter 3 provides more detail on these methods).

Energy requirements for walking or for wheelchair mobility do measure efficiency. The heart rate during the activity compared with the resting state is a simple way of assessing energy requirements for the individual patient. Measurements of oxygen consumption at rest and with activity are a more complex, but possibly more accurate, method of analysis (see Chapter 3).

In the patient who can stand unassisted, the objective measurement of balance should be relatively easy, with either pizoelectric force plates or strain gauge platforms linked with a computer program. We have developed this kind of instrumentation and computer analysis in the study of postural mechanisms in idiopathic scoliosis (Adler *et al.* 1985).

The World Health Organization has proposed a definition of terminology of impairment, disability and handicap (Alberman 1984*b*). All of the following definitions are used 'in the context of health experience':

(1) *Impairment*: any loss or abnormality of psychological, physiological or anatomical structure or function.

(2) *Disability*: any restriction or lack as the result of the 'impairment' of ability to perform an activity in a normal manner or within the range considered normal.

(3) *Handicap*: a disadvantage for a specific individual as the result of an 'impairment' or a 'disability', that limits or prevents the achievement of a rôle that is normal for age, sex, and socio-cultural milieu.

My conclusion is that all of our patients with cerebral palsy are impaired, and some are disabled. Our rôle is to help these individuals cope with their handicap so that they can lead as normal a life as possible.

Etiology

Because the consulting orthopaedic surgeon is often asked by parents to explain the cause of their child's disorder, I have included a brief review of the most common etiologies. Classifications based upon etiology were proposed by Sachs and Petersen in 1890 (Ingram 1984); but Freud objected, on grounds which are still valid today: (i) because of the frequent impossibility of identifying the time and nature of the brain damage; (ii) because a large number of patients had normal births, and no relevant family histories (in my own patient population seen during the past 30 years, 25 per cent have no known etiology), and (iii) knowing the etiology has little clinical value (Ingram 1984). As a broad generalization, a history of premature birth makes the diagnosis of spastic diplegia likely; and similarly a history of erthyroblastosis fetalis indicates that the diagnosis will be tension athetosis, with the associated defects of hearing loss and paralysis of the upward gaze.

The clinician must recognize the limitations of knowledge on etiology, and avoid pejorative speculative statements to parents such as: 'It's brain damage due to birth injury' or 'It's due to lack of oxygen at birth'. The latter statement usually comes from parents who want confirmation of their presumptions. My usual response is: 'On the contrary, we *used* to think these babies needed more oxygen. The result was administration of a lot of oxygen which caused blindness (retrolental fibroplasia).

This was indeed tragic because not only did the infant develop cerebral palsy, but had the additional handicap of blindness.'

Prematurity and low birthweight
Numerous studies have been done that demonstrate the relationship between a short gestation, low birthweight and cerebral palsy. Infants weighing less than 1501g, regardless of gestation, had a risk of cerebral palsy 27 times greater than for fullterm babies weighing 2500g or more (Ellenberg and Nelson 1979). Although the relationship between premature birth and cerebral palsy is close, other factors may be involved. It is not known if the cerebral damage is due to the effect of premature birth on the development of neurons, or to the risks of premature delivery which may result in intraventricular hemorrhage (Stanley and Alberman 1984).

Clearly the association of premature birth and low birthweight with cerebral palsy (usually spastic diplegia) is strong enough to suggest that prevention of preterm birth and low birthweights would eliminate almost half of the current caseload of children with cerebral palsy (in our analysis of 423 children with cerebral palsy, 43 per cent had premature births). The causes of prematurity are unknown, though many factors have been suggested: (i) social and cultural (Stanley 1984, Harel and Anastasiow 1985); (ii) racial (whites had a higher prevalence of cerebral palsy in Nelson and Ellenberg's 1979 study); and (iii) genetic and familial (Klebanoff *et al.* 1984). In an extensive review paper on the subject of low birthweight and its contribution to infant mortality and childhood morbidity, McCormick (1985) concluded that 'despite increased access to antenatal services, only moderate declines in the proportion of low birth weight infants has been observed, and almost no change has occurred in the proportion of those with very low birth weight at birth'.

Perinatal obstetrical problems
Prolonged and difficult labor, breech birth, prolapsed umbilical cord and birth trauma have all been shown to be commonly associated with cerebral palsy. Prenatal problems complicate the analysis of the etiology as well, so the examining physician should be cautious in assigning an etiology to a single event or entity occurring at birth.

Neonatal asphyxia
Birth asphyxia has been recognized as a cause of cerebral palsy. Nelson and Ellenberg (1981) studied the Apgar scores of 49,000 infants who they followed to the age of seven years. Apgar scores were recorded at one and five minutes, and in those with scores of less than 8 at five minutes, scores were also recorded at 10, 15, and 20 minutes. In Nelson and Ellenberg's study, 55 per cent of the children with cerebral palsy had Apgar scores of 7 at 10 minutes; 53 per cent of those with cerebral palsy had a score of 7 at five minutes. Of the 99 children who had scores of 0 to 3 at 10, 15, and 20 minutes, 12 per cent had cerebral palsy, and 11 per cent were

(Continued on page 14)

5

TABLE 1.I

Classifications of movement disorders

Type	Major clinical findings	Common etiology
I. PHYSIOLOGICAL (according to the movement disorder)		
1. *Spasticity (pyramidal)*	Increased stretch reflex in muscles, *i.e.* hypertonicity of 'clasp knife type' (Fig. 1.1)	Prematurity Perinatal hypoxia Cerebral trauma Rubella (maternal) Familial
	Hyperreflexia (deep tendon reflexes) Clonus Positive Babinski sign Esotropia or exotropia	
2. *Athetosis* (a) Tension type	Tension can be 'shaken out' of limb by examiner (Fig. 1.2) Extensor pattern (usually) Normal or depressed reflexes Paralysis of upward gaze Deafness (often)	Kernicterus due to Rh incompatibility
(b) Dystonia	Intermittent distorted posturing of limbs, neck, trunk (Fig. 1.3) No contractures Full range of joint motion when relaxed	

(Continued on page 8)

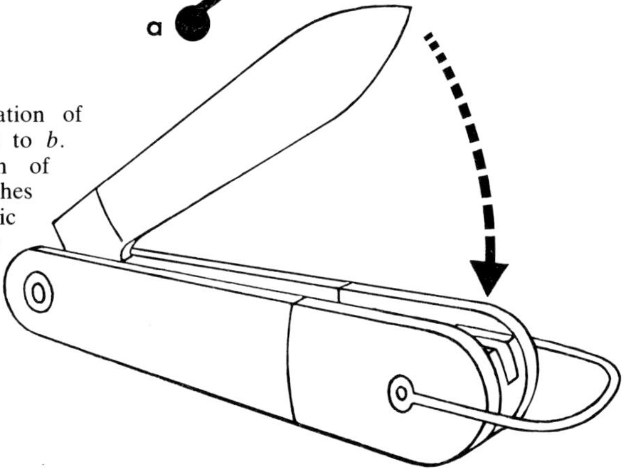

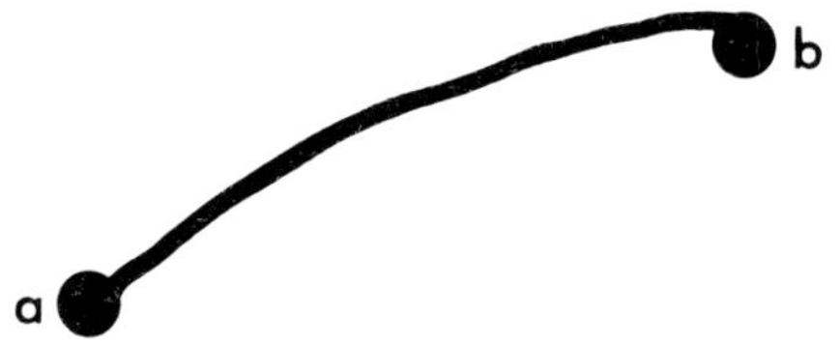

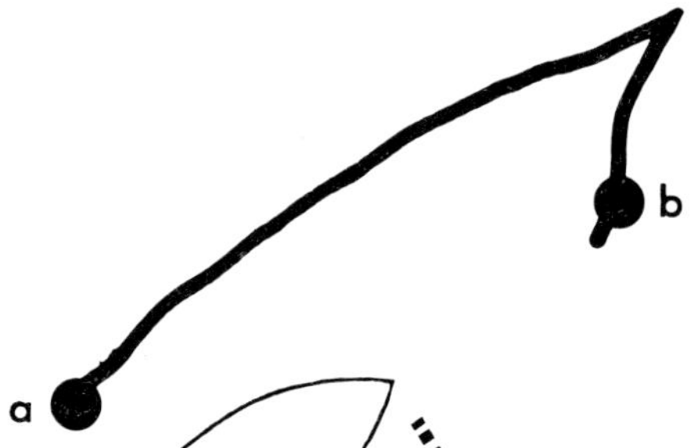

Fig. 1.1. *Above:* graphic representation of normal motor control from points *a* to *b*. *Above right:* graphic representation of spastic motor control—the patient reaches but overshoots the mark. *Right:* symbolic representation of characteristic spastic muscle which on stretch responds like a clasp knife (redrawn from Gesell and Amatruda 1947).

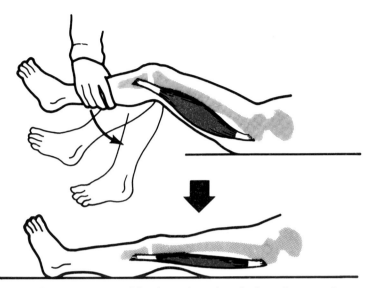

Fig. 1.2. In contrast to spasticity, in tension athetosis the resistance and response of the muscle to repetitive and fast stretch relaxes ('flails').

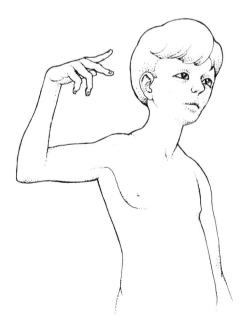

Fig. 1.3. Typical posturing of upper limb in hemidystonia. No contractures develop, and the limb will assume a normal posture when the patient relaxes completely (redrawn from Bleck and Nagel 1982).

Table 1.I contd.

Type	Major clinical findings	Common etiology
(c) Chorea	Spontaneous jerking of distal joints (fingers and toes) (Fig. 1.4)	Neonatal jaundice Hyperbilirubinemia Cerebral anoxia Encephalitis, meningitis, or both
(d) Ballismus (rotary, flailing)	Uncontrolled involuntary motions of proximal joints (shoulders, elbows, hips and knees) (Fig. 1.5)	
(e) Rigidity	Rigid limbs (i) Lead pipe type—continuous resistance to passive motion (Fig. 1.6) (ii) Cog-wheel type—discontinuous resistance to passive motion (Fig. 1.6)	

(Continued on page 10)

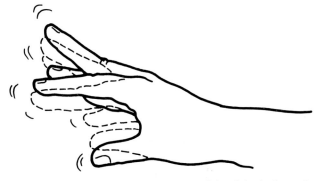

Fig. 1.4. Chorea—involuntary movements of the digits (redrawn from Bleck and Nagel 1982).

8

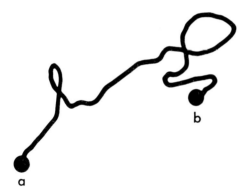

Fig. 1.5. Graphic representation of motor control in athetosis (redrawn from Gesell and Amatruda 1947).

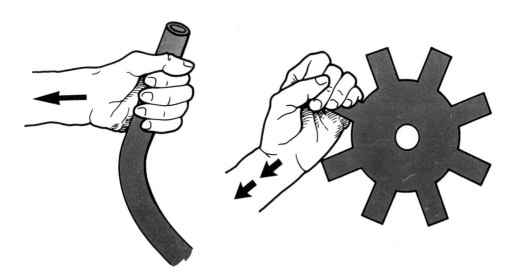

Fig. 1.6. Rigidity. *Left:* lead pipe type. *Right:* cog-wheel type.

Table 1.I contd.

Type	Major clinical findings	Common etiology
3. *Ataxia*	Lack of balance Unco-ordinated movement Dysmetria (Fig. 1.7) Dysarthria Wide-based gait (patient sways when walking) (Fig. 1.7) Pes valgus (flexible) common	Head injury Cerebral maldevelopment
4. *Tremor*	Rare Intentional or non-intentional (Fig. 1.8) Rhythmic or non-rhythmic	
5. *Atonia*	Rare Hypotonia of limbs and trunk (Fig. 1.9) Often evolves into athetosis as child matures	Cerebral anoxia
6. *Mixed types*	Spasticity and athetosis usual Total body involvement usual	Encephalitis Cerebral anoxia Birth trauma

(Continued on page 12)

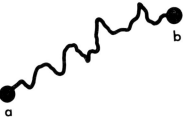

a

b

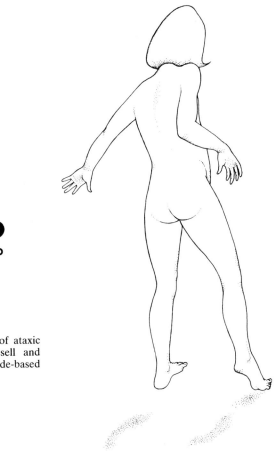

Fig. 1.7. *Above:* graphic representation of ataxic motor performance (redrawn from Gesell and Amatruda 1947). *Right:* typical ataxic wide-based gait (redrawn from Ducroquet 1968).

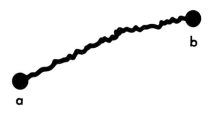

a

b

Fig. 1.8 (left). Graphic representation of tremor (redrawn from Gesell and Amatruda 1947).

Fig. 1.9 *(right)*. Graphic representation of hypotonia (or flaccid paresis). Motor control permits going from point *a* to point *b*, but weakness causes the limb to 'fall off' the terminal point (redrawn from Gesell and Amatruda 1947).

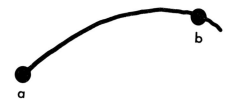

a

b

Table 1.I contd.

Type	Major clinical findings	Common etiology

II. TOPOGRAPHICAL

Type	Major clinical findings	Common etiology
Monoplegia	One limb involved Spasticity (usually) Patient should run to exclude hemiplegic pattern	
Hemiplegia	Spastic upper and lower limb on same side (Fig. 1.10)	
Paraplegia	Lower limb involvement only Rare in spastic type of cerebral palsy Common in familial type Spasticity	
Diplegia	Minor involvement of upper limbs (slight inco-ordination of finger movement) Major involvement of lower limbs (Fig. 1.11) Spasticity	
Triplegia	Three limbs involved Spasticity	
Quadriplegia or total body involved	Total body involvement (all four limbs, head, neck and trunk) (Fig. 1.12) Spastic, athetoid and mixed types	

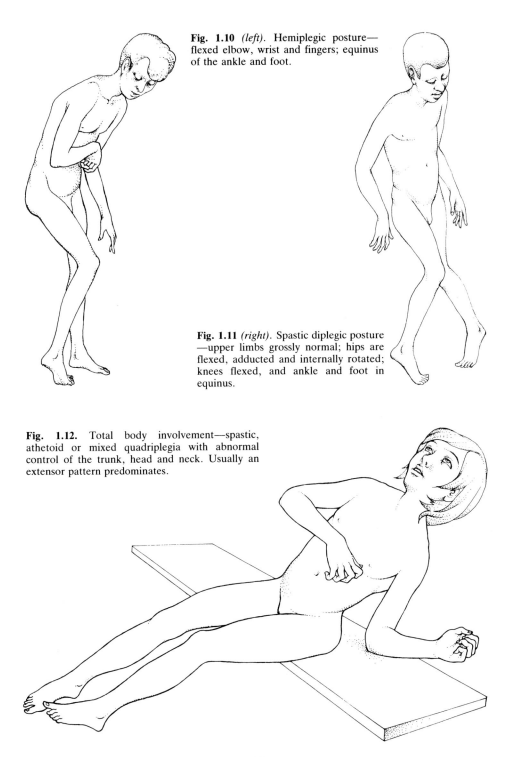

Fig. 1.10 *(left)*. Hemiplegic posture—flexed elbow, wrist and fingers; equinus of the ankle and foot.

Fig. 1.11 *(right)*. Spastic diplegic posture—upper limbs grossly normal; hips are flexed, adducted and internally rotated; knees flexed, and ankle and foot in equinus.

Fig. 1.12. Total body involvement—spastic, athetoid or mixed quadriplegia with abnormal control of the trunk, head and neck. Usually an extensor pattern predominates.

mentally retarded. However, three-quarters of the survivors of severe asphyxia had intact neurological functions when examined at the age of seven years.*

Kernicterus
Athetosis and associated deafness due to erythroblastosis fetalis with kernicterus has practically disappeared in Western countries (Stanley 1984). This tremendous advance in prevention is due to the advance of biomedical science in first discovering the Rh factor and the Rh antibody, immunization of Rh-negative women, intrauterine diagnosis and transfusion of the fetus, and the early diagnosis of neonatal jaundice with subsequent treatment by exchange transfusions and phototherapy. Cultural factors may also have contributed, because sensitized women may be having fewer children, and because of a general fall in multiparae.

Postnatal infections
The majority of cases of neonatal meningitis are due to gram-negative bacteria (Stanley and Blair 1984). In recent years, there have been more infections due to group B β-hemolytic streptococci (Haslam *et al.* 1977).

Postnatal central nervous system infections, either bacterial or viral, accounted for the etiology of cerebral palsy from 47 per cent to 63 per cent of the cases in New York, Chicago, and Western Australia (Stanley and Blair 1984).

Prenatal
Although in our own patient population, 25 per cent of the cases had no known etiology (the 1981 study by O'Reilly and Walertynowicz reported 19.1 per cent as 'idiopathic'), more and more prenatal causes of cerebral maldevelopment are being discovered. Even though the pathological lesions are being increasingly identified by the techniques of computerized axial tomography, magnetic resonance imaging and positron emission tomography, we are not certain of the reasons for abnormalities in the developing brain.

Rarely, cerebral palsy may be caused by genetically determined traits, most of which are autosomal recessive traits. Congenital ataxia is probably this kind of familial cerebral palsy (Stanley 1984). Familial spastic paraplegia has been reported, and I have seen two such patients (both of Armenian descent) whose pedigree strongly suggested an autosomal dominant trait.

Environmental influences which produce teratogens are known. Examples are endemic cretinism in New Guinea due to iodine deficiency, Minamata disease due to mercury contamination of food in Japan, and fetal alcohol syndrome. The viral infections of rubella and cytomegalovirus, and intrauterine toxoplasmosis, can also damage the developing brain. Smoking during pregnancy is now recognized as a cause of fetal growth retardation. Although I have seen no reports, it seems likely that drugs such as marijuana, cocaine and heroin could pass the placental barrier and adversely affect cerebral development.

*Experimental neonatal asphyxia in monkeys, and the resultant brain lesions, were studied by Ranck and Windle (1959). Asphyxia in these newborn monkeys beyond 25 to 30 minutes demonstrated brain damage in those who survived.

14

Postnatal

When the acute phase of a cerebral insult in a previously normal child has evolved into a non-progressive motor disorder, the child is then labeled as having cerebral palsy (neurologists seem to prefer the term 'static encephalopathy').

The leading cause of postnatal cerebral palsy is infection (60 per cent), followed by head injury (20 per cent). Cerebral anoxia due to near drowning, suffocation, and postoperative or intraoperative cardiac arrest account for 2 to 13 per cent of the cases reported. Cerebral vascular accidents vary with the location of the report from about 5 to 12 per cent. The residual brain damage from tumors in childhood were a cause of cerebral palsy in 8 per cent of the cases from New York. Heavy metal encephalopathy (lead) accounted for 2.4 per cent of 624 postnatal cases studied in Chicago (Stanley 1984).

Prevalence

The word 'prevalence' is chosen rather than the commonly used 'incidence' because of Alberman's recommendations (1984a): 'Prevalence is the number of cases of the disease present during a certain time-period'. Because cerebral palsy is by definition a permanent condition, birth prevalence is expressed as the number of cerebral palsy cases per 1000 neonatal survivors. Because the very early diagnosis of cerebral palsy is hazardous, due to the fact that infants who have some early neurological abnormality may have none by the age of seven years, over-interpretation of birth prevalence data needs to tempered (Nelson and Ellenberg 1982).

Epidemiological information is sometimes needed by clinicians when planning for services and special programs. Prevalence in school-age children, for example, can be used in a particular geographic area. Birth prevalence rates are remarkably similar in all Western countries—close to 2.0 per 1000 (Paneth and Kiely 1984).

REFERENCES

Accardo, P. J. (1982) 'Freud on diplegia—commentary and translation.' *American Journal of Diseases of Children*, **138**, 452–456.
Adler, N., Bleck, E. E., Rinsky, L. A., Young, W. (1986) 'Balance reactions and eye–hand coordination in idiopathic scoliosis.' *Journal of Orthopaedic Research*, **4**, 102–107.
Alberman, E. (1984a) 'Describing the cerebral palsies: methods of classifying and counting'. *In:* Stanley, F., Alberman, E. (Eds.) *The Epidemiology of the Cerebral Palsies. Clinics in Developmental Medicine No. 87.* London: S.I.M.P. with Blackwell Scientific; Philadelphia: J. B. Lippincott. pp. 27–31.
—— (1984b) 'World health initiatives.' *In:* Stanley, F., Alberman, E. (Eds.) *The Epidemiology of the Cerebral Palsies. Clinics in Developmental Medicine No. 87.* London: S.I.M.P. with Blackwell Scientific; Philadelphia: J. B. Lippincott. pp. 32–34.
Baird, H. W., Gordon, E. C. (1983) *Neurological Evaluation of Infants and Children. Clinics in Developmental Medicine Nos. 84/85.* London: S.I.M.P. with Heinemann; Philadelphia: Lippincott.
Bleck, E. E., Nagel, D. A. (1982) *Physically Handicapped Children: A Medical Atlas for Teachers, 2nd edn.* Orlando, Florida: Grune & Stratton.
Critchley, M. (Ed.) (1978) *Butterworths Medical Dictionary, 2nd edn.* London: Butterworths.
Ducroquet, P. (1968) *Walking and Limping.* Philadelphia: J. B. Lippincott.
Ellenberg, J. H., Nelson, K.B. (1979) 'Birthweight and gestational age in children with cerebral palsy or seizure disorders.' *American Journal of Diseases of Children*, **133**, 1044–1048.

Gesell, A., Amatruda, C. S. (1947) *Developmental Diagnosis, 2nd edn.* New York: Harper & Row.

Hallett, M. (1983) 'Analysis of abnormal voluntary and involuntary movements with surface electromyography.' *Advances in Neurology*, **39**, 907–917.

Harel, S., Anastasiow, N. J. (Eds.) (1985) *The At-Risk Infant.* Baltimore and London: Paul H. Brookes.

Haslam, R. H. A., Allen, J. R., Dorsen, M. M., Kanofsky, D. L., Mellito, E. D., Norris, D. A. (1977) 'The sequelae of group B β-hemolytic streptococcal meningitis in early infancy.' *American Journal of Diseases of Children*, **131**, 845–849.

Ingram, T. T. S. (1955) 'A study of cerebral palsy in the childhood population of Edinburgh.' *Archives of Disease in Childhood*, **30**, 85–98.

—— (1984) 'A historical review of the definition and classification of the cerebral palsies.' *In:* Stanley, F., Alberman, E. (Eds.) *The Epidemiology of the Cerebral Palsies. Clinics in Developmental Medicine No. 87.* London: S.I.M.P. with Blackwell Scientific; Philadelphia: Lippincott. pp. 1–11.

Jarvis, S., Hey, E. (1984) 'Measuring disability and handicap due to cerebral palsy. *In:* Stanley, F., Alberman, E. (Eds.) *The Epidemiology of the Cerebral Palsies. Clinics in Developmental Medicine No. 87.* London: S.I.M.P. with Blackwell Scientific; Philadelphia: Lippincott. pp. 35–45.

Klebanoff, M. A., Graubard, B. I., Kessel, S. S., Berendes, H. W. (1984) 'Low birth weight across generations.' *Journal of American Medical Association*, **252**, 2423–2427.

McCormick, M. C. (1985) 'The contribution of low birth weight to infant mortality and childhood morbidity.' *New England Journal of Medicine*, **312**, 82–90.

McMahon, T. A. (1984) *Muscles, Reflexes, and Locomotion.* Princeton: Princeton University Press.

Murray, M. P. (1976) *Personal communication.*

Nelson, K. B., Ellenberg, J. H. (1979) 'Neonatal signs as predictors of cerebral palsy.' *Pediatrics*, **64**, 225–232.

—— —— (1981) 'Apgar scores as a predictor of chronic neurologic disability.' *Pediatrics*, **68**, 36–44.

—— —— (1982) 'Children who outgrew cerebral palsy.' *Pediatrics*, **69**, 529–536.

O'Reilly, D. E., Walentynowicz, J. E. (1981) 'Etiological factors in cerebral palsy; an historical overview.' *Developmental Medicine and Child Neurology*, **23**, 633–642.

Paneth, N., Kiely, J. (1984) 'The frequency of cerebral palsy: a review of population studies in industrialised nations since 1950.' *In:* Stanley, F., Alberman, E. (Eds.) *The Epidemiology of the Cerebral Palsies. Clinics in Developmental Medicine No. 87.* London: S.I.M.P. with Blackwell Scientific; Philadelphia: Lippincott. pp. 46–56.

Ranck, J. B., Windle, W. F. (1959) 'Brain damage in the monkey Macacca mulatta by asphyxia neonatorum.' *Experimental Neurology*, **1**, 130–154.

Shepherd, G. M. (1983) *Neurobiology.* New York and Oxford: Oxford University Press.

Stanley, F. (1984) 'Prenatal risk factors in the study of the cerebral palsies.' *In:* Stanley, F., Alberman, E. (Eds.) *The Epidemiology of the Cerebral Palsies. Clinics in Developmental Medicine No. 87.* London: S.I.M.P. with Blackwell Scientific; Philadelphia: Lippincott. pp. 87–97.

—— Alberman, E. (1984) Birthweight, gestational age and the cerebral palsies.' *In:* Stanley, F., Alberman, E. (Eds.) *The Epidemiology of the Cerebral Palsies. Clinics in Developmental Medicine No. 87.* London: S.I.M.P. with Blackwell Scientific; Philadelphia: Lippincott. pp. 57–68.

—— Blair, E. (1984) 'Postnatal risk factors in the cerebral palsies.' *In:* Stanley, F., Alberman, E. (Eds.) *The Epidemiology of the Cerebral Palsies. Clinics in Developmental Medicine No. 87.* London: S.I.M.P. with Blackwell Scientific; Philadelphia: Lippincott. pp. 135–149.

Terver, S., Levai, J. P., Bleck, E. E. (1981) 'Les buts raisonnables que l'on peut fixer à un infirme moteur cérébrale gravement handicapé.' *Motricité Cérébrale*, **2**, 55–68.

16

2
NEUROLOGICAL AND ORTHOPAEDIC ASSESSMENT

The orthopaedist usually acts as a consultant upon referral of a pediatrician, family practitioner, neurologist or physiatrist, and consequently does not need to concentrate on the detailed examination of associated defects common to cerebral palsy. However, the surgeon does need to have at least a working knowledge of problems beyond the malfunction of the locomotor system. There are many excellent texts devoted to sensory and behavioral problems (Paine and Oppé 1966, Beadle 1982, Baird and Gordon 1983, Goble 1984).

Occasionally the etiology of an orthopaedic condition will not have been diagnosed: for example, a unilateral valgus deformity of the foot with peroneal spasticity. In these instances the orthopaedic surgeon will have to use all the diagnostic skills he or she can muster: being aware of the refinements of certain parts of the neurological examination, and as with all patients, doing a complete physical examination to collect the data necessary to form an opinion.

History

Where available, medical records should be scanned for pertinent information on the prenatal, perinatal and postnatal events, and the child's development. Records may contain useful information on past treatment, especially if surgery has been performed. In view of the common illusion by patients that not enough time has been spent with them, rather than read the record in isolation, I prefer to bring the past record with me to the examining room, and scan the record with the parents. In this way I can ask them questions to clarify certain parts of the history.

Too much importance can be attached to past records. Parents often exhibit considerable anxiety if records have not been received from referring sources. If they have not, I usually say that we can manage and do the job 'from scratch', and the physical examination should show us what surgery has been performed. Often physical or occupational therapists' records are lacking in systematic and serial recordings of the status of mobility, functional abilities in daily living, and verbal ability. Some system of recording the child's progress should be considered if physical, occupational and speech therapists' reports are to be of maximum value to the physician. For examples of serial checklists in recording function in one experienced center see Tardieu (1984).

Basic one-time historical data should be included in the consultant's record (Fig.2.1). A nurse or physician's assistant can obtain this information from the parents, and record it on a standard form. Birthdate, sex, and ethnic background is obviously required. The details of the prenatal, perinatal and postnatal histories are often clues to the etiology. The family history will indicate possible

(Continued on page 22)

17

BACKGROUND INFORMATION

Patient Identification:	Dates of Onset of Disease:

1. Name:

2. Chart #:

Write: 1 if present, positive
   0 if absent, negative

3. Birthdate:

50. Chief Complaints

4. Sex: male = 1   female = 0

5. Race:

     Caucasian 1   Indian 4
     Negroid 2   Mex-Am 5
     Oriental 3   Other 0

6. Age when complaint first noted:

7. Complaint first noted by:
     1 Patient   6 G.P.
     2 Parent   7 Pediatrician
     3 Relative   8 Orthopaedist
     4 Friend   9 Other M.D.
     5 Nurse   Specify

   Doctors consulted about complaint:
8.   Name:
     Address:
9.   Name:
     Address:

10. Referred by (agency or M.D.)
     Name:
     Address:

11. CCS _____   Medi-Cal_____
    Private ____   (check one)

12. Referred by staff of Medical Center
                   1 if yes
    _____   0 if no

CODES   DATES OF ONSET

(1) Poor posture   ____ ____ ____
(2) Backache   ____ ____ ____
(3) Leg ache, cramps   ____ ____ ____
(4) Night pain   ____ ____ ____
(5) Toe-in   ____ ____ ____
(6) Toe-out   ____ ____ ____
(7) Throws leg   ____ ____ ____
(8) Limps   ____ ____ ____
(9) Flat foot   ____ ____ ____
(10) Crooked foot   ____ ____ ____
(11) Club foot   ____ ____ ____
(12) Tip toes   ____ ____ ____
(13) Not walking   ____ ____ ____
(14) Weakness   ____ ____ ____
(15) Clumsy, falls   ____ ____ ____
(16) Spinal curvature   ____ ____ ____
(17) Cerebral palsy   ____ ____ ____
(18) Brain damaged   ____ ____ ____
(19) Dislocated hip   ____ ____ ____
(20) Other: ____ ____ ____

____
____

Fig. 2.1. Format for 'one-time' background information. Numbers on left-hand side of column are for computer data input as desired. *(Figure continued on following pages.)*

18

Past Medical History:

13. Past or Prior Treatment_____

    1 None   5 Corrective Shoes

    2 Exercises   6 Dennis-Browne Splint

    3 Milwaukee Brace   7 Surgery

    4 Casts

14. Progress_____

    1 improved   2 unimproved

    0 worse   3 don't know

       PAST SURGERY – Type & Dates

_____

_____

_____

_____

_____

Name of Surgeon or Institution:

_____

_____

General Past History
Childhood Diseases:

Allergies:

Family History:

    Mother_____

    Father_____

    Brother_____

    Sister_____

29. Scoliosis_____

30. Neurological or muscle disease_____

31. Flat feet_____

32. Pigeon toed_____

33. Diabetes_____

34. Hemophilia_____

    Bleeding Disorder_____

Pre- and Perinatal History:

43. Pregnancy_____

             NORMAL 1   ABNORMAL 2

15. Gestation (weeks)_____

16. Birth Weight (lbs./gms)_____

42. Labor_____

             NORMAL 1   ABNORMAL 2

    Duration of Labor (hrs)_____

17. Breech Birth_____

18. Caesarean Section_____

19. Cardiorespiratory Problem_____

20. Isolette_____

21. Convulsion (first week)_____

22. Rh – mother_____

    Rho Immunization – mother_____

23. Jaundice_____

    Fluorescent light Rx_____

    Bilirubin Serum_____

25. Abnormal Blood Chemistry_____

    Specify_____

              (e.g. hypoglycemia)

_____

Early Childhood Development:

Fussy Baby
26. Colicky ...._____
27. Convulsions............_____
   Sat alone................_____
   Stood up ...._____
28. Walked.................._____
   Talked ...._____

Immunizations:

	CHECK	DATES IF KNOWN
DPT	_____	_____
Smallpox	_____	_____
Polio	_____	_____
Rubella	_____	_____
Mumps	_____	_____
Measles	_____	_____
Other	_____	_____
Tetanus booster	_____	_____

Late Childhood Development:

Grade In School _____
35. Scholastic Achievement _____
                              AVERAGE 1

_____   _____
ABOVE AVERAGE 2 BELOW AVERAGE 3
36. Athletic Participation _____   _____
                         NONE 0   MINIMAL 1

_____   _____
AVERAGE 2   ABOVE AVERAGE 3
37. Special Classes or School _____
   Hand Use _____   _____
                 RIGHT 1   LEFT 2

_____
              AMBIDEXTROUS 3
38. Learning Disorder _____
39. Hyperactive _____
40. Takes Medication for Learning or
   Hyperactivity _____
   Name of Drugs and Dose _____
   _____
41. Takes Anticonvulsants _____
   Name and Dose _____
   _____

VISIT NUMBER / YEAR / DATE	DISEASE ONSET TO FIRST VISIT	1	2	3	4	5	6	7	8	9	10	11	12	13	14
VISIT NUMBER															
YEAR															
DATE															

INSTRUCTIONS: if an entire system is the "same" or "normal" then "S" or "O" may be placed in the system box (shaded) and will apply to all subheadings under the system.
KEY: S .... Unchanged; O .... Normal; (blank) .... Not Asked; +, 2+, 3+, 4+ .... Degrees of Abnormal

	VISIT NUMBER	Past	1	2	3	4	5	6	7	8	9	10	11	12	13	14
100	Height (cms)																
101	Weight (Kg)																
	BP—Systolic																
	BP—Diastolic																
	Temperature (°C)																
	Respirations/min.																
	Pulse Rate																
	ORTHOPAEDIC EXAM.																
	GAIT																
125	Normal																
850-851	Antalgic L / R																
852-853	Trendelenberg																
854-855	Tip-toes (equinus)																
129	Toes-in (degrees)																
130	Toes-out (degrees)																
860-861	Short Leg																
132	Spastic-Knee Flexed																
133	Spastic-Knees Hyperextended																
134	Spastic-Knees Normal																
135	Athetoid-dystonic																
136	Athetoid-choreiform																
137	Ataxic																
138	Base Gait-Heel to Heel (cms)																
139	Uses Crutches																
	Uses One Crutch or Canes																
	Uses One Cane																
140	Uses Walker																
141	Walks With Person Holding																
142	Cannot Walk																
143	In Wheelchair																
144	Transfers In & Out of Wheelchair																
102																	
	LIMB LENGTH																
158	Right Lower Limb (cms)																
159	Left Lower Limb (cms)																
	Right Upper Limb (cms)																
	Left Upper Limb (cms)																
	Leg Lengths Equal																

genetic factors. School achievement and placement may be relevant. When scheduling surgery, it is very important to know about past illnesses such as chickenpox (varicella), what the child is immune to, and recent exposure if not immune. A history of allergies (especially to antibiotics) is vital if surgery is contemplated. A knowledge of convulsive disorders and medications taken regularly is necessary for preoperative planning and postoperative care.

The physician's recording of the history (beyond the details from the past record and the one-time data base) is essential. After the usual introductions, which include talking directly to the child, the physician should ask what the problems are. The clinician can delve into the history in more detail and gain insight into the parent's perception of their child's behaviour: what their expectations might be, what fears they have and what hostilities are harbored. Some of this conversation might best take place without the presence of the child.

This process will not only establish an all-important rapport, but may also reveal the diagnosis. The late Douglas Buchanan (Professor of Pediatric Neurology, University of Chicago) taught that if you put the infant or young child on the mother's lap, and listened to the history, she would tell you the diagnosis (Buchanan 1967).

Orthopaedic neurological examination
The tools required are simple: toys, some small wooden blocks, round beads or pebbles, various objects of readily identifiable shape (triangles, circles and squares), a few coins, objects with differing textures, a tape measure, a goniometer, a small reflex hammer, a pocket flashlight, a wax pencil, a right-angled triangle, and a rule 5 to 8cm long. The wax pencil and right-angled triangle are useful for drawing on radiographs when explaining the findings to parents; the metric ruler can be used to measure discrepancies of anatomy (particularly the hip) visualized in radiographs. One instrument *not* needed in the examination of children with cerebral palsy is a sharp pin or needle! Loss of pain sensation in these children must be very rare.

If space is limited, it is more important to have a large corridor or waiting-room than a large examination room. Because cerebral palsy is defined primarily as a disorder of motion, the child must have adequate space in which to demonstrate movement. A corridor 2.5m wide and 9m long (I prefer 15m) is necessary for observational gait analysis. This corridor should be well lit, carpeted with a compact firm surface, warm and well ventilated. The examination room should be large enough to contain a padded table, 75cm wide, 75cm high and 185cm long. A step stool is important, to observe the child's climbing ability. There should be room for three chairs, for members of the family and observers (such as a social worker).

To be adequately examined, children should be undressed to their underwear, and socks and shoes removed. Gowns ought to be abolished! For 13 years we have used shorts for boys and girls, and a triangular halter for girls who want their modesty protected. If keeping cloth garments on hand is a problem, we have found disposable paper shorts and halters practical and cost-effective.*

The sequence of the examination described here is what I have evolved over the years. Others will have their own style of proceeding. The objective of the sequences, and the blend of the neurological with the orthopaedic examination, is to avoid shifting the child too often from one position to another as will occur when the orthopaedic examination is totally separate from the neurological. The purpose of the examination is to collect accurate data, effectively and efficiently, for the best possible analysis of the problem. It is the means by which the ends are achieved: a rationale for the recommended management, and a record that will permit subsequent evaluations.

The following sequences of the examination depend upon the age of the child and the status of his or her locomotor system. In infants and young children (under the age of six years), it is best to start with the assessment of the upper limbs while the child is in the security of the mother's lap.

In older children who can stand and walk (with or without external supports), I begin with assessing the standing posture, then the observational gait analysis, then (with the child sitting) the upper limbs are examined and tested for function and sensation, and finally the lower limbs are assessed. This is done with the child seated, knees flexed over the edge of the table, so that the deep tendon reflexes and the Babinski sign and its modifications can be elicited; in this sitting position the range of motion of the foot and its degree of axial rotation and tibial-fibular torsion are best determined. Then the lower limbs can be assessed with the child lying supine and prone on the table.

In children who cannot walk or stand, obviously the spine and sitting posture need to be examined in this position. The spine and pelvis alignments are most effectively observed with the child sitting (assisted by the parents) with legs over the edge of the table.

Studying the child's general appearance is appropriately termed 'the indirect examination' by Baird and Gordon (1983). This means we observe the behavior of the child, verbal ability, facial configuration and expression, eye contact, head control, drooling, general build, nutrition and mood. One can sense supportive, depressed or hostile parents. If the child is not sitting but moving about on the floor, movement disorders, postures, and hand preference can be ascertained. Appropriate toys should be available. During this time it should be possible to see how the child communicates.

Supine posture

Posture accompanies movement like a shadow; movement begins in posture and ends in posture (Sherrington, quoted by Rushworth 1964).

The supine posture of the infant and young child (less than seven years old) who cannot stand or walk, or the child older than seven years who has never walked, is

---

*Details about the purchase of these can be obtained from the Orthopaedic Clinic Nurse, Children's Hospital at Stanford, 520 Sand Hill Road, Palo Alto, CA 94304, USA.

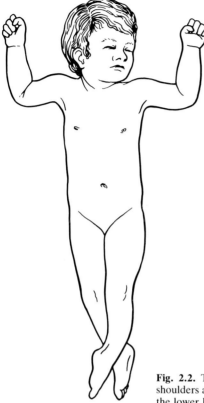

Fig. 2.2. Tonic labyrinthine reflex. When the baby is supine, the shoulders are abducted and elbows flexed, the spine is extended, and the lower limbs extended and abducted.

best examined *after* the upper limb and sitting posture assessments.

Retraction and abduction of the shoulders, elbow flexion, and an extension of the trunk and lower limbs is called the 'tonic labyrinthine reflex'. It is common in infants who have central nervous system lesions. When such infants are placed prone, the upper and lower limbs assume a flexed position. These postural abnormalities of a delayed development of the central nervous system were described by Magnus, and were thought to originate in the brainstem mediated through the upper cervical nerve roots (Bobath 1954) (Fig.2.2).

Infantile automatisms and postural responses can be tested while the infant or child is supine. Seven tests are considered valid for prognosis of walking, but only after the age of 12 months (Bleck 1975). The tests are performed in the following sequence (see Chapter 5 for the interpretation of these responses for the purpose of a locomotor prognosis).

1. *Asymmetrical tonic neck reflex.* With the child supine, turn the head to one side and then the other. A positive response is flexion of the upper and lower limbs on the skull side, and extension on the face side—the 'fencing' position. The reflex may be found to a minor degree in normal infants up to the age of seven months,

24

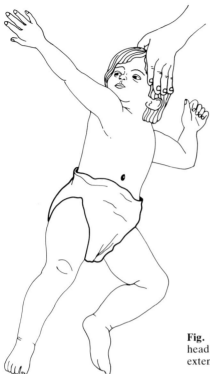

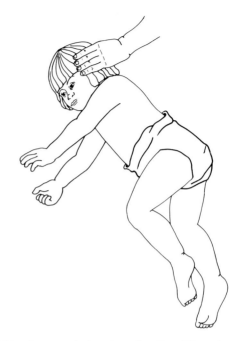

Fig. 2.3 *(left)*. Asymmetrical tonic neck reflex. When the head is turned, the limbs flex on the skull side (occipital) and extend on the face side.

Fig. 2.4 *(right)*. Neck-righting reflex. When the head is turned, the trunk and limbs turn to the same side.

but it is never normal if it can always be imposed and the child cannot move his or her limbs out of their position while the head is held turned to the side (Paine and Oppé 1966) (Fig. 2.3). In some children with cerebral palsy, only the upper limb may manifest the obvious reflex concomitant with lesser degrees of postural change in the lower limb; and the reflex may be positive with head turning to one side only.

2. *Neck-righting reflex*. This is positive if the shoulder girdle and trunk turn simultaneously when the head is turned. It is never normal if the child can be rolled over and over like a log (Fig.2.4). In its transient but imposable form it disappears in all normal infants by 10 months of age (Paine and Oppé 1966).

3. *Moro reflex*. This is precisely defined and should not be confused with the startle response, which is normal in infants and throughout childhood. A startle is a mass myoclonic movement which can occur during sleep, with a sudden noise or anything that evokes fear. It is thought to be a cortical release phenomenon that decreases with maturation (Baird and Gordon 1983). The Moro reflex is a sudden abduction and extension of the upper limbs with spreading of the fingers followed by an embrace. The best way to elicit the response is by lifting, gently with the right hand under the upper thoracic spine and the left hand under the head, and then dropping the left hand to allow neck extension (Baird and Gordon 1983). Suddenly jarring the examining table or making a loud noise is a more startling way to obtain

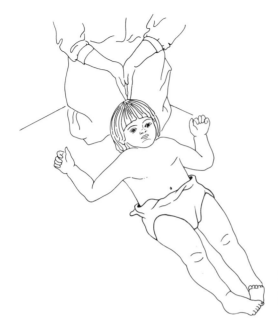

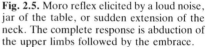

Fig. 2.5. Moro reflex elicited by a loud noise, jar of the table, or sudden extension of the neck. The complete response is abduction of the upper limbs followed by the embrace.

the Moro reflex. In normal infants it disappears by age six months (Fig.2.5).

4. *Symmetrical tonic neck reflex*. The child is placed in the quadriped (crawling) position. When the head is flexed ventrally, flexion of the forelimbs and extension of the hind-limbs results (Fig.2.6); extension of the head and neck causes extension of the forelimbs and flexion of the hind-limbs (Fig.2.6). A positive reflex is normal up to the age of six months.

5. *Parachute reaction*. The child is prone and lifted horizontally from the table and then quickly lowered to the table-top. With this movement, protective extension of the upper limbs and hands is automatic and is developed in all children

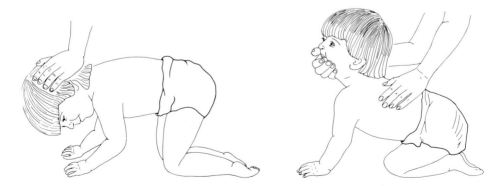

Fig. 2.6. Symmetrical tonic neck reflex. *Left:* flexion of head causes flexion of forelimbs and extension of hind-limbs. Hind-limb extension is often suppressed due to predominant flexor pattern of spasticity. *Right:* extension of head causes extension of forelimbs and flexion of hind-limbs.

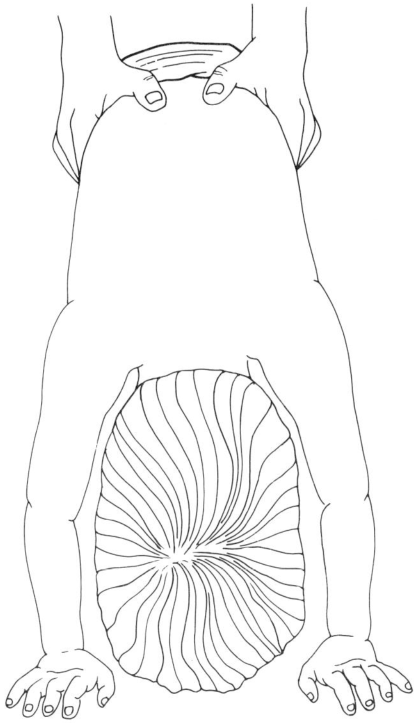

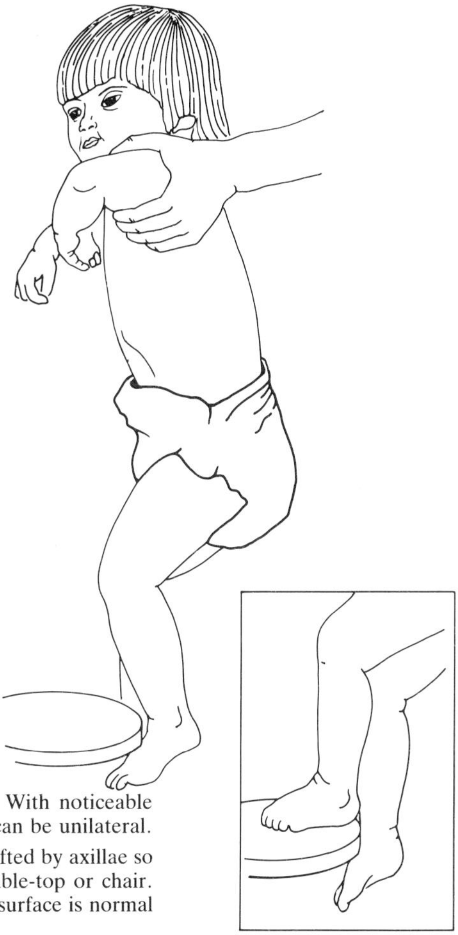

Fig. 2.7. *(above).* Parachute reaction. Child is lifted from table in prone position and suddenly lowered or tipped onto table-top. Normal response (after age 11 months) is automatic extension of the upper limbs and placement of hands on table's surface. With noticeable involvement of one upper limb, positive response can be unilateral.

Fig. 2.8 *(right).* Foot placement reaction. Child is lifted by axillae so that dorsa of feet come up against underside of table-top or chair. Symmetrical or asymmetrical placement of feet on surface is normal response.

by age 12 months (Paine and Oppé 1966) (Fig.2.7). If the child has severe involvement of one upper limb, the protective placement of the upper limbs may be unilateral; if so, the test is still valid and positive.

6. *Foot placement reaction.* With the child held by the chest and axillae, the dorsum of the feet are brought upward against the edge of the table-top or chair (usually the edge of a plain unpadded chair or table-top is best). Automatic foot placement on the table-top or chair surface occurs either symmetrically or asymmetrically. This response is normal in all infants. Suppression of it occurs with voluntary control, usually by the age of three or four years (Fig.2.8).

7. *Extensor thrust.* When the child is lifted by the axilla and suspended, and then lowered so that the feet touch the floor or table-top, it is always abnormal if there is definite and progressive extension of the lower limbs progressing upward into the trunk (Gesell and Amatruda 1947) (Fig.2.9). Normal infants will flex their legs with this maneuver.

27

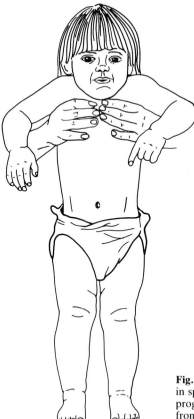

Fig. 2.9. Extensor thrust. When the child is suspended vertically in space and then lowered so that the feet touch the table-top, progressive extension of the lower limbs progressing superiorly from the feet to the trunk is abnormal.

The maneuvers used to obtain the *Landau reflex* are useful in documenting hypotonia. When the hypotonic infant (in cerebral palsy hypotonia often precedes athetosis) is raised in the horizontal prone position from the table, a collapse into the shape of an upside-down ∪ is classic. The true Landau reaction in normal infants is extension of the head and neck beyond the shoulder level, and extension of the spine. Spinal extension to form a concavity is not present in all infants until the age of 12 months (Baird and Gordon 1983). When the normal child is in this position, passive flexion of the head and neck causes loss of extensor tone. It has been used to assess the motor development of infants (Cupps *et al*. 1976).

The head
The head circumference should always be measured and compared with normal measurements (Fig.2.10). Measurement is easier if done when the child is supine and before s/he gets too tired and irritable. In babies, the fontanelles should be palpated for evidence of closure. I always auscultate the skull for a bruit. Rarely, one may find a vascular anomaly of the brain to explain the etiology of spastic hemiplegia.

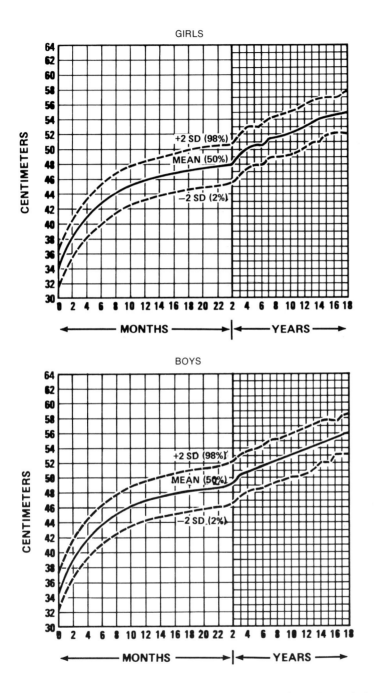

Fig. 2.10. Head circumference for girls *(top)* and boys *(bottom)*. Head circumference below −2SD almost always indicates mental retardation. If head circumference approaches −4SD, serious mental retardation is likely. Children with growth failure, but normal intelligence, have normal head circumferences (from O'Connell *et al.* 1965).

29

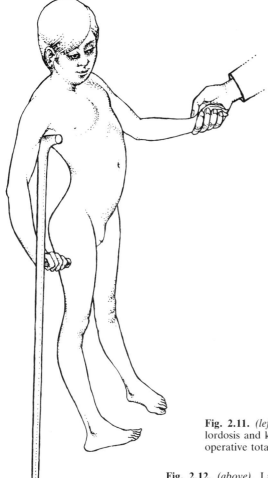

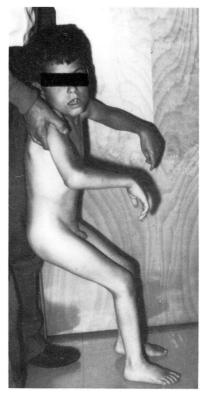

Fig. 2.11. *(left).* Lateral view of standing posture. Note lordosis and kyphosis. (Patient has spastic diplegia; postoperative total hamstring transfer.)

Fig. 2.12. *(above).* Lateral view of standing posture supported. Severe flexion of hips and knees, no lumbar lordosis (spastic diplegia).

Standing posture

The standing posture should be observed from three views: lateral, posterior, and anterior.

The *lateral* view permits observation of the head and neck position, thoracic kyphosis, lumbar lordosis, pelvic inclination and the position of the hip, knee, and ankle joints, and the feet (Figs.2.11, 2.12).

The extent of thoracic kyphosis and lumbar lordosis can be estimated by placing a meter rule against the mid-thoracic spine and sacrum. When significant thoracic kyphosis is suspected, the ruler deviates posteriorly from the perpendicular (Fig.2.13). Additionally, the distance between the edge of the ruler and the mid-lumbar spine is a clinical measurement of lordosis. In normal children, this distance is no more than 4cm (Fig.2.13).

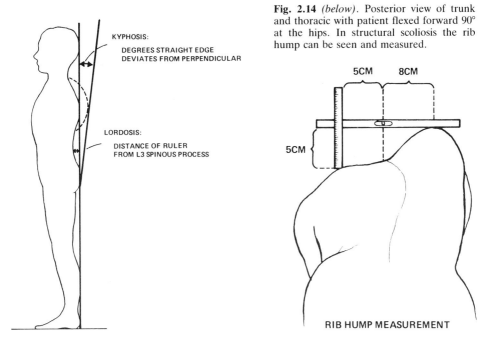

Fig. 2.14 *(below)*. Posterior view of trunk and thoracic with patient flexed forward 90° at the hips. In structural scoliosis the rib hump can be seen and measured.

KYPHOSIS:

DEGREES STRAIGHT EDGE
DEVIATES FROM PERPENDICULAR

LORDOSIS:

DISTANCE OF RULER
FROM L3 SPINOUS PROCESS

5CM   8CM

5CM

RIB HUMP MEASUREMENT

Fig. 2.13 *(above left)*. Assessment of standing posture with a ruler or yardstick placed against sacrum and thoracic spinous processes. With kyphosis, straight edge deviates posteriorly from perpendicular. The distance from straight edge to mid-lumbar spine is gross estimate of lordosis (normal 3 to 4 cm).

The *posterior* view will discern scoliosis, which is more frequent in cerebral-palsied than in normal children (Robson 1968, Balmer and MacEwen 1970, Samilson 1973, Madigan and Wallace 1981, Akbarnia 1984). Scoliosis is indicated by inequality in the height of shoulders or pelvis, and a shift of the trunk that creates unilateral loin fullness. A metal tape in a spool serves nicely as a plumb line which can be dropped from the tip of the first thoracic spinous process to delineate spinal alignment and balance. When the spine is perfectly balanced ('compensated'), the plumb line from the first thoracic vertebra will cross the mid-sacrum and the gluteal fold.

An essential test for structural scoliosis is to ask the child to flex the trunk forward 90° at the hips with the upper limbs extended downward and forward, and to avoid trunk rotation as much as possible, with palms together (as if at prayer.) With the examiner's vision directed level with the spine, asymmetry of the posterior thorax can be seen (Fig.2.14). A rib hump denotes rotation of the thoracic vertebra to the convex side of a structural scoliosis. The rib hump can be measured as indicated in Figure 2.14. Another and more recent type of measurement using degrees of tilt (with a 'Scoliometer') has been proposed by Bunnell (1984).

These findings of rib hump, unilateral loin fullness, shoulder height inequality and pelvic obliquity are indications for a radiographic examination. These same indications exist if the child can be examined only when seated.

31

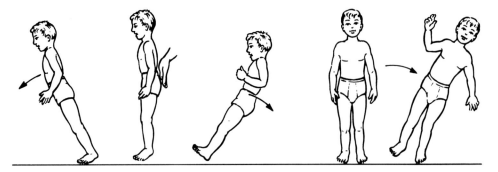

Fig. 2.15. Standing equilibrium reactions. The child is gently pushed forward, backward and from side to side. Lack of normal equilibrium reactions is easily demonstrated—the child topples over without normal stepping response.

A good way of measuring the range of spine flexion is with a tape-measure that spans the spinous processes from the first thoracic vertebra to a prominent spine of the sacrum. This distance is first measured with the patient standing erect, and then with the trunk flexed 90° at the hips. Normally the difference between the standing and the flexed distances is 10 to 13cm: a difference in measurement of 7cm or less indicates limited flexion of the spine.

From the posterior view the position of the heels should be recorded: neutral, varus (inverted) or valgus (everted) alignment.

In the *anterior* view of the posture the examiner can observe: (i) asymmetry of the chest (usually secondary to structural thoracic scoliosis with chest depression on the convex side of the curve); (ii) asymmetry of the limbs; (iii) the position of the femur whether internally, externally or neutrally rotated, adducted or abducted; (iv) the femoral-tibial alignment in varus (bowed) or valgus (knock-knee); (v) medial or lateral rotation of the foot; (vi) varus (inverted) or valgus (everted) position of the foot; and (vii) hallux valgus, flexion or clawing of the toes.

Equilibrium reactions
Presuming the child can stand without support, this is the time to test for the all-important standing equilibrium reactions (see Chapter 5 for their prognostic significance). The tests consist of pushing the child gently from side to side, anteriorly and posteriorly (Fig.2.15). Normal children will maintain their balance with ease, and with a prompt stepping response to regain stability, but children who have deficient equilibrium reactions will topple over like 'felled pine trees' (Hagberg *et al.* 1972) (Fig.2.16).

In children who have normal equilibrium reactions, but who seem to be clumsy or ataxic, the familar Romberg sign (performed with feet together and eyes closed) will document cerebellar ataxia (Baird and Gordon 1983).

The status of balance mechanisms can be further ascertained in those children who have good equilibrium reactions and negative Romberg signs if they can hop on one foot. If they can do this by the age of about six, proceed no further. If not, a child should be able to stand on one foot and then the other for at least 10 seconds;

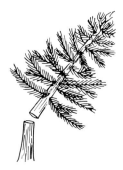

Fig. 2.16. The falling of the child who has abnormal equilibrium reactions has been likened to a 'felled pine tree' (Hagberg *et al.* 1972).

inability to do this by the age of five years is evidence of impaired motor function. Children with spastic diplegia or hemiplegia who can walk independently often fail the unilateral standing balance test, either on one side or both. This demonstration of ability to maintain balance with a compensatory lean of the trunk explains the frequently observed truncal sway during gait progression, and is often mistaken for a positive Trendelenberg sign which would connote weak hip abductor muscles.

Walking

The observation of the child's walking pattern is one of the most important parts of the examination, especially for the surgeon. The process is called 'gait analysis', with gait being defined as 'bipedal plantigrade progression'. 'It is distinctly human; it permits us to view the world in an upright manner, though not always acting in an upright way' (from lectures on gait by Vernon Inman MD, University of California, San Francisco, 1960-70).

The clinical examination of walking can be called 'observational gait analysis', which means describing what the examiner *sees*, as opposed to analysis by instruments and measurements. The terminology used should be the same as that used with instrumentation. Although accurate measurements cannot be made with careful observation alone, we need to remember that all laboratory findings must be correlated with clinical examinations. Indeed, most gait laboratories use videotape recordings of the patient's walking pattern as a check on the analog and digital data generated.

The type of motion disorder can often be diagnosed by observation of the gait, and applying the descriptive terminology delineated in Chapter 1. Spastic gait patterns are distinct from athetoid types of either the rotatory (ballismus) or dystonic forms. A purely ataxic gait is characteristic. A new and erudite term 'titubation' describes the shaking of the trunk and head with the staggering, reeling and stumbling gait of ataxia (Baird and Gordon 1983, p.100).

The base of the gait as measured from heel to heel can be estimated. In a normal person, the base of the gait as measured from heel to heel is 5 to 10cm (though in some individuals it can be as narrow as 1cm, which accounts for scuffing of the medial aspect of the heel counter of the shoes, or the wearing out of the inside cuffs of trousers).

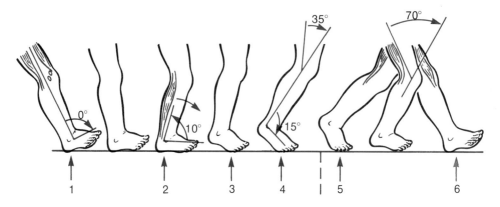

Fig. 2.17. Terminology of the events in the gait cycle (adapted from Perry 1967). *1:* heel strike. Ankle is flexed 0°; knee extended; hip flexed 30°; synchronous activity of hamstrings and quadriceps. *2:* mid-stance. Foot flat on floor; ankle dorsiflexed 10°; gastrocnemius-soleus contracts to prevent forward acceleration of the tibia. *3:* terminal stance ('roll-off'). This action is not a push, but rather a rocking action of the foot to advance the trunk. *4:* pre-swing, 35° to 40° of knee flexion. *5:* initial swing ('pick-up'). Knee flexion an additional 35° to prevent toe-drag; here hip flexion need be only 30° to 35°. After pick-up, the knee flexors relax. Ankle progressively dorsiflexes, and the ankle plantar flexes again (15° to 20°) when the limb passes the opposite supporting limb. Toe clearance is minimal and may be only 1cm. *6:* terminal swing ('reach'). Knee extends for maximum stride-length, hip flexes about 30° and ankle remains flexed. Knee extends primarily by passive swinging.

The *terminology* of the gait cycle can be used in clinical narrative descriptions of the position of the head, upper limbs, trunk, pelvis, femora, knees, ankles and feet while walking. Stance phase begins with heel contact and ends with toe-off. Stance is 60 per cent and swing is 40 per cent of the gait cycle.

To further improve observations, the gait cycle has been divided into several phases when describing joint and muscle function (Perry 1967, 1975) (Figs. 2.17, 2.18). Step length is the distance between the same point on each foot (right to left or left to right) during double-limb support; stride length is the distance traversed by the same point of the same foot during two successive steps (right to left or left to right). Cadence is the number of steps per minute, and velocity is meters traveled per minute.

Stride length can be estimated. Perry (1975) has pointed out that stride length is dependent on the stance rather than the swing limb during level walking. In spastic paralysis of the lower limbs, stride length can be limited by restrictions in the range of motion of the hip, knee and ankle; such limitations would account for the short swing of the opposite limb when the weight-bearing limb is in mid-stance. Our studies have confirmed that the majority of children with spastic diplegia had shorter stance phases and faster cadences than normal children (Bleck *et al.* 1975) (Figs.2.19, 2.20).

Other parameters of the normal gait cycle can be helpful. For example, when assessing the gait of the patient with a view to surgery or orthotics, it is useful to know that normally the knee flexes 35° at pre-swing and must flex 70° for the foot to clear the ground (Fig.2.17).

34

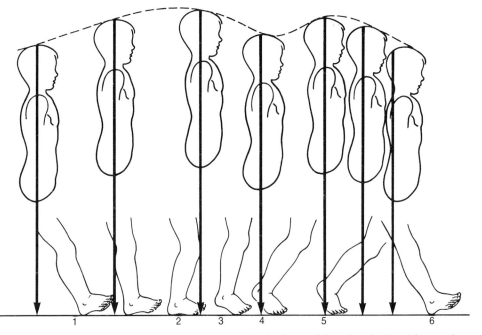

Fig. 2.18. Progression of trunk in relation to the foot in the six phases of the gait cycle. Trunk is posterior to the foot at point of heel contact *(1)*, and gradually progresses forward to mid-stance *(2)*. At terminal stance ('roll-off', *3*) the trunk is posterior to the foot again. Pre-swing *(4)* is followed by initial swing ('pick-up', *5*), and finally terminal swing ('rock', *6*). Broken line over head represents the normal vertical displacement of the body during walking on a level surface; this line is a low sinusoidal curve as described by Saunders *et al.* (1953).

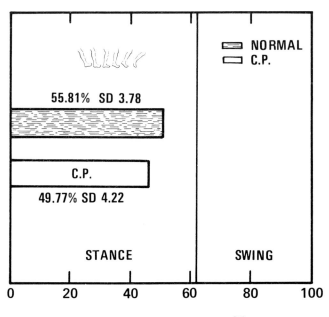

Fig. 2.19. Comparison of percent of gait cycle in normal children and in cerebral palsy (spastic diplegia). Stance phase is shorter in spastic gait patterns (Csongradi *et al.* 1979).

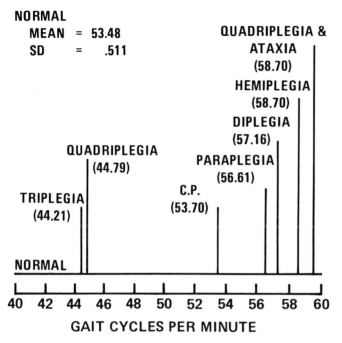

Fig. 2.20. Graphic description of cadence of normal gait compared with that of spastic gait. Normal child: 53.48 gait cycles per minute. With the exception of a few quadriplegics and triplegics who are slower than normal, most of the others are faster than normal—a confirmation of clinical observations that these children cannot slow down (Csongradi *et al.* 1979).

Gait mechanics

Conducive to astute observational gait analysis is an understanding of the accepted mechanical theories of walking based upon experimental evidence and principles of physics.

The ballistic walking model is comparable to a projectile moving through space, because once the swing phase begins, forward movement occurs entirely by the action of gravity (McMahon 1984).

The center of gravity is a fixed point in a body through which the force of gravitational attraction acts (Kelley 1971) (Fig.2.21). In the human body the center of gravity is located just anterior to the first and second sacral segments (Braune and Fischer 1898, cited by Brunnstron 1962). If the lower limbs are not considered, the center of gravity of the trunk only is just anterior to the 11th thoracic vertebra (Hellebrant 1938, cited by Brunnstrom 1962). In children, the center of gravity of the whole body is first located at about the level of the 11th thoracic vertebra, just anterior to the vertebral column where the vena cava enters the abdomen through the diaphragm; with maturation of the child, the center of gravity descends to its adult level anterior to the sacrum. The location of the center of gravity can be estimated as 55 per cent of the total height, measured from the soles of the feet.

Many of the postural abnormalities of patients with cerebral palsy seen during

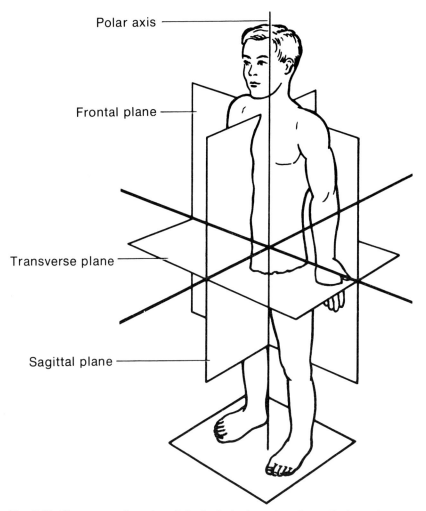

Polar axis

Frontal plane

Transverse plane

Sagittal plane

Fig. 2.21. The center of gravity of the body is the point where all planes (coronal, sagittal and transverse) converge, just anterior to the second sacral segment (redrawn from Kelley 1971).

walking are probably adjustments of the trunk and limbs to maintain the center of gravity when equilibrium reactions are deficient or when there are structural abnormalities of the trunk. Because the head, upper limbs and trunk represent 70 per cent of the bodyweight, this mass (HAT, standing for head, arms and trunk) has to be balanced and supported by the lower limbs. With anatomical shifts of the trunk, as might occur in scoliosis, balance is shifted and off-center. The lower limbs usually accommodate these changes by moving the feet wider apart (Perry 1975).

The vertical displacement of the center of gravity is at the core of mechanics. The most efficient instrument of motion on earth's surface is the wheel because its center of gravity remains perfectly level, horizontal to the ground and without oscillation in its path of motion (Fig.2.22). In human gait the vertical displacement

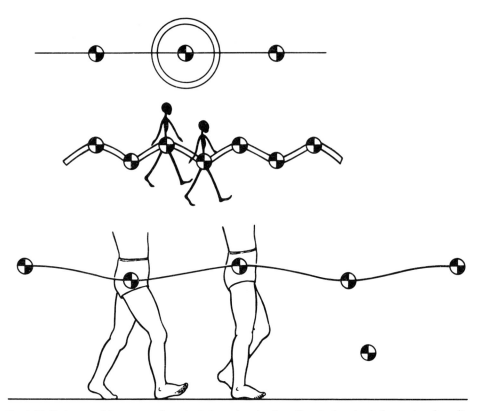

Fig. 2.22. Pathways of the center of gravity in lateral projection. *Top:* in the wheel, the center of gravity (the axis) remains horizontal, making it the most efficient instrument of forward motion. *Center:* in human walking, if the knee joint is eliminated, the center of gravity rises and falls precipitously. This increases energy expenditure. *Bottom:* in normal gait the oscillations of the center of gravity result in a low sinusoidal curve. The major determinants of gait (pelvis, hip, knee, foot and ankle) serve to keep the center of gravity as close as possible to that of the wheel, thus conserving energy.

of the center of gravity attempts to approximate the wheel by minimizing the displacement and tracing a trajectory as a low sinusoidal curve. This is to save energy. If the lower limbs in humans were unarticulated sticks, a 'compass gait' with high-amplitude oscillations of the center of gravity would result, with consequent increased energy expenditure (Fig.2.22).

The five major determinants of gait in the ballistic model of walking are responsible for maintaining the lowest possible sinusoidal path of the center of gravity (Saunders *et al.* 1953, McMahon 1984).

1. PELVIC ROTATION. At normal walking speed, the amplitude of motion of the pelvis in rotation is ±3°. Rotation increases at greater speeds. Pelvic rotation effects lengthening of the lower limb, and thus allows a longer step length and a greater radius for rotation of the hip. Walking racers exaggerate their pelvic rotation, which allows continued walking at high speeds rather than progression to running (McMahon 1984).

2. PELVIC TILT. Tilt of the pelvis in the coronal plane causes an angular displacement of 5° or more. The hip on the swing side falls lower than the hip on the stance limb. The lowering of the swing limb occurs just before toe-off, and accordingly the trajectory of the center of gravity is further lowered. As the pelvis dips, knee flexion of the swing limb must occur so that the advancing foot does not strike the ground on forward movement.

3. KNEE FLEXION in the stance phase further lowers the sinusoidal path of the center of gravity.

4. PLANTAR FLEXION OF THE STANCE ANKLE. At heel strike, the ankle plantar flexes and the knee flexes to shorten the limb. As the trunk passes over the stance limb, the knee then extends and the heel rises to effect lengthening of the limb.

5. LATERAL DISPLACEMENT OF THE PELVIS. The shift of the trunk is normally no more than 4 to 5cm during gait. Excessive displacement would occur if the lower limbs were parallel to each other. The normal anatomy of adduction of the femora and the resultant valgus angle between the femur and tibia prevents excessive displacement.

While the ballistic model of walking explains how gravity alone determines the dynamics of gait, the model assumes no muscular torques at the joints of the swing limb; hence it cannot represent running, or walking at very low or high speeds (McMahon 1984).

A moon-walk might demonstrate the low oscillations of displacement of the body's center of gravity. On the moon, the time of swing phase must be increased 2½ times; so the walking speed for a given step length can be only about 40 per cent of what it is on earth. This explains why the Apollo astronauts on the moon preferred to move about in a series of jumps rather than restrict their walking speed. The maximal jump height on the moon is said to be 4m (McMahon 1984).

Gait laboratory studies have shown that normally the pelvis and lower limb segments rotate internally throughout swing, and at mid-stance abrupt external rotation of these segments occurs. The function of the subtalar joint is to absorb the torques generated by the foot-floor reaction when these changes in rotation take place.

In spastic paralysis of the lower limbs, motion is often restricted in the joints that affect the major determinants of gait. If external rotation at the hip joint is limited, then pelvic rotation (the first determinant) will be restricted; the degree of pelvic rotation internally (*i.e.* anteriorly) is permitted by the degree of hip external rotation. With this kind of restriction, the path of the center of gravity would have higher peaks and valleys, and the gait would be less efficient. If knee flexion were limited (*e.g.* by a spastic quadriceps muscle), then the gait would be compass-like, the arc of the center of gravity would rise, and energy expenditure would increase. Compensation for restricted ankle motion can be accomplished by exaggerated movements of the hip and knee. These compensatory mechanisms are not often adequate in cerebral spastic paralysis, because neural integration may be deficient.

The lower limb movement patterns and ranges of joint motion during walking have been measured and standards are known; these standards of measurement are described in Chapter 3. The rôle of the muscles during gait has been determined by electromyography. The normative data derived from electromyography, and its possible applications in cerebral palsy, are also covered in the next chapter.

The effect of *deficient equilibrium reactions* on the abnormal gait pattern will be seen if a child is asked to walk without external support for a short distance. Crutches, parallel bars, and walkers are usually only compensations for the loss of balance mechanisms, and the abnormal dynamic postures during walking seem to be compensatory attempts to keep from falling. To test the possible effects of dysequilibrium on the gait pattern of children who walk unsupported, the examiner can stabilize the posture by securely holding the child's head from behind and walking with him. This kind of demonstration might dispel the prevalent idea of parents and some professionals (*e.g.* physical education teachers) that if the child would only 'exercise more' with a set of prescribed calisthenics, he would 'walk better'. We know of *no* exercises or treatments that can overcome defective central balance mechanisms.

Sitting posture
The sitting posture will be either supportive ('propped') or unsupportive. Children who are hypotonic, or who have cerebral damage, usually do not have the normal lumbar lordotic curve, so the spine is rounded. The lower limbs of the child who has total body involvement are frequently extended. When the manual supports of the seated child are removed, automatic protective placement of the extended upper limb and hand usually denotes good function of the hand and limb. Scoliosis, a posterior rib hump, and the levels of the pelvic brim can be discerned.

Deep tendon and plantar reflexes
Deep tendon reflexes and the plantar responses can be checked when the infant or young child is seated on the mother's lap, or when the older child sits with his knees flexed over the table edge. The biceps, triceps, and the periosteal-radial reflexes in the upper limb, and the quadriceps and Achilles reflexes in the lower limb, are hyperactive in spasticity and normal or absent in ataxia. While these responses are classical, variations occur according to age and severity of the spastic paralysis. In infants under one month of age, the predominant flexor pattern suppresses the triceps reflex, and the Achilles reflex may be weak or absent. Severe spasticity, rigidity, or a long-standing severe contracture of the triceps surae muscles may eliminate the ankle jerk response. The crossed adductor response, in which tapping of the patellar tendon results in adduction of the opposite hip, indicates severe spasticity. This crossed spread of the quadriceps reflex can be normal in infants up to the age of eight months, and in 2 per cent of infants at the age of 12 months (Paine and Oppé 1966, Baird and Gordon 1983).

The *Babinski sign* is best induced by gently stroking the lateral plantar aspect of the foot with a blunt instrument (*e.g.* a key or the handle of a reflex hammer). Joseph Babinski in 1896 noticed that the response was best obtained when the limb was slightly flexed and the muscles were well relaxed. Ordinarily, this state of the limb is achieved with the patient seated and the legs hanging over the table edge. The positive response consists of extension and spreading of the toes—usually strongest in the great and second toes (Baird and Gordon 1983). Many other ways of eliciting the Babinski sign have been described. I have found Chaddock's sign one of the better alternatives. The lateral aspect of the dorsum of the foot is gently stroked from the heel to the forefoot. Fanning and extension of the toes will occur if the sign is positive.

Associated defects: cranial nerves
Because the major associated defects (convulsive, learning and behavioral disorders excepted) are related to dysfunction of the cranial nerves, the examination of these nerves is presented. The sitting posture is the most practical for these observations.

III, IV and VI. Eye mobility is frequently affected in cerebral palsy. Esotropia or exotropia is easy to see. Esotropia is six times as common as exotropia (Perlstein 1960-66). Pupil inequality is uncommon, and most often seen in patients with hemiplegia due to cerebrovascular conditions, brain tumors, or after head injuries. Paralysis of the upper gaze is common in tension athetosis due to kernicterus. Nystagmus is sometimes seen in ataxia. The eye-righting reflex means that when the neck is flexed, extended and rotated, the eyes should follow the movement of the head. Absence of this reflex indicates brainstem injury. The absence of eye movements with rotation of the head, or turning of the eyes to the side opposite of head rotation, has been called 'doll's eyes'. The normal eye-reflex response may be delayed a few weeks in normal infants (Baird and Gordon 1983). Visual acuity testing and funduscopic examinations are best left to the ophthalmologist.

VII and XII. On inspection of the mouth and face, inequality of facial muscle function is sometimes seen in upper-motor neuron lesions. The corner of the child's mouth on the affected side may not move when crying or smiling, or he may not be able to wrinkle the forehead. In less severe unilateral lesions, the only finding may be a wide palpebral fissure on the affected side (Baird and Gordon 1983).

Athetoid movements of the orbicularis oris muscle, and muscles of mastication, are fairly common. They indicate a general motor disorder, rather than cranial nerve paralysis.

IX. If the child can open his mouth, paralysis of the pharyngeal muscles may be seen. The only manifestation of paralysis may be a slight dropping of the palatal arch. Despite paralysis, both sides of the arch may elevate when saying 'aah'. In his lectures on cerebral palsy, Meyer Perlstein (1960-66) gave some useful clinical tips: if swallowing is more difficult with fluids, spasm of the pharyngeal muscles should be suspected; if difficulty in swallowing is greater with solids, paralysis of these muscles may be present.

VIII. Gross hearing defects can be ascertained by asking the parents whether they think the child hears, and by watching the child's reaction to sounds out of his visual field *e.g.* by shaking a few grains of sand in a cardboard cylinder. In suspicious cases, referral for audiometry and otolaryngeal consultation is indicated.

Upper limb assessment
Where to position the infant or child for a good assessment of upper limb and hand

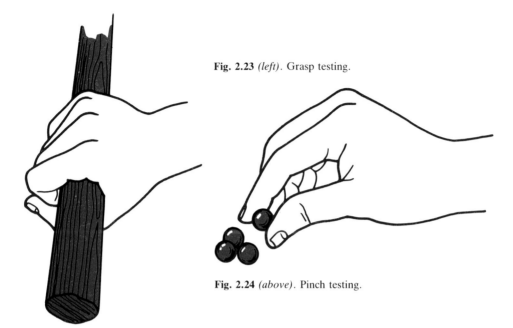

Fig. 2.23 *(left)*. Grasp testing.

Fig. 2.24 *(above)*. Pinch testing.

function depends on the age of the child, the status of his postural development, and the motor disorder. For the infant or toddler, the mother's lap is usually best; for the older child with hemiplegia, a desk and chair should be used; for the child who cannot sit unsupported and has gross involvement of one or both upper limbs, use a wheelchair with a seat insert and a lap tray. The child with no gross involvement of the upper limbs can be examined sitting with the knees flexed over the edge of the table; this particular child most often has spastic diplegia. For a more refined assessment of fine motor hand function, a chair and desk will be required.

Assessment of the upper limbs should include measurement of the passive and active ranges of motion of the shoulder and elbow; in this process spasticity, athetosis, dystonia, or ataxia can be recognized. Chorea will be demonstrated when the child is asked to hold his arms and hands extended forward; the sign of chorea is involuntary 'wormlike' movements of the fingers (Fig.1.4).

One good way to begin the assessment is to give the child an object that requires the use of both hands; wooden or plastic eggs within eggs or barrels within barrels are ideal. When the child grasps the object, one can see lateralization of hand function, the quality of grasp and release, and the ability of the hands to cross the midline. Gross grasp and release can be tested by handing the child a cylindrical stick or similar object (Fig.2.23). To test fine motion of the fingers and pinch, small wooden beads or hard-coated sweets are useful (Fig.2.24).

Gross spasticity of the wrist and digit muscles requires a more detailed examination, which must be precise if surgery is planned. Palpation of the spastic wrist flexors, as the wrist is extended, identifies which of these tendons is spastic and contracted (Fig.2.25). If the thumb is indwelling, measurement of the web

42

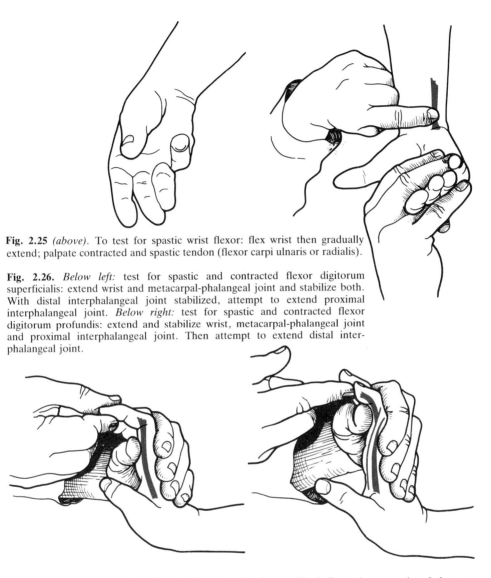

Fig. 2.25 *(above)*. To test for spastic wrist flexor: flex wrist then gradually extend; palpate contracted and spastic tendon (flexor carpi ulnaris or radialis).

Fig. 2.26. *Below left:* test for spastic and contracted flexor digitorum superficialis: extend wrist and metacarpal-phalangeal joint and stabilize both. With distal interphalangeal joint stabilized, attempt to extend proximal interphalangeal joint. *Below right:* test for spastic and contracted flexor digitorum profundis: extend and stabilize wrist, metacarpal-phalangeal joint and proximal interphalangeal joint. Then attempt to extend distal inter-phalangeal joint.

space while pulling the thumb into abduction will define the spastic abductor hallucis. Limited extension of the interphalangeal joint of the thumb, with the wrist held in the neutral position and the metacarpal-phalangeal joint in extension, indicates a spastic flexor pollicis longus muscle. If the fingers are consistently flexed in the palm, two maneuvers are necessary to determine if one or the other or both finger flexor muscles are spastic and contracted: (i) extend and hold the wrist in the neutral position, and extend and hold the metacarpal-phalangeal joints in neutral extension; the resistance to extension of the proximal interphalangeal joints while extending the distal joint will indicate the extent of spasticity and contracture of the flexor digitorum superficialis (Fig.2.26); (ii) with the wrist and metacarpal-

43

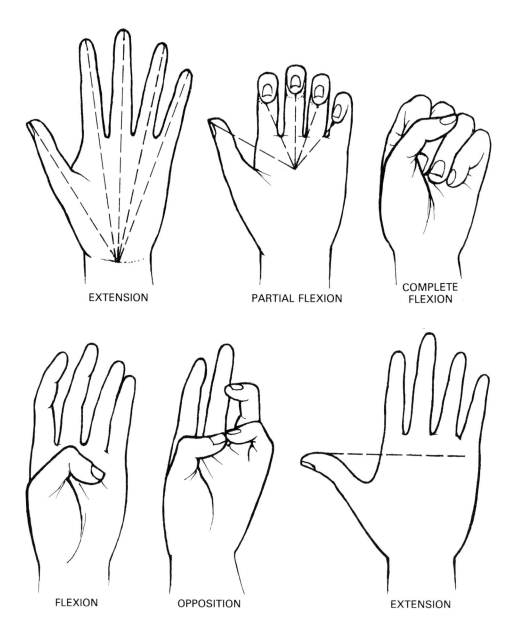

EXTENSION   PARTIAL FLEXION   COMPLETE FLEXION

FLEXION   OPPOSITION   EXTENSION

Fig. 2.27. Terminology to describe motion of the digits, and linear measurements to record ranges of motion. *Top:* for opening capacity of each finger, measure the distance from the extended finger to the distal flexion crease of the wrist. For closing capacity of the fingers, measure distance from tips of the fingers to the mid-palmar crease at the third metacarpal. *Bottom:* to measure opposing capacity of the thumb to the fingers, measure distance in centimeters between the tip of the thumb and the tip of each finger. (Note: this is 'pulp' pinch; 'key' pinch is just as useful and may be better—see Moberg 1984 and Chapter 7 in this volume.) To measure the opening and closing of the thumb in extension/abduction or flexion/adduction, measure distance from the tip of the thumb to the head of the fifth metacarpal in both extension and flexion.

phalangeal joints in the same position, stabilize the proximal interphalangeal joint in extension; flexion and resistance to extension of the distal interphalangeal joint implies a spastic and contracted flexor digitorum profundus muscle (Fig.2.26).

In patients who have wrist and finger flexion postures, the ability to extend the fingers voluntarily is tested by holding the wrist in extension; if active extension of the fingers occurs at the metacarpal-phalangeal joints, then the extensor digitorum muscles of the fingers have a good chance of functioning if the wrist and finger flexion contractures are relieved with surgery. If the fingers will extend only by dropping the wrist into flexion to open the grasp, then anything done to correct wrist flexion will seriously compromise function due to a permanent fist position. If there is doubt about voluntary control of wrist and finger extension, the median nerve can be blocked at the elbow with a local anesthetic to eliminate most of the flexor muscle function, and the quality of active wrist and finger extension will be evident.

For precision in terms describing active and passive motion of the thumb and digits, see Figure 2.27. Additional assessment techniques are described in the section on hand surgery in spastic hemiplegia (Chapter 7).

Fine motor inco-ordination of the hand is often seen in the child with spastic diplegia, ataxia, localized chorea, and the rare case of tremor. It can be discerned with the following simple tests: (i) ask the child to touch each fingertip to the thumb in as rapid a succession as possible; (ii) rapidly pronate and supinate the forearm to discover diodokinesis; (iii) with both hands resting, palms down on the desk or table-top, ask the child to mimic your own hand movements (*e.g.* tapping the fingers as if typing or playing the piano, or rapidly pronating and supinating one hand). With these latter movement tests, mirror movements in the opposite resting hand may be discovered. However, mirror motions can be normal in some children to the age of six or seven years. Mirror movements are fairly frequent in children who have hemiplegia on attempted voluntary manipulations with the hemiplegic hand.

Other tests for visual-motor co-ordination that can be useful are drawing tests. The simplest to use for a developmental estimate is the Slosson Drawing Co-ordination test. A three-year-old should be able to copy a circle and a vertical line, a 4½-year-old a square, a five-year-old an x, a 5½-year-old a triangle, and a six-year-old a diamond. With children six years of age or more, I usually start by asking them to copy a diamond. If they can, I proceed no further. More elaborate tests of hand function and visual-motor co-ordination are usually the province of the occupational therapist and psychologist, to whom the physician can refer the child when indicated (Baird and Gordon 1984).

The Elliott and Connolly classification of hand movements (1984) is a very recent innovation, based upon intrinsic movements of the digits in the hand. The descriptive terminology is appealing, *e.g.* 'pinch', 'dynamic tripod' (holding a pencil), 'squeeze' (compressing the barrel of a syringe), 'twiddle' (rolling a nut on a threaded bolt), 'rock' (holding a thin disc in the palm and rotating it, 'radial roll' (as in snapping the thumb), 'index roll' (rolling a pea-sized object between the pulp

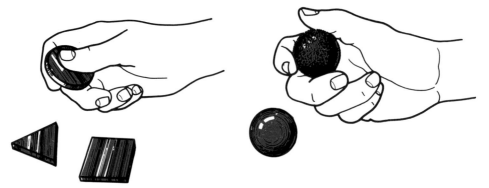

Fig. 2.28. Stereognosis test objects: 5mm plywood triangle, square and disc for shape recognition; smooth and rough (covered with flock paint) ping-pong balls for texture recognition.

of the thumb and index finger), plus combinations of manipulative movements termed 'steps' and 'slides'. For a complete detailed description of these tests, the original paper in *Developmental Medicine and Child Neurology* (1984) should be studied.

In children who have to use wheelchairs, hand use should be part of the assessment. We can observe whether or not the child can move a manual wheelchair independently and efficiently, and if so, whether with both hands or only one, and in what positions the hands and fingers are placed to propel the chair.

The *sensory* examination is frequently neglected in cerebral palsy, because of a failure to appreciate the all-important rôle of sensation in intellectual development.

In the hierarchy of the external senses touch was considered the most important in the philosophical discourses of Thomas Aquinas (1224-1274) (McInerny 1984). Aquinas saw touch wedded to a physical change. For example, when the hand feels a cold object and keeps it there for a time, the temperature of the body (37.5°c) gradually warms the cold object until the temperatures become equal. We hear such terms as 'deficient sensory perception', 'sensory retraining' and 'sensory integration' applied to the child with cerebral palsy, without knowing exactly what is meant or their implications for the child and attempts at remediation. Recognizing a deficiency in the sense of touch is important, to understand the possible limitations of hand function in the child.

One recent study on kinesthetic performance of children with spastic and athetoid cerebral palsy, when compared with age-matched normal children, demonstrated that those with spasticity had the greatest number of errors on kinesthetic tests (athetoids were less prone to error) when analyzed against the normal control's performance. The authors suggested that attempts to apply 'reafference theory' with methods using feedback of movement should not be done using the sense of touch in cerebral-palsied patients, but rather should use intact sensory systems, *i.e.* vision and hearing (Opila-Lehman *et al.* 1984).

Stereognosis is the most common defect. Generally, asterognosis in spastic hemiplegia seems to accompany the degree of atrophy of the upper limb. Testing for shape recognition with the hands is even more important if surgery is planned

46

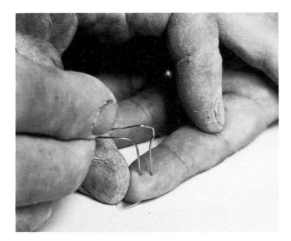

Fig. 2.29. *left:* Moberg's test instrument for the two-point discrimination test—a wire paper-clip reconfigured and bent. Tips can be spread apart to a measured distance (5mm). *Right:* to do the two-point discrimination test on the pulp of the fingers and thumb, both patient and examiners must be seated. The examiner uses free hand to stabilize the digit on the table-top (Moberg 1984). A measured 10g of pressure by the examiner is more accurate.

(Tachdjian and Minear 1958, Goldner and Ferlic 1966). The child has to be old enough to verbalize shape and texture (or if non-verbal, communicate with symbols or drawings). The child is asked to identify objects while blindfolded, or vision occluded with the examiner's hand. For shape identification we use pieces of wood cut into a triangle, square, and circle (or perhaps coins, for more sophisticated children); for texture recognition, use two ping-pong balls: one smooth and one rough (Goldner 1974) (Fig.2.28).

Another way to test for stereognosis is with dermographics. Again the child is blindfolded. The examiner traces an arabic numeral (1 to 9) on the palm of the hand, and the child is asked to identify it. As in the tests for shape and texture identification, in hemiplegic hands the opposite (presumed neurologically intact) hand can serve as a control.

The most sensitive test for adequate sensation is the two-point discrimination test as modified by Moberg (1984). It is used almost exclusively in the assessment of paralysis of the hands in spinal cord and peripheral nerve injuries. To my knowledge it has not been tried in cerebral palsy. If someone wants to compare Moberg's 'microsurgical' two-point discrimination test on the digits of cerebral-palsied children, it should be conducted according to his instructions (Moberg 1984). The examiner and patient are both comfortably seated so that the examiner's and the patient's hands can rest securely on the table or desk. The finger to be tested is held firmly against the table-top with the examiner's free hand. The test instrument is an ordinary paper-clip, unfolded so that the two free ends are at the same level, and then bent 90° in the middle of the reconfigured clip (Fig. 2.29). The ends of the clip can be spread 5mm for testing; the patient just has to say 'one' or 'two'.

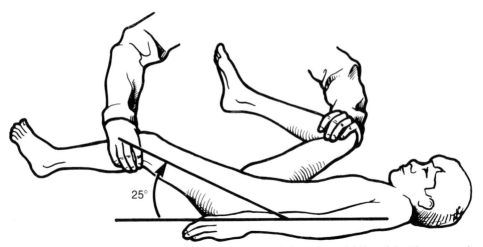

Fig. 2.30. *Above:* Thomas test for hip-flexion contracture. *Below:* the variability of the Thomas test in the same patient. Which one is the correct degree of contracture?

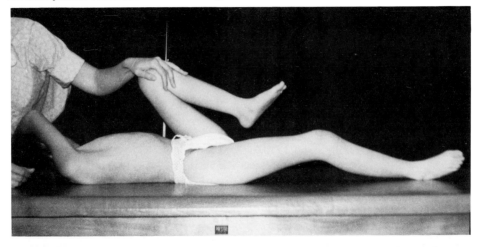

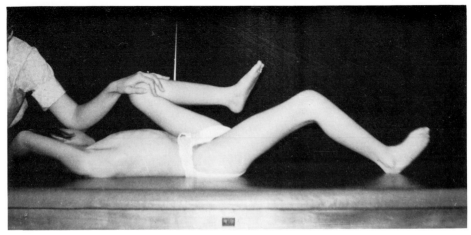

Lower limb assessment

Ranges of motion, measured with a goniometer of major lower limb joints, should be recorded methodically. Time-oriented serial examination forms are very useful when evaluating a patient over a period of years. The accepted ranges of motion in flexion and extension for normal individuals are placed in parentheses after the description of the passive range of motion to be tested. I recommend a recent publication by Staheli *et al.* (1985), based upon normal rotations of the lower limb anatomy.

Muscle testing, using the standards and grading originally developed for poliomyelitis, is too well known to be worth repeating here. While it is true that in cerebral palsy, muscle strength testing will be altered due to lack of voluntary control, or limited due to spasticity and/or contracture, at least some idea and explanation of the muscle function of a particular patient is gained.

Leg lengths should always be measured with the patient supine. I emphasize this because it is often overlooked. The proper way to measure leg length is with a tape measure (preferably a metal one) from the anterior superior iliac spine to the medial malleolus. If the patient has a flexion contracture of the knee joint, obviously this measurement will be affected. In such instances, the measurement can be from the anterior superior iliac spine to the medial joint space, and from the medial joint space to the medial malleolus. The addition of the two gives a reasonable estimate of the limb length. Asymmetrical adduction contractures of the hip result in the illusion of a short limb. Therefore measurement of the *actual* (rather than the apparent) limb length is important.

Hip. The range of abduction of each hip is measured with the hips flexed 90° and extended (normally 45° to 60°). The range of flexion varies in children (110° to 125°). Hip flexion contracture is common and is measured in two ways. In the classic Thomas test, the hip is flexed on the abdomen to flatten the lumbar spine, and the opposite hip is gently pushed to its maximum extension. The angle that the femur subtends with the table-top is a measure of the degree of hip flexion deformity (Fig.2.30). This test is unreliable. Varying degrees of hip flexion deformity can be produced in the same patient, depending on how far the hip is pushed onto the abdomen and how much pelvic femoral fixation is present due to spastic and contracted hamstrings (Fig.2.30). I believe that the Thomas test can identify spasticity and contracture of the iliopsoas by grasping the femoral condyles on the side which is to be measured, and attempting to rotate the femur externally. External rotation will be blocked when the iliopsoas is spastic. In contrast to spastic paralysis of the iliopsoas, the hip can be externally rotated easily in the Thomas test in patients whose hip flexion contracture is due to the iliotibial band. Contracture of this structure is most often seen in flaccid paralysis due to poliomyelitis or in muscle diseases (muscular dystrophy).

A second, more accurate, and preferred method of measuring the hip flexion contracture is that described by Staheli (1977). The patient is prone with the pelvis over the table's edge and the lower limbs hanging free in flexion. The examiner places one hand on the posterior superior iliac spines, while the other hand brings one lower limb gradually and slowly into extension. The point at which the pelvis

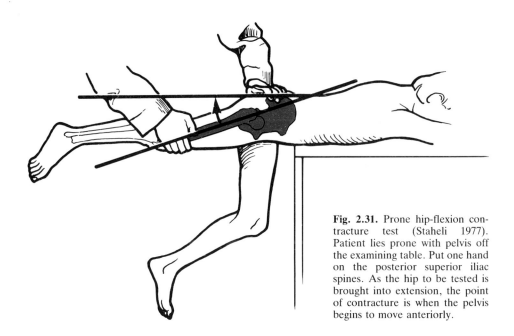

Fig. 2.31. Prone hip-flexion contracture test (Staheli 1977). Patient lies prone with pelvis off the examining table. Put one hand on the posterior superior iliac spines. As the hip to be tested is brought into extension, the point of contracture is when the pelvis begins to move anteriorly.

begins to move anteriorly is the point of the hip flexion deformity; the angle subtended by the femur and the horizontal plane is measured (Fig.2.31).

The normal range of hip extension (*i.e.* no flexion contracture) is at least zero, and may be as much as 20° in some children. All newborn infants have a flexion contracture of the hip with a mean value of 28° (Haas *et al.* 1973). At six weeks of age, the contracture decreases to a mean of 19°, and at three to six months to 7° (Coon *et al.* 1975).

With the patient still prone, internal and external rotation are measured (Staheli prefers the terms 'medial' and 'lateral'). The measurements are made with the knees flexed 90° and the pelvis stabilized by the examiner (or by a parent, nurse, or student) to avoid overestimation of hip rotation due to lateral rolling of the pelvis (Fig.2.32).

The recent study by Staheli *et al.* (1985) delineated normal ranges of medial and lateral hip rotation in children and adults. In infants and children up to the age of 15, medial rotation was greatest in infants less than one year old and gradually decreased from the age of seven or eight years to a mean value of 50° (range 25° to 65°) in males, and 40° in females (range 16° to 60°). Lateral rotation in infants had a mean value of almost 70° in infants less than one year old, and declined at about the same age found in medial rotation to a mean of 45° (range 25° to 65°). In contrast to the data on medial rotation where females had a greater degree of passive motion (mean 7°) than males, no sex difference was found in the measurements of lateral rotation.

With the patient still prone, spasticity of the quadriceps muscle can be estimated with the prone rectus femoris test, in which the knee is rapidly flexed and

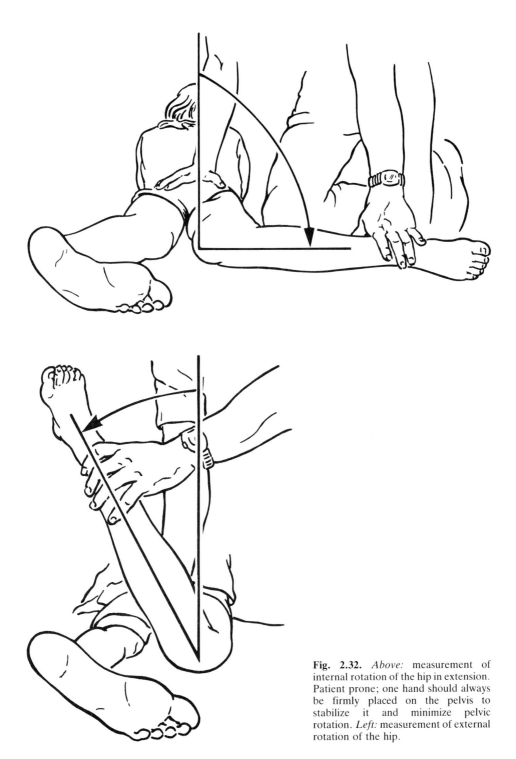

Fig. 2.32. *Above:* measurement of internal rotation of the hip in extension. Patient prone; one hand should always be firmly placed on the pelvis to stabilize it and minimize pelvic rotation. *Left:* measurement of external rotation of the hip.

51

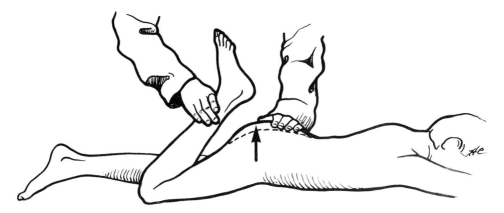

Fig. 2.33. Rectus femoris stretch test (Ely test). Patient prone; quick flexion of the knee causes buttock to rise if there is spasticity of the rectus femoris. Resistance to the flexion can be felt and represents quadriceps spasticity. This test also causes action potentials in the ilioposoas (Perry *et al.* 1976).

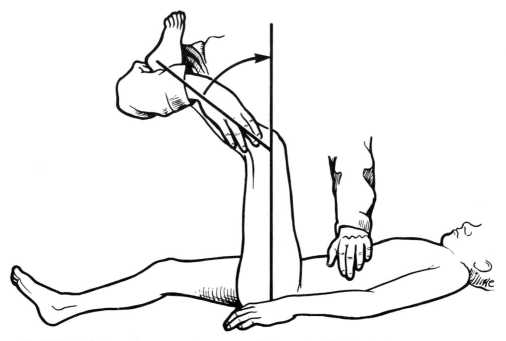

Fig. 2.34. Test for hamstring spasm and contracture. Patient supine; hip flexed 90° and knee extended to point of resistance. The angle between the neutral extended position of the knee and the tibia is the 'popliteal angle'.

its resistance to flexion is felt. Buttock elevation is supposed to be indicative of the complete positive test (Fig.2.33). This is not a pure rectus femoris test. Stretch electromyograms have shown that in this test the iliopsoas muscle has the same number of action potentials as the rectus femoris (Perry *et al.* 1976).

Stretch tests about the hips are limited in specificity (Perry *et al.* 1976), and the gracilis test* can be eliminated. Electromyographic data show that both the straight leg-raising and the gracilis tests induce the same amount of electrical activity of the medial hamstrings. The Thomas test produces similar amounts of electrical activity in both the iliopsoas and the rectus femoris. The adductors are sensitive to the hip adductor stretch tests (*i.e.* abducting the hips quickly) with the hips and knees flexed, or to the gracilis test, and also to the Thomas test.

Knee. Spasticity and contracture of the hamstrings are reliably measured with the straight leg-raising or the popliteal angle test. The hamstrings are almost exclusively active on electromyograms with straight leg-raising (Perry *et al.* 1976). To palpate the hamstrings and obtain a better estimate of contracture, I prefer to flex the hip 90° and then extend the knee to the limit permitted by the contracture. The degree of contracture is measured as the angle which the tibia subtends with the neutral and normal extension expected at the knee joint (0°); this angle is the popliteal angle (Fig.2.34). The mean popliteal angle in newborns was reported to be 27° (SD ±6.3°) in a range of 20° to 40° that decreased to zero by age one year (Reade *et al.* 1984). In children, Tardieu considered a 20° popliteal angle to be normal (Tardieu 1984). 'Tight hamstrings' are quite usual in the normal population.

The position of the patella is noted; whether it is riding above its normal location in the patellar-femoral groove (in the fashionable sporting terminology, 'patella alta', and the opposite: 'patella baja').

To discover the amount of flexion contracture of the knee joint, the limb is extended so it lies flat on the table. If firm pressure on the anterior aspect of the knee joint fails to extend the knee to the zero position, a flexion contracture of knee joint (posterior capsule) in addition to the hamstring contracture is likely.

Voluntary control of the quadriceps and its strength within the range allowed by a knee flexion contracture can be estimated with the child lying supine and his legs flexed over the table's edge (Evans 1975). Simultaneous extension of both knees seems easier for most patients. Those who have unilateral voluntary control of knee extension seem to have better walking patterns. With the patient in this same position, quadriceps spasticity might be elicited by quickly pushing the knees into flexion. Those patients who have severe quadriceps spasticity will not be able to have their knees passively flexed to 90°, and the increased stretch reflex can be seen easily.

Tibial-fibular torsion and foot rotation. For language purists, the normal degree of tibial-fibular rotation should be called 'version' and the abnormal 'torsion'. This fixed rotation of the tibia is measured as the expression of the angle between an imaginary line through the tips of the medial and lateral malleoli of the

*Phelps's gracilis test: with the patient prone, knees flexed and hips abducted, extend one knee. If the hip adducts on progressive extension of the knee, gracilis spasm and contracture are confirmed (Keats 1965).

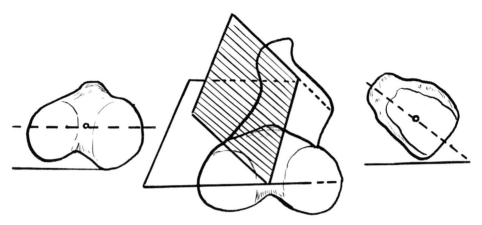

Fig. 2.35. Tibial torsion is the angle formed by the intersection of the two planes constructed between the proximal and distal ends of the tibia *(center)*. The coronal plane is through the proximal articular surface of the polar axis *(left)*. The other plane is through the distal articular surface of the tibia in a line which bisects the medial malleolus and the articular facet for the fibula *(right)*.

ankle and the polar axis of the proximal articular surface—the transmalleolar axis (Fig.2.35). Since Le Damany's treatise on torsion of the tibia (1909), many methods of measurement have been described together with anatomical and clinical studies (Hutter and Scott 1949, Dupuis 1951, Khermosh *et al.* 1971), McSweeny 1971, Staheli and Engel 1972, Engel and Staheli 1974, Ritter *et al.* 1976, Kobyliansky *et al.* 1979, Malekafzali and Wood 1979, Staheli *et al.* 1985). The results of all the different types of measurement show variations of a few degrees of normal tibial rotation, but all are generally in agreement on mean values.

Unless a formal and reportable study is planned by the examiner, it seems to me that elaborate instrumentation and calculations to measure tibial-fibular torsion are too time-consuming to be worthwhile. It is necessary to do some measurement, however. I have used the following method and the results seem to be comparable to those reported in the literature, with tolerable limits of inter-observer variance.

The patient sits with knees flexed over the table-edge and with the hip in neutral rotation. An imaginary line is visualized from the femoral condyles; this line would be roughly parallel to one through the polar axis of the proximal tibial surface. The second line is between the tips of the malleoli. One arm of the goniometer is placed parallel to the table edge and the other arm is placed in line with the oblique line constructed through the tips of the malleoli (Fig.2.36).

With this method of measurement, the normal mean angles with this method according to age were approximately as follows: 0 to 12 months, 7° (±4.1°); 13 to 24 months, 10° (±2°); 25 months to 13 years, 13° (±3°); and in the older children and adults the mean value was 22°. In the study by Staheli *et al.* (1985), in which a photographic method was used, the infant under age one year had a mean transmalleolar axis of about 0° (± 20°) and by age eight years had increased to 20° (range 0° to about 35°; and in the skeletally mature, the mean remained at 20° with a range of 0° to 45°.

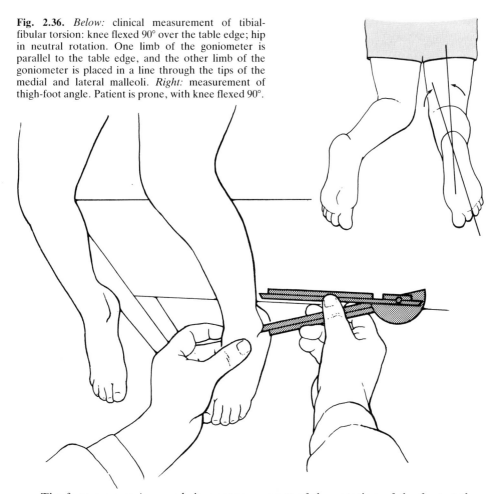

Fig. 2.36. *Below:* clinical measurement of tibial-fibular torsion: knee flexed 90° over the table edge; hip in neutral rotation. One limb of the goniometer is parallel to the table edge, and the other limb of the goniometer is placed in a line through the tips of the medial and lateral malleoli. *Right:* measurement of thigh-foot angle. Patient is prone, with knee flexed 90°.

The foot-progression angle is a measurement of the rotation of the foot at the ankle with reference to the mid-line of the thigh (Staheli *et al.* 1985). I have used this method since it was first described as the thigh-foot angle (Staheli and Engel 1972, Bleck 1982). The patient lies prone, and the knee is flexed 90°; the foot is dorsiflexed to neutral (the measurement is limited to those children who do not have equinus deformities of the ankle). In dorsiflexing the ankle, one has to avoid everting or inverting the foot. One arm of the goniometer is placed on a line that bisects the heel, and the other arm of the goniometer is placed directly over the visualized mid-line of the thigh. The medial or lateral deviation of the foot from the line on the mid-thigh is the angle of foot-progression or the thigh-foot angle. It is a lower angle than that for tibial torsion, but it does roughly parallel the angle of the transmalleolar axis with a mean of +10° and a range from −3° to +20°. It remains practically the same in children and adults (Fig.2.36).

Foot and ankle. The range of dorsiflexion of the ankle is measured with the heel held in inversion in order to get a true estimate of the dorsiflexion; holding the

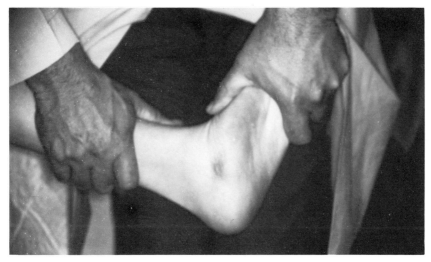

Fig. 2.37. For an accurate measurement of the range of passive dorsiflexion of the ankle, the foot must be held in varus (inversion) to stabilize the talonavicular joint and prevent dorsiflexion at the mid-tarsal joints.

foot in varus locks the midtarsal joints and prevents a false measurement of dorsiflexion of the ankle; simply dorsiflexing the entire foot as a unit can add dorsiflexion at the talonavicular joint (Fig. 2.37). The classical test to differentiate gastrocnemius muscle contracture from that of the soleus muscle was described by Silfverskiöld (1923). In this test, if dorsiflexion of the foot with the knee flexed is greater than that with the knee extended, then the gastrocnemius is implicated as the main site of the contracture (Fig. 2.38). If there is no change in dorsiflexion of the ankle with this maneuver, then contracture of both muscles is present. Electromyographic studies of these muscles in performance of the Silfverskiöld test demonstrated that both muscles show increased action potentials, regardless of the position of the knee joint (Perry *et al.* 1974). No clear-cut differences in gastrocnemius and soleus spasticity were found in three of Perry's eight cases, in spite of positive Silfverskiöld tests in all.

The only case in which I would implicate the gastrocnemius alone as the source of the equinus (and contracture), is when the foot (with hind-foot held in inversion) can be passively dorsiflexed with great ease when the knee if flexed 90°. If any force is required to dorsiflex the foot in this position, I consider the test negative.

Voluntary dorsiflexion of the foot is frequently absent. It is worth noting if the patient can dorsiflex the foot. Frequently active dorsiflexion can be obtained only with the flexor withdrawal ('confusion reflex'). This phenomenon is observed by flexing the knee 90° over the table-edge, and asking the patient to flex the hip actively while the examiner resists flexion of the thigh by manual pressure on the anterior portion of the mid-thigh (Fig.2.39).

Varus of the foot can be due to a spastic posterior tibial muscle which inverts the hind-foot, or an overactive anterior tibial muscle which inverts the mid-foot, or

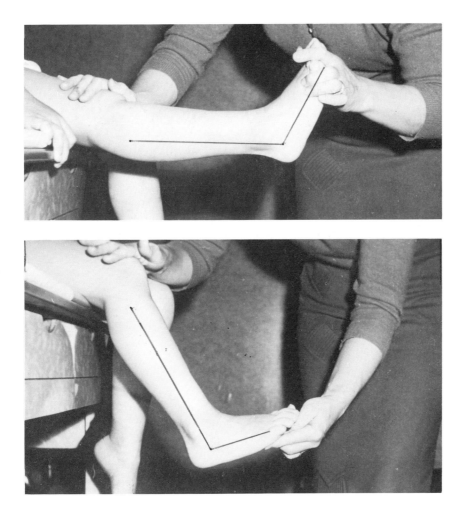

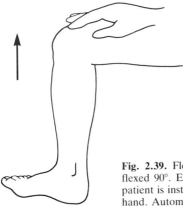

Fig. 2.38. Silfverskiöld test for gastrocnemius versus soleus contracture. *Top:* with knee extended and foot in varus, passively dorsiflex the ankle and note the limited range of ankle dorsiflexion. *Center:* the same maneuver is repeated with the knee flexed 90°. If the ankle dorsiflexes easily when the knee is flexed, gastrocnemius contracture alone is presumed.

Fig. 2.39. Flexor withdrawal reflex. Patient seated with hips and knees flexed 90°. Examiner's hand is on the anterior surface of the thigh. The patient is instructed to flex the hip against the resistance of the examiner's hand. Automatic dorsiflexion of the ankle occurs in a positive response.

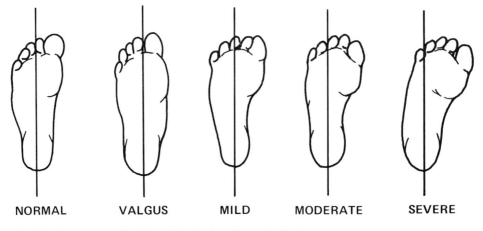

NORMAL   **VALGUS**   **MILD**   **MODERATE**   **SEVERE**

Fig. 2.40. Assessment of forefoot adduction based upon the heel bisector method in which the plantar aspect of the heel is visualized as an ellipse. The heel bisector is the major axis of the ellipse (Bleck 1971, 1982, 1983). Normal: bisects toes 2 and 3; metatarsus adductus: mild, toe 3; moderate, 3 and 4; severe, 4 and 5.

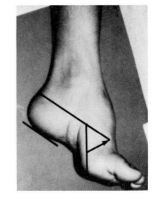

Fig. 2.41. Cavus deformity of the foot. The primary deformity is excessive forefoot equinus which can be measured as depicted with the foot dorsiflexed to its maximum amount, or with the patient standing.

Fig. 2.42. Measurement of forefoot equinus. The horizontal line is parallel to the weight-bearing surface of the heel. The normal angles range from 15° to 30°; +40° represents severe cavus.

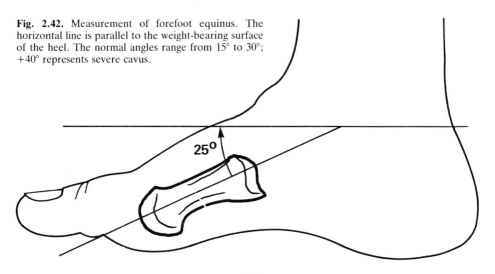

25°

both. If the varus position of the foot can be corrected passively, the deformity is 'dynamic' versus 'fixed'. Quick eversion of the heel may demonstrate an increased stretch reflex in the posterior tibial muscle; in this case, its tendon can be palpated and seen more prominently posterior to the medial malleolus.

Valgus of the foot appears to be due primarily to spastic peroneal muscles which over-power the inverters of the foot. A quick inversion of the foot may elicit the stretch reflex in the peroneal muscles which will offer resistance to this motion. The degree of 'fixed' valgus deformity should be ascertained by manipulating the foot into the corrected position. Usually equinus is a component of the valgus of the hind and mid-foot, and therefore to correct the deformity passively, the foot must be kept in equinus (see Chapter 8 for more details about preoperative assessment of equino-valgus deformities of the foot).

Forefoot adduction deformity (spastic metatarsus adductus) is found by inspection of the plantar aspect of the foot while the examiner holds the heel in one hand and the head of the first metatarsal medially is cupped by the palm and web space of the thumb; the forefoot is then abducted. Limited or no passive abduction of the forefoot indicates a fixed forefoot adduction deformity. One way to assess the metatarsal adduction deformity is to visualize the plantar weight-bearing surface of the heel as an ellipse; the major axis of this ellipse defines the center line of the foot (Bleck 1971, 1983; Bleck and Minaire 1983). In the normal foot, this line ('heel bisector') passes through the second and third toes; in moderate metatarsus adductus it passes between the third and fourth toes, and between the fourth and fifth toes in severe adductus (Fig.2.40). If dynamic metatarsus adductus has been noted during the gait examination, passive abduction of the forefoot is possible and the tendon of the spastic abductor hallucis can be palpated on the medial aspect of the head of the first metatarsal.

Deformities of the toes to be looked for are hallux valgus and toe flexion contractures. Hallux valgus rarely occurs in isolation, but rather is secondary to a valgus deformity of the foot.

A cavus deformity is excessive forefoot equinus and a fixed deformity. In ordinary terms it is a 'high arch'. The forefoot equinus can be compounded by a calcaneous deformity of the hind-foot (an excessive dorsiflexed position of the calcaneus) (Fig.2.41). The diagnosis is usually made by a perception of what constitutes a 'high arch'. To overcome too much subjectivity in this evaluation, I measure the angle between the horizontal weight-bearing surface of the head and the shaft of the first metatarsal (Fig.2.42). This angle should be measured on maximum passive dorsiflexion of the foot, or on photographs of the medial side of the foot when the patient is standing. In normal feet, this angle is between 15° and 30°, an angle of 40° or more denotes a cavus deformity.

Type of motion disorder
By the time this detailed orthopaedic and neurological examination has been completed, the examiner should have no difficulty in deciding whether the motion disorder can be classified as spastic, athetoid, dystonic, tension athetoid, ataxic, tremor or mixed. Even though there are patients who have mixed athetosis and

spasticity, we try to avoid taking this easy route, and prefer as much diagnostic precision as possible. Also based upon observations during the examination, one should have little difficulty in formulating an opinion on the geographic involvement—hemiplegia, diplegia, total body involved, and other refinements if desired, such as 'double hemiplegia' (Ingram 1984). The standard format for recording the diagnosis is, for example: 'cerebral palsy, spastic diplegia, etiology prematurity and low birthweight', or 'cerebral palsy, athetosis, total body involved, etiology, perinatal hypoxia' *etc.*

Summary

The sequence of the examination will be according to one's own style and thought process in data collection. I have resisted the temptation to be 'au courant' by constructing an algorithm*. These diagrams or little boxes with arrows pointing downward, sideways and obliquely, as a guide on what to do next in the diagnosis and treatment of cerebral palsy, are usually too complex to be useful. The diagnosis and management of cerebral palsy cannot be reduced to a simple road map with occasional detours: it is more like the maze at Hampton Court, and only repetition of the experience of examining children makes the process easier. *'Repetitio mater est studiorum'* (repetition is the mother of studies).

However, for those who have read the preceding pages and would like some guidance based upon my own style, I suggest the following order of the examination:

(1) For infants and children aged five years (± 2 SD):
   Begin with child sitting on mother's lap.
      upper limbs
      head
      associated defects
      deep tendon reflexes and plantar responses
      sitting posture
      supine posture
      lower limbs

(2) For older children (aged seven years, ± 2 SD) who cannot walk:
   Begin with child seated in the wheelchair.
      upper limbs
      head
      associated defects
      sitting posture
      deep tendon reflexes and plantar responses
      supine posture
      lower limbs

---

*Algorithm: a rule for solving a certain type of problem. Related to algorism—a method of computation with arabic figures. Arabic: *al* = the, and *Khwárizmi* (the surname of a ninth-century Muslim mathematician; *khwárism* (KHIVA + I + AN) (Urdang and Flexner 1968).

(3) For children who can stand and walk (with or without aids):
> standing posture
> equilibrium reactions
> walking
> sitting posture
> deep tendon reflexes and plantar responses
> head
> associated defects
> upper limbs
> supine posture (if walking is functional, no need to test locomotor prognostic signs)
> lower limbs

Physicians can only give their time, and no computer program has yet been devised to produce 'artificial intelligence' that will decrease the time needed for examination and data collection (Winograd 1985). The time for a complete assessment, recording all the data in a record, making necessary referrals, and above all talking with the parents will be at least 60 minutes. If the child has not been previously diagnosed, or if the condition is complex (*e.g.* total body involved, or spastic diplegia versus hemiplegia), 90 minutes will not be too long. If skeletal radiographs are necessary (excluding computerized axial tomography or magnetic resonance imaging *etc.*), another 30 to 45 minutes will be required, depending on the efficiency of the radiographic services. In the growing child, re-evaluations are almost always necessary every six months and will take at least 30 minutes. Parents usually have many questions and anxieties, which must be answered patiently.

In the United States there is a growing trend to make the physician 'more productive', by insisting that the time spent with patients must be restricted so that the volume of patients per physician can be increased. The proposed practice of medicine by 'Megacorporate Health Care' promises to exclude such luxuries as 'personal-consultation time with the practitioner'. Based upon what is known of these corporate practices, it is predicted that proper assessments of conditions such as cerebral palsy will be done only for 'relatively affluent individual consumers' (Freedman 1985). I hope that physicians will reject and dispel the illusion that a rapid screening process can replace proper medical diagnosis and advice.

Ironically, when things go wrong in patient care (usually due to errors in judgement), much more time is spent with attorneys and courts (or in societies less litigious than the United States, in explanations and filing reports) than was spent on the initial and subsequent assessments of the patient. Furthermore the fees paid, the money spent and the awards granted are considerably more than what was deemed to be the just fee on the first visit (Sanderson 1981).

The team approach arose after World War II, probably because of the greater interest by physicians in children with long-term orthopaedic impairments, and the growth of medical science and practice which permitted more effective management of complex conditions such as cerebral palsy and spina bifida. Many medical and paramedical specialists were educated to deal with the specific problems presented by such children. The public was not niggardly in providing funds to service the multiple needs of disabled children and their parents. The team approach meant that every child with cerebral palsy was seen by a member of the team: pediatrician, neurologist, ophthamologist, orthopaedic surgeon, physiatrist, audiologist, physical and occupational therapists, speech therapist, psychologist, and social worker (and in clinics within special schools, the teacher) regardless of the needs of the particular child. After some 25 years of this kind of team approach, it has been seriously questioned as a viable model. McCollough (1984) reported that such teams are inordinately expensive, and recommended a more rational and modified approach. The primary physician who assumes responsibility for the over-all patient management should refer only to those specialists who are required to assess a particular problem in a particular child. The medical and paramedical specialists should be available for consultation, but each child does not have to run through a mill with every member of the team taking a little piece of the child. In this regard, the advice of the late Dr Douglas Buchanan, Professor of Neurology, University of Chicago, is worth repeating: 'We have no routines in our clinic. When you have routines, everyone stops thinking'.

REFERENCES

Akbarnia, B. A. (1984) 'Spinal deformity in patients with cerebral palsy.' *Orthopaedic Transactions*, **8**, 116. *Developmental Medicine and Child Neurology*, **26**, 260. (*Abstract.*)
Baird, H. W., Gordon, E. C. (1983) *Neurological Evaluation of Infants and Children. Clinics in Developmental Medicine Nos. 84/85,* London: S.I.M.P. with Heinemann; Philadelphia: Lippincott.
Balmer, G. A., MacEwen, G. D. (1970) 'The incidence of scoliosis in cerebral palsy.' *Journal of Bone and Joint Surgery*, **52**, 134–136.
Beadle, K. (1982) 'Communication disorders'. *In:* Bleck, E. E., Nagel, D. A. (Eds.) *Physically Handicapped Children: A Medical Atlas for Teachers.* Orlando, Florida: Grune & Stratton.
Bleck, E. E. (1971) 'The shoeing of children: sham or science.' *Developmental Medicine and Child Neurology*, **13**, 188–195.
—— (1975) 'Locomotor prognosis in cerebral palsy.' *Developmental Medicine and Child Neurology*, **17**, 18–25.
—— (1982) 'Developmental orthopaedics. III: Toddlers.' *Developmental Medicine and Child Neurology*, **24**, 533–555.
—— (1983) 'Metatarsus adductus: classification and relationship to outcomes of treatment.' *Journal of Pediatric Orthopaedics*, **3**, 2–9.
—— Ford, F., Stevik, A. C., Csongradi, J. (1975) 'EMG telemetry study of spastic gait patterns in cerebral palsied children'. *Developmental Medicine and Child Neurology*, **17**, 307 (*Abstract.*)
—— Minaire, P. (1983) 'Persistent medial deviation of the neck of the talus: a common cause of in-toeing in children.' *Journal of Pediatric Orthopaedics*, **3**, 149–159.
Bobath, B. (1954) 'A study of abnormal reflex activity in patients with lesions of the central nervous system.' *Physiotherapy*, **40**, 259–289.
Brunnstrom, S. (1962) *Clinical Kinesiology*. Philadelphia: F. A. Davies.
Buchanan, D. (1967) *Lecture notes, Course in Pediatric Neurology, University of California Los Angeles School of Medicine.*
Bunnell, W. P. (1984) 'An objective criterion for scoliosis screening.' *Journal of Bone and Joint Surgery*, **66A**, 1381–1387.
Coon, V., Donato, G., Houser, C., Bleck, E. E. (1975) 'Normal ranges of motion of the hip in infants, six weeks, three months and six months of age.' *Clinical Orthopaedics and Related Research*, **110**, 256–260.

Csongradi, J., Bleck, E. E., Ford, W. F. (1979) 'Gait electromyography in normal and spastic children.' *Developmental Medicine and Child Neurology*, **21**, 738–748.

Cupps, C., Plescia, M. G., Houser, C. (1976) 'The Landau reaction: a clinical and electromyographic analysis.' *Developmental Medicine and Child Neurology*, **18**, 43–53.

Dupuis, P. V. (1951) *La Torsion Tibiale*. Paris: Masson.

Elliott, J. M., Connolly, K. J. (1984) 'A classification of manipulative hand movements.' *Developmental Medicine and Child Neurology*, **26**, 283–296.

Engel, G. M., Staheli, L. T. (1974) 'The natural history of torsion and other factors influencing gait in childhood. A study of the angle of gait, tibial torsion, knee angle, hip rotation, and development of the arch in normal children.' *Clinical Orthopaedics and Related Research*, **99**, 12–17.

Evans, E. B. (1975) 'The knee in cerebral palsy.' *In:* Samilson, R. L. (Ed.) *Orthopaedic Aspects of Cerebral Palsy. Clinics in Developmental Medicine, Nos. 52/53*. London: S.I.M.P. with Heinemann; Philadelphia: Lippincott.

Freedman, S. A. (1985) 'Megacorporate health care.' *New England Journal of Medicine*, **312**, 579–582.

Gesell, A., Amatruda, C. S. (1947) *Developmental Diagnosis, 2nd edn.* New York: Hoeber.

Goble, J. (1984) *Visual Disorders in the Handicapped Child*. New York: Marcel Dekker.

Goldner, J. L. (1974) 'Upper extremity tendon transfers in cerebral palsy.' *Orthopedic Clinics of North America*, **5**, 389–414.

—— Ferlic, D. C. (1966) 'Sensory status of the hand as related to reconstructive surgery of the upper extremity in cerebral palsy.' *Clinical Orthopaedics and Related Research*, **46**, 87–92.

Haas, S. S., Epps, C. H. Jr., Adams, J. P. (1973) 'Normal ranges of hip motion in the newborn.' *Clinical Orthopaedics and Related Research*, **91**, 114–118.

Hagberg, B., Sanner, G., Steen, M. (1972) 'The dysequilibrium syndrome in cerebral palsy.' *Acta Paediatrica Scandinavica, Suppl. 226.* 1–63.

Hutter, C. G., Scott, W. (1949) 'Tibial torsion.' *Journal of Bone and Joint Surgery*, **31A**, 511–518.

Ingram, T. T. S. (1984) 'A historical review of the definition and classification of the cerebral palsies.' *In:* Stanley, F., Alberman, E. (Eds.) *The Epidemiology of the Cerebral Palsies. Clinics in Developmental Medicine No. 87*. London: S.I.M.P. with Blackwell; Philadelphia: Lippincott.

Keats, S. (1965) *Cerebral Palsy*. Springfield, Illinois: C. C. Thomas.

Kelley, D. L. (1971) *Kinesiology, Fundamentals of Motion Description*. Englewood Cliffs, New Jersey: Prentice-Hall.

Khermosh, O., Lior, G., Weissman, S. L. (1971) 'Tibial torsion in children.' *Clinical Orthopaedics and Related Research*, **79**, 25–31.

Kobyliansky, E., Weissman, S. L., Nathan, H. (1979) 'Femoral and tibial torsion. A correlation study in dry bones.' *International Orthopaedics*, **3**, 145–147.

Le Damany, P. (1909) 'La torsion du tibia. Normal, pathologique, expérimentale.' *Journal à Anatomie et Physiologie*, **45**, 589–615.

Madigan, R. R., Wallace, S. L. (1981) 'Scoliosis in the institutionalized cerebral palsy population.' *Spine*, **6**, 583–590.

Malekafzali, S., Wood, M. B. (1979) 'Tibial torsion—a simple clinical apparatus for its measurement and its application to a normal adult population.' *Clinical Orthopaedics and Related Research*, **145**, 154–157.

McCollough, N. C. III (Chairman) (1984) Proceedings of the *Conference on The Critical Needs of the Child with Long Term Orthopaedic Impairment*. Washington, D.C. (*in press*).

McInerny, R. (1984) *St. Thomas Aquinas. 6 Lectures on the Saint and His Thought*. Notre Dame, Indiana: University of Notre Dame Press.

McMahon, T. A. (1984) *Muscles, Reflexes, and Locomotion*. Princeton, New Jersey: Princeton University Press.

McSweeny, A. (1971) 'A study of femoral torsion in children.' *Journal of Bone and Joint Surgery*, **53B**, 90–95.

Moberg, E. (1984) 'New facts on kinaesthesia. Role and examination of sensibility.' *Surgical Rehabilitation of the Upper Limb in Tetraplegia*. Second small group international conference, Hôpital Renée Sabran, Giens-Hyêres, France.

O'Connell, E. J. Feldt, R. H., Stickler, G. B. (1965) 'Head circumference, mental retardation and growth failure.' *Pediatrics*, **36**, 62–66.

Opila-Lehman, J., Short, M. S., Trombly, C. A. (1984) 'Kinesthetic performance of athetoid and spastic cerebral palsied and non-handicapped children.' *Orthopaedic Transactions*, **8**, 104. *Developmental Medicine and Child Neurology*, **26**, 241. (*Abstract*.)

Paine, R. S., Oppé, T. E. (1966) *Neurological Examination of Children. Clinics in Developmental Medicine Nos. 20/21*. London: S.I.M.P. with Heinemann.

Perlstein, M. D. (1960–66) Lectures in cerebral palsy. Annual meetings of the American Academy for Cerebral Palsy.

Perry, J. (1967) 'The mechanics of walking.' *Physical Therapy*, **4**, 778–804.

—— (1975) 'Cerebral palsy gait.' *In:* Samilson, R. L. (Ed.) *Orthopaedic Aspects of Cerebral Palsy. Clinics in Developmental Medicine Nos. 52/53.* London: S.I.M.P. with Heinemann; Philadelphia: J. B. Lippincott.

—— Hoffer, M. M., Giovan, P., Antonelli, D., Greenberg, R. (1974) 'Gait analysis of the triceps surae in cerebral palsy.' *Journal of Bone and Joint Surgery*, **56A**, 511–520.

—— —— Antonelli, D., Plut, J., Lewis, G., Greenberg, R. (1976) 'Electromyography before and after surgery for hip deformity in children with cerebral palsy.' *Journal of Bone and Joint Surgery*, **58A**, 201–208.

Reade, E., Hom, L., Hallum, A., Lopopolo, R. (1984) 'Changes in popliteal angle measurement in infants up to one year of age.' *Developmental Medicine and Child Neurology*, **26**, 774–780.

Ritter, M. A., DeRosa, G. P., Babcock, J. L. (1976) 'Tibial torsion?' *Clinical Orthopaedics and Related Research*, **120**, 159–163.

Robson, P. (1968) 'The prevalence of scoliosis in adolescents and young adults with cerebral palsy.' *Developmental Medicine and Child Neurology*, **10**, 447–452.

Rushworth, G. (1964) *The Role of the Gamma System in Movement and Posture.* New York: Association for the Aid of Crippled Children.

Samilson, R. L., Bechard, R. (1973) 'Scoliosis in cerebral palsy.' *In:* Ahstrom, J. P. (Ed.) *Current Practice in Orthopaedic Surgery Vol. 5.* St. Louis: C. V. Mosby.

Sanderson, R. R. (1981) 'Medical practice and malpractice.' *Legal Aspects of Medical Practice*, **9**, 1–7.

Saunders, J. B., Inman, V. T., Eberhart, H. D. (1953) 'The major determinants in normal and pathological gait.' *Journal of Bone and Joint Surgery*, **35A**, 543–558.

Silfverskiöld, N. (1923) 'Reduction of the uncrossed two joint muscles of the one-to-one muscle in spastic conditions.' *Acta Chirurgica Scandinavica*, **56**, 315–330.

Staheli, L. T. (1977) 'The prone hip extension test.' *Clinical Orthopaedics and Related Research*, **123**, 12–15.

—— Engel, G. M., (1972) 'Tibial torsion. A method of assessment and a survey of normal children.' *Clinical Orthopaedics and Related Research*, **86**, 183–186.

—— Corbett, B. S., Wyss, C., King, H. (1985) 'Lower-extremity rotational problems in children.' *Journal of Bone and Joint Surgery*, **67**, 39–47.

Tachdjian, M. O., Minear, W. L. (1958) 'Sensory disturbances in the hands of children with cerebral palsy.' *Journal of Bone and Joint Surgery*, **40**, 85–90.

Tardieu, G. (1984) *Le Dossier Clinique de L'Infirmité Motrice Cérébrale, 3rd edn.* Paris: Masson.

Urdang, L., Flexner, S. B. (1968) *The Random House Dictionary of the English Language.* College Edition, New York: Random House.

Winograd, T. (1985) 'Artifical intelligence may be over-sold.' *Campus Report, Stanford University: Stanford, California*, Feb. 27, pages 1 and 10.

3
SPECIAL ASSESSMENTS AND INVESTIGATIONS

In this chapter I have included only those special assessment methods which are of special interest to the orthopaedist. These are: the physical and occupational therapist's assessments which include developmental testing, radiology, photography, pedography, instrumented gait and motion analysis, myoneural blocks, and psychological testing. A little learning need not be a dangerous thing for orthopaedic surgeons or other physicians who care for children with cerebral palsy. I have not included special laboratory examinations such as blood, urine and cerebrospinal fluid for metabolic defects, chromosomal analysis, electroencephalography, or neurometric examinations. There is ample literature about these specialized subjects (Baird and Gordon 1983).

Physical and occupational therapist's assessments
A complete motor assessment includes the following examinations with the data recorded on special forms so that the status of the motor system can be followed as the child matures: (i) passive ranges of motion of the limb joints; (ii) manual muscle tests, particularly the delineation of selective motor control; and (iii) motor maturity evaluation. The motor age of the child is determined by the observations of postural and functional activities related to what is considered normal for age. For example, at seven months the infant assumes the quadruped position, at nine months pulls self to standing, at 13 months walks alone. The problem with motor age determinations is that normal children do not perform and develop on an exact timetable, and allowances must be made for individual variations. Another problem is that a motor age does not always tell us how a child functions, or what adaptations to function independently have occurred. Motor age determinations have been used for special studies and prognosis (Beals 1966). Testing for functional abilities is probably more important in evaluating and following children. Functions in eating, daily hygiene, toileting, dressing, mobility, and communication skills, when scored for independence and completion in a practical time, or performed with equipment and adaptations, are most informative. Most physical and occupational therapists have their own forms, and many have been published (Coley 1978, Bleck and Nagel 1982, Tardieu 1984).

A good simple developmental test for preschool children (ages two to five years) was published originally by Paine and Oppé (1966), and is reproduced in Table 3.I (from Baird and Gordon 1983).

Developmental screening tests
Due to the enormous interest in outcomes of infants born 'at-risk' (*e.g.* prematurity

TABLE 3.I

Check-list for assessment by observation of developmental level of preschool children

Age (yrs)	Historical (or observed) items	Items to be tested
2	Runs well Walks up and down stairs—one step at a time Opens doors Climbs on furniture Puts three words together Handles spoon well Helps to undress Listens to stories with pictures	Builds tower of six cubes Circular scribbling Copies horizontal stroke with pencil Folds paper once
2½	Jumps Knows full name Refers to self by pronoun 'I' Helps put things away	Builds tower of eight cubes Copies horizontal and vertical strokes (not a cross)
3	Goes upstairs, alternating feet Rides tricycle Stands momentarily on one foot Knows age and sex Plays simple games Helps in dressing Washes hands	Builds tower of nine cubes Imitates construction of bridge with three cubes Imitates a cross and circle

4	Hops on one foot
	Throws a ball overhand
	Climbs well
	Uses scissors to cut out pictures
	Counts four pennies accurately
	Tells a story
	Plays with several children
	Goes to toilet alone
		Copies bridges from a model
		Imitates construction of a gate with
		    five cubes
		Copies a cross and circle
		Draws a man with two to four
		    parts—other than head
		Names longer of two lines

5	Skips Names four colours Counts 10 pennies correctly Dresses and undresses Asks questions about meaning of words	Copies a square and triangle Names four colours Names heavier of two weights

From Paine and Oppé (1966).

and low birthweight, perinatal hypoxia), numerous developmental screening tests have been devised. These tests have been used in many clinical investigations of infants to determine the natural history of development of infants born 'at-risk' and to judge the efficacy of 'early intervention' for such infants (Nelson and Ellenberg 1982, Stanley and Alberman 1984, Harel and Anastasiow 1985). Recent national conferences have shown that there is no shortage of such studies (Biasini and Mindingall 1984, Bozynski *et al.* 1984, Hoffman-Williamson *et al.* 1984, Marquis *et al.* 1984, Nelson *et al.* 1984, Paludetto *et al.* 1984).

Most of these tests can be administered by therapists, especially the Denver Developmental Test. The Denver test is by far the most popular initial screening test used to identify suspected infants (Frankenburg and Dodds 1967, Frankenburg *et al.* 1971, Baird and Gordon 1983). This test has been standardized for infants born in other cultures and societies (Federal Republic of Germany: Flehmig *et al.* 1973; UK: Bryant *et al.* 1974; USA: Barnes and Stark 1975, Frankenburg *et al.* 1975; South Africa: Super 1976; Netherlands: Cools and Hermanns 1977; Japan: Ueda 1978; Israel: Shapira and Harel 1983).

More sophisticated developmental tests for the infant and child up to the age of three years have been published (Paine and Oppé 1966; Bayley 1969; Brazelton 1973, 1984; Sheridan 1975, 1978; Prechtl 1977; Saint-Anne Dargassies 1977; Touwen 1979; Amiel-Tison and Grenier 1983). Unless the therapist is very well trained and experienced in the techniques of a neurological examination, the assistance of a physician and/or a psychologist will be needed.

Developmental screening tests for the child over three years of age can be used for screening purposes. These tests are additions to the neurological examinations for gross and fine motor skills (Baird and Gordon 1983). Recommended and commonly used tests are: the Peabody Picture Vocabulary test, the Slosson Oral Reading test, the Draw-a-Person test, the Slosson Drawing Co-ordination test and the Bender-Gestalt test. This last test has given consistent results and has been judged to be dependable (Baird and Gordon 1983).

Special investigations that can be performed by the therapist include clinical photography, pedography and instrumented gait analysis; these can also help the physician in clinical examinations and investigations.

Because therapists usually have more intimate and day-to-day contact with the child and parents, they can inform the physician of the child's emotional and behavioral problems and parental concerns and expectations. Parenthetically, this indicates that therapists need to have training and some experience in psychology and interpersonal relations. Patients and parents need advice on coping with the handicap, and recommendations for adaptations and devices to compensate for functional loss. Such advice needs to be consistent with that of the physician who has assumed over-all responsibility for management.

The physician must recognize structural changes in the musculo-skeletal system that would impair function (*e.g.* subluxation of the hip, flexion contracture of the knee, scoliosis). Early discernment of such potential problems, and alerting the physician to them, assists the physician who can initiate appropriate clinical and radiographic investigations.

Special perceptual and visual-motor tests for the evaluation of learning disabilities have been very popular in the United States, parallel with the great interest and concomitant monies allocated to improve the education of children. The most widely applied tests (usually by occupational therapists) were those of Frostig (Frostig 1963, Frostig and Horne 1964) and Ayres (1972, 1978); they were often requested by the teachers. When these tests were positive, special remediation programs by therapists were initiated with the intent of improved academic performance. In follow-up studies much of this work has been discounted

(Feagans 1983). Based upon the evidence, I will not approve of these tests when a medical prescription is requested (in the USA written and signed 'prescriptions' for therapy tests and treatment are usually required).

Radiology
Plain radiographs are essential for the diagnosis and for surgical treatment of structural changes in the skeleton. Infants and children who have adduction and/or flexion spasticity of the hip musculature should have an anterior-posterior radiograph of the hips (with the hips held in the neutral abduction/adduction position) at approximately six-month intervals, in order to make the early diagnosis of subluxation. Based upon the clinical examination for the signs of scoliosis, a single anterior-posterior radiograph of the spine and pelvis (made with the patient standing or sitting) should be made. More projections will be necessary if orthotic or surgical treatment is planned. If a leg-length discrepancy of significance (more than 1cm) is found, special leg-length films are the only accurate way to document and then follow the shortening of the limb in the growing child. Radiographs of the other bones and joints are usually made when the history and clinical examination show they are necessary, most often in the preoperative evaluation, and postoperative follow-up.

In this nuclear age, and with the widespread publicity on the risks of radiation, parents today are rightly concerned about over-exposure to radiation. Despite the promise of magnetic resonance imaging to reduce the need for radiation, skeletal structures do not visualize as well as in radiographs; furthermore, the use of magnetic resonance imaging is contra-indicated in patients who have metallic implants in the spine or bones, due to the detrimental effects of the intense magnetic field (Kucharczyk *et al*. 1985). Therefore, although prudence in ordering radiographs in children is required, there is no other way for a correct diagnosis and treatment to be accomplished. Parents need to be more informed with objective information on radiographic dosages and risks of cancer. With special filters and modern radiographic equipment, the dosages per projection to various anatomical parts can be determined and related to what is deemed to be safe (see Appendix A). Since radiographic equipment differs, each radiographic unit would be advised to prepare its own data for publication. This kind of data has helped us give parents a perspective, and has reduced anxiety.

Computerized axial tomography (CAT) has revolutionized the diagnosis of suspected lesions of the brain (*e.g.* hydrocephalus, porencephalic cysts); invasive procedures such as pneumo-encephalography have practically disappeared. Because CAT necessitates more radiation than with plain radiographs, its use needs to be selective. This technology has been applied to various skeletal structures, and is especially useful in the analysis of abnormalities in the hip joint. It allows a better visualization of the femoral head in relation to the acetabulum, and the configuration of the acetabulum, so that surgical reconstruction can be more accurately designed and performed (Lasada *et al*. 1978, Weiner *et al*. 1978, Terver *et al*. 1982) (Fig.3.1). It has also permitted more accurate diagnosis of lesions of the cervical-occipital region in children (Fig.3.2).

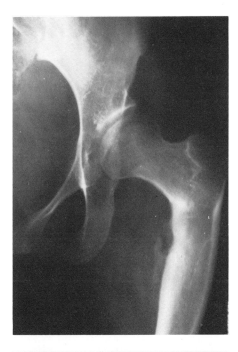

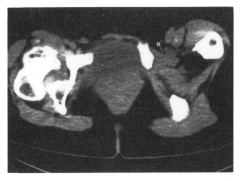

Fig. 3.1. *Left:* anterior-posterior radiograph of 19-year-old female with spastic diplegia, totally disabled because of hip pain. Was referred after femoral osteotomy and subsequent removal of the internal fixation device. *Above:* CT scan of patient's hip shows severe femoral torsion, erosion on the anterior femoral head, and an irregular acetabulum.

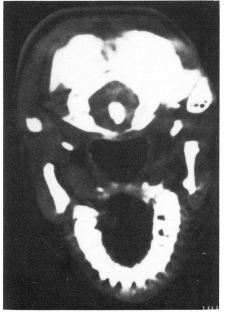

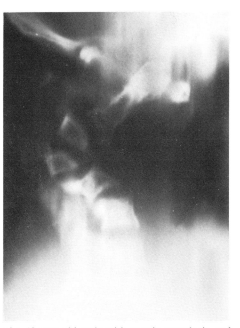

Fig. 3.2. *Left:* lateral tomograph of cervical spine of a 12-year-old male with spastic paraplegia and neurofibromatosis. Postoperative cervical laminectomy. *Left:* CT scan of base of skull and upper cervical spine of patient. The odontoid rests within the foramen magnum: occipitalization of the atlas. This was not noted at the time of his laminectomy; however, the tomograph *(right)* does demonstrate what appears to be a greatly elongated axis and suggests occipitalization of the atlas.

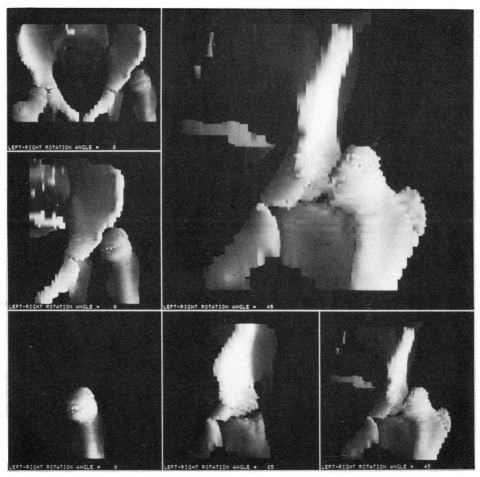

Fig. 3.3. Three-dimensional image reconstruction from CT scanning of 12-year-old with paralytic dislocation of the hip. *Top left:* 0° rotation; *center left:* close-up 0° rotation; *bottom left:* femur 'subtracted out' of image (note femoral torsion); *bottom center:* acetabulum and pelvis 'subtracted out' at 45° rotation; *bottom right:* femur and pelvis 45° rotation; *top right:* 45° rotation angle. Radiation dosage for this film was 3.5 rads. (Processor is Cemax-100 by Control Medical Systems Inc., Mountain View, California. Photo courtesy of S. T. Woolson MD, Palo Alto, California.)

A recent innovation has been three-dimensional construction of skeletal structures, from which plastic anatomical models can be fabricated (Woolson 1985) (Fig.3.3). This new technique will be limited to very special and complex surgical reconstructive problems of the joints, and possibly of the spine.

Radio-isotope imaging—brain scan, cisternography, single-photon-emission computed tomography (SPECT), positron-emission tomography (PET)—are techniques that enable more precise information on the structure and function of the brain, and thus are being used and developed for clinical neurological diagnosis (Baird and Gordon 1983, Ziporyn 1985*a*).

70

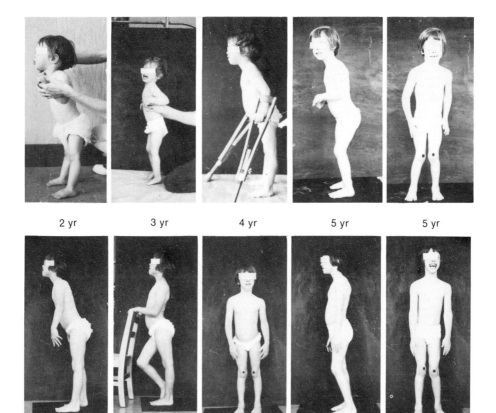

| 2 yr | 3 yr | 4 yr | 5 yr | 5 yr |

| 7 yr | 7 yr | 7 yr | 8 yr | 8 yr |

Fig. 3.4. Physical therapist's photographs of a child with spastic diplegia, demonstrating persistent hip-flexion deformities and hip internal rotation. After bilateral derotation subtrochanteric osteotomies at 10½ years, the hip-flexion deformities increased; to compensate for the severe hip-flexion contracture and remain erect, knee-flexion contractures developed. Serial black-and-white photographs of the patient's posture over the years can be a valuable record.

Magnetic resonance imaging (MRI), formerly called 'nuclear magnetic resonance (NMR), continues to be developed and applied apace primarily in the diagnosis of lesions of the spinal cord and brain (Kucharczyk 1985, Ziporyn 1985*b*). This technical advance will undoubtedly refine the diagnosis and anatomical lesions in cases of cerebral palsy and lesions of the spinal cord that cause paralysis.

Clinical photography

Black and white or color photographs continue to be useful for recording changes in posture as the child develops (Fig.3.4). We have found Polaroids useful in our clinics; they can be seen immediately, retaken if the views are not satisfactory, and mounted in the record. Tedious cataloguing of negatives, printing, sorting and finally mounting in the records is to be avoided.

71

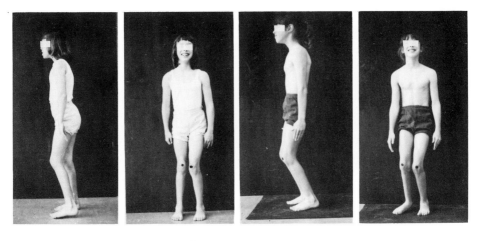

| 10 yr | 10 yr | 11 yr | 11 yr |

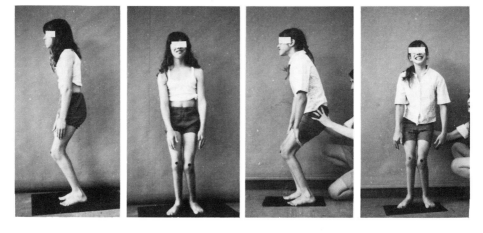

| 12 yr | 12 yr | 13 yr | 13 yr |

Fig. 3.4 *(continued)*.

To record gait patterns, mobility and upper limb functions, videotape recordings have replaced cinematography in many treatment units. As with photographic films, the major disadvantage is the need to splice serial tapes of one patient into a sequence. Special computerized video systems, which can search for and retrieve specific tapes, overcome this difficulty. Although the recording of walking and function can be of value in following a patient's progress (or lack of it), viewing films takes time (which always seems limited) over and beyond that required for a re-evaluation of the patient's status. Cinematography and videotape have been used for clinical studies, and while superior to written descriptions of walking, do remain somewhat subjective. Instrumented motion analysis permits more objective data. Cine and video films are effective for audio-visual education, but the effort is probably best left to academic centers which have the facilities and the funds.

Pedography

A simple and inexpensive way to record some elements of gait is to measure footprints made by walking. The method comprises a few sequences: (i) dip the plantar aspect of the feet in a pan of finely ground charcoal; (ii) walk on a strip of white paper 5m long and 1m wide; a mirror is placed about 2m beyond the end of the paper pathway so the patient may observe his/her gait; (iii) continue to walk off the end of the paper and onto the floor so that walking speed and pattern are not distorted.

From the resultant footprints, the extent of foot contact at the mid-stance (toe-walking will be evident) and in-toed or out-toed gait may be visualized.

Measurements are made according to the technique of Chodera and Levell (1973). Their method relates measurements to the continually changing direction of walking (Fig.3.5). From the measurements the following data can be obtained: (i) step length—the toe-to-toe distance between two successive footprints of the lower limbs, either right-to-left or left-to-right; (ii) stride length—a toe-to-toe distance between two successive footprints of the same foot; (iii) the base of the gait—the distance from heel to heel; and (iv) the angle of foot placement. Footprint analysis, although limited, can be used to determine the efficacy of treatment programs designed for a specific purpose, *e.g.* correction of equinus deformity, in-toeing, or limb adduction. We used pedographs as one of several measurements in evaluating the effects of a pharmaceutical proposed for the diminution of spasticity (Ford *et al*. 1976) (Fig.3.6).

Instrumented motion analysis

The measurement and analysis of human walking began in the latter part of the 19th century when Marey (1873, 1874) made records of running and walking. The development of photography permitted Muybridge (1901) to record with multiple exposure the gait of horses, humans and other animals. It has been claimed that he did the first gait analysis on the farm of Senator Leland Stanford in Palo Alto, California. Muybridge was able to prove Senator Stanford's contention that when a racehorse ran, there were times when all four feet were off the ground.

With increasingly sophisticated equipment, we can record not only muscle function during gait, but also motion of the lower limbs and trunk, forces generated between the feet and the ground, balance mechanisms and energy requirements.

The number of reports on motion analysis techniques has increased enormously in the past 20 years. A large number of papers on the study of pathological gait (especially due to cerebral palsy) have appeared in the North American and European literature; and lately reports from Asian countries have also been noted.

The physician needs objective criteria for analyzing problems of locomotion, to make rational decisions about surgery, orthotics, physical therapy and drug therapy. The decision not to treat is probably of more value than to treat. Furthermore, in cerebral palsy more objective assessments of outcomes of

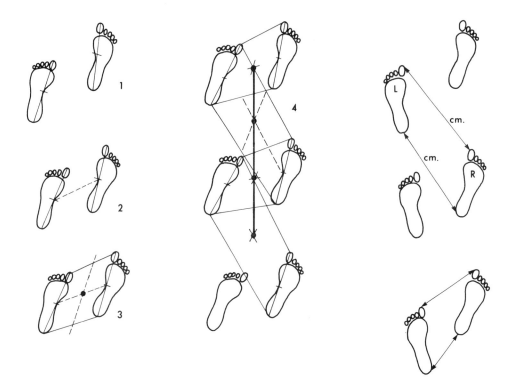

orthopaedic surgery should inevitably lead to better decisions on the selection of the surgical procedure. 'The patient with cerebral palsy who has orthopaedic surgery is not necessarily improved, but is certainly changed!' (Robert Salter MD).

Normative data for muscle activity, and the range of motion of the pelvis and lower limb joints during level walking, are now available (Murray 1967, Sutherland and Hagy 1972, Sutherland 1980, Chao *et al.* 1983). Publications and reports on their clinical usefulness have appeared in the last 10 years (Perry *et al.* 1976; Griffin *et al.* 1977; Perry and Hoffer 1977; Simon *et al.* 1978, 1984; Baumann 1980, 1984; Sutherland and Baumann 1981; Hoffer and Perry 1983; Knutsson 1983; Alder *et al.* 1984; Bose and Goh 1984; Gage *et al.* 1984; Mederios 1984; Simon *et al.* 1984; Skinner and Lester 1984).

While the initial costs of equipment are high, they do not seem astronomical when related to the cost of other technologies in relation to the benefits of accurate assessment and improved management of cerebral palsy. In fact initial equipment costs are not the major problem. I have found that the costs of computer programming and the continuing maintenance of the equipment by engineers and technicians are more important. However, with more automation of motion analysis and improved electronic circuitry, these costs should decrease considerably (as we have seen with computers in the past 10 years), and the number of people employed either full- or part-time by the laboratory should decrease. Our own

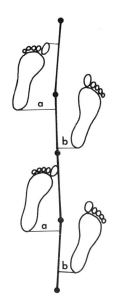

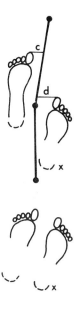

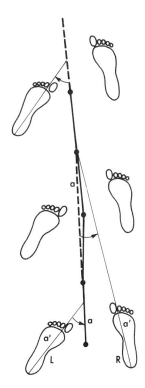

Fig. 3.5. Measurement of pedographs (from Chodera and Levell 1973). *Opposite, far left:* to find the centroid, in order to plot the progression of gait, (i) mark the footprint from tip of the great toe to the posterior border of heel and measure half the distance; (ii) connect the midfoot to the midfoot marks; (iii) mark toe-to-toe on opposite foot and heel to opposite heel—measure half this distance; (iv) connect centroids to find line of progression *(opposite center)*. *Opposite right:* step-length is the distance between two successive footprints: either right to left (left step) or left to right (right step). *Above left:* for stride-length, measure the distance between two successive footprints of the same foot: right to right and left to left. *Above center:* to find base of the gait, draw perpendicular lines from the center line to tip of great toe and to posterior border of the heel. Base of gait is sum of *a* + *b*. *Above right:* if a toe-walker, base of gait is sum of *c* + *d*. To find heel location of toe-walker, measure actual length of foot from toe to heel and transpose this measurement to the footprint, and mark posterior border of heel *(x)*. *Right:* measurement of angle of foot placement with reference to line of progression: construct a line which bisects the footprint from between the great and second toes and the posterior heel center. The left footprint *(L)* bisector, *a'* intersects the line of progression, *a;* the angle of toe-in can be measured. For the right footprint *(R)*, note that the angle formed by *a'* and *a* is constructed by extending the line of progression *(broken line)*.

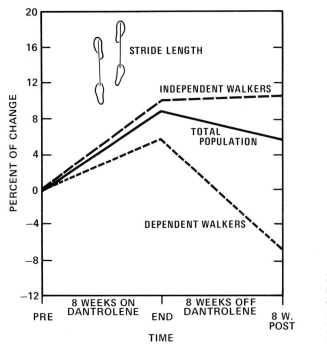

Fig. 3.6. Pedographic study of stride-length to assess the results of drug therapy in cerebral palsy (this was only one of the many parameters used in the study by Ford *et al.* 1976).

laboratory is staffed by one full-time physical therapist, one part-time relief therapist and on-call electronic engineers, technicians and computer programmers.

Electromyographic gait analysis
Equipment
Like most other laboratories, we use electromyographic (EMG) biotelemetry systems, to avoid the 'spaghetti effect' with wires from the patient to the recording instruments, and to allow freedom of movement. The action potentials of the muscles chosen for study (up to eight) are recorded from surface miniature electrodes or indwelling fine wire (50µ diameter nylon shielded copper wire). Intramuscular wire electrodes are used when recording of an isolated muscle is necessary (*e.g.* posterior tibial), and surface electrodes for large muscle groups (*e.g.* hip adductors). Most investigative studies have used wire electrodes for greater accuracy. However, for clinical use whenever possible, especially in children, surface electrodes are preferred.

The swing and stance phases of gait are simultaneously recorded with the electromyograms by compression of closing foot-switch sensors taped to the sole of the shoe over the heel, fifth metatarsal head and great toe regions. The EMG electrode wires and foot-switch lead wires are connected to a radio transmitter. In our system each muscle and the foot-switches have their own miniature transmitters that are battery-operated (Fig. 3.7).

The patient walks at least 10m on a walkway. Two photocells at each end of

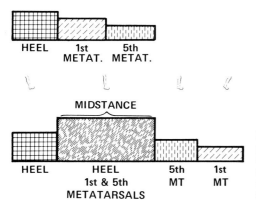

HEEL   1st   5th
METAT. METAT.

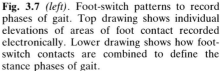

MIDSTANCE

HEEL   HEEL   5th   1st
1st & 5th   MT   MT
METATARSALS

Fig. 3.7 *(left).* Foot-switch patterns to record phases of gait. Top drawing shows individual elevations of areas of foot contact recorded electronically. Lower drawing shows how foot-switch contacts are combined to define the stance phases of gait.

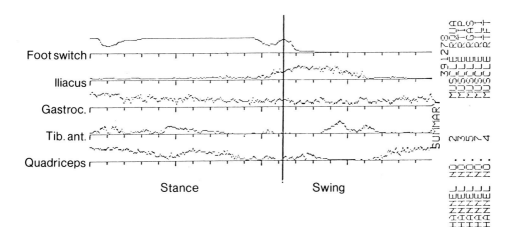

Foot switch

Iliacus

Gastroc.

Tib. ant.

Quadriceps

Stance   Swing

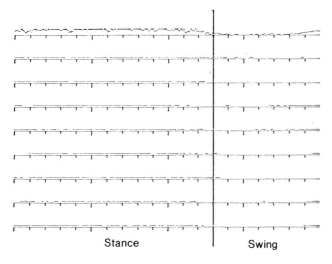

Stance   Swing

Fig. 3.8. *Above:* automated electromyographic record during gait of a 12-year-old male with spastic diplegia, postoperative iliopsoas recession. The grossly abnormal muscle activity is of the gastrocnemius and the quadriceps. This should be compared with the normal standards in Fig. 3.9. *Left:* the top line is a summary record of several gait cycles below. The automated electrotelemetry system records on-off firing; the EMG is not quantitative.

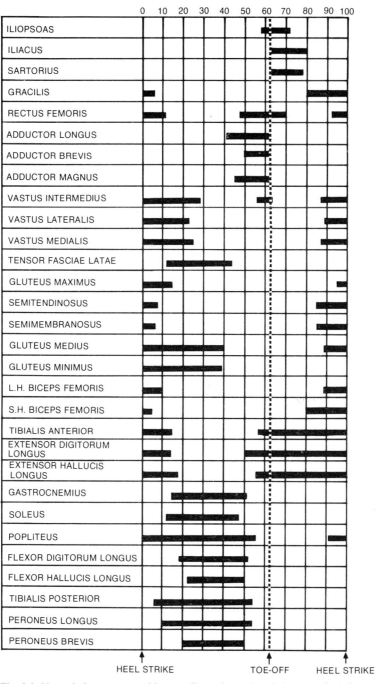

NORMAL ELECTROMYOGRAPHIC DATA

Fig. 3.9. Normal electromyographic recordings of muscles of the lower limb (courtesy of R. Mann and J. Hagy, Shriner's Hospital for Crippled Children, San Francisco, California).

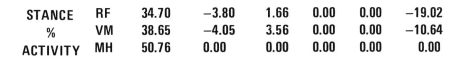

STANCE	RF	34.70	−3.80	1.66	0.00	0.00	−19.02
%	VM	38.65	−4.05	3.56	0.00	0.00	−10.64
ACTIVITY	MH	50.76	0.00	0.00	0.00	0.00	0.00

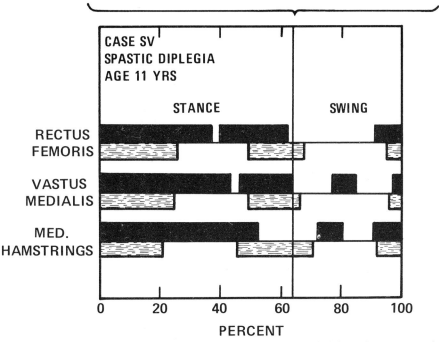

Fig. 3.10. Conversion of gait electromyogram of a patient into digital form *(top)* representing the percent of muscle activity during the stance and swing phases of gait. The lower record was drawn from raw records for clarity in publication. The black areas represent the abnormal firing of the patient's muscles; the shaded areas are the normal muscle firings.

the walkway act to trigger the start and stop of a timing device. The EMG and foot-switch signals are received by an antenna array, and are then transmitted into a bank of receivers (181 to 189MHz transmission band for the carrier frequencies). The amplified signals from the receivers are fed into an oscilloscope for visual monitoring, a light-beam oscillograph for permanent raw data recording on light-sensitive paper, a multiplexor for channel sampling, an analog to digital converter, and a minicomputer for recording and analysis. Data analysis by the computer detects the onset and termination of the EMG signals and foot-switches. A graphic printout of muscle activity timed with the stance and swing phases of gait completes the process. In this way, a report can be produced within an hour. The physician compares the patient's EMG with the normal data on muscle activity during gait (Figs. 3.8, 3.9). The EMG data can be presented in a variety of forms (Fig. 3.10). Clinical applications of gait EMGs of selected muscles in patients with cerebral palsy are displayed in Figures 3.11 to 3.14.

79

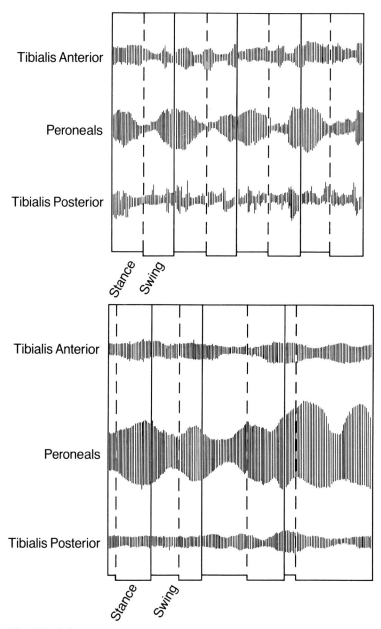

Fig. 3.11. Gait electromyograms redrawn from 'raw' recording by the optical method on photosensitive paper. Eight-year-old patient with spastic diplegia; postoperative subtalar extra-articular arthrodesis (Grice). *Top:* right foot; shows extent of muscle-action potentials co-ordinated with stance and swing phases of gait. Foot in balanced neutral position despite almost continuous low-level activity of the anterior and posterior tibial muscles. *Bottom:* left foot, now in varus. Note regularity of swing and stance phases contrasted with right foot. Has primarily stance-phase activity (rather than swing) of the anterior tibial and both swing and stance phase (normal is stance) of the posterior tibial muscles. Solution: split anterior tibial tendon transfer and lengthening of the posterior tibial tendon.

Fig. 3.12. Gait electromyogram re-drawn from 'raw' record. Quadriceps recording from vastus lateralis (fine wire electrode) and semitendinosus (fine wire electrode). Problem: knee-flexion posture of 30° during stance phase. EMG action potentials of quadriceps show fairly normal but somewhat prolonged stance-phase activity and normal activity at the end of swing. Medial hamstring activity in first two gait cycles depicted is fairly normal, with activity at the beginning of stance and end of swing. Solution: lengthening or tenotomy of

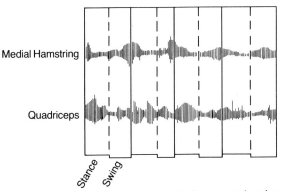

semitendinosus and fractional lengthening of semimembranosus aponeurosis with the expectation that almost normal knee function would be maintained. There is no need for elaborate procedures such as proximal hamstring release.

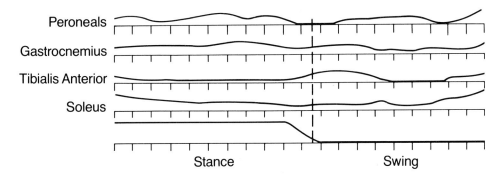

Fig. 3.13. Gait electromyogram drawn from automated recording (see Fig. 3.8). Fine wire electrodes in soleus and peroneal muscles; other muscles with surface electrodes. Problem was a dynamic equino-valgus deformity of the foot in a seven-year-old male with spastic hemiplegia. Positive Silfverskiöld test. EMG shows continuous activity of both gastrocnemius and soleus muscles; therefore Achilles tendon lengthening is indicated, rather than a gastrocnemius lengthening (Strayer) alone. Peroneal muscle activity throughout stance and most of swing phase. Anterior tibial activity is almost normal. Probably lengthening of the peroneus brevis tendon could be recommended in addition.

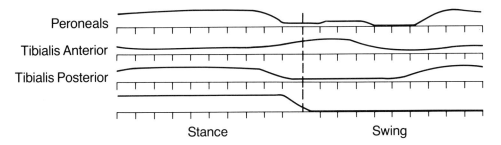

Fig. 3.14. Gait electromyogram drawn from automated recording. Fine wire electrode in posterior tibial muscle; surface electrodes on peroneals and anterior tibial muscles. Nine-year-old male with spastic diplegia. EMG is practically normal except for low-level continuous activity of the anterior tibial during stance.

81

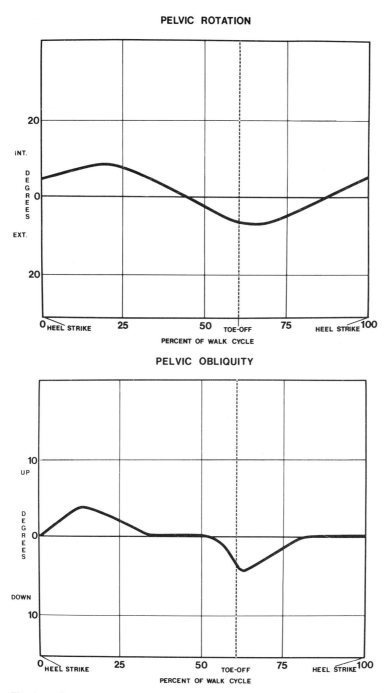

Fig. 3.15. Graphic representations of normal ranges of motion of segments of the lower limbs during level walking (courtesy of R. Mann and J. Hagy, Shriner's Hospital for Crippled Children, San Francisco, California). (*Figure continues opposite.*)

82

PELVIC TILT

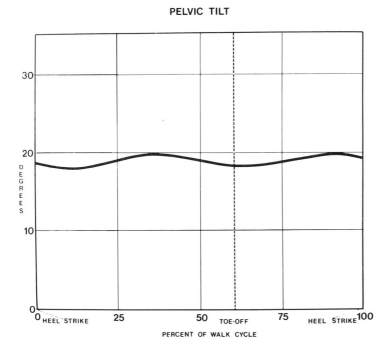

PERCENT OF WALK CYCLE

FEMORAL ROTATION

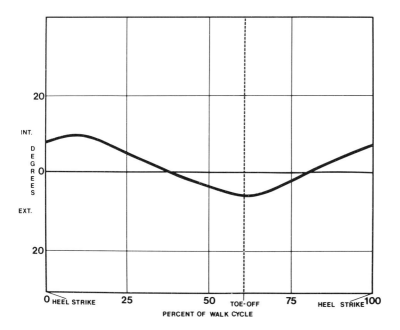

PERCENT OF WALK CYCLE

Fig. 3.15, *contd. (Figure continues over page.)*

83

HIP FLEXION-EXTENSION

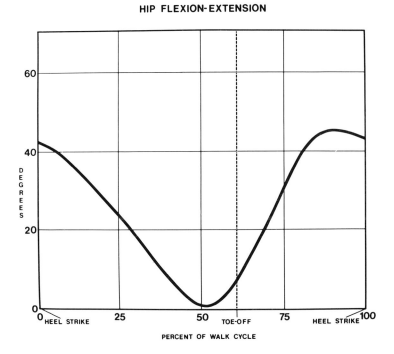

PERCENT OF WALK CYCLE

HIP JOINT ROTATION

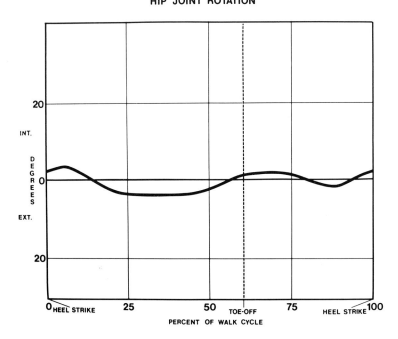

PERCENT OF WALK CYCLE

Fig. 3.15 *(continued)*.

84

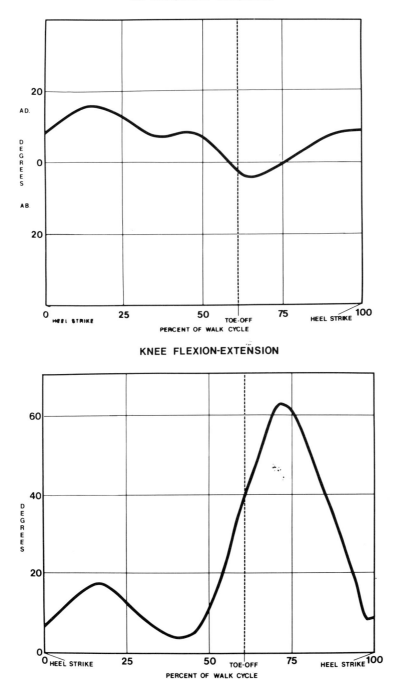

Fig. 3.15 *(continued)*.

85

KNEE JOINT ROTATION

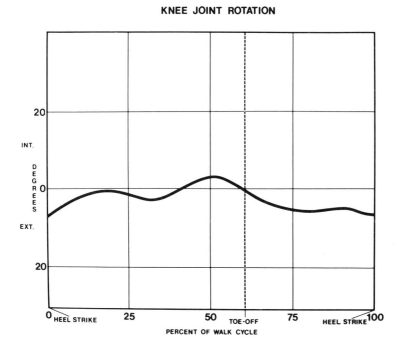

TIBIAL ROTATION

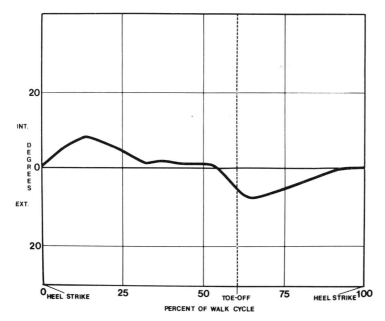

Fig. 3.15 *(continued).*

PLANTAR FLEXION-DORSIFLEXION

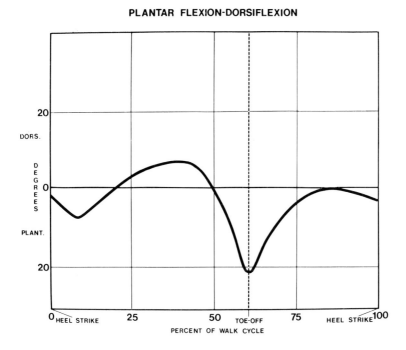

FOOT ROTATION

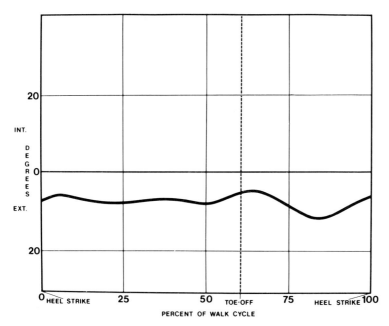

Fig. 3.15 *(continued)*.

87

Motion analysis
The technology of recording motion of the trunk and limbs during walking has progressed from photographic and cinematographic techniques to automated opto-electronic and television tracking systems. Most systems began with two-dimensional joint measurements in the saggital plane; now many systems have three-dimensional recording capabilities that include the transverse plane to record rotation. Some prefer systems that require hand digitizing; this is time-consuming, but is thought to produce accurate data (Tylkowski 1985). This preference will continue until the technology is sufficiently advanced to permit rapid automatic data output.

To record motion, all systems use targets fixed to the patient on anatomical points that show a relationship between the joints studied. Some systems use sticks, others use light-emitting diodes (Selspot), and others use reflective tape illuminated by near-infrared diodes at the cameras (Gage *et al.* 1984). Target locations can be on the arms, trunk, pelvis, thighs, knees, legs, feet or ankles.

Regardless of the method, standards of normal motion have been published and are effectively used to compare pathological with normal gait (Fig.3.15) (Sutherland *et al.* 1980).

Cadence, velocity and step-length
Normative data of linear measurements during gait for both adults and children have been published (Tables 3.II and 3.III).

Motion analysis seems more useful than electromyography in the over-all assessment of a gait problem in a child with cerebral palsy (Figs. 3.16, 3.17). Electromyograms before and after surgery appeared to be of limited value in two good studies (Waters *et al.* 1982, Gage *et al.* 1984). However, when planning specific surgery, electromyography of specific muscles (*e.g.* posterior tibial, anterior tibial) is helpful in making decisions.

Force-plate analysis is another component of gait assessment in some laboratories. A force-plate is a sensitive electronic scale which measures vertical, horizontal and lateral forces generated when the patient's foot hits the ground or floor. Force plates are rigid platforms, suspended on force transducers of either pizoelectric crystals or stiff springs instrumented with strain gauges. These instruments will measure forces and moments about joints, their trajectories and the potential and kinetic energies of each limb segment (McMahon 1984). Calculations of changes in mechanical energy of the center of mass of the body during walking, running, and other activities can be made (McMahon 1984). When used in gait analysis of young children with cerebral palsy, force-plate data become too irregular to be used because they frequently step off or miss the plate (Gage *et al.* 1984). Sutherland *et al.* (1981) used force-plate data in defining the pathomechanics of gait in children with Duchenne muscular dystrophy. Murray *et al.* (1975) used force-plate analysis to measure postural stability in men.

Balance (postural equilibrium) analysis
In patients who can stand alone, balancing ability should be measured to show the

TABLE 3.II

Linear measurements of the walking cycle for normal adults

Parameter	Right	Left
Opposite toe-off (%)	15.62	15.38
Opposite heel strike (%)	51.56	49.23
Single stance (%)	35.94	33.85
Toe-off (%)	65.62	64.62
Step length (cm)	60.30	60.70
Stride length (cm)	120.10	121.00
Cycle time (sec)	1.08	1.10
Cadence (steps/min)	109.85	109.84
Walking velocity (cm/sec)	110.43	110.43

% refers to percentage of the gait cycle.
From Gage *et al.* (1984).

TABLE 3.III

Average linear measurements of walking in children*

Age (years)	1	2	3	7	adult
Duration single-limb stance (per cent of gait cycle)	32.1	33.5	34.8	36.7	36.7
Toe-off (per cent of gait cycle)	67.1	67.1	65.5	62.4	63.6
Walking velocity (cm/sec)	63.7	71.8	85.5	114.3	121.6
Cadence (steps/min)	175.7	155.8	153.5	143.5	114
Step length (cm)†	21.6	27.5	32.9	47.9	65.5
Stride length (cm)	43	54.9	67.7	96.5	129.4
Ratio of pelvic span to ankle ('base of gait')	1–1.5	2		2.5	

*From Sutherland (1984). All measurements show a gradual increase with maturation except cadence which decreases. Most changes occur between the ages of one and four years.
†Step length has a linear relationship with leg length.
Note: Lower limb joint motions in children are only slightly different from adults. The same is true for gait electromyograms (Sutherland *et al.* 1980). For adult measurements of joint ranges of motion and electromyographic data, see Figures 3.5 and 3.15. For accurate graphs of lower limb joint ranges of motion in children, see Sutherland (1984).

integrity of the postural mechanisms. This kind of objective analysis allows a more accurate opinion on the status of a patient with ataxia due to a variety of causes. In cerebral palsy, defective equilibrium reactions seem more responsible than the spastic paralysis for the disabling gait of patients. During walking one must be able to support the trunk over only one limb as single stance shifts from limb to limb in forward progression. This means that lateral balance is essential as the body shifts about 2cm to the supporting limb (Perry 1975). If the patient lacks unilateral standing balance, due to the brain lesion, then the patient will fall to the swing limb when standing on one limb. This falling to one side is often confused with the Trendelenberg sign, which is due to insufficient hip abductor muscle function. It is not known if there is a relationship between the degree of defective equilibrium reactions and the abnormal and prolonged muscle contractions during the gait of a patient with cerebral palsy. Objective evaluation of ataxia should help to determine the efficacy of physiotherapy in such patients.

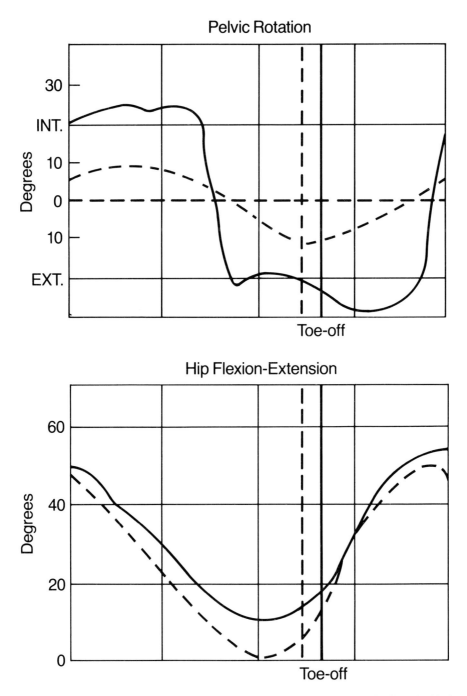

Fig. 3.16. Selected motion analysis records of 12-year-old female with spastic diplegia; hip internal rotation gait with equinus. *Top:* excessive pelvic rotation. Black line is the patient; broken line is the normal. *Bottom:* almost normal hip and knee flexion and extension.

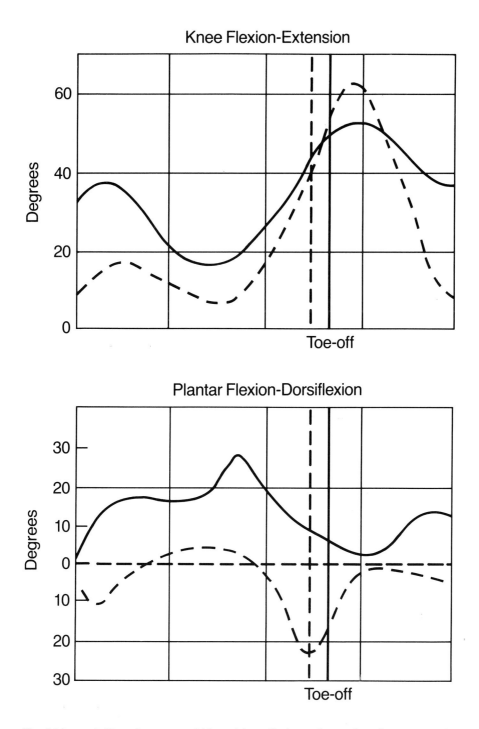

Fig. 3.16, *contd. Top:* almost normal hip and knee flexion and extension. *Bottom:* excessive ankle plantar flexion. (From the gait analysis laboratory of David H. Sutherland MD, San Diego Children's Hospital and Medical Center.)

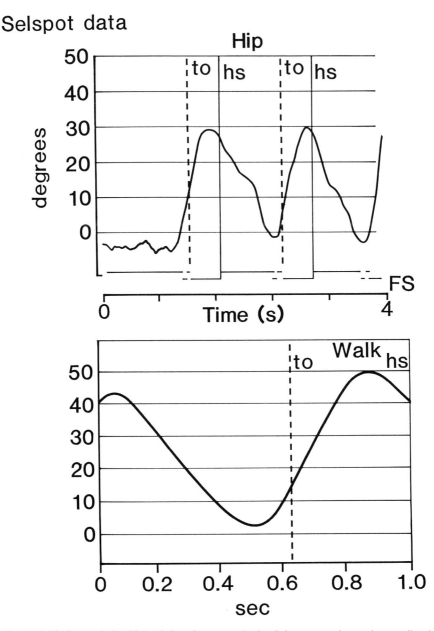

Fig. 3.17. Motion analysis with 'real-time data output' using Selspot opto-electronic recording (courtesy of Neil Alder MAS, RPT, John Mederios, PhD, RPT, and John Csongradi MD, of the Motion Analysis Laboratory, Children's Hospital at Stanford, Palo Alto, California). 10-year-old girl with spastic diplegia. Problem: is knee-flexion posture observed during stance significant? *Above:* plot of hip flexion extension. HS = heel strike; TO = toe-off; FS = footswitch. *Top* record is the patient; *bottom* is the normal. In this patient, maximum hip flexion is limited to 30° (normal 45° to 50°). Peak hip flexion occurs prematurely during late stance instead of early swing phase. Good hip extension and relatively normal pattern of hip flexion and extension exhibited by this patient. *(Figure continues opposite.)*

Selspot data

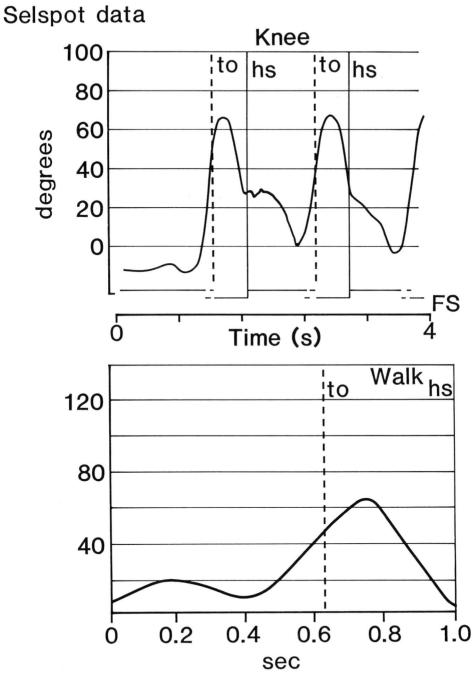

Fig. 3.17, *contd. Above:* Knee has excessive flexion during early stance phase; has 30° knee flexion (10° normal). Rapidly decreasing flexion to excessive extension during late stance. Peak flexion of 65° at mid-swing phase is near normal. (*Figure continues over page.*)

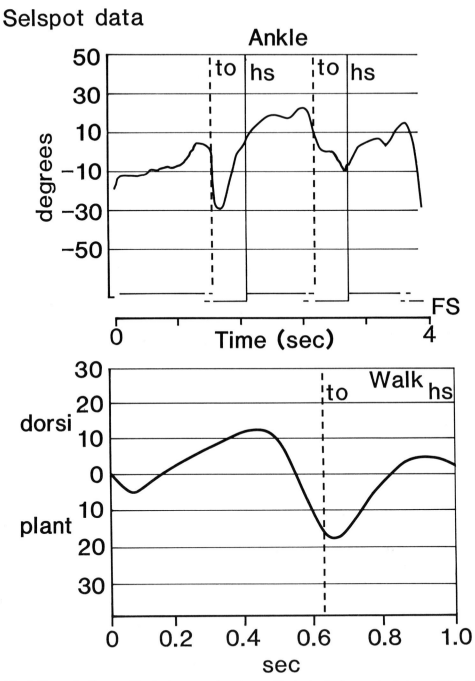

Selspot data

Fig. 3.17, *contd. Above:* ankle plot has normal contours with plantar flexion varying between 10° and 30°. Conclusion: excessive knee flexion during stance is 20° more than normal, and neither the hip nor ankle mechanisms appear to account for this. Inasmuch as the initial knee flexion decreases rapidly to extension in late stance, perhaps nothing need be done.

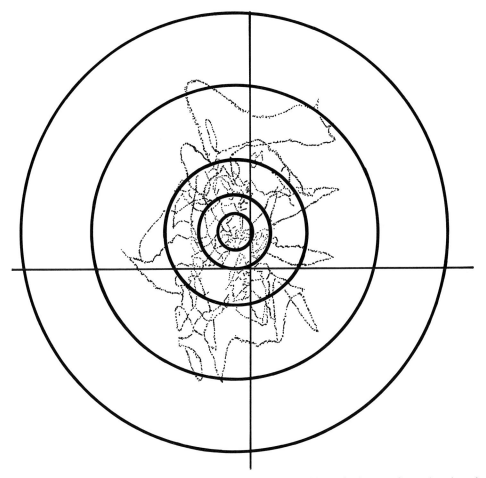

Fig. 3.18. Graphic display of extent of postural sway in patient with ataxia. See text for explanation of method.

The postural equilibrium measuring system we use was devised for a study of postural mechanisms in scoliosis (Adler *et al.* 1986). The system consists of two foot plates, with two strain gauges in each plate, interfaced to a minicomputer and printer plotter. The computer is programmed to display the center of foot pressure on the plates while the patient stands. An additional test is an 'instrumented Rhomberg sign' in which the platform is tilted sinusoidually 4° posteriorly eight times per minute. The test is done with eyes open and closed.

The computer program draws an X-Y axis and graphically displays the center of foot pressure and its change over time. The computer also calculates (as a function of bodyweight) the average center of foot pressure, and draws five concentric circles corresponding to 5, 10, 20, 40 and 60 per cent of the bodyweight around the average center. The printer provides a graphic display of postural sway (Fig.3.18).

TABLE 3.IV

Postural equilibrium measurements calculated by computer from instrumented foot-plate program described in text. Patient had cerebral palsy, ataxia; data are pre- and postoperative cerebellar stimulator implant

Test	Eyes	Tilt?	Standing base width (cm)	6/22 preop.	9/27 post o.	11/8 post o.	Control	Change* from 6/22 to 9/27	Change* from 9/27 to 11/8
					1982 dates				
				Average dispersion values					
A	open	no	16	4.97	7.33	10.43	6.2±1.6	−2.36	−3.10
B	close	no	16	3.63	7.80	5.33	7.6±2.0	−4.17	+2.47
C	open	no	7.5	6.95	5.20	5.70	6.2±1.6	+1.75	−0.50
D	close	no	7.5	5.50	4.60	7.15	7.6±2.0	+0.90	−2.55
E	open	yes	7.5	12.55	6.25	7.75	14.1±4.1	+6.30	−1.50

*+ = decreasing sway (improved); − = increasing sway (unimproved).

TABLE 3.V

Postural equilibrium measurements calculated by computer from instrumented foot-plate program described in the text. Patient with ataxia, age 6 years, cerebral anoxia from near drowning accident 3 months prior to tests

Test	Eyes	Tilt?	Standing base width standard (cm)	10/25	11/2	—	Control	Change* from 10/25 to 11/2
					1982 dates			
				Average dispersion values				
A	open	no	2	12.65	11.80		6.2±1.6	+0.85
B	close	no	2	16.60	13.55		7.6±2.0	+3.05
C	open	yes	2	13.15	16.40		14.1±4.1	−3.25
D	close	yes	2	21.90	20.20		20.3±4.5	+1.70

*+ = improvement; − = unimproved.

TABLE 3.VI

Heart rate and linear relationship to oxygen uptake

	Normal controls	Spastic diplegia
Age (yrs)	10.0±2.10	10.5±2.73
Velocity (m/sec)	73.2±1.0	42.6±0.21
Heart rate (beats/min)	113±12.10	138±24.5
Energy cost:		
ml O^2/kg/min	18.1±3.30	22.9±6.17
ml O^2/kg/m	0.247±0.045	0.862±0.85

From Waters *et al.* 1978.

Computer calculations of the number of times each concentric circle is crossed, and the time spent by the center of foot pressure within each zone, creates a digital analysis (Tables 3.IV, 3.V).

Energetics

The measurement of energy expenditure while walking can be useful, to evaluate the efficacy of walking aids, wheelchairs, orthotics, physical therapy and surgery in cerebral palsy.

Oxygen consumption measurements reflect the energy cost of activity. Oxygen consumption indicates aerobic energy-production by the muscles, in contrast to the anaerobic type in which glucose and phosphorus are metabolized without oxygen to convert adenosine diphosphate to adenosine triphosphate, with its high energy phosphate bonds. In anaerobic metabolism, lactic acid is the end product. Anaerobic metabolism is limited in energy production; almost 19 times more energy will be produced by the aerobic method (Waters *et al.* 1978).

Although oxygen consumption studies are important in clinical research, the methods are cumbersome particularly for children (Shephard 1975, Sutherland 1978, Ghosh *et al.* 1980). It is simpler to measure heart rate, and its relationship to oxygen consumption is linear from the resting state to the submaximal exercise levels in normal and disabled persons with the slope of the linear relationship differing in the two groups (Poulsen and Asmussen 1962, Ganguli and Datta 1978, Ghosh *et al.* 1980) (Table 3.VI).

The energetics of walking by spastic diplegic children were studied by Campbell and Ball (1978). In their study of six- to 13-year-old children, those with spastic diplegia had slower walking speeds than the normal controls, and their heart rates and energy costs were greater. Rose (1982) used an energy cost index derived from the average number of heartbeats per unit distance walked (heartbeats per minute divided by meters per minute). Each subject in this study was used as his or her own control by measuring the heartbeat in the resting state. Rose found that, in children with cerebral palsy, the energy cost was lower when wheeled walking aids were used rather than 'quad canes'. Wolfe (1978) measured the effects of floor surface on energy costs in wheelchair propulsion, and found that oxygen uptake per minute was higher on carpets; but it made no difference whether pneumatic or hard rubber tires were used.

Heart rate can be conveniently monitored by an electrocardiographic telemetry system, to allow walking to be as natural as possible. The heart rate is measured by walking a standard distance, and monitoring the heart rate for the last two minutes of a five-minute period of walking (Mederios 1984). This simple instrumentation is within the capabilities of almost any facility.

Myoneural blocks

The objective of myoneural blocks with alcohol, local anesthetics or phenol is to eliminate the stretch reflex of the spastic muscle temporarily by altering the sensitivity of the muscle-spindle receptors; the muscle is 'paralyzed'.

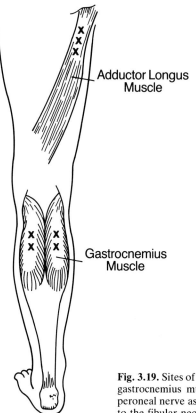

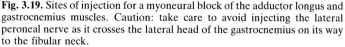

Fig. 3.19. Sites of injection for a myoneural block of the adductor longus and gastrocnemius muscles. Caution: take care to avoid injecting the lateral peroneal nerve as it crosses the lateral head of the gastrocnemius on its way to the fibular neck.

Alcohol

The pioneers in alcohol injection of muscles originally intended the method as a therapeutic modality (Hariga *et al.* 1964; Tardieu *et al.* 1964, 1971, 1975; Hariga 1966; Tardieu and Hariga 1972). It was hoped that the results of eliminating the stretch reflex in a specific muscle, primarily the gastrocnemius, would allow neurological restructuring so that correction of the deformity would be permanent. I believe these intentions have been modified now that more follow-up experience has been gained. As initiated by Carpenter and Mikhail (1972), the method is not useful so much for therapy as for diagnosis and evaluation.

Diluted alcohol of 45 to 50 per cent concentration is recommended in a dose of 5ml per kg bodyweight (Carpenter and Mikhail 1972, Carpenter 1983). Injection of 3 to 4ml of diluted alcohol into several areas of the muscle bellies is a simple procedure. The most common and accessible muscles which have been injected are the gastrocnemius and the adductor longus (Fig.3.19). The injection into the hamstrings is less reliable, and I no longer attempt it (Carlson *et al.* 1984). I perform these injections under brief general anesthesia. Hospitalization should usually not be required.

Preceding the myoneural blocks, it is important to record the gait on film or videotape. If motion analysis laboratory facilities are available, the gait electromyograph and one of the objective methods of recording lower-limb motion are ideal.

An additional refinement of the technique is to use a stimulating electrode injection needle before injecting the alcohol. With electric stimuli the action of the muscle can be observed (under general anesthesia), the alcohol injected, and the 'muscle put to sleep' (Campos da Paz 1981).

The effect of the block lasts two to six weeks, giving all observers ample time to determine if surgical treatment of the equinus or hip adduction deformity might improve gait function (Carpenter and Mikhail 1972, Carpenter and Seitz 1980, Carpenter 1983, Carlson *et al*. 1984). I have used 45 per cent alcohol myoneural blocks of the gastrocnemius in children (usually under age five years) who have a dynamic equinus and cannot tolerate an ankle-foot orthosis because of severe spasticity. In this way direct surgical intervention might be avoided and sufficient time can elapse to allow further development of the child's equilibrium reactions as the nervous system matures (to the age of three or four years). Another use of the gastrocnemius blocks has been in the rare case of disabling equinus in a child with hemidystonia. In this condition there is no contracture of the muscle, and a decision might be made after the block on whether or not a gastrocnemius neurectomy would partially relieve the disabling equinus, which is usually controlled with a plastic ankle-foot orthosis after the neurectomy. The myoneural block can demonstrate if an undesirable 'athetoid shift' of the dystonia to the ankle dorsiflexors might occur following the permanent gastrocnemius neurectomy.

Although some children will complain of muscle discomfort for a day or two after the blocks, no other complications have been reported. I have had one complication in which the lateral popliteal nerve, as it crossed over the lateral head of the gastrocnemius, was inadvertently infiltrated with the 45 per cent alcohol. When the child recovered from the anesthetic, she had an intractable dynamic varus deformity of the foot. Complete recovery occurred in three months. This complication might be avoided by mapping on the skin the course of the lateral popliteal nerve as it emerges from the popliteal fossa to become the peroneal nerve at the fibula neck before injection.

Local anesthetics
I have used lidocaine for a temporary (one to two hour) myoneural block of muscles in adolescents and adults who will tolerate needle injections. The dose of lidocaine should not exceed the toxic limits of about 1mg per kg of bodyweight. Excessive dosages can result in convulsions and cardiac arrest. If larger volumes of lidocaine are needed to infiltrate an entire muscle, a 0.5 per cent solution is safer. We no longer use bupivacaine (Marcaine r) because of its toxicity.

The problem with lidocaine is its relatively short duration of action, so effects must be observed at once. Lidocaine can also cause light-headedness and anxiety in children, which will preclude accurate observations and analysis of its effect on gait.

A contra-indication to the use of myoneural blocks with either alcohol or

TABLE 3.VII

Level of mental retardation according to IQ

Level	IQ scale	
	Stanford-Binet	Wechsler
(Borderline*)	(69–84)	(70–84)
Mild	52–68	55–69
Moderate	36–51	40–54
Severe	20–35	25–39
Profound	⩽19	⩽24

*Since the American Association on Mental Deficiency adopted its 1973 definition, persons who score in the borderline range are not considered mentally retarded.
(From Baird and Gordon 1983, p. 121.)

lidocaine is an obvious fixed deformity due to a definite contracture of the muscle. A deformity that is mainly dynamic can often be determined by clinical examination, if the child is relaxed and a slow stretch of the muscle is applied. When in doubt, only complete relaxation under general anesthesia can differentiate contracture from spasticity alone.

Phenol

Phenol has been used as a temporary but long-acting neurolytic agent in spastic paralysis. It has a short-term anesthetic effect, and a long-term destructive effect. Nerve fibers of all diameters are destroyed. Phenol blocks can last for six months to over a year. We have not used phenol because it is difficult to control the degree of tissue destruction. Direct injection into perineural tissue by open surgical exposure may result in undesirable and long-term overactivity of antagonistic spastic muscles. For example, a phenol injection of a motor point in the posterior tibial muscle could 'uncover' underlying spasticity of the peroneal muscles, with the result that a dynamic varus deformity of the foot would become a valgus deformity (Herman 1976). If phenol is inadvertently injected subcutaneously, skin necrosis and slough can occur (Samilson 1967).

Psychological tests

Even though the surgeon or physician is not trained or equipped to perform psychological testing, he or she will have to consider the intellectual functioning of the child when advising treatment or management in achieving functional goals. Consequently, some familiarity with the interpretation of psychological tests is advisable. Even though a high incidence of mental retardation was reported in cerebral palsy (Hohman 1953), the changing etiology of cerebral palsy should make us cautious in over-generalizing. Non-verbal ability is not necessarily an indication of mental retardation: witness the success of non-verbal communication techniques, from sign language to advanced computer technology and artificial voice devices. Mental retardation is not predictive of the ability to walk (Shapiro *et al.* 1979). Certainly, no child should be rejected for surgical treatment solely on the grounds of presumed intellectual status.

Table 3.VII is a guide for labeling the degree of mental retardation. Most persons with athetosis have normal intellects and some are superior; children who have spastic diplegia usually succeed in regular school although they may have some specific learning problems; those who have total body involved spastic paralysis (quadriplegia) seem to have a higher incidence of retardation; those with less motor involvement such as ataxia or spastic hemiplegia due to cerebral maldevelopment appear to have more mental retardation.

As pointed out by Baird and Gordon (1983), defining retardation can be based upon function. Cerebral-palsied children whose test scores show them to be ineducable—approximately 50 per cent according to Illingworth (1958) and Nelson and Ellenberg (1978)—can nevertheless learn a sufficient number of skills without formal 'schooling' to achieve reasonable independence for adult living. The increasing use of rehabilitation engineering technology and adaptive devices in recent years greatly enhances this prospect.

As any psychologist knows, referral of babies and toddlers for 'psychological testing' may be inappropriate because the estimate of intellectual performance is based mainly upon motor development and developmental tests, and may be inaccurate in terms of prognosis.

Good psychological testing at the appropriate age does have validity, even though there is lack of standardization for children with cerebral palsy. For groups of children the test-retest reliability is said to be 98 per cent, and 90 per cent for an individual child (Baird and Gordon 1983). I once looked at IQ test scores on 10 children with cerebral palsy who were tested initially between the ages of eight and 10 years, and again at age 16 to 18 years. I found no significant variance in these test scores over a period of eight years.

REFERENCES

Adler, N. T., Bleck, E. E., Rinsky, L. A., Young, W. (1986) 'Balance reactions and eye-hand coordination in idiopathic scoliosis.' *Journal of Orthopaedic Research,* **4,** 102–107.
—— Rinsky, L. A. (1984) 'Decision-making in surgical treatment of paralytic deformities of the foot with gait electromyograms.' *Paper read at Annual Meeting of American Academy for Cerebral Palsy and Developmental Medicine, Washington, D.C.*
Amiel-Tison, C., Grenier, A. (1983) *Neurological Evaluation of the Newborn and the Infant.* New York: Masson USA.
Ayres, A. J. (1972) 'Characteristics of types of sensory integrative dysfunction.' *Journal of Learning Disabilities,* **5,** 336–343.
—— (1978) 'Learning disabilities and the vestibular system.' *Journal of Learning Disabilities,* **11,** 18–29.
Baird, H. W., Gordon, E. C. (1983) *Neurological Evaluation of Infants and Children. Clinics in Developmental Medicine Nos. 84/85.* London: S.I.M.P. with Heinemann; Philadelphia: Lippincott.
Barnes, K. E., Stark, A. (1975) 'Denver Developmental Screening Test: a normative study.' *American Journal of Public Health,* **65,** 363–369.
Baumann, J. U. (1980) 'Gait analysis and its benefit to the patient.' *Progress in Orthopaedic Surgery,* Berlin and Heidelberg: Springer-Verlag, **4,** 103–107.
—— (1984) 'Clinical experience of gait analysis in the management of cerebral palsy.' *Prosthetics and Orthotics International,* **8,** 29–32.
Bayley, N. (1969) *Bayley Scales of Infant Development.* New York: Psychological Corporation.
Beals, R. K. (1966) 'Spastic paraplegia and diplegia: an evaluation of non-surgical and surgical factors influencing the prognosis for ambulation.' *Journal of Bone and Joint Surgery,* **48B,** 827–846.

Biasini, F. J., Mindingall, A. (1984) 'Developmental outcome of very low birthweight children.' *Orthopaedic Transactions*, **8**, 115. *Developmental Medicine and Child Neurology*, **26**, 260–261. (*Abstract*.)

Bleck, E. E., Nagel, D. A. (Eds.) (1982) *Physically Handicapped Children: A Medical Atlas for Teachers, 2nd edn.* Orlando, Florida: Grune & Stratton.

Bose, K., Goh, J. C. (1984) 'Gait analysis in clinical practice.' *Journal of Western Pacific Orthopaedic Association*, **21**, 57–62.

Bozynski, M. E. A., Nelson, M. N., O'Donnell, K., Genaze, D., Rosati-Skertich, C., Ramsey, R., Meier, W. A. (1984) 'Two-year follow-up of ≤ 1200 gram premature infants: long-term sequelae of intracranial hemorrhage.' *Orthopaedic Transactions*, **8**, 115. *Developmental Medicine and Child Neurology*, **26**, 259. (*Abstract*.)

Brazelton, T. B. (1973) *Neonatal Behavioral Assessment Scale. Clinics in Developmental Medicine No. 50.* London: S.I.M.P. with Heinemann.

—— (1984) *Neonatal Behavioral Assessment Scale. Clinics in Developmental Medicine No. 88.* London: S.I.M.P. with Blackwell Scientific; Philadelphia: Lippincott.

Bryant, G. M., Davies, K. J., Newcombe, R. G. (1974) 'The Denver Developmental Screening Test. Achievement of test items in the first year of life by Denver and Cardiff infants.' *Developmental Medicine and Child Neurology*, **16**, 474–484.

Campbell, J., Ball, J. (1978) 'Energetics of walking in cerebral palsy.' *Orthopaedic Clinics of North America*, **9**, 374–377.

Campos da Paz, Jr., A. (1981) *Personal communication.*

Carlson, W., Carpenter, B., Wenger, D. (1984) 'Myoneural blocks for preoperative planning in cerebral palsy surgery.' *Orthopaedic Transactions*, **8**, 111. *Developmental Medicine and Child Neurology*, **26**, 252–253. (*Abstract*.)

Carpenter, E. B. (1983) 'Role of nerve blocks in the foot and ankle in cerebral palsy: therapeutic and diagnostic.' *Foot and Ankle*, **4**, 164–166.

—— Mikhail, M. (1972) 'The use of intramuscular alcohol as a diagnostic and therapeutic aid in cerebral palsy.' *Developmental Medicine and Child Neurology*, **14**, 113–114. (*Abstract*.)

—— Seitz, D. G. (1980) 'Intramuscular alcohol as an aid in management of spastic cerebral palsy.' *Developmental Medicine and Child Neurology*, **22**, 497–501.

Chao, E. Y., Laughmann, R. K., Schneider, E., Stauffer, R. N. (1983) 'Normative data of knee joint motion and ground reaction forces in adult level walking.' *Journal of Biomechanics*, **16**, 219–233.

Chodera, J. B., Levell, R. W. (1973) 'Footprint patterns during walking.' *In:* Kenedi, R. M. (Ed.) *Perspectives in Biomedical Engineering.* Baltimore: University Park Press.

Coley, I. (1978) *Pediatric Assessment of Self-Care Activities.* St. Louis: C. V. Mosby.

Cools, A. T. M., Hermanns, J. M. A. (1977) *Denver Developmental Screening Test.* Amsterdam: Swets & Zeitlinger.

Feagans, L. (1983) 'A current view of learning disabilities.' *Journal of Pediatrics*, **102**, 487–493.

Flehmig, I., Schluun, M., Uhde, J., Van Bernuth, H. (1973) *Denver-Entwicklungsskalen (Denver Development Scales).* Stuttgart: Thieme.

Ford, F., Bleck, E. E., Aptekar, R. G., Collins, F. J., Stevik, D. (1976) 'Efficacy of dantrolene sodium in the treatment of spastic cerebral palsy.' *Developmental Medicine and Child Neurology*, **18**, 770–783.

Frankenburg, W. K., Dodds, J. B. (1967) 'Denver developmental screening test.' *Journal of Pediatrics*, **71**, 181–191.

—— Camp, B. W., Van Natta, P. A. (1971) 'The validity of the DDST.' *Child Development*, **42**, 474–485.

—— Dick, N. P., Carland, J. (1975) 'Development of preschool-aged children of different social and ethnic groups: implications for developmental screening.' *Journal of Pediatrics*, **87**, 125–132.

Frostig, M. (1963) 'Visual perceptual development and school adjustment programs.' *American Journal of Orthopsychiatry*, **33**, 367–368.

—— Horne, D. (1964) *The Frostig Program for Development of Visual Perception.* Chicago: Follett.

Gage, J. R., Fabian, D., Hicks, R., Tashmann, S. (1984) 'Pre- and postoperative gait analysis in patients with spastic diplegia: a preliminary report.' *Journal of Pediatric Orthopaedics*, **4**, 715–725.

Ganguli, S., Datta, S. R. (1978) 'A new method for prediction of energy expenditure from heart rate.' *Journal of the Institution of Engineers* (India) **58**, 57–61.

Ghosh, A. K., Tibarewala, B., Chakaraborty, S., Ganguli, S., Bose, K. (1980) 'An improved approach for performance evaluation in lower extremity involvement.' *Journal of Biomedical Engineering*, **2**, 121–125.

Griffin, P. P., Wheelhouse, W. W., Shiavi, R. (1977) 'Adductor transfer for adductor spasticity: clinical and electromyographic gait analysis.' *Developmental Medicine and Child Neurology*, **19**, 783–789.

Harel, S., Anastasiow, N. J. (Eds.) (1985) *The At-Risk Infant: Psycho/Socio/Medical Aspects*. Baltimore and London: Paul H. Brookes.

Hariga, J. (1966) 'Influences sur la motricité de la suppression des effecteurs gamma par alcoolisation des nerfs périphériques.' *Acta Neurologica Belgica*, **66**, 607–611.

—— Tardieu, G., Tardieu, C., Gagnard, L. (1964) 'Effets de l'application d'alcool dilué sur le nerf. Confrontation de l'étude dynamographique de l'étude histologique chez le chat décérébré.' *Revue Neurologique*, **111**, 472–474.

Herman, R. (1976) 'Postural control and therapeutic implications.' *In:* Murdoch, G. (Ed.) *The Advance in Orthotics*. London: Edward Arnold.

Hoffer, M. M., Perry, J. (1983) 'Pathodynamics of gait alterations in cerebral palsy and the significance of kinetic electromyography in evaluating foot and ankle problems.' *Foot and Ankle*, **4**, 128–134.

Hoffman-Williamson, H., Spungen, L., Farran, A., Georgieff, M., Bernbaum, J., Borian, F. (1984) 'Comparable developmental progress in infants of birth weights less than 1000 grams and 1001–1500 grams.' *Orthopaedic Transactions*, **8**, 115. *Developmental Medicine and Child Neurology*, **26**, 259–260. (*Abstract*.)

Hohman, L. B. (1953) 'Intelligence levels in cerebral palsied children.' *American Journal of Physical Medicine*, **32**, 282–290.

Illingworth, R. S. (1958) 'The early diagnosis of cerebral palsy.' *Cerebral Palsy Bulletin*, **2**, 6–8.

Knutsson, E. (1983) 'Analysis of gait and isokinetic movements for evaluation of antispastic drugs or physical therapies.' *Advances in Neurology*, **39**, 1013–1034.

Kucharczyk, W., Brant-Zawadski, M., Norman, D., Newton, T. H. (1985) 'Magnetic resonance imaging of the central nervous system—an update.' *Western Journal of Medicine*, **142**, 54–62.

Lasda, N. A., Levinsohn, E. M., Yuan, H. A., Bunnell, W. P. (1978) 'Computerized tomography in disorders of the hip.' *Journal of Bone and Joint Surgery*, **60A**, 1099–1102.

Marey, E. J. (1873) *La Machine Animale. Locomotion Terrestre (bipedes) et Aerienne*. Paris: Baillière

—— (1874) *Animal Mechanism: A Treatise on Terrestrial and Aerial Locomotion*. New York: Appleton.

Marquis, P. J., Ruiz, N. A., Lundy, M. S., Dillard, R. G. (1984) 'Primitive reflexes and early motor development in very low birth weight (VLBW) infants.' *Orthopaedic Transactions*, **8**, 108. *Developmental Medicine and Child Neurology*, **26**, 247–248. (*Abstract*.)

McMahon, T. A. (1984) *Muscles, Reflexes, and Locomotion*. Princeton, New Jersey: Princeton University Press.

Mederios, J. M. (1984) 'Clinical application of gait analysis.' Presented at *Pathokinesiology of Cerebral Palsy, Advances in Applied and Clinical Research*, Division of Physical Therapy, School of Medicine, University of North Carolina, Chapel Hill; and at the *Olympic Scientific Congress*, University of Oregon, Eugene.

Murray, M. P. (1967) 'Gait as a total pattern of movement.' *American Journal of Physical Medicine*, **46**, 290–322.

—— Seireg, A. A., Sepic, S. B. (1975) 'Normal postural stability and steadiness: quantitative assessment.' *Journal of Bone and Joint Surgery*, **57A**, 510–516.

Muybridge, E. (1901) *The Human Figure in Motion, an Electrophotographic Investigation of Consecutive Phases of Muscular Action*. London: Chapman and Hall.

—— (1955) *The Human Figure in Motion*. New York: Dover.

Nelson, K. B., Ellenberg, J. H. (1978) 'Epidemiology in cerebral palsy.' *Advances in Neurology*, **25**, 421–435.

—— —— (1982) 'Children who "outgrew" cerebral palsy.' *Pediatrics*, **69**, 529–536.

—— Bozynski, M. E. A., Genaze, D., Rosati-Skertich, C., O'Donnell, K. J. (1984) 'Comparative evaluation of motor development of ≤1200 gram infants during the first postnatal year using the Bayley scales versus the Milani-Comparetti.' *Orthopaedic Transactions*, **8**, 108. *Developmental Medicine and Child Neurology*, **26**, 247. (*Abstract*.)

Paine, R. S., Oppé, T. E. (1966) *Neurological Examination of Children. Clinics in Developmental Medicine Nos. 20/21*. London: S.I.M.P. with Heinemann.

Paludetto, R., Rinaldi, P., Mansi, G., Andolfi, M., De Curtis, M., Ciccimarra, F., Del Giudice, G. (1984) 'Behavioral evolution of 30 preterm infants from 35 to 44 weeks postconceptual age.' *Orthopaedic Transactions*, **8**, 119.

Perry, J. (1975) 'Cerebral palsy gait.' *In:* Samilson, R. L. (Ed.) *Orthopaedic Aspects of Cerebral Palsy. Clinics in Developmental Medicine Nos. 52/53*. London: S.I.M.P. with Heinemann; Philadelphia: Lippincott.

—— Hoffer, M. M., Antonelli, D., Plut, J., Lewis, G., Greenberg, R. (1976) 'Electromyography before and after surgery for hip deformity in cerebral palsy.' *Journal of Bone and Joint Surgery*, **58A**, 201–208.

—— —— (1977) 'Preoperative and postoperative dynamic electromyography as an aid in planning tendon transfers in children with cerebral palsy.' *Journal of Bone and Joint Surgery*, **59A**, 531–537.

Poulsen, E., Asmussen, E. (1962) 'Energy requirements of practical jobs from pulse increase and ergometer test.' *Ergonomics*, **5**, 33–36.

Prechtl, H. F. R. (1977) *The Neurological Examination of the Full Term Newborn Infant. Clinics in Developmental Medicine No. 63.* London: S.I.M.P. with Heinemann; Philadelphia: Lippincott.

Rose, J. (1982) 'Energy expenditure of children with cerebral palsy during assisted ambulation.' Masters degree thesis, Division of Physical Therapy, Stanford University School of Medicine, Stanford, California.

Saint-Anne Dargassies, S. (1977) *Neurological Development in Full Term and Premature Neonates.* Amsterdam: Excerpta Medica; New York: Elsevier North-Holland.

Samilson, R. L. (1967) *Personal communication.*

Shapira, Y., Harel, S. (1983) 'Standardization of the Denver Developmental Screening Test for Israeli children.' *Israeli Journal of Medical Science*, **19**, 246–251.

Shapiro, B. K., Accardo, P. J., Capute, A. J. (1979) 'Factors affecting walking in a profoundly retarded population.' *Developmental Medicine and Child Neurology*, **21**, 369–373.

Shephard, R. (1975) 'Efficiency of muscular work.' *Physical Therapy*, **55**, 476–481.

Sheridan, M. D. (1975) *Children's Developmental Progress from Birth to Five Years. The STYCAR Sequences 3rd edn.* Windsor: NFER.

—— (1978) *Sheridan Stycar Developmental Sequences.* Windsor: NFER.

Simon, S. R., Deutsch, S. D., Nuzzo, R. M., Mansour, J. M., Jackson, J. L. F., Koskinen, M., Rosenthal, R. K. (1978) 'Genu recurvatum in spastic cerebral palsy.' *Journal of Bone and Joint Surgery*, **60A**, 882–894.

—— Fernandez, O., Rosenthal, R. K., Griffin, P. A. (1984) 'The effect of heel-cord lengthening and solid ankle-foot orthosis on the gait of patients with cerebral palsy.' *Paper read at Annual Meeting of American Academy for Cerebral Palsy and Developmental Medicine.* Washington, D.C.

Skinner, S. R., Lester, D. K. (1984) 'Dynamic EMG findings in valgus hindfoot deformity in spastic cerebral palsy.' *Paper read at Annual Meeting of American Academy for Cerebral Palsy and Developmental Medicine.* Washington, D.C.

Stanley, F., Alberman, E. (1984) *The Epidemiology of the Cerebral Palsies. Clinics in Developmental Medicine No. 87.* London: S.I.M.P. with Blackwell Scientific; Philadelphia: Lippincott.

Super, C. M. (1976) 'Environmental effects on motor development. The case of African infant precocity.' *Developmental Medicine and Child Neurology*, **18**, 561–567.

Sutherland, D. H. (1978) 'Gait analysis in cerebral palsy.' *Developmental Medicine and Child Neurology*, **20**, 807–813.

—— (1984) *Gait Disorders in Childhood and Adolescence.* Baltimore and London: Williams and Wilkins.

—— Hagy, J. L. (1972) 'Measurement of gait movements from motion picture films.' *Journal of Bone and Joint Surgery*, **54**, 787–797.

—— Olshen, R., Cooper, L., Woo, S. K. (1980) 'The development of mature gait.' *Journal of Bone and Joint Surgery*, **62A**, 336–353.

—— Baumann, J. U. (1981) 'Correction of paralytic foot drop by external orthoses.' *In:* Black, J., Dumbleton, J. H. (Eds.) *Clinical Biomechanics.* Edinburgh: Churchill Livingstone.

—— Olshen, R., Cooper, L., Wyatt, M., Leach, J., Murbarak, S., Schultz, P. (1981) 'The pathomechanics of gait in Duchenne muscular dystrophy.' *Developmental Medicine and Child Neurology*, **23**, 3–22.

Tardieu, C., Tardieu, G., Hariga, J., Gagnard, L., Velin, J. (1964) 'Fondement expérimental d'une thérapeutique des raideurs d'origine cérébrale. Effect de l'aloolisation ménagée du nerf moteur sur le réflexe d'étirement de l'animal décérébré.' *Archives françaises de Pédiatrie*, **21**, 5–23.

Tardieu, G. (1984) *Le Dossier Clinique de l'Infirmité Motrice Cérébrale 3rd edn.* Paris: Masson.

—— Tardieu, C., Hariga, J. (1971) 'Infiltrations par l'alcool à 45° des points moteurs, des racines par voie épidurale ou du nerf tibial postérieur. Leurs indications et contre indications dans les divers modes de "spasticité" (expérience de dix ans).' *Revue Neurologique*, **125**, 63–68.

—— Hariga, J. (1972) 'Selective partial denervation by alcohol injections and their results in spasticity.' *Reconstructive Surgery and Traumatology*, **13**, 18–36.

—— Got, C., Lespargot, A. (1975) 'Indications d'un nouveau type d'infiltration au point moteur (alcool à 96°). Applications cliniques d'une étude expérimentale.' *Annales de Medicine Physique*, **18**, 539–557.

Terver, S., Dillingham, M., Parker, B., Bjorke, A., Bleck, E. E., Levai, J. P., Teinturier, P., Viallet, J. F. (1982) 'Étude de l'orientation réelle du cotyle grâce au tomodensitomètre axial ou scanner.' *Journal de Radiologie*, **63**, 167–173.

Touwen, B. C. L. (1979) *The Examination of the Child with Minor Neurological Dysfunction, 2nd edn. Clinics in Developmental Medicine No. 71.* London: S.I.M.P. with Heinemann; Philadelphia: Lippincott.

Tylkowski, C. H. (1985) *Personal communication.*

Ueda, R. (1978) 'Standardization of the Denver Developmental Screening Test on Japanese children.' *Developmental Medicine and Child Neurology*, **20**, 647–656.

Waters, R. L., Hislop, H. J., Perry, J., Antonelli, D. (1978) 'Energetics: application to the study and management of locomotor disabilities.' *Orthopaedic Clinics of North America*, **9**, 351–356.

—— Frazier, J., Garland, D. E., Jordan, C., Perry, J. (1982) 'Electromyographic gait analysis before and after operative treatment for hemiplegic equinus and equinovarus deformity.' *Journal of Bone and Joint Surgery*, **64A**, 284–288.

Weiner, D. S., Cook, A. J., Hoyt, W. A., Oravec, C. E. (1978) 'Computed tomography in the measurement of femoral anteversion.' *Orthopedics*, **1**, 299–306.

Wolfe, G. (1978) 'Influence of floor surface with energy cost of wheelchair propulsion.' *Orthopaedic Clinics of North America*, **9**, 367–370.

Woolson, S. T. (1985) *Personal communication.*

Ziporyn, T. (1985a) 'Medical News: PET scans relate clinical picture to more specific nerve function.' *Journal of the American Medical Association*, **253**, 943–949.

—— (1985b) 'Medical News: Magnetic resonance "sees" lesions of multiple sclerosis.' *Journal of the American Medical Association*, **253**, 949–951.

4
NEUROBIOLOGY

Ignorance is the fertilizer for the flowers of debate (Shepherd 1983).

In the past, the central nervous system was known only anatomically. How it functioned was a mystery for most; consequently the brain was thought to be a 'black box'. Due to the efforts of neuroscientists we now know much more. Debates have raged over the efficacy of various treatments for cerebral palsy—surgery, drugs, orthotics, plaster immobilization and physical and occupational therapy methods. Knowledge of scientific facts should provide us with a more reasoned judgement on treatments proposed from both theoretical and practical standpoints.

This is a brief review of some relevant neurobiological studies; it is not a comprehensive review of the whole and exploding field of neuroscience. I have discussed only those aspects that seem especially applicable to cerebral palsy. Those who wish more in-depth knowledge should consult the references at the end of the chapter.

Neurogenesis
It is well known now that the entire process of central nervous system development is under genetic control (also called 'innate'). In other words, humans, animals and insects have inherited the processes of their development.

Cell birth occurs from the precursor cells (neuroblasts) of the embryonic neural tube and crest. From the cells of the neural tube are derived the neurons, astrocytes, oligodendroglial and ependymal cells. Those that arise from the neural crest are the dorsal and autonomic ganglion, the bipolar auditory cells and the chromaffin cells of the adrenal medulla. Cells which share their origin from both the tube and the crest are the pia mater, arachnoid, microglial and Schwann (Shepherd 1983).

The neurons are all generated in 60 days in the monkey (gestation 165 days) and in 100 days in the human.

Cells migrate to their final destination by a process of growth cones which have ameboid movements. Nerve growth factor (NFG) is a protein (molecular weight of 130,000) that plays an important rôle in the development of some neurons.

Cell differentiation is the next step in development; however in some cells this begins before migration. It overlaps considerably with other stages of development. The evidence is that chemical factors (*e.g.* Ca^{2+}, acetylcholine) in the cell environment determine the differentiation.

Cell maturation time varies in different regions of the central nervous system, and in humans continues for some time after birth. Ramifications of the neuronal dendrites commence just after birth. By six months of age the rate of growth of

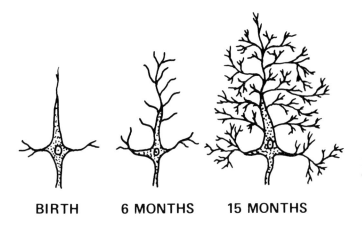

Fig. 4.1. Schematic drawing of dendritic arborization from birth to 15 months (from Schade and Von Groenigen 1961).

BIRTH   6 MONTHS   15 MONTHS

dendritic processes is striking. The dendrites increase in size and length but not in number up to the age of 15 months. By the age of two years, neuronal differentiation is essentially complete. After two years the growth continues, but at a reduced rate (Schade and Von Groenigen 1961) (Fig.4.1).

The brain regions do not develop synchronously. Cell multiplication is most rapid in the forebrain and is complete at 18 weeks gestation. Cell growth is rapid in the first three months of gestation but myelination continues until about the age of three years (Fig.4.2). Cerebellar growth starts about halfway through gestation and is complete by about 18 months (Dobbing and Sands 1973).

The acceleration of change in the developing brain has been compared to driving an automobile on a highway: the greater rate of acceleration, the

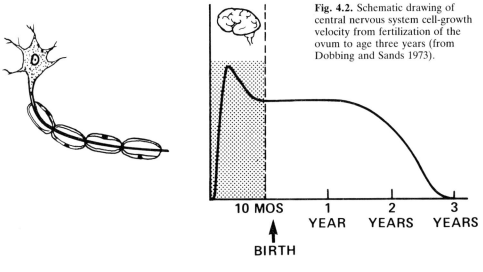

Fig. 4.2. Schematic drawing of central nervous system cell-growth velocity from fertilization of the ovum to age three years (from Dobbing and Sands 1973).

10 MOS   1   2   3
            YEAR   YEARS   YEARS

BIRTH

107

greater the stress on the controlling mechanism, and the greater chance for disaster when the mechanisms are blocked or side-tracked (Neligan 1974). Oda and Huttenlocher (1974) showed that when developing rats were administered corticosteroids, dendritic expansions were halted, and dendritic growth was irrecoverably stunted.

The limits of neurogenesis in primates have been shown by Rakic (1985). In an extremely detailed and tedious method of measuring DNA replication with radioactive [3H] thymidine, no evidence was found in 12 Rhesus monkey brains of any neuronal replication (regeneration). Furthermore, they previously demonstrated with these techniques that except for some granule cells of the cerebellum and hippocampus, the majority of neurons are produced in the first half of gestation. These findings are in striking contrast to neuron and axon regeneration in fish, amphibians and birds, which has provided hypotheses for various passive manipulations aimed at influencing the development of presumed or actual brain-damaged infants (infants at risk). The findings of Rakic have clinical importance. Why should neuronal stability be so important for us humans? 'One can speculate that a prolonged period of interaction with the environment, as pronounced as it is in all primates, especially humans, requires a stable set of neurons to retain acquired experience in the pattern of their synapses' (Rakic 1985).

Cell death is an established phenomenon in the development of the central nervous system as well as in non-neural tissues. Apparently death of up to 75 per cent of the cells occurs in some regions of the brain in a gene-programmed and regulated system. The hypothesis is that billions of neurons compete to innervate their targets, and some of them lose out (Shepherd 1983). The mechanisms of programmed cell death during fetal development, and the reasons for the phenomenon, are reviewed by Landmesser (1981) and by Cowan *et al.* (1985).

Neuroplasticity
In some ways the term 'neuroplasticity' is unfortunate because it can be used to justify various physical treatment regimes without the slightest basis in fact or a careful analysis of results. It seems as if used as a canard, 'neuroplasticity' can justify all sorts of experimental treatments and educational programs in children who have impairments of cerebral function.

Even though we have strong evidence that the nervous system degenerates irreversibly after a specific injury (Ramon y Cajal 1928, Windle 1956, Clemente 1964), we do know that some humans make a partial recovery from brain injury. Adults have sometimes recovered remarkably from cerebral vascular accidents (Rosner 1974). Some process accounts for the clinical observations of recovery of apparent brain insult. Probable mechanisms of recovery continue to be the subject of intense study.

The mechanism of recovery is not regeneration of a dead neuron, but is due almost entirely to the capability of synapses to modify their function, be replaced, and to increase or decrease in number when necessary (Cotman and Nieto-Sampedro 1985). Liu and Chambers (1958) were the first to prove that neurons

108

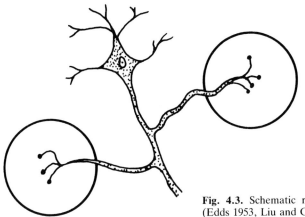

Fig. 4.3. Schematic representation of axonal sprouting (Edds 1953, Liu and Chambers 1958).

have an innate ability to form new connections when other cells are lost (Fig.4.3). They demonstrated axonal sprouting in the cat spinal cord after experimental transection of the spinal cord. Since then other investigators have confirmed the ability of uninjured axons to sprout extra or collateral connections with the denervated structures (Cotman and Nieto-Sampedro 1985). Growth of dendrites and axons into the neuritic plaques of the brain of patients who had Alzheimer's disease have been demonstrated. Other areas of the brain show dendritic atrophy. As stated by Cotman and Nieto-Sampedro (1985), this capacity for growth is 'expressed in a pathologic manner but can be expressed nonetheless'.

The time-lapse for synaptic replacement is between one and five days in mammalian adults; however, *in vitro* experiments show that a neuron which has lost its axon can sprout a new axon growth cone in 15 minutes and synapses can form in less than one day (Cotman and Nieto-Sampedro 1985). The rate of growth is hindered by the need to remove products of degeneration after brain injury.

Transplantation of neurons, and their growth with the formation of synapses, has been demonstrated when fetal brain tissue was used. Adult neuronal transplantation was poor. Axons from embryonic central nervous system transplants seem to be guided to their correct targets in adult central nervous systems, but adult axons need signals from neurons in the immediate environment which is provided by either peripheral nerves or the embryonic transplants. The specificity of synapse formation appears to be due to the particular neurotransmitters in both the transplanted and host target cells. Some types of lost function have been restored with transplants such as dopamine neurons which restore motor deficits caused by lesion of the substantia nigra or loss due to ageing. Transplants into the mature central nervous system do not seem to restore completely the original circuitry; instead they appear to serve as endogenous chemicals to supply the proper area (Cotman and Nieto-Sampedro 1985).

The molecular basis of neuronal plasticity is receiving much attention by neuroscientists. The numerous studies show an extremely complicated chemical

109

process consisting of nerve growth factors, neuropeptides, gangliosides and many other substances (Nirenberg *et al.* 1985). The neurotransmitters themselves are apparently capable of change to accomplish 'neuroplasticity'. The functional implications of this research at the molecular level have yet to be determined (Black *et al.* 1985).

The status of functional plasticity of the damaged nervous system was recently reviewed by Freed *et al.* (1985). The best example of functional recovery due to neuritic growth is in the resuturing of severed peripheral nerves. Experiments have shown that axonal growth can be enhanced by refinements in suturing the cut ends, freezing and then cutting the stumps before suture, and soaking the nerve ends in a modified Collins fluid to chelate or counteract intracellular calcium (calcium is thought to disrupt neurofilaments and initiate degeneration). Scar formation after injury appears to preclude regeneration, and attempts have been made to minimize scarring when the spinal cord has been transected in animals. Trophic and growth substances that promote neuronal growth (*e.g.* nerve growth factor, ganglioside, glycoproteins, heart-conditioned medium, neuronotrophic factors induced by the lesion) have been investigated and found to promote regeneration. Recently Müller *et al.* (1985) have identified a specific 37,000 Dalton protein in both the central and peripheral nervous systems of week-old rats. This same protein was also accumulated at the site of severed sciatic nerves but not in the adult central nervous system. These differences in quantity of the specific protein were thought to represent a critical molecular difference between peripheral nerves and the central nervous system—an explanation of why central axons fail to regenerate, in contrast to the well-known regeneration of peripheral nerves after injury.

Artificial bridges to reduce the interposition of scar tissue in experimental central nervous system injuries have been used (*e.g.* bovine collagen); differences exist between the neurons in their capacity for growth.

Brain-tissue grafts have been used experimentally to replace damaged cells such as those of the nigrostriatal dopamine system and the adrenal medulla. Embryonic grafts survive better, and it is possible that the response to grafts varies among species.

Electronic devices to aid or replace function of damaged neurons have become a reality—the cardiac pacemaker and the cochlear implant. Microchips to monitor single neuronal units and to stimulate the same neuron are being developed.

Recovery in immature nervous systems has been presumed to be superior to that in adults. Most of this presumption has been based upon the greater regenerative ability of lower vertebrates such as amphibia and reptiles (Kerr 1975). Research indicates that the immature nervous system may be less plastic than originally envisaged (Goldman 1972, 1974; Lawrence and Hopkins 1972; Berman and Berman 1973). In experimental animals, hemisection of the spinal cord in adults and neonates indicated that the timing of the lesion is important; true sparing of function may have been restricted to motor patterns not directly affected by the lesion because in young animals these patterns had not yet developed at the time of the injury (Bergman and Goldenberger 1983). Although axonal sprouting in experimental animals can be demonstrated, the extent of functional recovery is

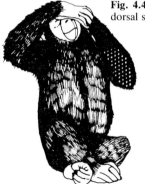

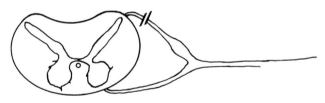

Fig. 4.4. Deafferentation of one upper limb of monkey produced by cutting dorsal spinal roots. Motor system is left intact.

IF INHIBIT USE OF NORMAL SIDE, RECOVERY.
IF USE NORMAL SIDE, INHIBIT RECOVERY.

unknown and thus unproven (Tsukahara and Murahami 1983). Apparent recovery of damaged neurons seems to occur not so much by regeneration as by development of behavioural maneuvers which mask the less specific motor functions. The experimental data indicates that damage to the central nervous system during its period of rapid growth may result in more destruction of ultimate function than injury during the more stable phases of brain development (Teuber 1971; Goldman 1972, 1974; Brunner and Altman 1974; Goldberger 1974; Neligan 1974; Schneider and Jhavery 1974).

The masking of neurological deficits can be spectacular. Reports abound in clinical and laboratory reports (Geschwind 1974). Recovery of near-normal behaviour after hemispherectomy is well known, and recovery of normal speech after ablation of cortical areas for speech has been observed. Despite these examples of dramatic recovery, there are patients who do not recover from brain lesions. Small lesions have produced large functional deficits. What are the possible reasons for these results?

Past experiments suggested that function might be recoverable, but inhibited by the remaining intact system. When a single upper limb of a monkey was deafferented by cutting of the dorsal spinal roots, permanent impairment of all spontaneous limb movement resulted (Mott and Sherrington 1895, Lassek 1953, Twitchell 1954). In addition, reflex activity unrelated to the dorsal-root sensory nerves was impaired, *e.g.* the static labyrinthine reflexes (Denny-Brown 1966). If both limbs were deafferented, functional recovery occurred spontaneously (Knapp *et al.* 1963, Taub and Berman 1968). In a monkey in which the dorsal-root afferent nerves were cut in only one limb and the opposite limb restricted in movement, recovery of the deafferented limb was enhanced (Fig.4.4). With this evidence we might conclude that forced use of the deafferented limb discouraged recovery, and that the intact sensory system in the normal limb selectively inhibited recovery of the normal intact limb (Taub *et al.* 1973). One might be tempted to use this experimental data clinically while forgetting that the lesions were of the spinal-cord nerve roots and not of the brain.

Similar phenomena have been observed in pyramidal-tract lesions in which

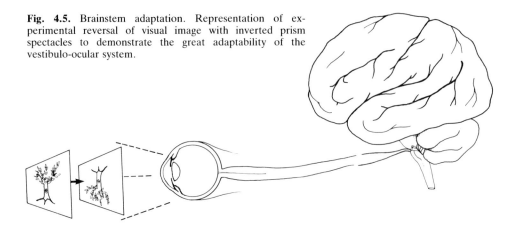

Fig. 4.5. Brainstem adaptation. Representation of experimental reversal of visual image with inverted prism spectacles to demonstrate the great adaptability of the vestibulo-ocular system.

recovery was enhanced by secondary lesions of the contralateral cerebral hemisphere (Bard 1938, Semmes and Chow 1955) and also of the ventrolateral funiculus of the spinal cord (Goldberger 1969). These findings implied an inhibitory process in the contralateral hemisphere. Amphetamines were thought to improve recovery by suppression of some of the inhibitory cortical areas (Beck and Chambers 1970).

Classic operant conditioning methods have achieved near-normal function in deafferented limbs (Bossom and Ommaya 1968). Liu and Chambers (1971) reported that monkeys could be trained to perform accurate and complicated maneuvers with their deafferented limbs without visual guidance. These maneuvers were performed with little or no feedback from the limb. Thus it was concluded that training methods 'unmasked' latent abilities in the central nervous system.

Leonard *et al.* (1984) performed cortical ablations in neonatal and adult cats. They analyzed the function of the cats with neurological tests and motion analysis. They found that the neonatal cats had a more prolonged emergence of reflexes and had fewer deficits than the adult cats. Motion analysis (kinematics) of the neonates showed that abnormalities of their locomotion were compensated for during a later phase of development, and the deficit was masked. These results indicated two possible mechanisms: (i) behavioural plasticity, which means masking of the deficits by movements different from the normal; and (ii) neurological plasticity, *e.g.* axonal sprouting.

The vestibular system appears most adaptable. The vestibulo-ocular system and its reflex can be easily altered by visual training with inverted prisms. In human experiments, when people wore spectacles that inverted their visual field (Fig.4.5), they were initially helpless: but with time they recovered and could move about normally. The synaptic circuits in the vestibular reflexes seem to be easily rearranged (Miles and Fuller 1974; Gonshor and Melvill-Jones 1976*a, b*). We have known for a long time that lesions of the vestibular system due to unilateral labyrinthectomies or neuronitis do not produce long-lasting symptoms, and compensation readily occurs. As with conditioned motor behaviour, these

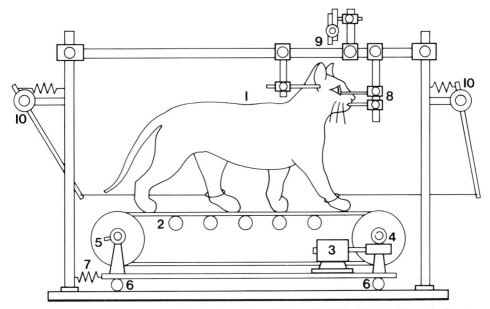

Fig. 4.6. Mesencephalic cat preparation (redrawn from Shik *et al.* 1966). (1) cat with cerebral cortex removed; (2) treadmill to record gait; (3) electric motor; (4) break; (5) belt-speed marker; (6) rollers; (7) dynamometer; (8) stereotaxic instrumentation; (9) electrodes; (10) pick-ups to measure horizontal displacement of limbs.

brainstem systems are almost independent of cortical control and are influenced primarily by lesions of the cerebellum and its nuclei (Llinas *et al.* 1975)

The effects of weightlessness on the vestibular system have been reported by astronauts during and after space flight. After returning to earth they were unable to stand on a narrow rail with eyes open on the first day, but recovered later. Standing was almost impossible with eyes closed, and this deficit in balance lasted longer before returning to normal. The data clearly show that postural mechanisms are affected by weightlessness; the hypothesis is that a 'pattern center' of the CNS changes to adapt during space flight, and then reverses upon return to earth. This is an example of central nervous system 'plasticity' (Shepherd 1983).

Motor behaviour

More and more research clearly indicates that we have genetically inherited 'innate' movement patterns (Grillner 1985). These patterns are co-ordinated neural circuits in the brain and spinal cord; despite being innate, they can be modified by experience and by sensory inputs in order to adapt to the immediate environment.

Wilson (1968) first suggested that there might be built-in circuits for motor behaviour. To study the flight-control system of the locust, he cut the sensory nerves to the wings and then stimulated the central nervous system with a noise pattern. With the noise he was able to obtain replicas of the flight pattern from the motor neurons of the locust. Flight for the locust is thus a 'motor score' written in the brain, and there is no need for direct stimulation and sensory input from its wings. Shik *et al.* (1966) provided additional evidence of an innate central program for gait in the cat. These Soviet scientists prepared a mesenchephalic cat by surgical decerebration and then applied gradations of electrical current to the remaining brain. With varying degrees of electrical stimulation (10 to 20μA) the cat walked, trotted and ran (Fig.4.6). Corresponding brainstem areas for locomotion have been found in primates, reptiles and fish.

Experimental data indicates that even when movement-related afferent input from the limb or body has been abolished, the locomotor circuits can be activated. The current view is that locomotor output is produced by the central nervous system and spinal cord which house central program generators (CPGs). Sensory feedback from muscle and joint receptors in the limbs is important; without this the system breaks down.

The decision to take a step is sufficient to begin walking. Signals are channeled through the basal ganglia to the spinal cord CPGs. While the loss of equilibrium sensation severely compromises walking, this loss can be compensated for by a treadmill which prevents the animal from falling; experimental animals adapt the speed of locomotion to that of the treadmill.

The brainstem centers control the spinal rhythm generators by spontaneous and modulating discharges which facilitate the phases of the gait cycle. Although the cerebellum is very important for the perfection of the movement patterns, it has no direct connections with the spinal cord. In the hierarchy of the central nervous system it is in the middle between the spinal cord and the cortex. It controls muscle tone, balance and sensorimotor co-ordination, and modulates sensory feedback from the limbs.

Grillner's (1985) experiments with the lamprey formed the hypothesis that individual CPGs exist to be used alone or in combination. If we wish to walk, we call on an ensemble of CPGs; but if we only want to move the big toe, we just call on one. Other evidence of 'hard-wired' motor synergies was suggested by Ghez *et al.* (1983). The onset of contraction of different muscle groups reflected the property of the total system. Further evidence of an innate central system of locomotion was provided by Forssberg and Svartengren (1983), who found retention of the extensor pattern in the cat gastrocnemius after it had been surgically transposed to a dorsiflexor action. They concluded that the spinal motor network had little plasticity.

The 19th-century concept of the cerebral cortex as the supreme commander is no longer tenable. Rather it is one part of a 'distributive system'—a combination of cortical and subcortical centers. It is often the middle of signal processing. Any cortical region can be significant for its synaptic connections and its connections to other cortical and subcortical regions. These synaptic circuits generate the special functions. The human attributes we have are in the organization of the synaptic circuits of the cortex (Shepherd 1983).

Environment

The cortical synapses are sensitive to environmental influences. For example, the removal of a rodent's eye reduces the number of spines (which make synapses) on apical dendrites in the visual cortex; in these newborn rodents, either the spines are lost or the dendrites fail to mature. When animals are raised in enriched environments, with toys to play with and mazes to run in, their cortices are thicker and synapses larger than those raised in barren cages. Cortices of wild animals may be 30 per cent thicker than domesticated ones. Dendritic spines are reduced in some types of human mental retardation. In monkeys when one eye is closed at birth, there is expansion of the ocular-dominance columns of the cortex of the normal eye. This expansion depends upon noradrenaline in the cortex, which opens the field to further study of the importance of neurochemicals (Shepherd 1983).

Held and Hein (1963) placed kittens in a circular room in which the walls were painted with stripes. One kitten was linked to the other by an apparatus in which one kitten walked and pulled the other kitten in a gondola. This arrangement permitted constant visual stimulation for both kittens, and a comparison between the influence of active and passive movement. The kittens spent three hours per day in the apparatus; the remainder of the day was spent in darkness. After 30 hours of this trial, the kitten that walked and pulled the gondola had normal responses to visually guided tasks, blinked when approached by an object, had placing reactions when dropped downward, and avoided the steep side of a cliff. The passive kitten in the gondola at first failed to show any of these normal behaviours, but eventually recovered. The obvious conclusion is that active movement is necessary to integrate visual motor control mechanisms.

In studies of single-unit recordings, as well as depth electrode electro-encephalographic records of the hippocampus in monkeys, it has been shown that pyramidal neurons will fire impulses when the monkey is in a certain corner of the cage but not another. Most importantly, this activity is recorded only when the animal actively moves to the locations. The cell is silent if the animal is passively placed.

Self-controlled movement is important for the development of the central nervous system (Connolly 1969). Goldberger (1969) pointed out that although monkeys who had lesions and then passive manipulations to assist recovery performed well under test conditions when conditioned stimuli were applied, they exhibited little improvement in spontaneous behaviour. For example, a monkey in which only the pyramidal tract cortex has been preserved may be trained to feed itself or to grasp an object if the conditioned stimulus is applied, but is unable to perform the task voluntarily. Conditioned motor behaviour is patterned, and therefore inaccessible to cortical volition when the cortex is damaged. Hepp-Reymond (1970) reported that conditioned behaviour remained unchanged despite extensive cortical and pyramidal tract lesions.

Cerebral cortex and human behaviour
A complete description of this complex subject is not possible here. However, some general remarks seem pertinent, because in the past 25 years there has been an explosion of manipulative educational and infant treatment programs for cerebral palsy. Many of these programs have been presumptuous and based on speculation.

Contemporary evidence dispels our old concepts that all intelligence, cognitive abilities, affective behaviour and temperament reside solely within the billions of cells of the cerebral cortex. Instead the new idea is that these functions are mediated by a system of cortical and subcortical centers. We used to accept the evolutionary idea that the size of the forebrain and cortical development was linear. We were taught that the neocortex first appeared in amphibians; in reptiles and birds sensory systems were projected through the thalamus from the cortex; and finally, in mammals, the cortex grew larger with the inputs from the thalamus and basal ganglia. One new idea is that the forebrain and cortex have not undergone gradual and linear evolutionary change, but that species have developed their forebrains independently. We also know that the functions of neuritic tracts are mediated differently among species. Various animal species have neither a typical tract nor a center for a given function. These independently evolving structures are termed 'homoplastic' (Shepherd 1983).

Psychological development in infants appears to be 'canalized' (Kagan 1982)—a term describing the common behavioural changes and developmental milestones in infants between the ages of 17 and 24 months. These include the sense of right and wrong, emergence of speech, self-awareness in actions and in recognition, memory for the past and maintenance of an active memory. These behavioural events occur in parallel as the central nervous system matures. In the rat, a sevenfold increase in the number of synapses was found in the parietal cortex between the 12th and 26th days after birth. Similar increases in synaptic connections occur in the primate and human after birth. Programmed cell death and synaptic remodeling occur at the same time. All of these events take place under genetic regulation. The neuron reaches maturity under the influences of *its own* environment.

The old belief that developmental milestones in cognition, emotion and behaviour were determined almost solely by the social interactions of parents and children, meant that differences of behaviour had to be due to differing family experiences. Although we cannot deny the importance of family experiences in human development, we also need to recognize the effects of innate characteristics that appear on a biologically determined timetable. Even Freud eventually recognized that innate maturational forces in infants would have common developmental profiles (Kagan 1982). Thus parents are not the sole and only sculptors of their children. Anyone who has raised more than one child or has observed children in other families and cultures can acknowledge the common developmental profiles of infants and children as well as their inherited behavioural traits.

Kagan gives numerous examples of canalization of infant development. One is the anxiety of infants between the ages of eight and 12 months when separated from the mother. This is true in infants worldwide including blind infants, infants in kibbutzim in Israel, villages in Guatemala, in Indian villages in Central America, in day-care centers and in nuclear families. All have maximum distress at about 15 months, but by the third birthday they no longer fuss or cry on separation.

Eight-month-old infants show no fear of infants the same age. However, by the middle of the second year they become inhibited, circumspect and timid, and cling to the mother. Again this characteristic mood disappears in the third year. This fearfulness has been observed in all social classes, races and groups. This fear is probably due to the new cognitive functions resulting from the growth of the central nervous system.

Cerebral cortical functions are not compartmentalized in local regional centers. The cortical area is one part of a larger interconnecting system. For example, seeing an object requires connections from the occipital lobe to the motor outputs in the parietal and frontal lobes; grasping it requires additional connections to the eye fields in the frontal cortex to co-ordinate eye movements with our fingers. Neurochemicals are also important for the function of cortical systems. When dopamine was selectively suppressed in the frontal cortex of monkeys by injections of 6-hydroxydopamine, the monkeys could not remember the location of a test object; these results were comparable to those obtained by prefrontal lobotomy. The effects of dopamine depletion were reversed by dopamine agonists.

Techniques for mapping the workings of the cortical systems in humans have been developed. An example of the results of such techniques can be found in the mapping obtained when a person is asked to name a seen object. Shepherd (1983) reported that the visual information was first received in area 17, further processed in areas 18 and 19, and then the image was transferred to a posterior speech area which include areas 39 and Wernicke's. From area 39 the visual representation was sent to auditory area 22; from area 22 the signals went to Broca's speech area to obtain the motor programs of speech. These motor programs were interpreted by the face area of the motor cortex, where the co-ordination of the muscles used in speech lie. The final result of this complex processing was the spoken word (Shepherd 1983).

Clinical implications

Given the complexity and distribution of central nervous system functions that make us human, it seems clear that a highly localized cerebral lesion does not usually explain the motor, sensory and cognitive defects commonly observed in cerebral palsy.

The biological evidence that neurons are irreplaceable should assist our understanding of the prognosis in cerebral palsy. The existence of innate central motor programs within the spinal cord and brain ought to make us wary of passive manipulative treatments presumed to restore locomotor ability in infants. The data on maturation of the neurons, and their connections during the first three years of life, might temper our zeal in ascribing developmental progress to special educational programs or treatment methods. The scientific data clearly indicate that passive activities and manipulations do not create synaptic connections or account for neuronal growth. Doing and perfecting the task by active self-controlled activity has a firm neurobiological basis. 'Enriched environments' for developing children at the appropriate time, consistent with maturation of the nervous system, would seem more logical.

While the administration of brain-altering drugs, electrical stimulation and neuron transplants are fascinating experiments in animals, there is only limited scope for their direct clinical application to solve the problem of cerebral palsy. Much more research needs to be done. Meanwhile, we will have to be content to manage the child with cerebral palsy based upon realities, and not upon wishes and dreams to treat the brain as a computer which we can 'program' by experimental manipulations.

ACKNOWLEDGEMENT

Much of the literature on neuroplasticity was abstracted from lecture notes of Wise Young, MD, PhD, in the 1979 edition and retained in this text.

REFERENCES

Bard, P. (1938) 'Studies on the cortical representation of somatic sensibility.' *Harvey Lectures*, **33**, 143–169.
Beck, C. H., Chambers, W. W. (1970) 'Speed, accuracy and strength of forelimb movement after unilateral pyramidotomy in rhesus monkeys.' *Journal of Comparative and Physiological Psychology*, **70**, 1–22.
Bergman, B. S., Goldenberger, M. E. (1983) 'Infant lesion effect: II. Sparing and recovery of function after spinal cord damage in newborn and adult cats.' *Brain Research*, **285**, 119–135.
Berman, A. J., Berman, D. (1973) 'Fetal deafferentation: the ontogenesis of movement in the absence of peripheral sensory feedback.' *Experimental Neurology*, **38**, 170–176.
Black, I. R., Adler, J. E., Dreyfus, C. F., Jonakait, G. M., Katz, D. M., LaGamma, E. F., Markey, K. M. (1985) 'Neurotransmitter plasticity at the molecular level.' *In:* Abelson, P. H., Butz, E., Snyder, S. H. (Eds.) *Neuroscience*. Washington: American Association for the Advancement of Science. pp. 30–39.
Bossom, J., Ommaya, A. K. (1968) 'Visuo-motor adaptation in prismatic transformation of the retinal image in monkeys with bilateral dorsal rhizotomy.' *Brain*, **91**, 161–172.
Brunner, R. L., Altman, J. (1974) 'The effects of interference with the maturation of the cerebellum and hippocampus on the development of adult behavior.' *In:* Stein, P. G., Rosen, J. J., Butters, N. (Eds.) *Plasticity and Recovery of Function in the Central Nervous System*. New York: Academic Press.
Clemente, C. D. (1964) 'Regeneration in the vertebrate central nervous system.' *International Review of Neurobiology*, **6**, 257–301.
Connolly, K. (1969) 'Sensory motor coordination: mechanism and plans.' *In:* Wolff, P. H., MacKeith, R. (Eds.) *Planning for Better Learning. Clinics in Developmental Medicine No. 33*. London: S.I.M.P. with Heinemann; Philadelphia: Lippincott.
Cotman, C. W., Nieto-Sampedro, M. (1985) 'Cell biology of synaptic plasticity.' *In:* Abelson, P. H., Butz, E., Snyder, S. H. (Eds.) *Neuroscience*. Washington: American Association for the Advancement of Science. pp. 74–88.
Cowan, W. M., Fawcett, J. W., O'Leary, D. D. M., Stanfield, B. B. (1985) 'Regressive events in neurogenesis.' *In:* Abelson, P. H., Butz, E., Snyder, S. H. (Eds.) *Neuroscience*. Washington: American Association for the Advancement of Science. pp. 13–29.
Denny-Brown, D. (1966) *The Cerebral Control of Movement*. Liverpool: University of Liverpool Press.
Dobbing, J., Sands, J. (1973) 'Quantitative growth and development of the human brain.' *Archives of Disease in Childhood*, **48**, 757–767.
Edds, M. V. (1953) 'Collateral nerve degeneration.' *Quarterly Review of Biology*, **28**, 260–275.
Forssberg, H., Svartengren, G. (1983) 'Hardwired locomotor network in cat revealed by a retained motor pattern to gastrocnemius after muscle transposition.' *Neuroscience Letters*, **41**, 283–288.
Freed, W. J., Medinaceli, L. de, Wyatt, R. J. (1985) 'Promoting functional plasticity in the damaged nervous system.' *Science*, **227**, 1544–1552.
Geschwind, N. (1974) 'Late changes in the nervous system: an overview'. *In:* Stein, P. G., Rosen, J. J., Butters, N. (Eds.) *Plasticity and Recovery of Function in the Central Nervous System*. New York: Academic Press.

Ghez, C., Vicario, D., Martin, J. H., Yumiga, H. (1983) 'Sensory motor processing of target central control motor programs.' *Advances in Neurology*, **39**, 61–92.

Goldberger, M. E. (1969) 'The extrapyramidal systems of the spinal cord. II: Results of combined pyramidal and extrapyramidal lesions in the macaque.' *Journal of Comparative Neurology*, **135**, 1–26.

—— (1974) 'Recovery of movement after central nervous system lesions in monkeys.' *In:* Stein, P. G., Rosen, J. J., Butters, N. (Eds.) *Plasticity and Recovery of Function in the Central Nervous System.* New York: Academic Press.

Goldman, P. S. (1972) 'Developmental determinants of cortical plasticity.' *Acta Neurobiologiae Experimentalis*, **32**, 495–511.

—— (1974) 'An alternative to developmental plasticity: heterology of central nervous system structures in infants and adults.' *In:* Stein, P. G., Rosen, J. J., Butters, N. (Eds.) *Plasticity and Recovery of Function in the Central Nervous System.* New York: Academic Press.

Gonshor, A., Melvill-Jones, G. (1976a) 'Short term adaptive changes in the human vestibulo-ocular reflex arc.' *Journal of Physiology*, **256**, 361–379.

—— —— (1976b) 'Extreme vestibulo-ocular adaptation induced by prolonged optical reversal of vision.' *Journal of Physiology*, **256**, 381–414.

Grillner, S. (1985) 'Neurobiological bases of rhythmic motor acts in vertebrates.' *Science*, **228**, 143–149.

Held, R., Hein, A. (1963) 'Movement-produced stimulation with development of visually guided behavior.' *Journal of Comparative and Physiological Psychology*, **56**, 872–876.

Hepp-Reymond, M. C., Wiesendanger, M., Brunnert, A., Mackel, A., Unger, R., Wespi, J. (1970) 'Effects of unilateral pyramidotomy on conditioned finger movement in monkeys.' *Brain Research*, **24**, 544.

Kagan, J. (1982) 'Canalization of early psychological development.' *Pediatrics*, **70**, 474–483.

Kerr, F. W. L. (1975) 'Structural and functional evidence of plasticity in the central nervous system.' *Experimental Neurology*, **48**, 16–31.

Knapp, H. D., Taub, E., Berman, A. V. (1963) 'Movements in monkeys with deafferentated limbs.' *Experimental Neurology*, **7**, 305–315.

Landmesser, L. (1981) 'Pathway selection by embryonic neurons.' *In:* Cowan, W. M. (Ed.) *Studies in Developmental Neurobiology.* New York: Oxford University Press. p. 53.

Lassek, A. M. (1953) 'Inactivation of voluntary motor function following rhizotomy.' *Journal of Neuropathology and Experimental Neurology*, **12**, 83–87.

Lawrence, D. G., Hopkins, D. A. (1972) 'Developmental aspects of pyramidal motor control in the rhesus monkey.' *Brain Research*, **40**, 117–119.

Leonard, C. T., Robinson, G. A., Goldberger, M. E. (1984) 'Development and recovery of function in brain damaged neonates of cats.' *Orthopaedic Transactions*, **8**, 105. *Developmental Medicine and Child Neurology*, **26**, 243. (*Abstract*.)

Liu, C. N., Chambers, N. W. (1958) 'Intraspinal sprouting of dorsal root axons.' *Archives of Neurology and Psychiatry*, **79**, 46–61.

—— —— (1971) 'A study of cerebellar dyskinesia in bilaterally deafferentated forelimbs of the monkey (Macca mulatta and Macca speciosa).' *Acta Neurobiologiae Experimentalis*, **31**, 263–289.

Llinas, R., Walton, K., Hillman, D. E. (1975) 'Inferior olive: its role in motor learning.' *Science*, **190**, 1230–1231.

Miles, F. A., Fuller, J. H. (1974) 'Adaptive plasticity in the vestibulo-ocular responses of the rhesus monkey.' *Brain Research*, **80**, 512–516.

Mott, F. W., Sherrington, C. S. (1895) 'Experiments on the influence of sensory nerves upon movement and nutrition of the limbs.' *Proceedings of the Royal Medical Society of London*, **57**, 81–88.

Müller, H. W., Gebicke-Härter, P. J., Hangen, D. H., Shooter, E. M. (1985) 'A specific 37,000-Dalton protein that accumulates in regenerating but not in nonregenerating mammalian nerves.' *Science*, **228**, 499–501.

Neligan, G. A. (1974) 'The human brain growth spurt.' *Developmental Medicine and Child Neurology*, **16**, 677–678.

Nirenberg, M., Wilson, S. P., Higashida, H., Rotter, A., Krueger, K. E., Busis, N., Ray, R., Kenimer, J. G., Adler, M. (1985) 'Modulation of synapse formation by cyclic adenosine monophosphate.' *In:* Abelson, P. H., Butz, E., Snyder, S. H. (Eds.) *Neuroscience.* Washington D.C.: American Association for the Advancement of Science. pp. 118–129.

Oda, M. A. S., Huttenlocher, P. R. (1974) 'The effect of corticosteroids in dendritic development in the rat brain.' *Yale Journal of Biology and Medicine*, **47**, 155–165.

Rakic, P. (1985) 'Limits of neurogenesis in primates.' *Science*, **227**, 1054–1056.

Ramon y Cajal, S. (1928) *Degeneration and Regeneration of the Nervous System* (Translation by May,

R. M.), London: Oxford University Press.

Rosner, B. S. (1974) 'Recovery of function and localization of function in historical perspective.' *In:* Stein, D. B., Rosen, J. J., Butters, N. (Eds.) *Plasticity and Recovery of Function in the Central Nervous System.* New York: Academic Press.

Schade, J. P., Von Groenigen, W. B. (1961) 'Structural organization of the human cerebral cortex. I. Maturation of the middle frontal gyrus.' *Acta Anatomica*, **47,** 74–111.

Schneider, G. E., Jhaveri, S. R. (1974) 'Neuroanatomical correlates of spared or altered function after brain lesion in the newborn hamster.' *In:* Stein, P. G., Rosen, J. J., Butters, N. (Eds.) *Plasticity and Recovery of Function in the Central Nervous System.* New York: Academic Press.

Semmes, J., Chow, K. L. (1955) 'Motor effects of lesions of the precentral gyrus and of lesions sparing this area in monkeys.' *Archives of Neurology and Psychiatry*, **73,** 546–566.

Shepherd, G. M. (1983) *Neurobiology.* New York and Oxford: Oxford University Press.

Shik, M. L., Severin, F. C., Orlovskii, G. N. (1966) 'Control of walking and running by means of stimulation of the mid-brain.' *Biofizika*, **11,** 659–666.

Taub, E., Berman, A. J. (1968) 'Movement and learning in the absence of sensory feedback.' *In:* Freedman, S. J. (Ed.) *Neuropsychology of Spatially Oriented Behavior.* Homewood, Illinois: Dorsey Press.

—— Parella, P., Barro, G. (1973) 'Behavioral development after forelimb deafferentation on day of birth in monkey with and without blinding.' *Science*, **181,** 959–960.

Teuber, H. L. (1971) 'Mental retardation after early trauma to the brain: some issues in search of facts.' *In:* Angle, C. R., Bearing, E. A. Jr. (Eds.) *Physical Trauma as an Etiological Agent in Mental Retardation.* Bethesda, Maryland: National Institutes of Health.

Tsukahara, N., Murahami, F. (1983) 'Axonal sprouting and recovery of function after brain damage.' *Advances in Neurology*, **39,** 1073–1084.

Twitchell, T. E. (1954) 'Sensory factors in purposive movement.' *Journal of Neurophysiology*, **17,** 239–252.

Wilson, D. M. (1968) 'The flight control system of the locust.' *Scientific American*, **218**(5), 83–90.

Windle, W. F. (1956) 'Regeneration of axons in the vertebrate central nervous system.' *Physiological Reviews*, **36,** 427–440.

5
PROGNOSIS AND STRUCTURAL CHANGES

The prognosis for function of a child with cerebral palsy is uppermost in the minds of parents who consult the physician or therapist. Parents want to anticipate and plan. Prognosis and natural history are also extremely important in assessing the outcome of treatment: whether this is surgery, physical or occupational therapy or drug administration.

For this we need to understand the structural changes that have occurred in the brain, and the changes in the muscles, bones and joints due to the motor disorder as the child grows into adulthood. If possible, we also need to know what further disability the changes in the musculoskeletal system will cause in adult life.

Motor prognosis
Walking prognosis tests
When a child is diagnosed as cerebral palsied, the first question asked by the parents is always 'Will he walk?', the second is usually 'When?', and the third is 'What can we do to make him walk?'

To answer these questions we have to deal with probabilities (better than an 80 per cent chance) and not possibilities. To try to answer these questions with something more than a shrug or a categorical 'Never!', I did a prospective study of infants and children with cerebral palsy. The study was based upon testing for retained infantile automatisms which should not be present at age 12 months or later and postural reflexes which should be present at that time (Bleck 1975). 73 infants and children who were 12 months of age or older and not walking were tested, a prognosis for walking was given, and then they were followed to the age of at least seven. The oldest patient still being studied was born in 1962.

The following seven tests (Fiorentino 1963, see also Chapter 2) were done and one point assigned if the automatism was definitely and unequivocally present or the normal postural reflex was absent:
(1) Asymmetrical tonic neck reflex—1 point
(2) Neck right reflex—1 point
(3) Moro reflex—1 point
(4) Symmetrical tonic neck reflex—1 point
(5) Extensor thrust—1 point
(6) Parachute reaction (should be present)—1 point if absent
(7) Foot placement reaction (should be present)—1 point if absent.
A score of two points or more gave a poor prognosis for walking, a one-point score was a guarded prognosis ('might walk'), and a zero score indicated a good prognosis.

The results were analyzed after the child's seventh birthday. To qualify as walkers, children had to walk a minimum of 15m without falling. Those who could walk with crutches were also considered functional walkers in the study. Children

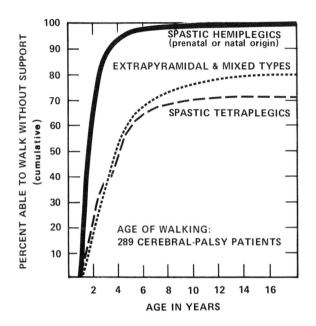

Fig. 5.1. Percentage of cerebral-palsied patients able to walk, according to age. Note that the ability to walk ceases for all groups at about the age of seven years (redrawn from Crothers and Paine 1959).

who walked only with the aid of a mobility device or only in parallel bars were not considered functional walkers. The accuracy of these predictions was 94.5 per cent.

Of the 73 children, 13 never walked, 16 had been given a poor prognosis (2 points or more), and all had total body involvement with either spastic paralysis in all four limbs or athetosis. In subsequent follow-up of seven children who had a score of one point and a guarded prognosis, all eventually did walk with crutches; but generally by the age of 10 to 12 years, most depended upon their wheelchairs for anything but short distances in the home. These patients had a strong extensor thrust, and although their lower limbs were in extension posture, the absence of flexion of the knee precluded efficient walking.

Age of walking
In our study we observed that walking ability reaches a plateau by the age of seven years. Crothers and Paine's data on walking ability (1959) show practically the same age when no further walking occurred (Fig.5.1). A study by Beals (1966) also showed that motor performance in spastic diplegic children reached a plateau at age seven years. An interesting coincidence comes from the data on development of mature gait by Sutherland *et al.* (1980), which showed that all gait electromyograms, major determinants of gait and linear measurements were of the adult type at age seven years.

All of our children with hemiplegia walked between the ages of 18 and 21 months. Most children with spastic diplegia were walking by 48 months. In another study by Robson (quoted by Chaplais and MacFarland 1984) the mean age of walking for hemiplegic children was 15 months, and 24 months for spastic diplegia.

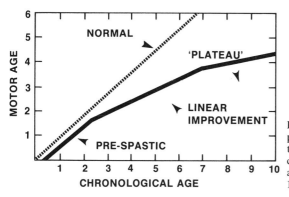

Fig. 5.2. Graphic representation of improvement in motor performance of spastic diplegic children. Note plateau (no change in motor performance) beginning at age seven years (redrawn from Beals 1966).

Generally parents become concerned if their child is not walking by 18 months. In a detailed study of 242 late-walking children (Chaplais and MacFarland 1984), 5.8 per cent were found to have some neurological abnormality (3.5 per cent having cerebral palsy). Late walkers otherwise were called 'idiopathic'; 48 per cent of these children had bottom shuffling as their method of locomotion. A positive family history for delayed walking was found in 50 per cent of their first-degree relatives. The age of walking was 19.5 months in 50 per cent and 24 months in 97 per cent. These idiopathic and probably genetically determined late walkers had general hypotonia and increased joint laxity. I have seen similar children, and they had these same findings. The prognostic test scores based upon the seven tests were zero in all cases giving a good prognosis.

The prognosis of at-risk infants before the age of one year demands great caution. The 1982 study by Nelson and Ellenberg, who examined 32,000 children before age one year and again at seven years, showed that the diagnosis of cerebral palsy was made early in 229, but at age seven years 118 of these were free of motor handicaps. In this group, about 20 per cent had early-intervention physical therapy. This study clearly demonstrates children who 'outgrew' cerebral palsy. Motor prognosis should not be made before the age of 12 months. This is not surprising, given what we know about central nervous system development (see Chapter 4).

Other prognostic indicators for walking
Molnar and Gordon (1974) studied 233 non-walking children with cerebral palsy, and found that under the age of two years the ability to sit independently was not a good predictor of walking; inability to sit alone after the age of four years did predict non-walking.

To predict walking in children who had spastic diplegia, Beals (1966) devised a motor quotient and a severity index. The motor quotient was derived by division of the chronological age divided by the motor age. Motor age was determined by standard tests such as those referenced in Chapter 3. The prognosis according to the motor quotient was as follows: if 30 or more, free walking would occur; if 16 or below, no ambulation could be expected. The test results were uniform up to the age of two years; at later ages (to the age of five) they had increasing variability. A

TABLE 5.I

Walking prognosis in spastic diplegia

Severity index	Prognosis
12 or more	Free walking by 7 years
10-11	Lowest score consistent with free walking
9	Crutch walking
9-0	No walking

From Beals (1966).

major finding of this study was that motor gains reached a plateau or ceased between the ages of six and seven years (Fig.5.2).

Beals (1966) also devised a severity index based upon the motor age in months for three-year-old children (Table 5.I). These scores were applied to the anticipated locomotor functional goals when considering orthopaedic surgery. If the severity index was 0 to 9, surgery was not recommended for the goal of free walking; an index of 10 to 11 indicated that walking was a reasonable goal to be enhanced by surgery. If the severity index was 12 to 18, free ambulation was thought possible, but surgery was recommended only to improve gait.

Bose and Yeo (1975) proposed a scoring system to determine severity of gross motor function at any age. Their objective was to select children who might benefit most from treatment and to assess the results of treatment programs. Similar scoring methods were devised by Forbes and McIntyre (1968) and Reimers (1972). All of these systems used demerit points (*e.g.* sitting impossible, −30; standing impossible, −30; and a total score below 25 indicating that walking was possible). These methods of scoring described the extent of the disability, but had limited predictive value. In my literature search I found no further references to these scoring methods in predicting ambulation. Numerical scores have been helpful in assessing potential for functional goals and in assessing results of management to achieve goals by us. These methods and results are described in Chapter 6.

Mental retardation has little if any effect on the ability to walk (Molnar and Gordon 1974). Shapiro *et al.* (1979) studied 152 profoundly mentally retarded children (IQ below 25) who had neither an acquired nor a progressive degenerative disease, and found that walking began at a mean age of 30 months. The majority (95.2 per cent) of the children who had no major neurological disability walked by age six years. Walking occurred in 63.6 per cent of those who had both mental retardation and seizure disorders, and in only 10 per cent who also had cerebral palsy. These authors concluded that 'cognition is a less important determinant of the ability to walk than is the basic neurological integrity'. It is evident that motor assessment alone cannot determine mental retardation.

Equilibrium reactions
Standing equilibrium reactions, the testing for which was described in Chapter 2, are important to determine whether or not the child needs external support to walk. Children may have good prognostic signs for walking, but be unable to do so

TABLE 5.II

Equilibrium reactions and need for walking aids*

Walking status	Standing equilibrium reactions			Per cent
	Poor in all planes	Poor posterior Poor anterior Good lateral	Poor posterior Good anterior Good lateral	
Not walking	10			8.6
Walker (4-point ambulator)	5			4.3
Crutches		18		15.5
Independent			83	71.5
Totals	15	18	83	99.9

*Based on a study of 116 spastic diplegic children (Miranda 1979).

without external aids to compensate for the lack of balance. I have found that if the standing equilibrium reactions are good from side to side (lateral reactions) but deficient fore (anteriorly) and aft (posteriorly), crutches are required for support. Four-legged walkers are needed for those who have deficient equilibrium reactions in all directions. Children with spastic diplegia usually have good side-to-side and fore reactions but are poor aft. They fall backward easily with the slightest push. Despite this, they can walk independently. Table 5.II is a study of equilibrium reactions in 116 spastic diplegic children.

Of all the motor problems in cerebral palsy, deficient equilibrium reactions interfere the most with functional walking. The need to balance on one foot and then the other in walking stresses all of their lower-limb and trunk muscles. When external support is added, the gait immediately becomes more smooth and even. Even holding the head of such children and following them while they walk is often an impressive demonstration that the major disability is not the spastic paralysis or the athetosis but the lack of balance. Because the loss of normal equilibrium reactions is due to the brain lesions, muscle-strengthening exercises often enforced by parents (particularly by athletic fathers) are not often useful. If we can find some way of correcting the defects in the postural mechanisms, we will have reached a milestone in therapy. I have noted on follow-up that some spastic diplegic children who needed crutches were able to do without them in the household after about the age of 10 years. Orthopaedic surgery will not necessarily alter the need for crutches or walkers—a point that needs to be emphasized to both child and parent preoperatively. Indeed crutches or walkers improve the results of lower-limb surgery, and can cover a multitude of sins.

Prognosis for upper-limb function

Beals (1966) used his severity index (determinations of motor age at three years) to predict upper-limb function. The tests included the upper limbs. The severity index scores and the prognosis for upper-limb function are in Table 5.III. The most significant finding in this study was that intelligence paralleled the upper-limb severity index.

TABLE 5.III

Upper-limb function prognosis

Severity index	Prognosis
0-6	Profound disability
7-11	Moderate disability
12-17	Mild disability

*From Beals (1966).

In children younger than three years, some generalizations appear valid. The prognosis for upper-limb function is poor when the child has no limb dominance (lateralization of hand use), or when the upper limbs are unable to cross the mid-line of the trunk. When stereognostic sensation in the hand is deficient, function will always be compromised. The child will have to use visual feedback exclusively to control the hands.

Structural changes

Structural changes in the anatomy are all acquired. Those in the brain, of course, occur either prenatally, perinatally or postnatally. Those changes firstly in the muscles and secondarily in the bones and joints occur most often as the result of the spastic paralysis, and occasionally in athetosis. Spinal curvature may be the result of defective postural mechanisms. Structural change, unless prevented by orthopaedic surgery, occurs with the passage of time and may not cause serious disability until the child becomes obsolete—*i.e.* an adult. Therefore, we should have some idea of what can happen to compromise function as the child matures and becomes an adult. This looking ahead is part of the prognosis too.

Brain

The structural changes in the brain can arise from prenatal, perinatal and postnatal causes. The major source for the following brief description is Wigglesworth (1984).

Prenatal lesions such as porencephaly, encephalomalacias and hydrocephalus represent the effects of intrauterine damage which might be due to cytomegalovirus, toxoplasmosis or cerebral ischemia. Wigglesworth found pathological evidence of acute anoxic damage in stillborns. The basal nuclei and brainstem showed dead neurons and reactive gliosis. In some of these cases he found histories of maternal respiratory arrest during the second trimester of pregnancy. The infants died because of damage to the respiratory center. This may be the case in infants who survive episodes of maternal hypoxia *in utero* and after they develop cerebral palsy, which is thought to have a genetic origin. Placental infarction due to pre-eclampsia or antepartum uterine hemorrhage may cause fetal cerebral ischemia.

Genetic and chromosomal defects or teratogenic agents do not ordinarily result in severe malformations of the brain. Genetically determined metabolic defects result in subtle changes which often are not seen at the structural level.

Perinatal causes are the familiar direct trauma at birth and resultant tearing of

126

the tentorium or vein of Galen. With such tears it is the hemorrhage from the veins which will impair the cerebral circulation, resulting in anoxic brain damage.

Neonatal hypoxia produces variable effects. The pattern of cerebral damage is affected by those regions of the brain that have higher metabolic activity and require greater bloodflow. In the infant up to term, the areas with the greatest metabolic activity are the nuclei of the spinal cord, brainstem, midbrain, thalamus and basal ganglia. The effects of hypoxia vary from infant to infant and depend upon the status of the infant's circulatory system and cerebral perfusion.

Brain hemorrhage in the newborn is the most common phenomenon in both premature and term infants, although it has been recognized in 40 to 50 per cent of all newborns with birthweights less than 1500g. Bleeding is from the microcirculation and arises in the subependymal cell plate near the head of the caudate nucleus. Bleeding occurs with greater frequency in the respiratory distress syndrome, which is characterized by hypercapnia and metabolic acidosis. Bleeding can break through to the ventricles. Recent research suggests that eliminating the fluctuating cerebral bloodflow velocity in preterm babies with respiratory distress syndrome can reduce the incidence and severity of intraventricular hemorrhage (Perlman *et al.* 1985). The extent of cerebral damage due to subependymal and intraventricular hemorrhage can be quite variable. There might be a small or large ventricular clot, or extensive spread of blood into the brain tissue, or CSF obstruction with secondary hydrocephalus.

It is thought that hemorrhage and ischemia often coexist. Ischemia results in the pathological change of periventricular leukomalacia. This structural change in the brain is believed to be responsible for cerebral palsy, which is more frequent in premature infants. The majority of premature infants who do develop cerebral palsy have spastic diplegia. At postmortem, the areas of affected brain show softening and early coagulation necrosis. In later stages white spots due to areas of fat-laden histiocytes are found, and still later after birth glial scars and cystic areas are found.

Bilirubin encephalopathy is due to the cellular effects of bilirubin. It alters cell function by depressing cell respiration, by affecting the mitochondrial chemistry of oxidative phosphorylation and inhibiting the formation of protein from the amino acids. The pathological postmortem findings are bilirubin stains of brain regions similar to those affected by cardiac arrest: thalamus, basal ganglia, midbrain and brainstem.

Wigglesworth (1984) says that after 28 weeks of gestation, the capacity of the fetal brain for remodeling is greater than that of older fetuses and infants. At this age only rudimentary connections are present. Recovery from fetal cerebral ischemia may be greater than at a later age. In general, large lesions produce significant neurological signs. However, there are reports of infants who have small brain lesions yet have major handicaps, and conversely infants with large lesions have had minor difficulties. All we can conclude from these accounts is that as cerebral imaging techniques become more and more feasible, clinicians need to be prudent in predicting the eventual severity of the neurological manifestations based solely upon presumed cerebral damage depicted in the brain images.

Muscle

Muscle neurophysiology, growth and contracture

In spastic paralysis in children, there is excessive contraction of the involved muscles: and with growth, some muscles become contracted. Excessive contractions of the muscles are due to increased stretch reflexes, which are a function of the spinal cord reflex arc. If the nerve supply to a muscle is cut experimentally, stretch of the muscle produces only a small increase in tension, due to the inherent elastic properties of the muscle and its tendon. Muscles can be stretched about 3 per cent of their length before breaking down, and tendons about 6 per cent of their length before rupturing (Alexander 1984). So the stretch reflex is responsible for the greatly increased tension in muscle action. The elastic properties of the muscle and tendon probably serve as springs to conserve energy during walking and running (Alexander 1984).

Within the muscles are sense organs called muscle spindles, which contain small muscle fibers (intrafusal fibers). These intrafusal fibers are arranged in two different ways: in a sacular central location called nuclear bag fibers, and in a chain called nuclear chain fibers. Each has its own innervation and its own axons of small diameter, which have been named gamma fibers to distinguish them from the large axons of the muscle itself (extrafusal muscle fibers and alpha axons). The muscle spindles are sense organs, which provide afferent feedback for the control of fine movements and which maintain posture in certain muscles (*e.g.* the soleus muscles have many spindles while the shoulder muscles have few). Afferent fibers from the spindle primary ending (Ia) travel at the rate of 70 to 120 m/sec and detect the phasic stretch of the muscle—the stretch or myotatic reflex. Afferent fibers from spindle secondary endings (II) have a slower speed of 30 to 70 m/sec, and detect the steady stretch of the muscle. Their postural function is to contribute both to the extensor reflexes (myotatic) and flexor reflexes. The flexor reflex arises from cutaneous endings in the skin whose afferents (II, III, IV) are very much slower in time (0.5 to 70 m/sec) and have the function of detecting harmful stimuli so that the limb automatically withdraws from harm.

The tendons have their own sensory receptors, the Golgi tendon organ, located at the musculotendinous junction. The Golgi tendon organs detect active stretch of the tendon, and through their afferents (Ib fibers; 70 to 120 m/sec) they control muscle force and stiffness and may prevent overstretching of the tendon.

All of these muscle sense organs (kinesthetic sensors) are part of the gamma motor system. In normal mammals (and presumably in the human) the gamma system is active continuously due to increased afferent impulses from the primary endings in the contracting intrafusal fibers, and when stretching of the muscle occurs there is increased sensitivity of the receptors. During active contraction of a muscle, the tendon organ is also subjected to increased tension, while the muscle spindle becomes slack due to the parallel arrangement of the muscle fibers (extrafusal) with the spindle muscle fibers (intrafusal). The separate gamma innervation system to the nuclear bag and to the nuclear chain fibers allows these sensory endings in the muscle spindle to be controlled independently; this adds precision.

128

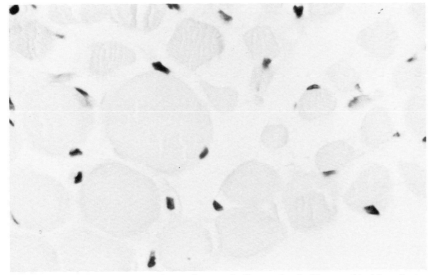

Fig. 5.3. Photomicrograph 43X. Biopsy of sacrospinalis muscle of a 12-year-old with scoliosis and spastic total body involvement. Note variation in size and shape of muscle fibers (hematoxylin-eosin stain).

We now know that there is cortical representation of the kinesthetic sensations from the muscles. Originally it was thought that kinesthesia was only a subcortical function. However, if all skin afferents from the arm are blocked with local anesthesia, the fingers retain their sense of position. Such observations have confirmed that cortical representation is present.*

We are still uncertain of the nature of spastic paralysis, except that it occurs experimentally when higher brain centers are cut off from the lower ones (as was done by Sherrington by cutting across the midbrain of cats). Spasticity has been thought of as an alteration in the gamma nervous system which overloads the muscle spindles and makes them hypersensitive, particularly to stretch of the muscles. Burke (1983) re-examined this concept of the fusimotor system involvement in disorders of muscle tone, and found no evidence to suggest that this system is solely involved. In his studies, local anesthesia did not produce a selective fusimotor block. In mammals, movement is mediated by the final common pathway, the alpha motorneurons. The fusimotor system contributes to the control of movement.

Where is the contracture in spastic muscles? We observe that prolonged spasticity in the muscle of a growing child often leads to a shortening of the muscle ('myotatic contracture'). Histological studies with ordinary staining techniques and light microscopy fail to show fibrosis, and show few significant changes. In three patients out of 279 who had biopsies of the limb muscles we found a mixture of dystrophic and neurogenic changes. In patients who had cerebral palsy and scoliosis, we found neuropathic changes on both sides of the curve (Fig.5.3). We

*Muscle neurophysiology, abstracted from Shepherd (1983).

found similar changes in spinal muscle biopsies in cases of idiopathic scoliosis (Bleck *et al.* 1976). These changes were alterations from normal of fiber types visualized by histochemical staining techniques. Castle *et al.* (1979) used histochemical techniques in their study of muscle biopsies of limb muscles in children with cerebral palsy; changes in fiber types from normal controls were noted. It is uncertain whether these abnormalities of fiber type in scoliosis and in the limb muscles are secondary or primary to the deformation of the spine or limbs.

From the work of Tardieu (Tardieu *et al.* 1971, 1977, 1979, 1982; Tardieu 1984), it appears that in normal cats the length of the sarcomere in the muscle fiber remains constant for a given angle of ankle dorsiflexion, irrespective of the age or size of the animal, and is an adaptation to skeletal growth. When the cat's triceps surae muscle is immobilized, the tension-extension curve is more abrupt; the muscle has decreased strength, histological evidence of atrophy, and (with electron microscopy) a decrease in the number of sarcomeres. This decrease in the number of sarcomeres is also noted in the muscle biopsies of the ankle extensor muscles in children with cerebral palsy. The continued studies by these French physicians indicated that there were two different types of spastic contracture ('hypoextensibility') in children with cerebral palsy: (i) defective 'trophic' regulation—the sarcomeres failed to increase in number during skeletal growth, and (ii) normal growth regulation. In type (i), plaster-casting to stretch the muscle had no effect, but surgery did effect elongation of the muscle; in type (ii) plaster-casting was more effective when tolerated. Tabary *et al.* (1971) in his study of biopsies of the spastic triceps surae muscles in 17 patients who had lengthenings of these muscles found notable increases in the length of the sarcomeres with light and electron microscopy.

From the above studies it might be concluded that muscles normally grow along with the bones of the child. In children with spastic paralysis something interferes with the growth of sarcomeres in number and shortening occurs. Ziv *et al.*'s (1984) experimental studies in mice who have a genetic spasticity of the lower limbs suggested that muscle growth occurs at the musculo-tendinous junction which they termed the 'growth plate' of the muscle.

Effects of immobilization
Because immobilization of joints and limbs is so commonly used as a method of treatment, to overcome or prevent contractures and for postoperative care, the histological effects on muscle fibers merit review. Cooper (1972) studied the effects of plaster immobilization in the adult cat soleus, gastrocnemius and flexor digitorum longus muscles. With two weeks of immobilization, the muscle nuclei became more prominent. In four weeks the nuclei were centrally located; muscle fibers were irregular in shape and size, and vacuolar degeneration of fibers was evident. After six to 22 weeks of immobilization, there was hyaline and granular degeneration but the sarcolemmic tubes were preserved. When the data were combined with those of other experiments, Cooper concluded that complete regeneration would occur in three months. Cooper also noted an increase in the contraction and relaxation times of muscles during immobilization. These

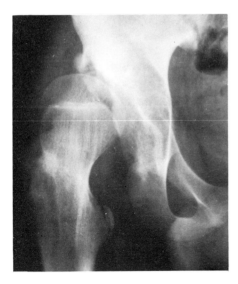

Fig. 5.4. A 'silent' subluxation of the hip which pain made evident in an 18-year-old man with spastic diplegia; walked independently with crutches.

experimental results seem clinically applicable. Should the immobilization of the limbs of patients who have had tendon lengthenings or tenotomies of spastic muscles be for only three weeks whenever possible? And it is probable that the good results reported after plaster immobilization for equinus deformities were due to the muscle atrophy and degeneration which occurs with immobilization?

Joints

Hip

The most common and serious structural change is subluxation and dislocation of the hip. This is an acquired deformity, as can be appreciated by serial radiographs of the hip beginning in the six-month-old infant who has spasticity of the hip musculature. The configuration of the hip is normal. Due to the combination of the abnormal pull of spastic muscles, femoral torsion and the status of weight-bearing subluxation is generally apparent about the age of three years, with secondary acetabular dysplasia occurring after the age of five years. An exception would be the infant who has both a congenital dislocation of the hip and cerebral palsy; these patients' radiographs will show acetabular dysplasia very early in life. However, the incidence of congenital dislocation of the hip is only about one per 1000 livebirths; consequently it is not often observed in cerebral palsy. The genesis of the acquired dislocation of the hip will be discussed more fully in Chapter 9.

In patients who walk with crutches, subluxation of the hip will be 'silent' without pain for many years. Eventually, in the adolescent or young adult years, pain ensues and becomes disabling due to degenerative arthritis (Figs.5.4, 5.5). Later, subluxation of the hip results in secondary deformities of the femoral head (Fig.5.6); the lateral aspect of the head is flattened due to the pressure of the

131

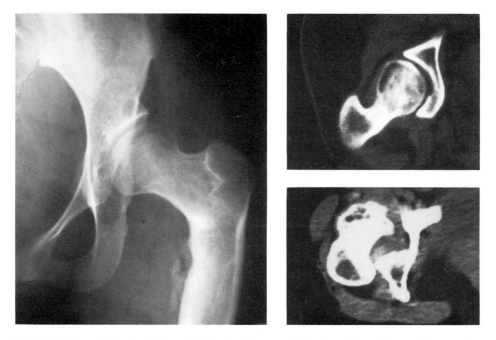

Fig. 5.5. 19-year-old female with spastic diplegia who was crutch walker. *Above left:* anterior-posterior radiograph of the hip. Approximately 30 per cent of the femoral head lies outside the acetabulum. One year postoperative subtrochanteric varus-derotation osteotomy; patient complaining of constant hip pain and unable to walk. *Top right:* computerized tomographic image in transverse plane of the hip. There is apparent femoral torsion. Anteriorly and laterally the femoral head is not contained, and subchondral osteolysis is seen. *Bottom right:* computerized tomographic image. This section is through the inferior portion of the femoral head. Note extensive irregularities of the anterior and medial portions of the head of the femur, indicative of degenerative arthritis.

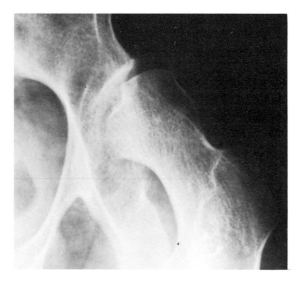

Fig. 5.6. Anterior-posterior radiograph of the hip in an 18-year-old male with spastic diplegia and independent walking with crutches. Subluxation of the hip and acetablular dysplasia. The femoral head is flattened laterally and osteoporotic. The notch in the medial central portion of the head is due to the pressure of the ligamentum teres.

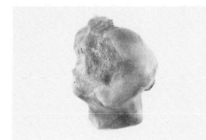

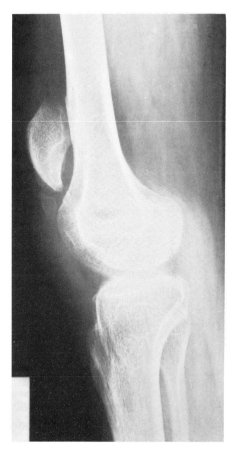

Fig. 5.7 *(above)*. Photograph of femoral head and neck removed in 20-year-old patient with spastic total body involvement and dislocation of the hip. Hip pain became disabling, whether in bed or wheelchair. In this anterior view of the femoral head, note extensive erosion of cartilage on the anterior and medial surfaces, and irregular contour and flattening of lateral surface. Head and neck excised because reconstructive surgery was impossible given the extensive degenerative changes.

Fig. 5.8 *(right)*. Lateral radiograph of knee of 35-year-old man with spastic triplegia; independent walking with crutches. Had severe flexed knee gait up to the age of 12 years when he had correcion with bilateral hamstring lengthening. A spastic quadriceps has maintained his knee posture in extension on stance phase with ability to flex 40° on swing phase. Note cephalad displacement of patella and severe structural changes. Patient with severe and unremitting knee pain. Now he has a university degree and works full time. Solution: patellectomy. The articular surface of the patella was totally covered with shredded cartilage.

gluteal muscles, and the ligamentum teres produces a deep groove in the femoral head medially (Samilson *et al*. 1972). In dislocated hips, the femoral head articular cartilage will undergo degeneration as well as deformation (Fig.5.7).

Knee

Patients who walk with flexed knees develop a cephalad displacement of the patella ('patella alta'). In older patients this can cause disabling pain due to cartilage degeneration (chondromalacia patellae, see Fig.5.8). Deformations of the patella are common in patients who have flexed knee postures (Lottman 1976). In young patients, ranging in age from 10 to 14 years, I have noted knee pain with tenderness at the inferior pole of the patella. Lateral radiographs of the knee show fragmentation of the lower pole of the patella. This lesion is comparable to the sporting disability 'jumper's knee'. In cerebral palsy it is probably the constant pull of the patellar tendon on the distal pole of the patella that produces the symptoms and the radiographic findings (Cahuzac *et al*. 1979).

I have seen in consultation patients who can no longer walk due to disabling degenerative arthritis of the knee induced by long-standing flexion contractures of the knee beyond 20°. These are patients who were asymptomatic with their flexed knee gaits until the age of 35 to 40 years.

Ankle

Equinus of the ankle is the most common deformity in spastic cerebral palsy. It is not known whether the persistence of a significant ankle equinus (beyond 10°) causes disabling symptoms in adult life, because almost all patients have correction of equinus before adulthood. It seems logical that prolonged tiptoe walking would result in painful areas over the metatarsal heads.

Valgus deformities of the ankle joint can accompany as a secondary change to severe pes valgus. Although I have not followed patients with valgus deformities of the distal tibial articular surface through adult life, it seems likely that these ankle joints would undergo painful degenerative arthritis. Orthopaedic surgeons who have followed adult patients with malunited fractures of the distal tibia could no doubt confirm this prediction. The abnormal tilt of the ankle joint and weight bearing will cause degenerative joint changes eventually.

Foot

Foot varus and valgus deformities are due to subluxations at the talonavicular and calcaneocuboid joints. In the case of varus deformities, the secondary and painful condition is increased pressure with callosities on the lateral border of the foot over the base of the fifth metatarsal. In valgus deformities, the abnormal pressure is over the medial aspect of the first metatarsal head and the great toe, which is secondarily displaced into valgus. Usually adults with severe valgus deformities have to wait until past the age of 50 years before they notice disabling symptoms. These are usually due not only to the callosities on the medial border of the forefoot and great toe, but also due to degenerative arthritic changes in the talonavicular joint. Severe pes cavus does cause symptoms, usually beginning about the age of 12 years, and metatarsus adductus and hallux valgus with bunion become troublesome in adolescence. Painful flexion contractures of the toes seem to develop in the late adolescent or young adult years. The mechanisms of these foot deformities are amplified in Chapters 8 and 9.

Upper limbs

The most notable skeletal change in the upper limb in patients with spasticity of the elbow flexors and the pronator teres is a posterior subluxation and (in some) a dislocation of the head of the radius. Posterior bowing of the ulna may accompany this displacement of the radial head. This change can explain the limitation of elbow extension and the futility of gaining complete elbow extension with passive stretching or surgery.

Articular cartilage

Cartilage degeneration occurs when the opposing articular surfaces are not in contact. This certainly seems to be the case in a paralytic dislocation of the hip of

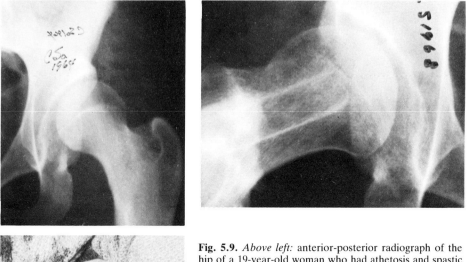

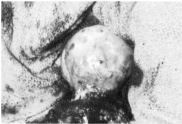

Fig. 5.9. *Above left:* anterior-posterior radiograph of the hip of a 19-year-old woman who had athetosis and spastic paralysis of the lower limbs and walked independently. Complained of severe hip pain and a crunching sound in the hip on movement. *Above right:* lateral radiograph of the same patient, after a derotation and varus subtrochanteric osteotomy had failed to relieve symptoms. *Left:* femoral head of the same patient at time of arthroplasty. Large areas of the femoral head were eroded and not visible in the plain radiographs as shown.

long duration. Complete disappearance of large segments of the articular surface of the femoral head is often seen. Similar destruction of cartilage occurs in subluxation and may be quite difficult to discern with radiographic studies until much later, when joint margin osteophytes and narrowing of the joint surface become obvious (Fig.5.9). Experimental studies have demonstrated joint cartilage degeneration in non-contact opposing surfaces (Bennett and Bauer 1937, Hall 1969). In addition, cartilage needs movement of the joint for its nutrition from the synovial fluid; the nutrition of the cartilage cells is by diffusion, which occurs with movement (Ingelmark and Saaf 1948, Maroudas *et al.* 1968, Sood 1971, Freeman 1972). Articular cartilage needs movement to survive and to repair itself; Salter (1984) showed the positive effects of continuous passive motion in surgical defects of the articular cartilage of the rabbit knee joint. The clinical application of this work has been the increasing use of continuous passive motion machines in postoperative knee surgery where the integrity of the cartilage has been defective.

Compression of articular cartilage will also cause degeneration. In experimental animals, joints subjected to continuous compressive forces show gross and histological degenerative changes (Salter and Field 1960, Salter and McNeil 1965). Evidence of compression of the articular surface of the talus and degenerative changes have been noted in cases of talipes equinovarus when forced manipulations of the foot with plaster casts were applied to correct the equinus deformity. It has been said that 'ligaments are hard and cartilage is soft', which should subdue enthusiasm for attempts to correct a contracture by forced positioning of the joints in plaster or orthoses.

Joint contracture

Joint capsule contracture is superimposed on the myostatic contracture if the latter is unrelieved for several years. The major joints affected are the elbow, hip, knee and ankle. Contracture is thought to happen because of reorganization of the connective tissue, preventing the collagen fibers from gliding (Kottke 1966). Swinyard and Bleck (1985) believe that the lack of joint motion in the developing fetus causes the well-known severe joint contractures in children with arthrogryposis (multiple congenital contracture syndrome).

Experimental immobilization of rat knee joints demonstrated proliferation of subsynovial intracapsula fibers in the infrapatellar and intercondylar spaces of the knee. Connective tissue extended between joint surfaces to form adhesions and the cartilage degenerated (Evans *et al.* 1960). Parallel changes in human knee-joint immobilization for prolonged periods have been described (Enneking and Horowitz 1972).

Bones

Osteoporosis of the bones does occur in cerebral palsy, but practically always in total body involved patients who are dependent on their wheelchair and spend much of their time in bed. These patients are unable to be helped in and out of a chair. These effects are overwhelmingly due to the lack of the stress of weight bearing, and thus the effects of gravity on the bones. Since the work of Dalen and Olsson (1974), who clearly demonstrated the effects of physical activity on bone mineral content, there have been many other reports on calcium loss from the bones due to the lack of gravity. Definite loss of bone calcium has been shown in astronauts during their anti-gravity periods in flight.

It is not known how to prevent osteoporosis in these severely involved patients, who often have deformities of the limbs and trunk that preclude supportive standing. Furthermore, we do not know how many hours they should have supportive standing to prevent bone mineral loss. It is well known that they are prone to fractures (McIvor and Samilson 1966, Bleck and Kleinman 1984).

The shafts of the long bones are rarely if ever deformed in spastic paralysis. Anterior bowing of the femoral shaft cannot be attributed to the spasticity of the hip flexors. Measurements of the femoral shaft with lateral radiographs of the hip and femur in normal children, compared with 27 children who had spastic hip flexion deformities, failed to demonstrate any significant change from the normal anterior bow of the femur which had a mean of 7° and a range of 1° to 20° (Bleck 1968).

Torsional deformation of the bones is their major structural change. There is significant abnormal femoral anteversion for age in children with subluxation and dislocation of the hip, as well as with spastic hip-flexion internal rotation gait patterns (Lewis *et al.* 1964, Beals 1969, Bleck 1971, Baumann 1972, Fabry *et al.*

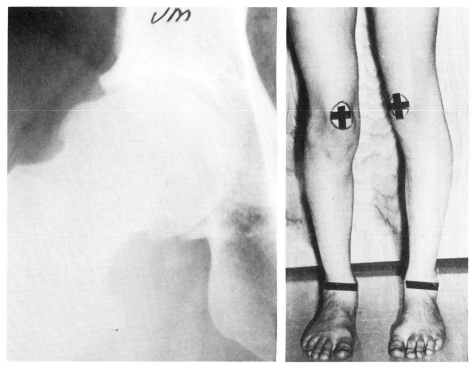

Fig. 5.10. *(left).* Anterior-posterior radiograph of the hip of a 25-year-old woman with spastic diplegia. Walked independently; complained of intermittent, but not yet disabling, pain in both hips. Examination showed a 35° hip-flexion contracture bilaterally and an increased range of hip internal rotation to 75°, and decreased external rotation to 15° consistent with the usual findings of femoral torsion. Radiographs show clear signs of early degenerative arthritis.

Fig. 5.11. *(right).* Photograph of lower limbs of a 14-year-old boy with spastic diplegia and a hip internal rotation gait. The line of progression of the feet is almost normal in appearance due to compensatory excessive external tibial-fibular torsion of 45°.

1973). It is uncertain whether persistent and excessive femoral anteversion of the proximal femur (femoral torsion) in independently ambulatory patients results in late degenerative arthritis. Hip pain affects some adults with spastic diplegia, hip-flexion contractures and femoral torsion; radiographs of their hip joints often show evidence of early degenerative arthritis (Fig.5.10).

Excessive external tibial-fibular torsion (beyond the mean of 23°) has often been observed in patients who have internally rotated hip-walking patterns (Le Damany 1909). This external tibial-fibular torsion apparently develops as a compensatory change to the gait associated with internal femoral torsion (anteversion) (Somerville 1957) (Fig.5.11).

Spine and pelvis
Scoliosis is the most common and serious structural change in the spine of patients with cerebral palsy, and is more frequent and severe in non-walkers with total body

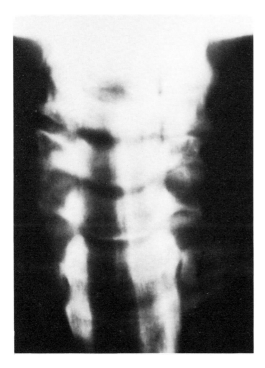

Fig. 5.12. Anterior-posterior tomogram of the cervical spine in a young adult woman with total body athetosis and continuous rotation of the head to the right. Complained of constant neck pain radiating into the right upper limb. Note widening and chondral erosion of the right articular facet between the fifth and sixth cervical vertebrae. Solution: anterior cervical spine fusion.

involved. Pelvic obliquity often accompanies the scoliosis, though not necessarily due to asymmetrical adduction contractures of the hips or dislocation. The subject of scoliosis in cerebral palsy will be dealt with more fully in Chapter 9.

Kyphosis without scoliosis is seen in cerebral palsy but rarely progresses to a severe degree (> 60°). It begins as a postural defect and is flexible. If it persists throughout growth it can become a fixed structural deformity.

Lordosis is usually due to increased anterior pelvic inclination secondary to a flexion contracture of the hips in patients who stand and walk. Like kyphosis it is initially flexible, but as the child grows it becomes structural and fixed due to lack of mobility at the lumbosacral articulation. Young adult patients who have fixed flexion contractures of the hip (usually > 20°) develop an almost horizontal sacrum, and complain of low back pain when erect. Hip flexion contractures in growing children should be treated surgically, to relieve disabling low back pain.

Fulford and Brown (1976) proposed that position in infancy and childhood might be responsible for deformities in cerebral palsy. They described children who had windswept lower limbs, facial asymmetry, a 'bat' ear and plagiocephaly. They suspected that these deformities have a positional etiology, and suggested that somehow asymmetrical postures and positions should be prevented.

Degenerative arthritis of the cervical spine has occurred in patients who have athetosis. The constant involuntary movements of the neck seem responsible for the arthritic changes in the intervertebral facet joints. These patients can have disabling symptoms due to constant neck pain, often accompanied by radicular pain in an upper limb (Fig. 5.12.) I have performed an interior spine fusion at the c5–c6 level in the case of a 20-year-old athetoid woman who had unremitting neck pain and unilateral upper-limb radicular pain. She became asymptomatic immediately postoperatively and had remained so for 10 years. Angelini *et al.* (1982) reported an unusual cervical myelopathy in a 12-year-old girl who had a dystonic and spastic quadriplegia. Radiographic examination revealed an anterior slipping of the fourth cervical vertebra, which was eliminated with general anesthesia. These authors concluded that her signs and symptoms were due to intermittent spinal cord compression due to the subluxation which was secondary to the torsion dystonia. Fortunately athetosis is becoming rare, at least in the USA.

Summary
The data on the development of the musculoskeletal system in cerebral palsy shows that structural change does occur frequently, despite the efforts of therapists and orthotists. Most of these skeletal deformities cause few symptoms in the growing child. Disabling pain develops many years later in adult life—long after the child has left the special treatment unit, the physical therapist, social worker, school, pediatrician and family. It is for this reason that orthopaedic surgery in cerebral palsy has been developed and applied in children—to prevent serious structural change and decreasing function due to disabling symptoms in adult life. At times, orthopaedic surgery has created another deformity. However, progress in surgical treatment will depend upon the proper analysis of the problem and exactly the right surgery in both quantity and quality. Life does not end at 16; and follow-up and access to care should be available to adults with cerebral palsy.

REFERENCES

Alexander, R. McN. (1984) 'Walking and running.' *American Scientist*, **72**, 348–354.
Angelini, L., Broggi, G., Nardocci, N., Savoiardo, M. (1982) 'Subacute cervical myelopathy in a child with cerebral palsy. Secondary to torsion dystonia?' *Child's Brain*, **9**, 354–357.
Baumann, J. U. (1972) 'Hip operations in children with cerebral palsy.' *Reconstructive Surgery and Traumatology*, **13**, 68–82.
Beals, R. K. (1966) 'Spastic paraplegia and diplegia: an evaluation of non-surgical and surgical factors influencing the prognosis for ambulation.' *Journal of Bone and Joint Surgery*, **48A**, 827–846.
—— (1969) 'Developmental changes in the femur and acetabulum in spastic paraplegia and diplegia.' *Developmental Medicine and Child Neurology*, **11**, 303–313.
Bennett, G., Bauer, W. (1937) 'Joint changes resulting from patellar displacement and their relation to degenerative hip disease.' *Journal of Bone and Joint Surgery*, **19**, 667–692.
Bleck, E. E. (1968) 'Observations and treatment of flexion, internal rotation, and bone deformities of the hip in cerebral palsy.' (*Thesis*) American Orthopaedic Association.
—— (1971) 'The hip in cerebral palsy.' *In:* Instructional Course Lectures. American Academy of Orthopaedic Surgeons, St. Louis: C. V. Mosby.
—— (1975) 'Locomotor prognosis in cerebral palsy.' *Developmental Medicine and Child Neurology*, **17**, 18–25.
—— Koehler, J. P., Dillingham, M., Trimble, S. (1976) 'Histochemical studies of thoracis spinalis and sacrospinalis muscles.' *American Academy of Neurology*, (*Program Abstract.*)
—— Kleinman, R. G. (1984) 'Special injuries of the musculoskeletal system.' *In:* Rockwood, C. A., King, R. E. (Eds.) *Fractures. Vol. 3: Fractures in Children.* Philadelphia: Lippincott. Ch. 3.
Bose, K., Yeo, K. Q. (1975) 'The locomotor assessment of cerebral palsy.' *Proceedings* (Singapore), **10**, 21–24.

Burke, D. (1983) 'Critical examination of the case for or against fusimotor involvement in disorders of muscle tone.' *Advances in Neurology*, **39**, 133–150.

Cahuzac, M., Nichil, J., Olle, R., Touchard, A., Cahuzac, J. P. (1979) 'Les fractures de fatigue de la rotule chez l'infirme moteur d'origine cérébrale.' *Revue de Chirurgie Orthopédique*, **65**, 87–90.

Castle, M. E., Reyman, T. A., Schneider, M. (1979) 'Pathology of spastic muscle in cerebral palsy.' *Clinical Orthopaedics and Related Research*, **142**, 223–233.

Chaplais, J. De Z., MacFarland, J. A. (1984) 'A review of 404 late walkers.' *Archives of Disease in Childhood*, **59**, 512–516.

Cooper, R. R. (1972) 'Alterations during immobilization and degeneration of skeletal muscle in cats.' *Journal of Bone and Joint Surgery*, **54A**, 919–953.

Crothers, B., Paine, R. S. (1959) *Natural History of Cerebral Palsy*. Cambridge: Harvard University Press.

Dalen, N., Olsson, K. E. (1974) 'Bone mineral content and physical activity.' *Acta Orthopaedica Scandinavica*, **45**, 170–174.

Enneking, W. F., Horowitz, M. (1972) 'The intra-articular effects of immobilization on the human knee.' *Journal of Bone and Joint Surgery*, **54A**, 973–985.

Evans, E. B., Eggers, G. N. W., Butler, J. K., Blumel, D. (1960) 'Experimental immobilization and remobilization of rat knee joint.' *Journal of Bone and Joint Surgery*, **42A**, 737–758.

Fabry, G., MacEwen, G. D., Shands, A. R. (1973) 'Torsion of the femur.' *Journal of Bone and Joint Surgery*, **55A**, 1726–1738.

Fiorentino, M. R. (1963) *Reflex Testing Methods for Evaluating Central Nervous System Development*. Springfield, Ill.: C. C. Thomas.

Forbes, D. B., McIntyre, J. M. (1968) 'A method for evaluating the results of surgery in cerebral palsy.' *Canadian Medical Association Journal*, **98**, 646–648.

Freeman, M. A. R. (1972) *Adult Articular Cartilage*. New York: Grune & Stratton.

Fulford, G. E., Brown, J. K. (1976) 'Position as a cause of deformity in children with cerebral palsy.' *Developmental Medicine and Child Neurology*, **18**, 305–314.

Hall, M. C. (1969) 'Cartilage changes after experimental relief of contact in the knee joint of the mature rat.' *Clinical Orthopaedics and Related Research*, **64**, 64–76.

Ingelmark, B. E., Saaf, V. (1948) 'Über die Ernährung des Glenkknorpels und die Bildung den Glenkflüssigkeit und der verschiedenen funktionellen Verhältnissen.' *Acta Orthopaedica Scandinavica*, **17**, 303.

Kottke, F. J. (1966) 'The effects of limitation of activity upon the human body.' *Journal of the American Medical Association*, **196**, 825–830.

LeDamany, P. (1909) 'La torsion du tibia, normal, pathological, experimental.' *Journal d'Anatomie et Physiologie*, **45**, 589–615.

Lewis, F. R., Samilson, R. L., Lucas, D. B. (1964) 'Femoral torsion and coxa valga in cerebral palsy—a preliminary report.' *Developmental Medicine and Child Neurology*, **6**, 591–597.

Lottman, D. B. (1976) 'Knee flexion deformity and patella alta in spastic cerebral palsy.' *Developmental Medicine and Child Neurology*, **18**, 315–319.

Maroudas, A., Bullough, P., Swanson, S. A. V., Freeman, M. A. R. (1968) 'The permeability of articular cartilage.' *Journal of Bone and Joint Surgery* **50B**, 166–177.

McIvor, W. C., Samilson, R. L. (1966) 'Fractures in patients with cerebral palsy.' *Journal of Bone and Joint Surgery*, **48A**, 858–866.

Miranda, S. (1979) 'A study of 119 spastic diplegic children.' *Unpublished study at Children's Hospital at Stanford, Palo Alto, California*.

Molnar, G. E., Gordon, S. V. (1974) 'Predictive value of clinical signs for early prognostication of motor function in cerebral palsy.' *Archives of Physical Medicine* (1976), **57**, 153–158. *Albert Einstein College of Medicine of Yeshiva University, Bronx, New York. Paper submitted for the scientific program of the American Academy for Cerebral Palsy in 1975.*

Nelson, K. B., Ellenberg, J. H. (1982) 'Children who "outgrew" cerebral palsy.' *Pediatrics*, **69**, 529–536.

Perlman, J. M., Goodman, S., Kreusser, K. L. Volpe, J. J. (1985) 'Reduction in intraventricular hemorrhage by elimination of fluctuating cerebral blood-flow velocity in preterm infants with respiratory distress syndrome.' *New England Journal of Medicine*, **312**, 1353–1357.

Reimers, J. (1972) 'A scoring system for evaluation of ambulation in cerebral palsied patients.' *Developmental Medicine and Child Neurology*, **14**, 155–165.

Salter, R. B., Field, P. (1960) 'The effects of continuous compression in living articular cartilage: an experimental investigation.' *Journal of Bone and Joint Surgery*, **42A**, 31–49.

—— McNeil, R. (1965) 'Pathological change in articular cartilage secondary to persistent deformity.'

Journal of Bone and Joint Surgery, **47A**, 185–186. (*Abstract.*)

—— Hamilton, H. W., Wedge, J. H. (1984) 'Clinical application of basic research on continuous passive motion for disorders and injuries of synovial joints: a preliminary report of a feasibility study.' *Journal of Orthopaedic Research*, **1**, 325–342.

Samilson, R. L., Tsou, P., Aamoth, G., Green, W. (1972) 'Dislocation and subluxation of the hip in cerebral palsy.' *Journal of Bone and Joint Surgery*, **54A**, 863–873.

Shapiro, B. K., Accardo, P. J., Capute, A. J. (1979) 'Factors affecting walking in a profoundly retarded population.' *Developmental Medicine and Child Neurology*, **21**, 369–373.

Shepherd, G. M. (1983) *Neurobiology*. New York and Oxford: Oxford University Press.

Somerville, E. W. (1957) 'Persistent foetal alignment of the hip.' *Journal of Bone and Joint Surgery*, **39B**, 106–113.

Sood, S. C. (1971) 'A study of the effects of experimental immobilization on rabbit articular cartilage.' *Journal of Anatomy*, **188**, 497–507.

Sutherland, D. H., Olshen, R., Cooper, L., Woo, S. K. -Y. (1980) 'The development of mature gait.' *Journal of Bone and Joint Surgery*, **62A**, 336–353.

Swinyard, C. A., Bleck, E. E. (1985) 'The etiology of arthrogryposis (multiple congenital contracture).' *Clinical Orthopaedics and Related Research*, **194**, 15–29.

Tabary, J. C., Goldspink, G., Tardieu, C., Lombard, M., Chigot, P. (1971) 'Nature de la rétraction musculaire des I.M.C. mésure de l'allongement des sarcomères du muscle étiré.' *Revue de Chirurgie Orthopedique et Reparatrice de l'Appareil Moteur (Paris)*, **57**, 463–470.

Tardieu, C., Tabary, J., Huet de la Tour, E., Tabary, C., Tardieu, G. (1977) 'The relationship between sarcomere length in the soleus and the tibialis anterior and the articular angle of the tibiacalcaneum in cats during growth.' *Journal of Anatomy*, **124**, 581–588.

—— Tardieu, G., Colbeau-Justin, P., Huet de la Tour, E., Lespargot, A. (1979) 'Trophic muscle regulation in children with congenital cerebral lesions.' *Journal of the Neurological Sciences*, **42**, 357–364.

—— Huet de la Tour, E., Bret, M. D., Tardieu, G. (1982) 'Muscle hypoextensibility in children with cerebral palsy: I. Clinical and experimental observations.' *Archives of Physical Medicine and Rehabilitation*, **63**, 97–102.

Tardieu, G. (1984) *Le Dossier Clinique de L'Infirmité Motrice Cérébrale. 3rd edn.* Paris: Masson.

—— Tabary, J. C., Tardieu, C., Lombard, M. (1971) 'Rétraction, hyperextensibilité et "faiblesse" de l'I.M.C., expressions apparement opposées d'un même trouble musculaire. Consequences thérapeutiques.' *Revue de Chirurgie Orthopédique et Reparative de l'Appareil Moteur* (Paris), **57**, 505–516.

—— Tardieu, C., Colbeau-Justin, P., Lespargot, A. (1982) 'Muscle hypoextensibility in children with cerebral palsy: II. Therapeutic implications.' *Archives of Physical Medicine and Rehabilitation*, **63**, 103–107.

Wigglesworth, J. (1984) 'Brain development and its modification by adverse influences.' *In:* Stanley, F., Alberman, E. (Eds.) *The Epidemiology of the Cerebral Palsies. Clinics in Developmental Medicine No. 87.* London: S.I.M.P. with Blackwell Scientific; Philadelphia: Lippincott.

Ziv, I., Blackburn, N., Rang, M., Koveska, J. (1984) 'Muscle growth in normal and spastic mice.' *Developmental Medicine and Child Neurology*, **26**, 94–99.

6
GOALS, TREATMENT AND MANAGEMENT

This chapter is intended to define the goals or aims of what used to be called the 'treatment' of cerebral palsy. Because we now recognize the realities, 'management' is now more acceptable. After half a century of sincere and intense effort by professionals to 'treat' cerebral palsy, most now acknowledge that these remedial efforts have been unsuccessful in achieving function (Bobath and Bobath 1984, Goldkamp 1984, Scrutton 1984).

To gain a perspective on management of cerebral palsy, this chapter will delineate the goals, review the many and varied treatments of the past, discuss how the goals might be achieved in the most severely involved patient, suggest the rôle and timing of orthopaedic surgery, relate current experience and efficacy of drugs, and conclude with the rôle of the family and its importance in effecting the desired outcome óf management.

Because orthopaedic surgeons and physicians who assume responsibility for the care of cerebral-palsied children are often asked about the value of neurosurgical procedures, I have reviewed the recent published reports of brain and spinal-cord surgery for motor disorders. Parents and teachers often ask about what can be done for intractable drooling. They expect a surgeon to know about surgery. Accordingly, I have included a brief review of the surgical procedures for this annoying problem.

Goals

The child with cerebral palsy becomes the adult with cerebral palsy (Sylvain Terver).

If we can accept this reality, then it should be possible to develop goals based upon the needs of adults for optimum independent living. In order of priority these are:

1. *Communication*. There is an obvious human need to express our wants, thoughts and feelings. We now know that communication need not be exclusively oral or verbal, and that non-oral methods can be equally effective. The use of sign-language by the deaf is the best example of such communication. Non-verbal communication outputs can be writing, symbols or electronic synthetic voice devices.

2. *Activities of daily living (ADL)*. The basic need is to care for oneself in feeding, toileting, bathing, grooming and dressing. Beyond these elementary activities are meal preparation and household maintenance. In non-industrial societies, daily living tasks might include growing your own food supply, making clothing and constructing shelter.

3. *Mobility* is essential for independence, social integration and, if possible, employment. It is particularly important in modern urban mobile environments. If someone cannot walk independently or efficiently, mechanical substitutes are

required. Able-bodied persons regularly extend their mobility beyond walking with mechanical devices: bicycles, motor vehicles, trains and aircraft.

4. *Walking*, although often perceived initially as the highest priority for children with cerebral palsy, becomes the last priority as maturation occurs and independence and social integration needs predominate. Walking ability in cerebral palsy can be classified as it was for spina-bifida patients (Hoffer *et al.* 1973):

(a) community walker—can get about the whole community with or without walking aids (*e.g.* crutches).

(b) household walker—can move about the household, but a wheelchair is required outside the home.

(c) physiological walker—can walk only in a physical therapy department (or at home) with parallel bars or with assistance of another person. A wheelchair is required in all other locations.

(d) non-walker—needs a wheelchair for all activities. The wheelchair-dependent person can be functionally classified as: (i) independent—able to get in and out of the chair without help; (ii) assistive transfer ability—needs help of one person to get in and out of the chair; and (iii) dependent—unable to do assistive transfers and must be lifted in and out of the chair.

Methods of assessment, goal setting and results

Aim- or goal-oriented management requires that the child's problem be analyzed consistent with the priorities of needs for independent living. This will depend upon the extent of the physical and mental impairment and the most accurate prognosis possible in the areas of communication, activities of daily living, mobility and walking. This approach demands a careful and detailed examination of the child.

We believe that a reasonably accurate prognosis in the major areas of function can be made based upon reported studies and a knowledge of the natural history. For example, we know that the prognosis for independent function, normal schooling and social integration is generally good for those with spastic diplegia or hemiplegia if not compromised by severe mental retardation.

From the examination, the prognosis and the list of problems, we can then try to determine which might be eliminated, ameliorated or compensated.

Scrutton (1984) also wisely advises an analysis of the 'child's situation': where and with whom s/he is living, the composition of the family and its responsibilities, the status of the child's education and where it occurs, day and night behaviour and what activities engage the child beyond schooling. When this comprehensive assessment is completed, a list of practical goals can be made and given priority.

To turn the focus of the parents from the disease to the goal-oriented approach always takes much discussion and time. It is vital that the referring physician, paramedical persons, therapists and teachers have the same perspective.

In order to study the effectiveness of prospective goal-setting in 85 children who had total body involvement, Terver devised a system of numerical scores to record the functional status of the child and to set the goals to be achieved (Terver *et al.* 1981). Table 6.I defines the numerical score for each function in

TABLE 6.I

Numerical scores for functional assessment (from Terver *et al.* 1981)

INDEPENDENCE
 1 = total dependence on others
 2 = partial dependence on others
 3 = independence from others but dependent on a technical device to accomplish the task
 4 = total independence but the activity is not normal in its execution, energy level or appearance

EFFICIENCY
 Communication (verbal or non-verbal)
  1 = ability to indicate 'yes' or 'no' by any means
  2 = ability to express needs only (*e.g.* call for help)
  3 = ability to engage in a dialogue of direct questions and answers only
  4 = ability to initiate and sustain a conversation, retain information and communicate at a distance
 Activities of daily living
  1 = ability to assume simple needs of eating, dressing, cleansing face and hands
  2 = ability to completely assume all personal needs
  3 = ability to assume household activities and needs
  4 = ability to assume all of the above and have a social life
 Mobility
  1 = has mobility but unable to utilize effectively
  2 = able to move about household only
  3 = able to travel beyond the household within the immediate neighbourhood
  4 = able to travel everywhere in the community
 Walking
  1 = physiological walker, but can transfer in and out of wheelchair
  2 = household walker
  3 = household and immediate neighbourhood
  4 = community walker

0 = no activity, 5 = normal

TABLE 6.II

PULSES monitoring system (from Goldkamp 1984)

P = general, systemic or imposed conditions
U = upper limbs
L = lower limbs
S = special senses and speech
E = excretory functions
S = cerebration

Scores
 1 = no disorder
 2 = disorder with no activities of daily living deficiency
 3 = needs some assistance
 4 = needs maximum help
 (any patient with a score of 3 or 4 is dependent)

Example
 P U L S E S
 — — — — — —
 1 2 3 2 1 1

In this patient with cerebral palsy there is no systemic or other condition; the patient has no activities of daily living deficiencies in the upper limb but has deficiencies due to lower-limb impairment, no problems in speech or the special senses and has normal excretory functions and normal intelligence. This profile seems to describe the person who has spastic diplegia.

independence and efficiency. It is always possible to be independent but inefficient in task performance.

Other methods of defining the child's problems have been proposed (Maloney *et al.* 1978). Goldkamp (1984) used a numerical system (PULSES Monitoring System—Table 6.II) to define independence in activities of daily living in a follow-up study on the efficacy of treatment in cerebral palsy. Probably no system of assessment and recording function will satisfy all who work in this field, but at least these methods encourage us to think about the needs of the child rather than our own needs in attempting treatment.

The problem and the challenge of the goal-oriented approach is in the total body involved or quadriplegic child. This group represents approximately 40 per cent of our patients with cerebral palsy. The other 60 per cent who have spastic diplegia or hemiplegia generally have a good prognosis for functional goals. For this latter group the needs are mainly educational and social. Orthopaedic surgery for this group might be helpful in preventing and correcting deformities of the lower limb, so that walking ability will be facilitated and sustained.

A study of goal-oriented management
MATERIALS AND METHODS
To determine if the goal-oriented approach was successful and to determine at what age goals could be set, we conducted a prospective study of 85 children who had total body involvement and spastic quadriplegia (Terver *et al.* 1981). We had two groups of patients: group 1 consisted of 14 children in whom goals were set by age four years and followed for a minimum of eight years; group 2 comprised 71 children in whom goals were set after age four years (mean age—seven years) and who were followed up for an average of 14 years.

The initial and follow-up assessments used the numerical scoring methods as detailed in Table I. Based upon the initial assessments and prognosis, goals were set and scored.

Prognosis for communication in the non-verbal child was thought to be good if there was any means of eliciting a 'yes' or 'no' response, by symbol recognition and with psychological tests. The prognosis for activities of daily living depended upon voluntary control of at least one hand and upper limb. Assessment of hand function was often deferred until adequate sitting balance could be secured with appropriate seating. Mobility prognosis was highly dependent upon the ability to control some part of the body voluntarily—toes, foot, forearm, head, chin or tongue. Walking prognosis, including transfer ability from a wheelchair, was determined by the tests for locomotor prognosis (Bleck 1975) and equilibrium reactions.
The findings were as follows:

1. *Communication.* The goal of independent communication was set at 3, which meant the ability to communicate independently with a technical device. It was achieved by all except four total body involved children who were severely mentally retarded. Those who achieved independence in communication also had scores between 4 and 5, which indicated their ability to initiate and sustain a conversation.

2. *Activities of daily living.* Initial scores in this function in both independence and efficiency were 1. The children were totally dependent on others to fulfil basic needs. We set minimal goals of 3 (independent with a technical device and able to do household tasks). Except for those who were mentally retarded (N=4), all achieved this goal at follow-up.

3. *Mobility.* Initially the scores were 2, which meant partial dependence on others for only household mobility. The goal of independence with a technical device (score 3) and the ability to travel beyond the household (score 4 in efficiency) was achieved, and in patients over age 18 it included mobility in the community. Again lower scores were achieved by those few who were mentally retarded, which indicated continued partial dependence on others in the ability to move about the household.

4. *Walking.* In those below six years, walking was initially physiological and dependent. Although the goal set was independence with the assistance of a technical aid for household walking only (score 3) walking was not deemed efficient in a final follow-up of those over age 14 years, and they reverted to the physiological dependent walker.

Our conclusions were that the major factor in goal achievement in this group of patients was engineering technology and adaptive equipment, including environmental adaptations (*e.g.* home architectural modifications). Most significantly, goals could be set as early as age four years.

Employment and independence
Positive indicators for employment and independence have been reported:

1. Regular schooling and completion of high school (Bachman 1972, O'Reilly 1975).

2. Independence in mobility with ability to travel beyond the home, $p=0.01$ (Bachman 1972).

3. Good hand function and skills, $p=0.05$ (Bachman 1972)

4. Niche employment for the handicapped was best found in small towns rather than large cities (Ingram *et al.* 1964).

5. Spastic paralysis was more favourable for employment than athetosis (O'Reilly 1975). Not surprisingly, spastic hemiplegia and diplegia were most often associated with full-time employment (Ingram *et al.* 1964, Hassakis 1974, Soboloff 1981).

Our own study of 119 adolescents and young adults with spastic diplegia confirmed the good prognosis of this group for independence in all areas. None were in a day-care centre, only 3 per cent were in a sheltered workshop, and 97 per cent were either still in high school, more advanced education or working. Of the 30 per cent over age 21 years and working, the jobs varied: some were housewives and mothers, computer programmers, bankers or salesmen, and one is the mayor of his California town.

Negative factors for independence and employment have been suggested:

1. Intellectual retardation (Ingram *et al.* 1964, Hassakis 1974, O'Reilly 1975, Cohen and Kohn 1979).

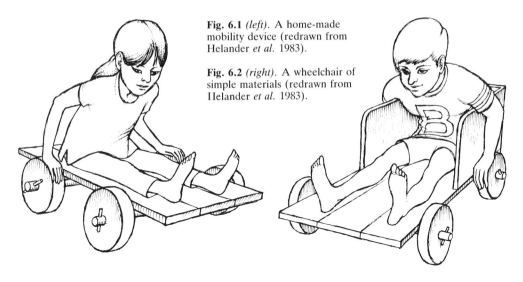

Fig. 6.1 *(left).* A home-made mobility device (redrawn from Helander *et al.* 1983).

Fig. 6.2 *(right).* A wheelchair of simple materials (redrawn from Helander *et al.* 1983).

2. Severity of the handicap (Ingram *et al.* 1964, Cohen and Kohn 1979).

3. Prolonged treatment programs have not been effective in achieving maximum independence (Cohen and Kohn 1979, Goldkamp 1984). Indeed, prolonged treatment programs and special schools may have been detrimental in permanently segregating the handicapped from the community (Taft 1972). To demonstrate the action behind the rhetoric, Milani-Comparetti (1979) was instrumental in closing some 13 special schools in Florence, Italy.

4. The family could act as a barrier to achievement by not accepting the child's disability and allowing the child to accept responsibility (Cohen and Kohn 1979, Soboloff 1981).

5. Social, cultural and economic factors are also undoubtedly responsible for unemployment. The needs of adults with cerebral palsy have been overlooked. Attention to adult needs, and the reality that adults are more than 'obsolete children', is being drawn by special reports and editorials (Bleck 1984, Thomas *et al.* 1985), and by the handicapped themselves and their organizations.

Cherpin has argued that the environment defines the extent of the handicap (Cherpin *et al.* 1985, Cherpin and Weber 1985). They conducted a detailed study of function of almost all 500 inhabitants of a small village near Lyon, France.

Goal-oriented approach in developing countries
The United Nations has designated 1983–1992 the decade of disabled persons. Apparently the World Health Organization has wisely adopted the goal-oriented approach, as evidenced by their training manual for disabled persons (Helander *et al.* 1983). This comprehensive manual is written with only 1600 English words to allow easy translation. Its illustrations demonstrate how to use local material for rehabilitation aids (Figs. 6.1, 6.2). The recommended techniques for rehabilitation are clearly focused on primary functions: communication, activities of daily living and mobility. These functional goals are combined with education in the

147

community schools, with the ultimate goal of employment to assist the family and the community. All World Health Organization programmes are community-based rather than based on elaborate central rehabilitation centres in the capital cities.

Especially pertinent is the clear statement by the World Health Organization that no more studies of incidence and numbers of handicapped people are needed. The drive to register handicapped people is totally unjustified unless those who register can immediately receive services. 'Every dollar spent on further investigations is a dollar mis-spent' (*World Health*, May 1984). From this same journal, the quotation of an African might be heeded by those of us in developed countries: 'We disabled people are fed up with being registered, censused, surveyed and photographed. We want services—now!'

Life expectancy
In considering how one has to live beyond childhood and what our management should be in children who will become adults, life expectancy of cerebral palsy is pertinent. Only two studies give some indication of longevity in cerebral palsy (Schlesinger *et al.* 1959, Cohen and Mustacchi 1966). Cohen and Mustacchi found that in 1416 persons with cerebral palsy the cumulative survival rate was 83 per cent, compared with 98 per cent for the normal population. Those who had the spastic type of cerebral palsy had the lowest mortality rate and a survival rate of 93 per cent. As expected (Schlesinger *et al.* 1959, Cohen and Kohn 1979), those who died early were severely involved and probably had been confined to long-term care institutions. For the child who is mildly or moderately involved we can expect a normal lifespan, which has now been extended in developed countries to 70 to 75 years. Even those who are total body involved and have achieved optimal function, combined with good nutrition and medical care, probably will have a normal lifespan. The statistics from the studies quoted should be interpreted with caution, and overgeneralization about mortality in cerebral palsy avoided.

Treatment

> *Tout ce qui est excessif est superflu* (Paul Valery, Académie Francaise)

'All that is excessive is superficial' is a statement that might be applied to the treatment of cerebral palsy as a disease. After Freud wrote his monograph, 'Les diplégies cérébrales infantiles' for *Revue Neurologique*, he felt he had reached a dead-end in his studies of cerebral palsy and thought it an intolerable burden: 'I am fully occupied with children's paralysis, in which I am not the least interested' (Accardo 1982). He then founded the new discipline of psychiatry. With the exception of orthopaedic surgery, medicine turned away from cerebral palsy as a 'wastebasket category' (Accardo 1982).

Interest in taking care of children with cerebral palsy was rekindled by Phelps, an orthopaedic surgeon, when he established his famous residential institute for cerebral palsy in Maryland (Slominski 1984). When the success of the poliomyelitis immunization seemed assured in the 1950s, it was perhaps natural for professionals to concentrate their efforts on other handicapping conditions in children. Cerebral palsy was and remains the predominant condition. Many sincere, serious and often zealous efforts to 'treat' the disease were promoted.

In the following paragraphs I will review the majority of the treatments proposed that might have continuing popularity. I will attempt to describe the rationale of treatments and offer a critique of each, based upon reported results or lack of them. In this way the physician who assumes responsibility for the management of the child may become familiar with various methods, and be able to counsel parents on appropriate management.

Central nervous system surgery

A direct attack on the altered brain function to alleviate the signs of cerebral palsy has obvious appeal. Two main types of brain surgery have been and apparently continue to be performed.

Stereotactic surgery

The methods of locally destroying a region of the brain by electrical current or freezing (cryosurgery) to alleviate the motor disorder of cerebral palsy seems to have waned in popularity in North America. Gornall *et al.* (1975) reported 10 cases of athetosis or spasticity in which stereotactic surgery created a lesion in the thalamus or dentate nucleus. In their results, six out of seven children with spastic hemiplegia or diplegia benefited; one child became worse in one limb. Two severe cases of the total body involved were said to have improved by a reduction in tone.

Vasin *et al.* (1979) performed similar surgery on the cerebellar dentate nuclei in 92 patients. Improvement in hyperkinesia and hypertonia was reported; however, they emphasized proper rehabilitation as the most important and decisive factor in achieving a satisfactory result. Broggi *et al.* (1980) reported satisfactory results with stereotactic thalamotomy in 24 patients with cerebral palsy. The side-effects after surgery were motor or sensory impairments and autonomic or mental disturbances. These undesirable side-effects were transient and were thought to be due to cerebral edema. In 1983, Broggi *et al.* reported longer term results of thalamotomy in 33 patients who had a one- to four-year follow-up. The best results were in those with tremor or hyperkinesis who had unilateral involvement. Spasticity tended to recur.

Ohye *et al.* (1983) performed similar stereotactic surgery in six children with tremor and athetosis, and in two with tremor and dystonia. They also thought that tremor and motor performance improved. These Japanese neurosurgeons, like the Soviets, emphasized the great importance of postoperative physical therapy.

Given the evidence of the diffuse nature of brain damage in many children, and the complexity of the interneuronal network, it seems unlikely that stereotactic surgery to destroy one or several spots in the brain will be successful in significantly alleviating the motor disorder. When weighed against the risks, such surgery will continue to be considered experimental.

Cerebellar stimulation

The principle of electrical stimulation of the cerebellum is derived from

Sherrington's observation of decerebrate animals. He noted a decrease in extensor hypertonia with stimulation of the anterior lobe of the cerebellar cortex (Davis *et al.* 1980). The method of implanting a self-controlled stimulator on the surface of the cerebellum ('cerebellar pacemaker') was introduced by Cooper *et al.* (1976). Some improvement was noted in 50 cases of cerebral palsy, and judicious use was deemed warranted.

The largest series of cases in which cerebellar stimulation was used has been reported by Davis *et al.* (1980). Of 262 patients with cerebral palsy (ages three to 53 years), a decrease in the tone of the spastic muscles was noted in 90 per cent after six months of use of the stimulator. In 40 per cent the device malfunctioned; the authors considered these blind controls. Assessments were entirely clinical. 61 per cent of the patients were said to have benefited, and 18 per cent had no benefit. In their assessment of results, the authors did state that in the future they hoped to use more objective methods of assessment in a bio-engineering laboratory. One patient who died had atrophy in the underlying folio of the cerebellum, with a focal loss of Purkinje and granule cells, and a reactive gliosis. The reason given for this change was over-use of the electrical stimulation, with an excessively high frequency of electrical current.

Robertson *et al.* (1980) noted improved sound and speech related to better intra-oral breath control in 10 children with cerebral palsy examined two months and six months after cerebellar stimulation. Among the changes considered significant were increased vowel phonation by two seconds, and improved articulation in four who had moderate dysarthria.

No significant benefit from cerebellar stimulation was claimed by Bensman and Szegho (1978), Whittaker (1980), and Ivan *et al.* (1981).

It would appear that the 'jury is still discussing its verdict' on the cerebellar pacemaker. A new method of alleviating athetosis and dystonia has been by electrical stimulation of the cervical spinal cord (Waltz and Davis 1983).

Spinal surgery for spasticity
Another attempt to alter spastic paralysis is by a direct cutting of the posterior nerve roots. Posterior lumbar rhizotomy was performed in 46 patients with cerebral palsy by Benedetti and Colombo (1981) and Peacock and Arens (1982). Both reported good results, except for six recurrences in the 46 patients of Benedetti and Colombo. Benedetti *et al.* (1982) reported a follow-up of four months to 3.5 years in 18 patients who had a mean age of 9.3 years. Three with spastic quadriplegia had first cervical to third cervical rhizotomies; the other 15 who had spastic paraplegia had lumbar rhizotomies. No mortality or major complications occurred, and generally good results were claimed. Results were said to be related to the motivation of the patient, the extent of the perceptual deficit, and intellectual impairment.

As we have seen in the chapter on neurobiology, cutting the posterior nerve roots in monkeys did result in a flail arm from which the monkey eventually recovered. Rhizotomy in the human apparently is an attempt to reproduce these experimental results, by interruption of the afferent input from the muscles in the

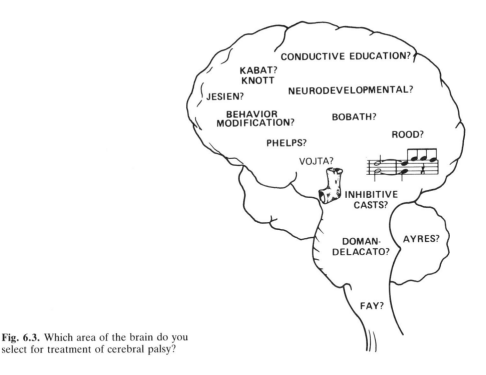

Fig. 6.3. Which area of the brain do you select for treatment of cerebral palsy?

hope of reducing the spasticity. Judging from the literature review since 1978, the operation is not popular in North America or Asia as an effective treatment. I believe that this type of neurosurgery for cerebral palsy should also be considered experimental.

Physical therapy

> *All physiotherapy can be decoded to become experience of life, instead of encoding life into therapeutic exercise (*Milani-Comparetti 1979).

Thompson (1977) surveyed 233 cerebral-palsy treatment units in the United States by questionnaire. The responses indicated that most therapists used a combination of 'methods' or 'systems' (Gillette 1969). The most commonly used methods were Ayres sensory integration (1971, 1972, 1977, 1978) and the Bobath neurodevelopmental treatment (1954, 1958, 1966, 1967, 1980, 1984). Other methods were Rood (1954), Phelps (Slominski 1984), Kabat (Kabat and Knott 1953, Kabat 1977), Fay (1958, 1977) and Doman-Delacato (1960). In more recent years the Vojta method has been widely adopted in Europe (Jones 1975, Kanda *et al.* 1984, Vojta 1984). Rolfing has enjoyed some popularity (Perry *et al.* 1981). More unusual forms of therapy reported have been 'mud therapy' (Kvashnik *et al.* 1978) and 'rhythmic psychomotor music therapy' (Gollnitz and Schulz-Wulf 1973). Skinnerian behavioural modification was suggested as an occupational therapy method for cerebral palsy (Hollis 1974) (Fig.6.3).

151

Two structured educational methods have become well known: 'conductive education' (Cotton 1974) and the 'Portage Project Model' (Jesien 1984). These systems both combine therapeutic efforts with goal-oriented approaches.

'Early intervention' has become the primary emphasis and by-word with most proponents of therapy methods or systems, because the best results in alleviating the condition are thought to be with very early treatment (*i.e.* under the age of six or eight months).

In the following discussion a brief description of each method will be attempted and then followed by a critique of the methods. Finally, I will discuss the use of traditional physical therapy skills and the rôle of the contemporary therapist. I have included these details because the physician is usually responsible for approval of the methods used, and in many regions of the United States a written 'prescription' is required by State agencies, as if therapy were a controlled drug. In the past 30 years, physicians and orthopaedists have not worried too much about prescribing therapy—allowing the therapists to 'do their thing' without asking too many questions. The language of the therapies has become complex and riddled with abstract neurophysiological terms, which may have intimidated some physicians. The disease-oriented approach was accepted.

The advice of Golden (1980) seems most apt. The burden of proof is on the proponents of the treatment. Critics need not prove ineffectiveness but can insist on positive data. Ethically, controlled studies are demanded. Golden quotes Bronowski (1978): 'Magic is a technology, technology without science'.

I feel that in 1986 and beyond, physicians who are being held accountable for increasing health-care costs need to be more aware of proposed methods of treatment and to be critical of the costs-benefits related to the outcome of the treatment. Is it effective?

Ayres sensory integrative therapy
This received its main impetus with the discovery of 'learning disorders' which affected the child's functional abilities (White 1984). Ayres (1972) devised tests which were used to determine the child's perceptual and visual-motor deficits. Because most of these tests required use of the hands, the testing procedures and treatment became the territory of the occupational therapist.

The theory behind the method is that children who have cerebral palsy are unable to integrate the sensory inputs (tactile and proprioceptive) from their trunk and limbs. Because of this defect, the vestibular system fails to provide correct information about the movement and posture of the limbs and body; consequently the movement disorder in cerebral palsy persists. Thus primitive reflexes persist, and the child is unable to motor plan. This theory is based upon dysfunction of the brainstem centres, which are considered the primitive sites of massive patterned responses. Evolutionary progression of the cerebral hemispheres allowed individual and discrete motor patterns.

The treatment is one of passive and active tactile and proprioceptive stimulation, which should capitalize on the 'remarkable plasticity' of the brain and its connections after damage; reprogramming and new connections by the

152

treatment are presumed. All sorts of tactile stimuli can be used: the only limit is the imagination of the therapist. Examples of the method include swinging in a hammock or a playground swing, and whirling in a swivel chair. As White (1984) pointed out, the equipment used looks very much like that found in an ordinary park playground.

Bobath neurodevelopmental treatment

This has become so established that the abbreviation 'NDT' is standard physical therapist jargon. It has been one of the oldest and most widely applied methods worldwide. The rationale for this treatment of cerebral palsy is a defect which interferes with normal postural control against gravity (Bobath 1980, Bobath and Bobath 1984). The original treatment program concentrated on an analysis of tonic reflexes, such as the tonic neck reflex and the tonic labyrinthine reflexes, as well as the positive supporting reaction to explain the motor patterns of the child with spastic paralysis.

The treatment program consisted mainly of passive positioning of the child in postures devised to reduce spasticity. At the same time it tried to give the child a sensation of normal movements (facilitation of automatic righting reactions). With the knowledge of development of normal babies, neurodevelopmental therapy attempted to follow and implement the stages of normal development in the child with cerebral palsy. Some therapists appeared to adhere to this protocol as a rigid dogma. They insisted that the child go through all stages of motor development, beginning with rolling before sitting, kneeling before standing, then crawling, standing, and finally walking. Even though the child had a great desire to stand and walk with external aids, therapists dissuaded them because they believed that walking with support before the child was developmentally ready was detrimental.

As with most therapies the parents were instructed to do the various postural positionings and exercises at home. Formal therapy sessions in a treatment unit varied from 30 to 60 minutes, one to five times a week. When the 'infant-at-risk' was discovered, this therapeutic program became popular as a method of 'early intervention'.

Mrs Bobath contributed a great deal to my management of cerebral palsy when she visited our treatment unit in 1956–57. She encouraged me to eliminate the constricting full-control braces (now called orthoses) which were standard equipment for many children. Instead she advised tennis shoes for most children, and we became more selective in advising orthotics. I was also introduced to the postural reflexes and infantile automatisms. I did not use these for treatment but as a way to determine locomotor prognosis more accurately (Bleck 1975).

The Rood method

This was an attempt to reduce spasticity and activate contraction of antagonist muscles by tactile stimulation with heat, cold and brushing. Hagbarth and Eklund (1977) seemed to propose a similar but more sophisticated method of stimulation with a muscle vibrator. The basis of this suggestion was animal experiments which presumed that vibration of muscles stimulated primary endings of the muscle spindle, the Golgi tendon organ and secondary spindle endings. The principle was to relieve certain motor neuron pools from excessive excitation and others from excessive inhibition.

The Children's Rehabilitation Institute

The Phelps method began at his institute in 1936. It was an eclectic approach and applied to each child individually according to the child's needs. Various standard physical treatments were used: passive and active assisted motion, relaxation therapy and massage. Therapists worked on individual muscles and gross movement patterns. These exercise programs were combined with learning specific skills, on the principle that normal people needed training in skills; therefore retraining to learn self-help skills seemed logical. Extensive bracing was also used, to control abnormal movement patterns. Phelps was insistent that the treatment program be in parallel with the educational one. The focus remained on self-help (Slominski 1984).

The Phelps program was thoroughly integrated in the residential centre, the Children's Rehabilitation Institute at Cockeysville, Maryland. Phelps was an orthopaedic surgeon, and used orthopaedic surgery as one aspect of necessary management. He was the original physician who established the principle that children who had cerebral palsy could and should be helped to achieve their full potential as persons. With a few other physicians he raised the national interest in cerebral palsy.

Kabat and Knott

Kabat and Knott (1953) introduced the idea of using a summation of facilitation of motor centres for neuromuscular education. They used active, active assistive, and resistive mass movement patterns for therapeutic exercise. They advocated manual resistance to muscle contraction. This exercise excluded individual muscles and used total movements of the limb (Kabat 1977).

Evolution of the brain

Fay's method (1958, 1977) was based upon the then accepted evolution of the human crawling: crawling first as an amphibian, then progressing to the crossed movement pattern of reptiles, lizards and alligators. His treatment was to elicit these early evolutionary forms of locomotion. He recommended use of spinal automatisms in spastic paralysis at the primitive level of function. An example of one spinal automatism was elicited by flexing the toes quickly, while at the same time pressing the knee outward; the resultant automatism was spontaneous flexion of the knee. His method implied passive manipulation to obtain progressive evolution of the damaged brain, thereby ameliorating the motor disorder. Fay's ideas were adopted by Doman and Delacato (1960).

The Doman-Delacato method (1960) consists of passive exercises designed to repeat the evolutionary progression of movement in evolution from fish, to amphibian, to reptile and finally to primates (Fig. 6.4). The theory postulates that the brain is organized in a series of evolutionary layers, each of which corresponds

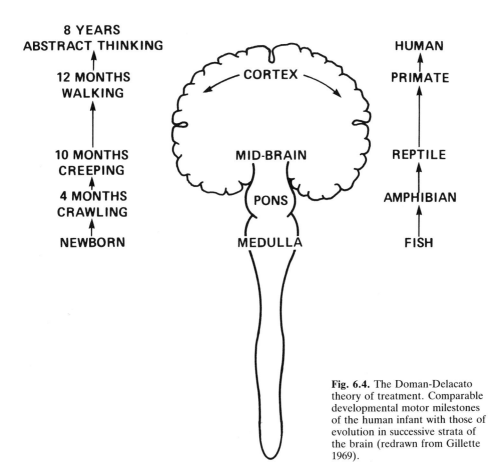

8 YEARS
ABSTRACT THINKING

12 MONTHS
WALKING

10 MONTHS
CREEPING

4 MONTHS
CRAWLING

NEWBORN

CORTEX

MID-BRAIN

PONS

MEDULLA

HUMAN

PRIMATE

REPTILE

AMPHIBIAN

FISH

Fig. 6.4. The Doman-Delacato theory of treatment. Comparable developmental motor milestones of the human infant with those of evolution in successive strata of the brain (redrawn from Gillette 1969).

to a form of locomotion specific for the species. The theory of cerebral dominance and treatment directed towards this end is another feature. Usually parents are instructed on the passive exercises ('patterning') in which two-person teams alternately flex and extend the upper and lower limbs in a cross pattern. These exercises are to be done several hours per day. Families organized teams from the neighbourhood and volunteers to do these passive movements for hours at a time. As might be imagined, the method entails total dedication, belief, zeal and a great deal of the parent's time away from normal household family and social activities. Many parents through the popular press have expressed their faith in the method over the past 25 years.

The Vojta method
This theory holds that the child with cerebral palsy has the same reflex movements that can be provoked in the normal newborn. These movements 'have a common neurogenic pattern in the subcortex, not in the motor cortex' (Vojta 1984, p.75).

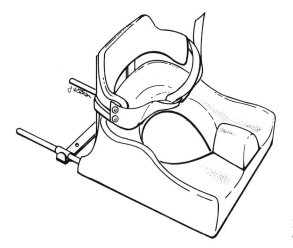

Fig. 6.5. The Memphis potty seat (reproduced by permission from Kohn 1982).

The treatment program elicits patterns of reflex motion by manual pressure on 'trigger zones' (*e.g.* the medial epicondylar area of the elbow). Vojta has delineated nine such 'trigger zones' to induce reflex creeping and turning, nine other zones for side-lying patterns and combinations and variations of sequences to excite these points of pressure. He states there are 'thousands of possibilities of activating the central nervous system' (Vojta 1984, p.81). These patterns of motion are then supposed to be 'imprinted' in the central nervous system (particularly in the cerebral hemispheres), stored within the brain, and apparently used by the infant.

The storage of the normal induced reflex patterns in the child with cerebral palsy presumably allows normal rather than pathological patterns of locomotor function to emerge. Parents are instructed in the method, so that the therapist needs to see the child no more than two to four times a month, and once every four to six weeks for older children. Vojta advised that if no improvement is seen in one year, then the treatment has no more to offer.

Jones (1975) reported the results of Vojta's treatment programs as reported by him in the European literature. Of 207 children with presumed cerebral palsy, 199 were normal on discharge. The treatment was also applied to 344 infants-at-risk, who were apparently defined as such by the tests devised by Vojta. Of these, 149 needed no treatment; 38 were said to have needed treatment but did not receive it. In a group of 67 infants treated, 43 had 'minimal cerebral dysfunction'. The method presumably was not used exclusively in cerebral palsy; other conditions treated were mental retardation and epilepsy.

Conductive education
Hari and Tillemans (1984) admit that this method is 'difficult to understand'. It is an educational system for children who have cerebral palsy. The 'conductors' are licensed generalists who have a four-year college training in what medicine, psychology, education, physical and logo therapy have to offer in the education of physically handicapped children. This seemingly structured and intensive in-patient

program, founded by Dr Petö in Budapest, is located in the Institute for the Motor Disabled in Budapest and administered by the Ministry of Education of Hungary.

The system is basically educational and goal-oriented towards maximum independence. They have no special techniques, but there are principles: *e.g.* 'rhythmic intention', which means involving the children in their own learning directed by their 'inner voice'; all learning must be relevant to that particular child, who obtains feedback on his/her performance so that the brain can restructure itself; in learning tasks the child finds the most efficacious way for him or her—this is called 'orthofunction'.

Equipment often pictured in demonstrating this method is a 'plinth' which consists of a platform of slotted boards around which the children can fit their hands and grab to transfer, turn over and adjust their posture (Hari and Tillemans 1984). Old-fashioned iron or brass-rail bedsteads have been used to assist self-transfer into and out of bed (Cotton 1977). The conductor is a generalist and uses whatever equipment or therapy that seems to work best for the child (Fig. 6.5). Special equipment, however, is deemed a last resort and only a temporary expedient to learn the task.

The Portage Project

The Portage Project (Jesien 1984) derives its name from the town of founding, Portage, Wisconsin, USA. It is a home educational program, directed and encouraged by a home teacher who visits the family weekly. An initial assessment is based upon 580 developmentally sequenced skills which occur from birth to six years. This assessment is used as a guide for an individual curriculum, in which one can select four to seven possible ways to teach the 580 skills. Despite the seeming rigidity of the skill-learning lists, they are not applied in this way for every child, and require modification depending upon the child's motor and intellectual involvement.

Parents are taught to become the educators, after the teacher has collected the baseline data from the assessment and demonstrated the activity to be performed (called 'modeling'). Regular review of the activity is done by the teacher with the parents during the weekly home visit. The method insists on weekly progress: otherwise the objectives are modified. The teacher or 'home visitor' acts as a counselor and supporter of the family. The originator of this program insists that the program must be flexible and easily suited to the family's needs.

The home visitor sees 10 to 15 families per week; visits range from 60 to 90 minutes each. The visitor's rôle is reinforced by weekly half-day conferences with the supervisor, to discuss problems and plan the next week's activities. The visitor also assists the family in arranging clinic visits to evaluate the child.

The Portage Project system has been translated into 12 languages and implemented in 20 countries (Jesien 1984). To be successful, Jesien insists on 'strict adherence' to the model, while still adapting the specific procedures to the needs of the child and the parents. Maximum involvement of the parents seems to be the essential ingredient in this early childhood educational method.

157

Evaluation of therapy methods and management techniques

The advantage of one treatment over another can be proved only by careful clinical evaluation. Knowledge of the neurophysiological mechanisms that could be involved is irrelevant to this process (McLellan 1984).

Early intervention of 'high-risk' infants with various therapies became the paradigm of the 70s and 80s. This concept of 'reprogramming' the assumed 'plasticity' of the infant brain gave rise to the identification of infants-at-risk. In questioning the efficacy of early intervention programs, Ferry (1981) wrote: 'Premature infants in neonatal intensive care units are being cuddled, patted, stroked with vibrators, and rocked in water beds and motorised hammocks; they are exposed to flashing lights, dangling birds and toys, piped-in heart beat sounds and music ("This Old Man"). We have home-based parent-oriented programs, home-based child-oriented programs, centre-based child-oriented programs, and centre-based parent- and child-oriented ones'. Infant stimulation and developmental therapy programs have, as Ferry stated, become a major industry.

Do these programs unwittingly convey to parents that the brain cells will grow or reform with this sort of special intervention? Tizard (1980) took to task those who screen alleged infants-at-risk because more parental misery is caused by uncertainty than when the diagnosis is certain. The effect of much early treatment has been to enhance its reputation. Tizard is correct in criticising the rôle of the popular press in promoting therapies 'mostly in periodicals intended, sometimes rather insultingly, for a female readership'.

The Bobaths (1984) now recognize that very early treatment presents a problem because the diagnosis of cerebral palsy is usually impossible under the age of four months and often under the age of eight months. Parmelee and Cohen (1985) have also found it impossible to predict outcomes of suspected infants-at-risk, except those with immediate and catastrophic neurological problems. Their studies showed no correlation between perinatal factors and later development. Michaelis *et al.* (1985) studied infants who had serious abnormal findings during the first year of life but did not show any developmental abnormalities later in childhood. Amiel-Tison (1985) also noted that most cases of perinatal origin had mild cerebral palsy that mimicked spastic hemiplegia or diplegia, and that these signs often disappeared by age six to eight months. This neurologist thought that brain plasticity was overrated; normalization was related more to maturation.

Weber (1983) discussed the inevitability of treating a considerable number of unaffected infants when the diagnosis is in doubt. He posed a pertinent and often disregarded question: are there adverse psychological effects from treatments such as that promulgated by Vojta?

Early treatment was sometimes thought to raise the intelligence quotient (Köng 1966), but others have disputed this (Bobath 1967). Intelligence may be related to gains from therapeutic intervention programs (Parette and Hourcade 1983, 1984). Scherzer *et al.* (1976) also noted a trend towards positive change in children who had higher intelligence.

While perinatal asphyxia with low Apgar scores might predict neurological handicaps later in childhood, data on 49,000 infants who did not achieve a score of higher than 8 at five minutes (Nelson and Ellenberg 1981) does not make us certain of identifying all infants-at-risk for cerebral palsy. In this study of infants who survived severe asphyxia, three-quarters had no apparent neurological problem at age seven years. In another prospective study of 51,285 pregnancies and births of babies weighing more than 2500g (Nelson and Ellenberg 1984), there was no increased risk of cerebral palsy after obstetrical complications in those with high five-minute Apgar scores. The final capstone to early identification of infants who might have cerebral palsy is the study of 32,000 infants assessed for risk factors at four months and then again at age seven years. The majority 'outgrew' their presumed cerebral palsy (Nelson and Ellenberg 1982).

Despite the impossibility of clearly identifying infants who will later have serious handicaps, is early intervention effective? Denhoff (1981) reviewed the data on 1000 infants in the United Cerebral Palsy Association collaborative study. These infants had intensive therapy and enrichment programs. The only parameter to show significant improvement on test-retest was the measurement of social-emotional interaction.

Amiel-Tison (1985) perhaps offers the best perspective about these infant programs. She suggests that any attempt to help parents to accept their infant and reinforce interaction is also early intervention. Anastasiow (1985) suggests that these programs are primarily interventions with the parents; the objective should be to raise them to the level of adult functioning. Bax (1983) surmised that if such programs decreased child abuse they would be worthwhile. Even so, it seems to me that prudence is necessary to avoid an over-elaborate infant program, particularly one that projects resolution of the neurological problem by a system of passive physical or occupational therapy.

When early therapy is labelled with a name or an abbreviation (*e.g.* NTD), something more than parent support and education is connoted. In our population, about 60 per cent of the infants enrolled in these programs evolve with mild cerebral palsy (spastic hemiplegia or diplegia), walk, and go on to regular school. The other 40 per cent are the severely involved children. Then their parents either demand more therapy to achieve the 'cure' observed in the milder involved, feel guilty because they did not do the 'home' program exercises, or accuse the therapy or therapist of being inadequate.

The real value of preschool nursery programs (Bleck and Headley 1961) seems to be the opportunity for sorting out the children according to their potential and directing them and the parents to the appropriate next step, where they can best achieve their potential. The major part of the process is parent education and counseling, with appropriate referral to the community educational resources (Fig. 6.6). Whether this needs to be accomplished in a school-like setting with a team of professionals, or only in the home with one professional visitor-counselor (as in the Portage Project (Jesien 1984)), depends primarily on the parents' needs, and secondarily on the size, location and resources of the community. A parent-centred home program for children with cerebral palsy in sparsely populated northern

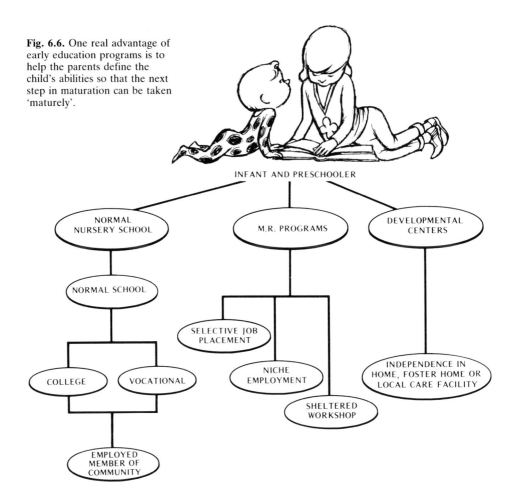

Fig. 6.6. One real advantage of early education programs is to help the parents define the child's abilities so that the next step in maturation can be taken 'maturely'.

INFANT AND PRESCHOOLER

NORMAL NURSERY SCHOOL

M.R. PROGRAMS

DEVELOPMENTAL CENTERS

NORMAL SCHOOL

SELECTIVE JOB PLACEMENT

COLLEGE

VOCATIONAL

NICHE EMPLOYMENT

INDEPENDENCE IN HOME, FOSTER HOME OR LOCAL CARE FACILITY

SHELTERED WORKSHOP

EMPLOYED MEMBER OF COMMUNITY

Sweden was deemed successful by 21 of the 26 families who responded to a questionnaire. But five of these families (25 per cent) thought that there were too many exercises, and another five thought that the exercises were inadequate (Von Wendt *et al.* 1984).

Evaluation of specific therapy systems
'Systems of therapy' have been described in books (Gillette 1969), published in journals, and been the subject of many conferences and seminars. It would seem that after 15 years of intensive trials, at least some data on the effectiveness would be forthcoming. Other than generalisations to confirm hypotheses, most clinical studies have been either negative or questioning. Perhaps it is time to give up trying to 'cure' the neurological deficits by remedial methods, stop looking for positive studies, and get on with the task of helping children and their parents in the management of the motor disorder to allow optimum function for independent living.

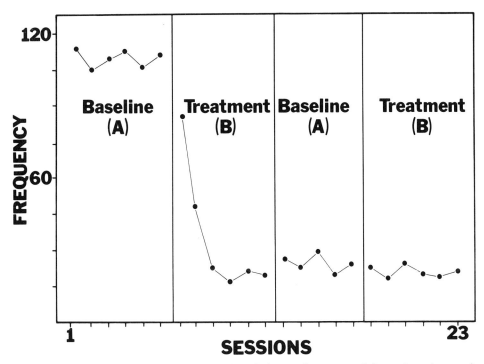

Fig. 6.7. Graphic representation of single-subject design studies suggested for various therapeutic endeavours. (Reproduced courtesy of Leonard Epstein, Auburn University, Texas, from Martin and Epstein 1976.)

As long ago as 1962, Paine questioned the value of treatment in cerebral palsy by comparing a group of 74 patients who had had no therapy with 103 children who had had intensive physical therapy, bracing, and orthopaedic surgery. He found that those who had mild spastic hemiplegia improved both with and without treatment. More severely involved spastic patients, who had various forms of treatment, did have a better gait and fewer contractures. But physical therapy did not reduce the need for orthopaedic surgery and made no difference in patients with athetosis.

Specific therapy programs have not often been evaluated by their proposers because it is claimed that there are too many variables in the patient population. This is true enough. Furthermore, controls are difficult to impose. A possible solution to this problem was suggested by Martin and Epstein (1976), who devised methods of evaluation of a single patient. Figure 6.7 explains their methods. I have not seen any reports which used this method for therapies. We have used a similar method in the study of a drug intended to reduce spasticity (Ford *et al.* 1976). Harris *et al.* (1985) used this single-subject design to evaluate the effects of 'tone reducing' and standard short-leg plaster casts in two patients with spastic equinus.

Bobath neurodevelopmental therapy had one good clinical study by Wright

161

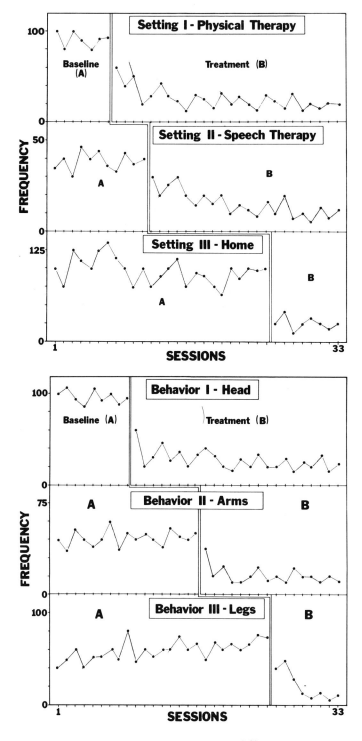

Fig. 6.7. *(contd.)*

162

and Nicholson (1973), who conducted a prospective controlled study in two groups of children. They found no significant differences after 12 months between treated and untreated children, when analyzed with regard to motor function, range of movement or joints, and loss of primitive reflexes.

Goldkamp (1984), in a study of 53 children according to an ADL scoring system, found no significant improvement as the result of therapy (more than 50 per cent had Bobath treatment). He concluded that 'management' would be a more appropriate term than 'treatment', and 'adaptation' more acceptable than 'improvement'. Adaptation could be facilitated by assistive devices, environmental modifications, and even practice.

The Bobaths have written (1984) that they grossly overrated the tonic reflexes in explaining abnormal patterns in the spastic child and no longer include them in their assessments. They also reported the inadequacy of concentrating on automatic righting reactions, and the detrimental effects of absent or insufficient balance reactions which remain 'one of our greatest problems' (p.8). They go on: 'Indeed it was wrong to try to follow the normal developmental sequence too closely'. They now know that children do not need to go rigidly through a developmental sequence of rolling over, sitting, kneeling and half-kneeling before progressing to standing. Finally, the Bobaths observed that their treatment program had not carried over into activities of daily life as they had expected. Their treatment 'now incorporates systematic preparation for specific functions... There is no time to waste on unspecific, general, developmental treatment, for we cannot expect that such treatment will automatically carry over into functional skills later on' (p.11). These honest, intelligent and dedicated professionals, who have lived only for the improvement of care of the child with cerebral palsy, deserve our gratitude for having the temerity to admit their mistakes and their desire to learn from their experience. I only hope that some of our more zealous NDT therapists have similar humility, and are willing to modify their ideas which were originally derived from the Bobaths.

Sensory integrative therapy has been investigated in a few studies. Montgomery and Richter (1977) reported on the results in mentally retarded children in whom cerebral palsy was excluded. The control group consisted of 25 children who had no special program except for physical education. The experimental groups consisted of 25 children in two groups: (i) developmental physical education, and (ii) therapeutic sensorimotor education. Gains, albeit small, were made in gross and fine motor skills in the sensorimotor-treated children. They noted that negative changes occurred during the summer in the sensorimotor group, and explained that this might be due to the lack of repetition of these activities during the summer months—because 'repetition over a period of months is necessary for integration to become firmly established, it is possible that these responses were not well integrated' (Montgomery and Richter 1977, p.805). In contrast, the children in the developmental physical education program improved over the summer in reflex test items. This improvement was thought to be due to the first half year of the program, when there was an emphasis on 'reflex items reflecting brain stem responses, those integrated by floor activities'.

These studies were accompanied by elaborate statistical analysis, to prove the point of treatment efficacy. It was stated that none of the 118 test items were practised or mentioned by the teacher during the year of the study. A sample of tests performed seems so ordinary that I wonder about the practice. Some test items were: number of beads laced within 30 seconds, number of blocks transferred within 30 seconds, the distance jumped in a standing broad jump, the number of times the child changed body position in 20 seconds, the number of sit-ups in 30 seconds, and the number of steps on a balance beam. One could wonder about the effects of ordinary maturation or, as the authors implied, whether there was a higher functioning in one group than the other.

Kanter *et al.* (1976) tried to show the efficacy of vestibular stimulation accomplished by spinning Down's syndrome children in a swivel chair one minute per day. The experimental group had two children with Down's syndrome, aged six and 24 months; in the control group were three normal infants, six to nine months of age, and two with Down's syndrome. One normal child and one with Down's syndrome increased their motor abilities, 21.5 and 16 points respectively. The authors concluded that the improvement in these two children were the result of advancement of vestibular inhibitory mechanisms.

My reason for dwelling on these reports of sensorimotor integration is that the tests and the method was promoted by Ayres (1978) for learning disabilities. The tests were rapidly learned and adopted, mainly by occupational therapists, and then were applied to children with cerebral palsy—usually spastic diplegia or hemiplegia—and in whom fine motor-skill defects could easily be found in hand function. However, the official position of the American Association of Occupational Therapists is still that the educationally related (occupational therapy) service is, with purposeful use of activities, to increase functional performance of independent living skills (American Association of Occupational Therapists 1981). The 'cure' prescribed was often (and still may be in some treatment units) the sensory integration therapy method. It would appear that these sensory integration therapies for learning disabilities and improving motor function are experimental. Without controls, random samples, or even single-subject designs, the results have been equivocal or questionable.

Controlled studies that adjust for normal maturation have been negative. Sellick and Over (1980) reported negative results in vestibular stimulation to alleviate motor development in cerebral palsy, in a controlled study which adjusted for normal maturation of the child. A careful study of vestibular dysfunction in normal and learning-disabled children in Toronto (Polatajko 1985) revealed no consistent evidence of vestibular dysfunction in the learning-disabled child. I conclude that the concept of vestibular dysfunction in these children should be abandoned, and the practice of sensory integrative therapy re-evaluated.

A recent review of the management of learning disabilities was provided by Feagans (1983). Treatment programs have not generally been effective in preventing academic problems, nor has a learning disability disappeared. The basis of these special treatment methods for perceptual-motor problems was the presumption of a neurological mechanism. This concept has been discounted. The idea that a learning disability is the same mechanism as in brain-damaged children has been discarded. So the application of these methods to the management of children with cerebral palsy is probably not reasonable. Consequently, physicians have little justification for prescribing these special therapy techniques unless they are to be used as part of a research project, with review by a human subjects' investigation committee and informed parental consent, similar to any other biomedical study involving the use of humans.

Patterning treatment (Doman-Delacato) is based upon the concept of brain development that ontogeny recapitulates phylogeny (Fay 1977). While it was an attractive and easily understood concept, it is not supported by present knowledge of central nervous system development (Cohen *et al.* 1970). The Institute for Achievement of Human Potential have used their own instrument, the Doman-Delacato Developmental Profile, to prove the efficacy of the method. This profile showed some improvement in program-related responses (Holm 1983).

One controlled study by Sparrow and Zigler (1978) had negative results in 43 retarded children. In a policy statement, the American Academy of Pediatrics (1982) concluded that the patterning treatment had no special merit and that the claims of its advocates were unproven. Furthermore, the demands on the family were very great. The policy statement stated that the well-designed study of the method, which was publicly and privately funded in 1967, was in the final planning stage when the Institute for Achievement of Human Potential withdrew their original agreement to participate.

The *Vojta* method has achieved considerable worldwide popularity with therapists (Vojta 1984). Schutt (1981) reported the case of a cerebral-palsied girl whose subluxation of the hip was reduced after three years of the Vojta treatment.

Kanda *et al.* (1984) used this method in eight spastic diplegic children treated early and in 21 treated late. They based the assessment of severity of the cerebral palsy on the CT scans of the brain. All walked by age three years, but steadier walking occurred in the early-treatment group. It was difficult to change the pattern of walking in the late group. In this study the more severe cases were in the early-treatment group, as judged from the CT scans which showed varying degrees of cortical atrophy and ventricular dilatation. In view of the well-known lack of correlation between the anatomical change in the brain and the severity of the motor disorder, one would have to be cautious in utilizing the CT scan alone to judge severity in infants presumed to be at risk.

In view of Vojta's paper (1981) which assessed the results of his treatment, the Bobaths are cautious in ascribing the treatment to the good results claimed (1984). In a statistical analysis of 207 babies diagnosed and treated between one week and four months of age (Vojta 1981), 199 became normal in motor and intellectual function. Vojta then wrote that perhaps about half of these babies (infants-at-risk) might have been treated unnecessarily. This is probably true, given the careful study by Ellenberg and Nelson (1981) who examined 32,000 infants at age four months and again at seven years. At four months the suspected cerebral palsy rate was about 1 per cent; of those with definite abnormal neurological signs, only one of seven developed cerebral palsy at school age. In the entire group at follow-up, the incidence of cerebral palsy dropped to 1:1000. Thus, as with so many special therapy methods, treatment always looks better if you begin it before a diagnosis can be made with certainty.

The effectiveness of *Rolfing* in cerebral palsy was studied by Perry *et al.* (1981). After the pressure massage, which was thought to break up adhesions between tendons to allow better sliding, it was thought that mildly involved subjects improved in the velocity, stride-length and cadence of gait; the moderately involved made only slight gains, and the severely involved were not improved. In no cases was muscle strength or the electromyographic pattern altered.

Neuromuscular facilitation, as originated by Kabat (1977), was based on the principle of summation by facilitation in the motor centres through mass movement patterns against resistance. Its use in cerebral palsy has not been popular. One report by Carlsen (1975) of its use in 12 children, age one to five years, showed improvement in the Denver Developmental and Bayley test scores, when compared with a functional treatment approach (Carlsen 1975).

Behaviour modification has been tried and found effective in forcing reverse tailor sitting in children with cerebral palsy (Bragg *et al.* 1975). It was not reported whether this reduces the range of hip internal rotation in children, or whether it creates a continuing battle between parent and child.

Behaviour modification was reintroduced by Skinner in 1971, 50 years after the same approach was first introduced by Watson in 1920 and then abandoned in the 1930s due to the influence of Freud, Dewey and other followers. It seemed natural for physical therapy in cerebral palsy, but now seems to be on the wane again—though it may return. This is why I have included it in this text. The editorial commentary on 'the modification of behaviour modification' (Schowalter 1977) offered a perspective and a caution—'child-rearing is a trendy, cyclical business'. As Schowalter wisely points out, behavioural schedules (and I would add any kind of home-therapy schedules) may be so energy-consuming that they may destroy the parent-child relationship through the busy work recommended by the therapist. The busy work may absorb the parent's anger, or the hostility may be increased.

Prescribing physical and occupational therapy
After this review of questionably effective methods, it is obvious that a special therapy is impossible to prescribe or approve.

In an effort to improve the communication between physician and therapist, Levine and Kliebhan (1981) suggest that this communication be written (called a 'prescription' in the USA), including the diagnosis, the family picture, the motor abnormalities, the functional goals, the precautions and the intensity (*e.g.* for maintenance—one hour per month; moderately active intensity—one hour per month to half an hour per week; active—one to two hours per week; intensive—more than two hours per week).

This sort of precision in measuring time seems unrealistic because it presumes a result. These authors then advise that much depends on the 'faithfulness with which the family carries out the home program'. Although they advise functional goals in general, the major thrust was towards recommending Bobath neurodevelopmental treatment.

Levine and Kliebhan (1981, p.209) highlight the dilemma of the physician who wants to be rational in this matter: 'We recognise that therapy services are being provided even though uncertainty exists about the efficacy of some of the specific therapy techniques. However, therapy will continue because it is mandated by law' (in the USA).

Mandating and enshrining any medical treatment by law surely could not have been the intention of our legislators.

The way out of this dilemma is to change the terms. We do not 'treat' cerebral palsy, any more than we treat spina bifida; we manage it. We manage it to allow optimum fulfilment of that child's potential for adult living. This means the goal- or aim-oriented approach as recommended by us and Scrutton (1984).

In the aim-oriented management , Scrutton's guidelines are the best (Scrutton 1984). In 1985 the Committee on Children's Disabilities of the American Academy of Pediatrics advised that the proper therapy prescription should meet the functional needs of the child and include necessary adaptive equipment. The essential features of Scrutton's (1984) program are:

(1) The most accurate possible prognosis in all areas
(2) An assessment of the problems which might be eliminated or alleviated
(3) An assessment of the child's daily life situation
(4) The assessment forms the framework for listing a priority of aims and how these might be accomplished
(5) A time frame and review date is set.

In this new framework, which calls for management rather than treatment, no hourly or weekly 'therapy' sessions should need to be specified. The therapist and parents decide on how to accomplish the tasks for function and how much time need be spent. This will often entail special positioning, seating and adaptive equipment.

A major principle of management should be that it does not become more burdensome to the patient and family than the disability itself.

The rôle of the modern therapist

The therapist discusses functions of everyday life instead of mystifying neurophysiological problems avoiding mysterious and irrelevant concepts such as muscle tone, reflexes, and spasticity (Milani Comparetti 1979).

Rather than just following a cook-book of therapy recipes, the modern therapist has a much more demanding task as analyst, catalyst and family adviser. Management involves the home and the family. The modern therapist needs training and skill in interpersonal relationships, and must not inadvertently disturb the delicate relationships that exist within most families.

The modern therapist is a professional, with a knowledge of normal and abnormal motor and psychological behaviour, the entire range of compensatory devices from the fields of science and technology, and the realities of life in both

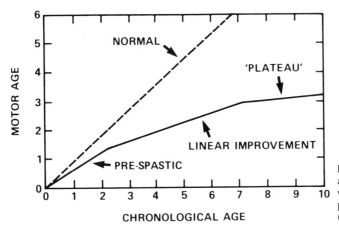

Fig. 6.8. Motor development and maturation of the child with spastic diplegia. Note the plateau at age seven years (redrawn from Beals 1966).

urban and rural communities. The therapist works with the physician towards the common goal of all rehabilitation—independence consistent with the extent of the handicap.

After orthopaedic surgery, intensive short-term therapeutic exercise, gait restoration, and confidence-building is invaluable. It need not continue indefinitely—just to the point of maximum improvement anticipated. Usually, after major orthopaedic lower-limb surgery in ambulatory patients, this intensive program is no longer than six months: and usually three months is sufficient.

Stopping therapy
When to stop seeing the therapist? When the child is outdoors playing with his/her peers, then this is the therapy and it is time to halt. Some parents and children like to visit the therapist once a week or once a month. This is not really a therapeutic session but a physician assistant's check-up and perhaps a psychological help. Each patient's and family's needs in this regard have to be ascertained. If they perceive no need, then no physical or occupational check-up is necessary.

In order to integrate the cerebral-palsied child into regular school (providing intellectual functioning is satisfactory), it is usually essential for the physician and therapist to state that optimum benefits of 'therapy' have been obtained. Certainly by the age of seven years, motor improvement of children with spastic diplegia levels off (Beals 1966) (Fig. 6.8). Walking patterns in normal children are normally mature by the age of seven; Burnett and Johnson (1971) showed that the adult walking pattern is achieved 55 weeks after walking begins. The elegant instrumented gait analysis of children by Sutherland *et al.* (1980) confirms that adult gait patterns are fixed by age seven years.

More severely involved children who do not walk can have goals set by the age of four years (Terver *et al.* 1981). Goal achievement entails the co-operation of the therapist and rehabilitation engineers and orthotists to achieve communication, optimum self-care and mobility. Much of this program can be accomplished by the age of eight years. Its success depends on the extent of the motor disability, and especially on the intellectual function of the child.

Sports

There's no play like snow play (Arnoff 1973).

Even though for several generations medicine took a dim view of anything that might be fun, sports programs for the handicapped have proliferated and have been rapidly advanced in North America and Europe. In Brasilia, after 10 years of passive physical therapy to effect change in the motor disorder of cerebral palsy in 2000 patients, this approach was abandoned in favour of fun and games (Campos da Paz Jr 1980). As expected, some have attempted to demonstrate therapeutic value in sports such as 'hippotherapy' (Tauffkirchen 1978) and 'therapeutic horseback riding for cerebral-palsied children' (Hengst 1976, Feldkamp 1979). These attempts are perhaps the natural outgrowth in countries with liberal medical care insurance schemes—an indirect approach to finance recreation for children whose parents cannot afford it. But these attempts at the medicalization of sports have come under suspicion: 'If horseback riding and swimming are good for the atheotid, this does not make the horse a therapist nor the swimming pool a medical appliance' (Milani-Comparetti 1979).

For children with cerebral palsy, swimming is one of the best activities. A recent publication by Campion (1985) is an excellent and detailed guide to swimming pool programs for the handicapped. The National Handicapped Sports and Recreation Association has become a focal point for many national organizations and sports programs.*

Children who have total body involvement with spastic quadriplegia seem to get more relaxation from a heated whirlpool spa or tub than any other modality or medication I have ever recommended. Alpine and cross-country skiing is another sport well suited to many children and adults who have cerebral palsy. In the USA this program was founded under the auspices of the Children's Hospital Medical Center, Denver, Colorado (Messner 1976). As a result, other winter sport programs for the handicapped have evolved.

Soccer is a popular sport for young people who have spastic diplegia or hemiplegia and are independent walkers; another is golf, and tennis may be possible with proper instruction. The wheelchair Olympics and the Olympic games for the disabled are now national institutions.

Given the growing recognition and success of sports for the handicapped, physicians and therapists have every reason to encourage and assist children with cerebral palsy in learning and preparing for a lifelong sporting activity rather than a life of therapeutic exercise and passive manipulation. If adults who have normal motor control want to visit a health club regularly, why not a health club for the handicapped rather than a recurring prescription for physical therapy at a medical rehabilitation unit or hospital?

*Farragut Station, PO Box 33141, Washington DC 20003.

Plaster casting

When the only tool you have is a hammer, everything looks like a nail (Paul H. Hirshman).

Plaster immobilization to reduce muscle hypertonicity may have been first suggested by Australian therapists (Hayes and Burns 1970). Yates and Mott (1977) reported their results in the application of bilateral short-leg walking plasters in 49 children who had a spastic dynamic equinus due to cerebral palsy. They termed this method of immobilization in plasters 'inhibitive casts' because 100 per cent of their patients exhibited changes in 'tone', and all but four walking patients improved their gaits; the posture and movement of non-walkers improved, and it was said that upper-limb tone was reduced. The unexplained neurological mechanism responsible for the change towards relaxation of the muscles was called 'inhibition'.

In a follow-up report, Mott and Yates (1981) reported that only nine patients had surgery post-casting: six had plantar fasciotomies and only three had an Achilles tendon lengthening.

The inhibitive casts were modified to include a prefabricated wooden footplate with a ridge of felt or other material to provide pressure under the metatarsal heads and to extend the toes. Felt padding was placed posterior to the ankle malleoli and with the usual cast padding a plaster-plastic polymer short leg cast was applied. It was then bivalved and Velcro fastening straps affixed. The child wore the casts for several hours a day; the average duration of this treatment was 10 months.

Since 'inhibitive casts' were first introduced in 1977, they have been recommended and applied by therapists to increasing numbers of infants and toddlers who have spastic paralysis and equinus, as a 'method' to reduce 'tone' throughout the body and to obtain improved function, particularly in children who have not yet begun walking and have no actual shortening of the triceps surae (*i.e.* no contracture). Therapists who are specially trained in the technique are referred patients by other therapists. The practice of inhibitive casts seems to have displaced 'neurodevelopmental therapy' as a treatment of choice in many young children: so much so, that in 1984 I observed that the majority of new patients referred for consultation had not just one set of bivalved plasters but two other appliances. And one child who had a bilateral spastic calcaneus deformity (excessive dorsiflexion of the ankle) also had 'inhibitive casts'.

Sussman and Cusick (1979), in an enthusiastic report of 99 cerebral palsy patients who had this cast treatment, stated that the casts effected 'tone reduction', increased postural stability, and were useful in improving weight-bearing activities and walking. Sussman (1983) suggested that these casts are not inhibitive but more like a rigid plastic ankle-foot orthosis. Indeed, these orthoses seem to be applied after the casts have been worn for unspecified periods of time.

Duncan and Mott (1983) wrote that the theory of inhibitive casts was to control reflex-induced foot deformity by reduction of the hypertonus of co-contracting musculature. The hypothesis is that early balance of the infant is facilitated by inborn supporting reflexes, righting reaction and four superficial foot reflexes which can be elicited in the first year of life in normal infants (Duncan 1960). There

170

are four specific areas which respond to skin stimulation: head of the first metatarsal, head of the fifth metatarsal, ball of the foot, and plantar aspect of the heel. If the centre of gravity is displaced forward, for example, pressure on the ball of the foot evokes the toe grasp reflex with contracture of the toe flexors, the triceps surae, hamstrings, gluteal muscles, and spine musculature in a proximal cascade in the attempt to counteract the continuing displacement.

Duncan and Mott warn that cast application is contra-indicated in a fixed contracture. While the cast is on the child, the physical therapist can help the child in establishing normal movements. Inhibitive casts as described by Mott and Yates (1977) were used for three to 12 months; the weaning process included the use of plastic ankle-foot orthoses. In the analysis of their results in 111 children, 68 per cent were predicted to be non-walkers; but after this treatment, 64 per cent were walking independently, 20 per cent were cruising or walking with aids, and only 14.4 per cent were not walking. The mean follow-up time was eight years; 23 per cent required surgery or an orthosis.

A prospective study of inhibitive casting was done by Watt *et al.* (1984) in 34 children who had spastic dynamic equinus due to cerebral palsy. They used the method of Yates and Mott (1977); the casts were applied for three weeks. Statistically significant improvement in the range of ankle dorsiflexion was found immediately after and five weeks post-casting, with deterioration to the pre-casting ranges at six months. They found no changes in the quadriceps reflex, the Babinski response or ankle clonus, and neurodevelopmental milestones did not change other than accounted for by natural maturation.

A positive report on the use of the inhibitive cast was a single-case report by Zachazewski *et al.* (1982) of a 25-year-old man who had a positive support reaction (*i.e.* spasticity of the extensor muscles of the lower limb) due to a skull fracture and an intracerebral haematoma. After four weeks of cast immobilization his gait improved considerably. This was followed by a 'molded polypropylene tone-inhibiting AFO' for the right leg. He continued to improve in his gait, but reached a plateau until a cranioplasty was performed. Three days after this surgery, dramatic improvement in the gait pattern was observed. But a recent report by Otis and colleagues (1985) found too much variability in results to draw any positive conclusions.

Plaster cast treatment was used to stretch the spastic triceps surae muscle in the majority of Westin's patients (Westin and Dye 1983) over a period of 27 years (1952–1979). The plasters were used repeatedly throughout the growth of the child. Surgery was performed only in patients whose equinus deformity could not be managed by plaster alone. Of 194 patients, 61 per cent were treated by plaster alone and 23 per cent had plaster and surgery. Westin pointed out that one disadvantage of plaster was 'problems with atrophy' (p.162).

This observation of induced muscle atrophy after plaster immobilization is probably one explanation why inhibitive or any other immobilization reduces 'tone'. Anyone who has treated children or adults in lower-limb plasters knows that weakness of the triceps surae is an inevitable result. Cooper (1972), in a landmark paper on the effects of immobilization on muscle in cats, clearly demonstrated distinct degeneration of muscle fibres, which began to regenerate one week after immobilization was discontinued.

Tabary *et al.* (1972) found structural changes in the cat soleus muscle after experimental immobilization. Herbison *et al.* (1978) also documented fibre atrophy in the gastrocnemius, soleus and plantaris muscles in rats after cast immobilization. Rosemeyer and Stüz (1977) studied 40 patients in whom one lower limb was immobilized in plaster in periods from three to 12 weeks. Mechanical and electrical investigations of the muscles showed changes after immobilization. After 12 and 24 weeks of remobilization the muscle mass remained diminished. Sziklai and Grof (1981) measured energy metabolites in the skeletal muscles of rabbits whose limbs were immobilized in plaster for one and six weeks. They noted lower energy levels at one week, and then a steady state reflected by the measurements of the high-energy phosphate content.

Although short-leg walking plaster casts have been successfully used in reversing the gait pattern of habitual toe-walkers (Griffin *et al.* 1977), we cannot transfer this experience to that of spastic paralysis. Habitual toe-walkers have no clinical or electromyographic evidence of spastic paralysis. I have not used plaster-cast treatment in children with cerebral palsy. The method seems tedious and time-consuming, and has the usual risks of skin pressure sores and blisters (Westin and Dye 1983).

Is there a neurological explanation for the claimed results? Conrad *et al.* (1983) used electromyographic gait analysis, and found that bilateral local anaesthetic blocks of the plantar nerves had no effect on the normal electromyographic pattern of the gastrocnemii. The conclusion was that afferents have no effect on the gait pattern itself, and the CNS stabilizes balance at the expense of walking speed.

In children who have dynamic equinus, I prefer to use rigid plaster ankle-foot orthoses; if the orthosis cannot resist the degree of spasticity, myoneural 45 per cent alcohol blocks of the gastrocnemius muscle have been helpful. As the child develops better equilibrium reactions, improvement in foot equinus can occur. If the hamstring muscles are very spastic, posterior stability is threatened and balance is achieved by tiptoe posture which brings the centre of gravity of the trunk (located just anterior to the tenth thoracic vertebra—see Brunnstrom 1962) anterior to the base of support between the ankle joints. If there is a contracture of the triceps surae, I perform a sliding Achilles tendon lengthening rather than inducing atrophy by immobilization and stretching in plaster.

This long explanation and critique of 'inhibitive casts' has been written for the benefit of the orthopaedic surgeon who is asked to approve of such treatment and to engage in a discourse and not a polemic with the proposing therapist. It has become a very popular method in the USA and may have spread to other continents, since most therapy systems seem to be disseminated quite rapidly.

Walking aids
Walkers
Four-post aluminium frames, usually with small wheels in the front, are most commonly used in children who have dysequilibrium in all four planes (see Chapter

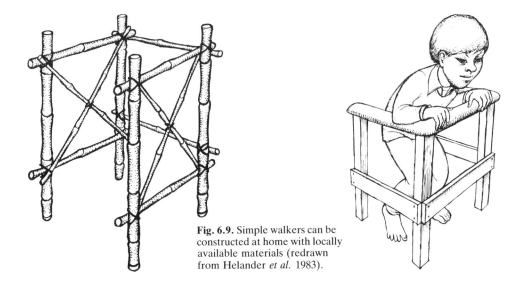

Fig. 6.9. Simple walkers can be constructed at home with locally available materials (redrawn from Helander *et al.* 1983).

5), and who can grasp the top sides of the frame. Most children prefer to have the walker in front of them (Fig. 6.9). Innovative therapists at one of our local medical therapy units have found the gait and posture better in some children when the walker is constructed with the closed end at the back, so that it follows the child.

The ring walkers have four wheels; the child sits on a seat or sling in the centre of the walker, or can be erect while using a reciprocal gait pattern. Many children seem merely to lean into such walkers: for children who cannot walk with aids, this may be a good way to gain some sense of self-mobility.

Holm *et al.* (1983) caution against the use of the walker in 'high-risk infants', because theoretically it might interfere with the development of more mature balance reactions and should be deferred until such are established. They also worry that the walker may threaten success with the neurodevelopmental therapy (Bobath) by not allowing inhibition of abnormal reflexes (though as we have seen, the Bobaths are no longer so worried about such inhibition). Accidents due to infant walkers were reported by Kavanagh and Banco (1982).

The weight-relieving walker, first designed by Wally Motloch at the Rehabilitation Engineering Center at Stanford, was used for children with osteogenesis imperfecta. We subsequently found that it was very useful to provide hands-free walking in children who had minimal athetosis or spasticity but mainly ataxia (Fig.6.10).

Crutches and canes
Crutches are essential for cerebral-palsied children who have good lateral equilibrium reactions but deficient anterior and posterior ones (see Chapter 5). So crutches are used not so much for weight-bearing as to compensate for lack of balance. Because the need for balance is primary, the usual axillary crutches used by patients for non-weightbearing (as in a limb fracture) are not necessary in

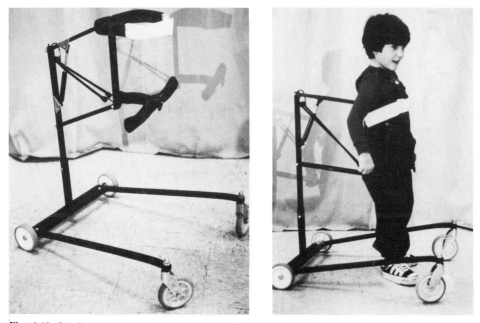

Fig. 6.10. Stanford weight-relieving walker provides walking with support. It is especially useful for primary ataxia.

cerebral palsy. Most use either a triceps cuff crutch with a hand support, or the Lofstrand-type crutch.

Quad canes have great stability and stand alone because of the four-post base. Patients generally walk more slowly with quad canes, but these are useful in those who seem to be borderline on balance ability.

Rose *et al.* (1985) studied the energy requirements in children with spastic diplegia and quadriplegia using either a walker or quad canes. By monitoring the heart rate, they found the mean heart rate while walking with walkers was 164 beats per minute, and with quad canes 157 beats per minute (compared to 114 beats per minute in normal children without assistive devices). With this measure of energy requirements, some of the children were more efficient with walkers and others with quad canes. The heart rate was closely correlated with the energy cost as measured with oxygen consumption.

The children in the heart-rate study had slower mean walking speeds (27 metres per minute with walkers and 20 metres per minute with canes, compared to the normal mean of 70 metres per minute). These slow walking speeds and high heart rates suggest a high physiological work-load. These data indicate how impractical it is to encourage (or force) disabled children to walk long distances with assistive devices. They need to avoid undue fatigue in order to accomplish other tasks of daily living as well as school work, learning, social life and community integration.

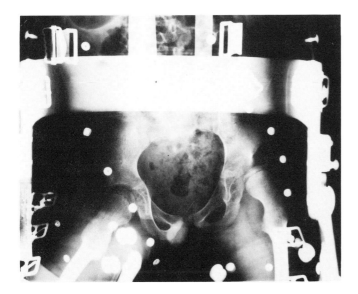

Fig. 6.11. Hip dislocation despite a 'full-control' brace.

Orthotics

Experience in the management of cerebral-palsied children with or without bracing leads to the conclusion that a brace has very little place in the management of cerebral palsy, provided the child is given adequate physiotherapy and the fixed deformity is prevented by good combined physiotherapy and surgery (Sharrard 1976).

Full-control bracing was popular 25 years ago (Stamp 1973). It has been abandoned by most experienced professionals in cerebral palsy. Although it was hoped that the child with cerebral palsy would eventually 'learn' how to walk correctly in the brace, no carry-over was ever noticed or reported. Nor did bracing prevent serious structural change. Hips dislocated even though the hip-control brace was worn all day (and presumably at night too, when this was the fashion) (Fig. 6.11).

In a study of 25 symmetrically spastic diplegic or quadriplegic children, in whom one limb only was braced, Sharrard (1965) found that the brace delayed deformity, but no longer than one year. The deformity then became as severe as the opposite unbraced limb (Sharrard 1976).

Lee (1982) reviewed 204 cerebral-palsied children and classified them according to the motor disorder and the extent of involvement. Regardless of spastic hemiplegia, diplegia or athetosis, bracing versus non-bracing was ineffective in preventing the need for surgery to correct deformities, in preventing recurrences after surgery, or improving the gait.

Very few, if any, adults continue with orthoses—especially in the case of athetosis, in which an orthosis seems logical to control involuntary movements (Sharrard 1976). And we had the identical experience as Sharrard when full-control

175

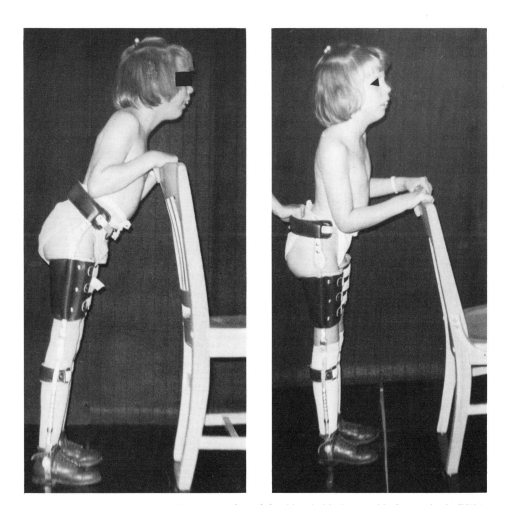

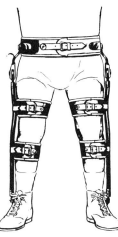

Fig. 6.12. *Above left:* old-style hip-knee-ankle-foot orthosis (HKA-FO) used to control hip flexion, adduction and internal rotation. With hip joint unlocked, hip-flexion spasticity pulls trunk forward. *Above right:* with hip-joint locked, posture adapted to the hip-flexion contracture by increased anterior inclination of pelvis and lumbar lordosis.

Fig. 6.13. Outmoded cable twister orthosis. It fails to control or correct hip internal rotation deformities.

and extensive bracing was imposed on children. When the parents were assured of our non-punitive attitudes, the majority removed the braces after school so that the child 'could play and run about'. I have not used night splinting in an attempt to prevent structural change (*e.g.* contracture of the triceps surae or hamstrings). Our analysis of recurrence of the triceps surae contracture after Achilles tendon lengthening, in patients in whom we did not use day or night splinting postoperatively, is convincing evidence that this added management is not often necessary (Lee and Bleck 1980). Our recurrence rate of 9 per cent after Achilles tendon lengthening compared favourably with others (usually stated to be about 6 per cent). This means that if we had enforced night splinting we would have imposed unnecessary management 91 per cent of the time!

Sharrard (1976) reported a study of spastic equinus in 50 children, none of whom had bracing and all of whom had similar physical therapy. A correlation between the development of deformity and the degree of calf-muscle spasticity was not significant. He found a correlation between the weakness of ankle dorsiflexor power and the development of equinus.

Another tool to help overcome equinus was a sort of short aluminium ski attached to the plantar aspect of the shoe with French leather ski bindings. It appeared to be successful in stretching contractures of the triceps surae (Hanks and MacFarlane 1969). So why not try cross-country skis, or Swedish roll skis when there is no snow, and practise on paved roads or fibre-glass tracks through the forest?

The Forestown boot, described by Craig and Mathias (1977), is another way to control equinus. Although the boot is leather, it seems sufficiently rigid to restrain plantar flexion similar to plaster.

Hip-knee-ankle-foot orthoses (HKAFO)

Occasionally we have used a Garrett temporary hip-abduction orthosis in an infant or toddler, in whom the signs of spasticity seem to be diminishing and who have no contracture but only dynamic adduction (Garrett *et al.* 1966). The 'abduction pants' described by Hare (1977) seem adequate for this purpose; the pants are a large H-shaped diaper with a foam centre of maximum width to obtain abduction of the hips. This appears similar to the Friejka pillow splint, which was used for congenital dysplasia of the hips.

Hip-flexion contracture has not been controlled with hip-knee-ankle orthoses which can be locked at the hip and knee in extension. The only change this orthosis will make is on the pelvis, as it is forced into anterior inclination, and concomitant lumbar lordosis to compensate for the hip-flexion contracture (Fig. 6.12).

Cable twister orthotics have not corrected a hip internal-rotation deformity in cerebral palsy (or for that matter in a non-paralytic hip internal-rotation due to excessive femoral anteversion). Instead the orthosis may only reinforce the tendency to develop excessive external (lateral) tibial fibular torsion (Fig. 6.13).

Knee-ankle-foot orthoses (KAFO)

The knee-ankle-foot orthosis with a drop-lock at the knee joint is occasionally

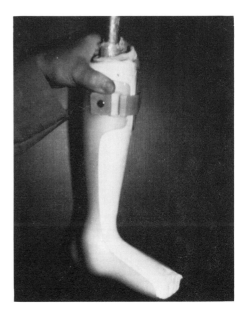

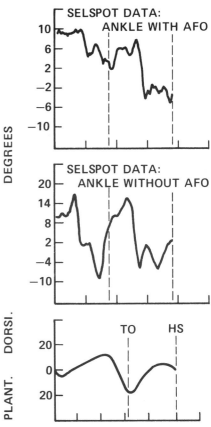

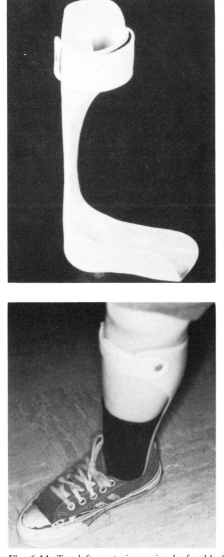

Fig. 6.14. *Top left:* posterior spring-leaf ankle-foot
orthosis (AFO). Not very useful if gastrocnemius-
soleus muscle is very spastic; more useful for
foot-drop due to flaccid lower motoneuron paralysis. *Top right:* rigid plastic ankle-foot orthosis
constructed from a positive mold of limb with foot
in desired position. *Above:* plastic ankle-foot orthosis can be worn with any shoe. *Right:* measurement
of ankle plantar and dorsiflexion by photoelectronic
method during level walking with and without
ankle-foot orthosis. Orthosis effectively stops
stance-phase plantar flexion (to left of center
broken line). Bottom is normal range of motion.
TO = toe-off; HS = heel strike.

178

useful in a child who has just begun to walk and whose knees are flexed more than 15° during the stance phase of gait, and in whom the hamstring spasticity and contracture can possibly be tolerated for function and counterbalanced by increasing spasticity of the quadriceps.

After hamstring lengthening and posterior capsulotomy of the knee joint in older children, knee orthoses are useful to control excessive flexion: particularly if little quadriceps spasticity seems to be present. An orthosis like this is usually used from six to 12 months postoperatively until the patient regains quadriceps strength and confidence during gait. Once walking can be done with the knee unlocked, and extension of the joint occurs in the stance phase, the orthosis is no longer required.

Knee hyperextension deformity (*genu recurvatum*) can sometimes be managed with a rigid plastic ankle-foot orthosis with the foot dorsiflexed, providing the ankle does have a sufficient range of dorsiflexion (at least 5° or more with the knee extended and the foot held in varus—see Rosenthal 1975).

Ankle-foot orthosis (AFO)

The plastic molded ankle-foot orthosis is the commonest support in cerebral palsy (Staros and LeBlanc 1975, Hoffer and Koffman 1980, Rosenthal 1984, Taylor and Kling 1984). The plastic should be rigid in spastic paralysis, rather than the flexible or posterior spring-leaf type which is used in flaccid paralysis for a 'drop foot'.

The modern plastic orthosis is so useful because all motions of the foot and ankle can be controlled; and if the spasticity is not too great, equinus, varus and valgus can be controlled. The orthotist makes the orthosis from a negative plaster shell made with the foot held in the corrected position. A positive plaster mold is made from this, and the heat-softened plastic sheet is drawn over it by vacuum and then trimmed to the finished product. It can be worn over a stocking in an ordinary shoe (Fig. 6.14).

I have not found the plastic ankle-foot orthosis useful in severe spastic valgus deformities. I have had some success in holding a severe valgus deformity in the old-style single medial tubular steel upright fitted into the channel of a high-top shoe (Bolkert 1979) (Fig. 6.15). Even if the deformity does not correct, it might be held until the child is old enough for surgical correction (usually not before six or seven).

Foot orthoses (FO)

ARCH SUPPORT TYPES

Plastic, felt or metal arch supports have not been useful in correcting either valgus or varus deformities in spastic or athetoid types of cerebral palsy. The University of California Biomechanics Laboratory (UCBL) plastic shoe insert has not been successful in correcting spastic valgus deformities (Bleck and Berzins 1977). The popular sports medicine type of 'orthotic' has not been useful in children with cerebral palsy, although I have seen a few children who had these prescribed by foot-problem practitioners.

179

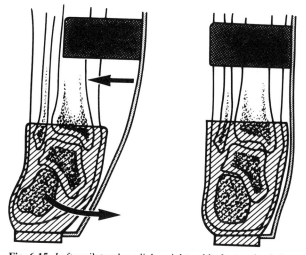

Fig. 6.15. *Left:* unilateral medial upright ankle-foot orthosis for pes valgus. The mechanism of the brace is demonstrated. As the medial upright (which can be bent more medially for more correction) approximates the calf, a valgus force is exerted on the heel through the channel in the shoe. A lateral T-strap exerts no correction; it holds the upright in the shoe channel. A lateral upright is used for a varus foot. *Right:* orthosis fixed to leg by the calf band, to correct the foot position.

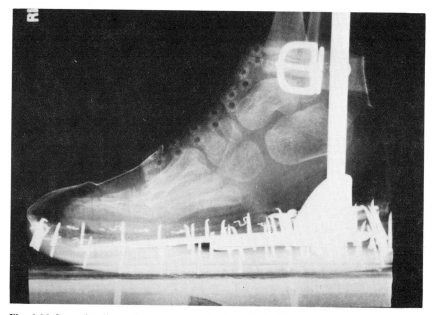

Fig. 6.16. Lateral radiograph of foot and ankle in a child with spastic equinus and wearing a 90° ankle stop to dorsiflexion. The equinus is conveniently hidden in the high top shoe.

180

Sneakers (tennis shoes, 'trainers' or jogging shoes) provide good ground-contact and possibly force more muscle co-ordination. Hiking-boots with crêpe or heavy rubber soles seem to help ankle stability, possibly by decreasing the range of ankle plantar and dorsiflexion so that postural adaptation and control by the anterior tibial and the gastrocnemius-soleus muscles need not be as great; boots also add a bit of weight, and might help control balance.

I have found no use for corrective or orthopaedic shoes (Bleck 1971). The high-top 'orthopaedic' shoe, so often forced on the children of yesteryear with all sorts of orthopaedic disabilities (real or imagined), is ideal to hide the deformity (Fig. 6.16). The theory of the orthopaedic shoe is best explained by Perry (1974): 'If you don't see it, it's not there'.

What is so bad about cerebral-palsied children going barefoot? Quite a few children have never gone without shoes, even in the home on thick pile carpets! As a result, I find these children's feet super-sensitive to touch; they often complain of painful feet when barefoot, and the plantar skin is devoid of callous. The soles of their feet are like a baby's buttocks. Shoes are to feet what gloves are to the hands. When the ground environment is safe, going barefoot in the home, in the sand at the beach and on the lawn, seems a rational and natural way to stress the plantar skin and fat so that hypertrophy occurs and sensitivity decreases. European grandmothers may not like such advice, even though it would seem unnecessary and obvious to people in South-East Asia and Polynesia. Standing and walking barefoot does not cause 'fallen arches'!

Biofeedback devices
Biofeedback means that the patient by some mechanical-electrical device is able to monitor the action performed. Auditory feedback is more correctly called augmented feedback. In the past decade the technique has captured the imagination of professionals who deal with locomotor system disorders (Russell *et al.* 1976, Harrison 1977). Biofeedback devices have been used for a variety of problems in children with cerebral palsy. The Ontario Crippled Children's Centre has been at the forefront of clinical investigations into head and joint position, jaw closure and postural alignment (Woolridge and McLaurin 1976). It was thought that the majority of patients could be trained with this technique, and that in some cases it carried over for sustained performance. Long-term clinical results have been lacking.

I can only report a few long-term anecdotal results. One was the behavioural training helmet used to control consistent neck-flexed posture in an eight-year-old boy who had spastic diplegia. When he flexed his head and neck, a telemetry control switch attached to the helmet automatically shut off his television screen. After about six months of such training, head control was maintained in a one-year follow-up.

Conrad and Bleck (1980) reported their results with auditory augmented feedback for dynamic equinus. The device was a pressure-sensitive on/off switch inside the shoe and under the heel (Fig. 6.17). The switch was connected to a

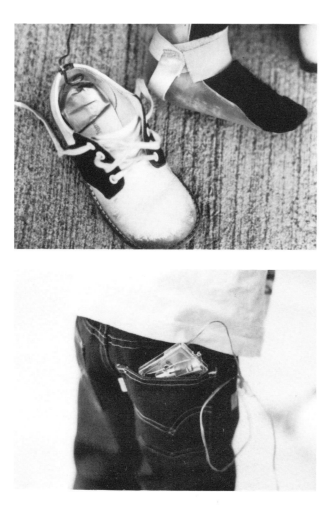

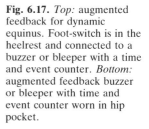

Fig. 6.17. *Top:* augmented feedback for dynamic equinus. Foot-switch is in the heelrest and connected to a buzzer or bleeper with a time and event counter. *Bottom:* augmented feedback buzzer or bleeper with time and event counter worn in hip pocket.

battery-powered bleeper. When the bleep was heard, the child knew that heel contact occurred. After instruction by the physical therapist, the device was used three hours per day for three months at home. This regimen appeared more effective than daily visits to a physical therapist for 'stretching' and 'gait training', or nagging by parents. All patients had dynamic equinus, *i.e.* no contracture of the triceps surae so that the ankle could be dorsiflexed with the foot in varus at least to neutral. The results in eight children (six with cerebral palsy, two idiopathic toe-walkers) were carefully analyzed with time and event counters, pedographs, and measured ranges of motion. Immediate follow-up at three months showed improvement in all when compared with the untreated foot: the range of dorsiflexion improved ($p<0.001$), the total accumulated heel-down position was 90 per cent ($p<0.001$) and the total heel strikes increased ($p<0.01$). At longer follow-up of three months to one year (mean:5.7 months) without the auditory signal, the total heel-down time improved 45 per cent from the pretreatment status. We think this method is worthwhile in patients over four years of age, who have mild spasticity of the triceps surae and no contracture of the muscle—a highly selected group to be sure.

Seeger *et al.* (1981) reported a practically identical auditory feedback device for dynamic equinus in four girls with spastic hemiplegia. All had good results. But Seeger and Caudry (1983) reported on the long-term efficacy of this method, and found that the results were not maintained after 24 to 28 months.

Kassover *et al.* (1984) used essentially the same method in four patients with spastic diplegia and equinus. They reported significant and dramatic improvement within three weeks of this treatment.

Unless there are more clinical outcome studies than have been published to date, we can conclude that biofeedback methods have not fulfilled their initial promise in motor behavioural modification of cerebral palsy. But I think it is worthwhile as a trial in cases of dynamic equinus—it does no harm and is inexpensive as a therapeutic modality.

Rehabilitation engineering

The application of science and technology to the needs of the physically handicapped has grown and become more and more accepted as the best means to achieve functional goals in severely handicapped persons, such as those with total body involvement (spastic or athetoid). For some patients, simple adaptive equipment designed and recommended by an occupational therapist will be sufficient. In the more severely disabled, a team of electrical and mechanical engineers or special rehabilitation engineers, occupational therapists, speech pathologists, and orthotists are required to analyze the patient's functional capacity and the ability to utilize various standard commercially available devices and the necessity to custom-design appropriate interfaces and controls (Bleck 1977*a*, *b*, 1978, 1979, 1982, 1984, 1985).

Non-verbal communication methods

Communication is a basic human need. In those individuals who cannot verbalize, the solution has been the rapid development of non-oral methods of communication.

THE HAND

The simplest method of non-oral communication has been with sign-language developed for the deaf. However, most non-verbal children with cerebral palsy do not have the finger dexterity necessary to use sign-language.

SYMBOL LANGUAGE

Credit goes to Mrs Shirley McNaughton for demonstrating that non-verbal children had inner language to be tapped by the use of symbol language devised by Bliss

183

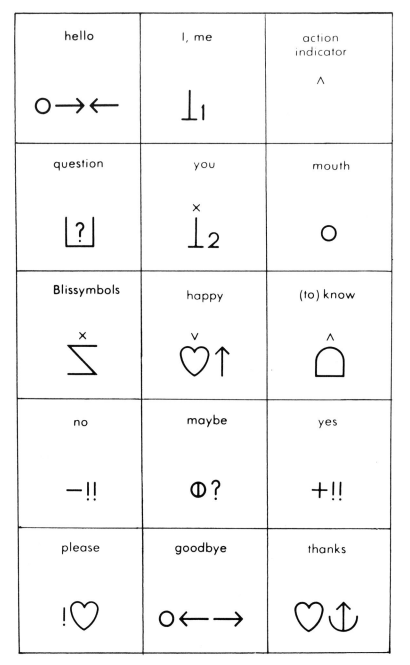

Fig. 6.18. Example of Bliss symbol language (reproduced by permission from McNaughton 1982).

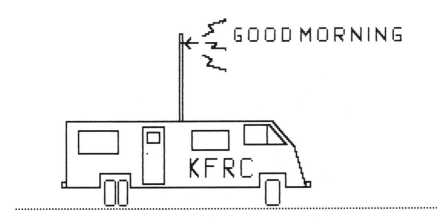

The song is true. Only the Good Die Young. Because 2 of my good friends died in the past 2 years.

My first friend died in the fall of '81'. He went to school with me at Fremont Older. I remember that he could walk , but I didn't know him very well. When we went to Monroe Jr. High he got hassled from the other kids from Chandler Tripp. I felt sorry for him. I got to know him very well..
....

At the High School they had a wheelchair soccer team, he and I were one it. He was the best player on the team. We went to some of the High School footb all games together. In his last year of High School he died. When I go to bed I think of all the good times we had. I will get sad and tears start forming in my eyes and I wish that he didn't die, because he was my best friend .

Fig. 6.19. *Top:* computer-generated drawing by 17-year-old who is total body involved, non-verbal, and uses head controls. *Bottom:* first written communication by the 17-year-old total body involved man, generated by him on his special system which included an Apple II plus computer.

(1965) and modified by McNaughton and her group at the Ontario Crippled Children's Centre in Toronto, Canada (McNaughton 1977, 1982) (Fig. 6.18).

COMMUNICATION DEVICES
Communication aids are commercially available, and new ones continue to appear on the market. These can be categorized as providing (i) visual outputs, (ii) printed outputs, and (iii) speech outputs.

The latter is a synthetic voice which satisfies the psychological needs of many non-verbal children and adults (LeBlanc 1982). The computer has revolutionized the ability of children to communicate their thoughts and feelings; some have also exercised their latent artistic talents (Fig. 6.19), and newsletters are available on the state of this technology and its availability.

Activities of daily living aids
Adaptive equipment and devices have proliferated for eating, toileting and

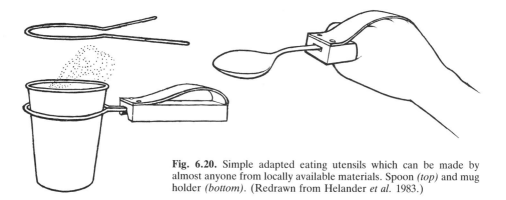

Fig. 6.20. Simple adapted eating utensils which can be made by almost anyone from locally available materials. Spoon *(top)* and mug holder *(bottom)*. (Redrawn from Helander *et al.* 1983.)

bathing; commercially available devices can be found in catalogues, trade literature and central data bases. Some simple aids can be made at home or in the local community by almost anyone with a minimum of manual skills (Fig. 6.20).

Architectural and community barriers (*e.g.* curbless street crossings) continue to be eliminated in North America and European countries. Patients just need the expertise of a rehabilitation engineering team to advise them on appropriate equipment, to make required adaptations, and (of great importance) to advise them on financial considerations (McCollough 1985).

Mobility devices
Mobility is vital for community integration. While walking is the least complicated means of mobility, we know it is not practical for many who have cerebral palsy.

For play and exercise, special devices are useful for some children who have insufficient balance mechanisms and require compensation (Letts *et al.* 1976). Steerable walkers and special backward-peddling tricycles, to make use of the dominant extensor pattern, may be practical for some children. All sorts of innovative mobility play equipment have been designed and made. Bicycles with training wheels are the most common adaptation for children who can pedal but lack adequate postural balance.

WHEELCHAIRS
Due to the growing awareness of the handicapped as part of our society and humanity, and their need for mobility in order to achieve social integration, there has been a rapid increase in the acceptability of the wheelchair in Western countries. Urbanization and concrete paving have also made the wheelchair feasible. This may not be the case in less developed countries.

Wheelchairs can be either hand-driven or power-driven. Hand-driven types are for children who have good function in both upper limbs and can move the chair with efficiency and speed. Many children who use walkers or crutches for household and neighbourhood mobility find wheelchairs essential for traveling longer distances. A wheelchair conserves energy; crutches use it (Campbell and Ball 1978, Fisher and Patterson 1981). The energy expended when using a manual

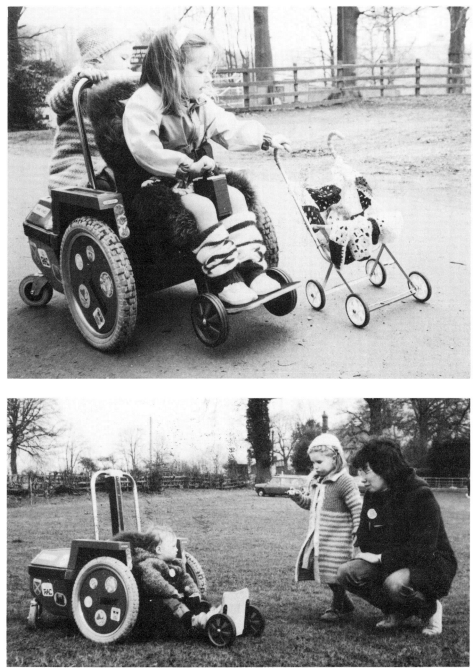

Fig. 6.21. A new powered wheelchair for children, adjustable from age 19 months to 12 years. *Top:* note heavy-duty tires. This chair can handle uneven ground, muddy roads, gravel and grass, and is ideal for rural areas as well as cities. *Bottom:* seat can be lowered to near the ground with power controls, so that child can get out of the chair. (Courtesy of Everaids Ltd., Cambridge, England.)

187

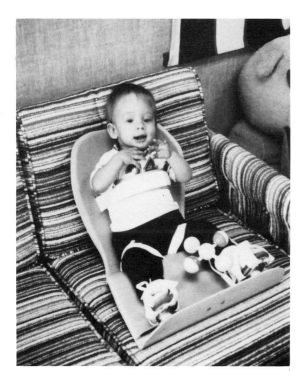

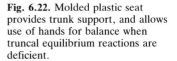

Fig. 6.22. Molded plastic seat provides trunk support, and allows use of hands for balance when truncal equilibrium reactions are deficient.

wheelchair is comparable to that used by normal persons when walking on level surfaces (Cerny 1978).

A great choice of manual wheelchairs is available, depending on personal needs. There are lightweight sport chairs for play and games, and heavy-duty chairs for large-bodied people who are very active. Two chairs are often desirable: one for sport and quick transport into an automobile, and the other for everyday school or work. We do not recommend a manual chair for those who have use of only one upper limb. Alternating control between the right and left upper limbs is necessary to drive a manual chair. The adaptive chair for one-hand operators (a 'hemiplegic' chair) is complex, cumbersome and generally not optimally functional. For these individuals we unequivocally recommend an electrically powered wheelchair.

ELECTRIC WHEELCHAIRS

Electric-powered wheelchairs now come in a variety of designs and sizes. Portable electric wheelchairs for children were first produced by ABEC*, and were responsible for giving independence and mobility to total body involved children with cerebral palsy. We have prescribed electric carts for small children, as young as age three and four years. All children learn control of the chair, usually within an hour. All chairs come with joystick controls. Those who cannot use a joystick can

*(Registered trademark) ABEC Electric Wheelchair Inc., USA and United Kingdom.

188

have pressure-sensitive hand- or finger-control switches. In fact any part of the body that the patient can move voluntarily can be linked to a control of the powered chair (and also to control communication devices). Improvements in powered chairs continue apace (Fig. 6.21).

SEATING

Children who have no trunk control must constantly use their upper limbs for balance; this necessity precludes the functional use of their hands. Seat-inserts for wheelchairs have become an accepted technology for children and adults with cerebral palsy. Many different designs and methods of construction have been developed (Cristarella 1975, Motloch 1977, Barber 1978, Carlson and Winter 1978, Carrington 1978, Ring *et al.* 1978, Trefler *et al.* 1978, Holte 1980, Fulford *et al.* 1982, Nwaobi *et al.* 1983, Craig *et al.* 1984). We prefer a modular plastic seat-insert, padded with foam material and upholstered with fabric (Fig. 6.22).

Formerly most seats were constructed to flex the hips beyond 90° in varying slopes, to reduce the extensor pattern in total body involved children and thus improve hand function. Seeger *et al.* (1984), in a sophisticated analysis of hand function by the ability to control a joystick and target an object, found that the hip-flexion position made no significant difference. They concluded that stability and comfort were more important.

COSTS

The cost of a powered wheelchair and seating system for severely disabled persons were analyzed by Kohn *et al.* (1983). The mean use time was 10 hours per day for 30.9 months. The cost per patient was $1.50 per day. The system provided was judged optimal by 79 per cent of the 196 patients in the study; and the remaining 21 per cent, who thought the effectiveness was suboptimal, could think of no other choice to accomplish the mobility desired. The cost-effectiveness of their mobility and seating was assessed in human terms and cannot be ignored: 'Family enjoys more social life' (81 per cent); 'more contact with peers' (67 per cent); and 'allows more normal function' (62 per cent). These costs have to be weighed against the costs of long-term ineffective (and generally not cost-accountable) therapies which hope somehow to reprogram the brain and stimulate the child to walk. The cost to a parent who has to attend the child day-in and day-out (including weekends when the medical team is off) is another calculation missing in cost considerations by fiscal administrators. If, by use of comfortable and effective seating and mobility equipment, a child can remain at home rather than in a State long-term care institution, the argument about cost should become moot.

TRAVEL AND TRANSPORTATION

Of all the factors that limit adult independence and employment, the inability to get out of the home is the most important (Bachman 1972). Root (1977) found that only 16 per cent of the total body involved persons with cerebral palsy had the capability or means for independent travel.

Public transport presents many obstacles for the severely handicapped

(Bourgeois *et al.* 1977). Even though there has been much pressure to improve access to public transport, the cost will probably always preclude widespread alterations of public systems to accommodate all handicapped persons. In small villages the powered electric wheelchair and all sorts of small electric-powered vehicles may provide all the local transportation necessary for the individual person. In this regard, it is probably true that the environment does determine the extent of the handicap (Cherpin *et al.* 1985).

We have found that modern autovans and buses equipped with ramps or hydraulic lifts are the best mode of travel for urban and inter-urban transportation. Not all persons with cerebral palsy will be able to operate a motor vehicle independently. Special testing for depth perception, direction sense and motor control are required and need to be done in special motor-vehicle operation assessment centres. If the tests confirm a person's potential to operate a vehicle, special instruction is essential. Persons who have major spastic involvement of the lower limbs but minor motor inco-ordination in the upper limbs (spastic diplegia or hemiplegia) can usually be successful and safe drivers, with hand controls that can be adapted to any automobile. Such adaptations are usual and customary for persons who have traumatic spinal paraplegia or quadriplegia, various types of flaccid paralysis, rheumatoid arthritis and osteogenesis imperfecta.

Orthopaedic surgery

Today the orthopaedic surgeons seem to have got it just about right (Tizard 1980).

We accept the compliment, despite what seemed like a negative comment in Goldkamp's (1984) paper on treatment effectiveness in cerebral palsy. He studied the functional outcomes of 53 children with cerebral palsy who began treatment at age 3.9 years and were followed to the age of 18.8 years. Physical therapy treatments (mainly neurodevelopmental) did not improve function for activities of daily living, and the surgery results were reported as 'less than good' in 24 per cent. But even in this small sample, 76 per cent seem to have had good results from surgery. With careful preoperative analysis, correct selection of surgical procedure, proper surgical technique and follow-up care, and when the aims of surgery are clearly defined, good results should be greater than 80 per cent and probably 90 per cent.

In a study of 3460 records of patients who had surgery for cerebral palsy from 1966 to 1983 in Brasilia, Brazil (Campos da Paz Jr *et al.* 1984), 274 post-surgical patients were found for follow-up study. The relapse rate of deformity, after soft tissue procedures such as hamstring lengthening, varied from 40 to 67 per cent. Interestingly, adductor tenotomies had good results up to four years in the follow-up study. They speculated that a complex interaction occurs between the deformity, altered perception and brain processing. Theoretically, new mechanisms of compensation could be triggered due to operative treatment. Their question was how far we should go in interfering with 'the natural course' of the condition.

At the risk of generalizing, my own follow-up studies make me more optimistic

190

TABLE 6.III

Recurrence and overcorrection of deformities after orthopaedic surgery, eight- to 18-year follow-up (mean 12 years)
Spastic diplegia—ambulatory

Type of surgery	N	Recurrence	Overcorrection
Adductor longus and gracilis myotomy, anterior branch obturator neurectomy	92	0 (<20° abduction*)	1 (>10° abduction during stance**) = 1%
Hamstring lengthening	79	4 (>15° flexion during stance) = 4%	5 (>10° recurvatum of knee) = 6%
Achilles tendon sliding lengthening (Hoke)	50	5 = 9%	1 (calcaneus) = 2%
Iliopsoas recession	25	1 = 4%†	0

*Passive range of hip abduction with hip extended
**Stance phase of the gait cycle
†One had no correction of the hip flexion deformity: 60° preoperatively and postoperatively.

about the effects of orthopaedic surgery. From 1955 to 1979 we had 693 patients who were being followed. This group included patients who had orthopaedic surgery. By 1984 we had follow-ups of surgery that ranged from eight to 18 years (mean 12 years). The recurrence rates for specific surgeries and overcorrections are delineated in Table 6.III.

In the study by Campos da Paz Jr *et al.* (1984), 40 per cent developed *genu recurvatum* after hamstring transfer. It did not take me long (two cases) to realize that transferring too many of the hamstrings might cause overactivity of the spastic quadriceps and a non-functional knee gait—straight but stiff. This means that outcome studies depend not only upon the type of surgery chosen, but also on the indications for surgery, the preoperative analysis for decision-making, and the type of patient (45 per cent were quadriplegic in the 1984 report by Campos da Paz *et al.*). Campos da Paz is probably correct to say that sudden alteration of a long-standing deformity does disturb the person's self-perception.

Studies and writings on the development of body-image strongly suggest that it is not fully developed in normal children until late childhood (Eiser and Patterson 1983, van der Velde 1985). Body-image may have important clinical implications (Bauman 1981). Apparently its importance in paediatric orthopaedic surgical procedures has been recognized by at least one orthopaedic service in a children's hospital (Letts *et al.* 1983). They have implemented a program of preoperative play with puppets and dolls, to prepare the child for loss of part of a limb or its sudden alteration by surgery. If at all possible, orthopaedic surgery should probably not be delayed in cerebral palsy until skeletal maturity has been reached and adolescent body-image and concern is at its height. To my knowledge, body-image studies have not been done in children with cerebral palsy.

The progression of structural changes in the joints, despite assiduous therapy and bracing, has been evident when patients have been followed for long periods. If a child is followed only to age 15 or 16 years, physicians and therapists might have an illusion that structural changes in childhood and early adolescence are not significant. Those who have followed patients for longer periods know that a painless subluxation of the hip in a crutch-walking child may not jeopardize mobility due to the pain of degenerative arthritis until after age 18 years. Similarly, a dislocated hip may not be painful until after age 15 years. Orthopaedic surgery deferred until later adolescence is more difficult, more complicated and has a greater incidence of postoperative psychological problems (Williams 1977). In Goldkamp's follow-up study (1984), 17 of the 53 patients with cerebral palsy needed psychiatric assistance (32 per cent). The reason for this high incidence of psychiatric problems with and without surgery in adolescent patients is not explained. It may be that overemphasis on the disease-oriented and ineffective treatments in their childhood years has thwarted their psychological development. Reality occurs when the cerebral-palsied child becomes an adult with the same cerebral palsy. The struggle to overcome the disease may then be recognized as time wasted.

Timing of orthopaedic surgery
THE PRESCHOOL CHILD
I recommend that surgery for intended functional improvement of gait be deferred until the child with a good prognosis for walking is actually walking independently or with walking aids. Samilson and Hoffer (1975) made the valid point of deferring surgery in the first three to four years because it was difficult to know what the main problem would be. They also advised against upper-limb surgery until age five or six years, so that selective control and sensation could be ascertained.

If the child has a good prognosis for ambulation, surgery will not hasten its development: although if one fortuitously performs the operation just when central nervous system maturation occurs, walking may begin very shortly after the surgery. If the surgeon wants to be a 'miracle worker', this is the time to do surgery. For example almost all spastic hemiplegic children walk by age 18 to 21 months.

The preschool child may be operated on, however, if structural changes develop—especially in the hip. Early subluxation can be prevented in most cases from developing into persistent subluxation and secondary acetabular dysplasia or dislocation (almost always in children who are non-walkers) if surgery is done before the age of five years. Another example of structural change for which surgery would be considered is a contracture of the hamstring muscles with a contracture of the knee joint; these indications are as rare as those for lengthening of the Achilles tendon in these young children.

The locomotor prognosis has to be kept in mind when considering the type of surgery in subluxation of the hip. If the child has a good prognosis, an iliopsoas lengthening or recession might be preferable to an iliopsoas tenotomy, which could permanently weaken hip flexion. But if the prognosis is poor, then iliopsoas tenotomy could be the best choice because hip-flexion weakness may have no long-term functional significance in a child who will be dependent upon a wheelchair.

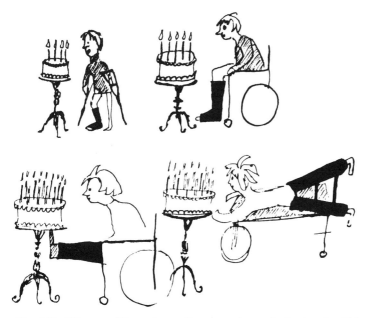

Fig. 6.23. When possible, orthopaedic surgery in cerebral palsy should be done at one stage. This cartoon depicts the life of the cerebral-palsied child—an operation and a plaster cast, with birthdays. (Courtesy of the artist, Mercer Rang MD, Toronto.)

THE SCHOOL-AGE CHILD

The optimum time for lower-limb surgery in the ambulatory child seems to be between the ages of five and seven years. At this time the gait pattern can be analyzed and decisions made on the basis of desired functional improvement. For example, a passive stretch test may indicate contracted hamstring muscles. But when the child walks, knee flexion during stance phase may be less than 10° due to the counterbalancing effect of the spastic quadriceps. As a result of such observations, hamstring lengthening need not be considered.

With careful and repeated analysis by examinations and recognition of potential structural skeletal changes, most soft-tissue surgery can be performed at one time and at as many levels as required (Norlin and Thaczok 1985) (Fig. 6.23). When the postoperative immobilization entails limited time in a plaster (usually three to six weeks), and early mobilization even in plaster within two to five days postoperatively, postoperative rehabilitation has not been unduly prolonged (Sussman and Cusick 1981). Three to six months of supervision by a physical therapist is often all that is necessary. Short-term intensive supervised therapeutic exercise and functional training by the therapist is more effective than long-term rehabilitative training sessions once a week.

THE ADOLESCENT AND ADULT

In skeletally mature persons, fixed contracture and permanent skeletal changes are

193

the most frequent indications for surgery. We have found good responses to soft-tissue surgery in adults with spastic cerebral palsy, particularly for improved gait function (Goldner 1985). The principles and practice of surgery in these cases are identical to that used in children. Adults who have no flexion contracture of the knee beyond 10° are amazed at the functional improvement in their gait due to increasing stride-length following fractional hamstring lengthening. The same has held true for adductor myotomy. Adults who have flexion contractures of the hip, resultant compensatory anterior inclination of the pelvis and constant low back pain due to the lumbar lordosis, have obtained relief of the back pain after iliopsoas tendon lengthening.

Severe skeletal changes in adults (*e.g.* subluxation of the hip and degenerative arthritis or flexion contracture of the knee beyond 15° and painful patellar-femoral arthritis) need bone surgery combined with tendon lengthenings or tenotomies to restore function.

In a small study referred to in a recent publication by Thomas *et al.* (1985) on the needs of physically handicapped adults, 11 per cent required orthopaedic surgery.

Indications for orthopaedic surgery
The major indication for orthopaedic surgery in children with cerebral palsy is to prevent structural changes of the limbs and trunk which may become disabling in later life.

The indications for surgery to improve function needs more discernment. For those who walk either independently or with aids, surgery for functional improvement is usually in the hip, knee and foot. For those who do not walk, the functional goal will be to maintain or improve the ability for either assistive or self-transfer from the wheelchair. Straightening a knee-flexion contracture is justifiable in these cases, as is a corrective arthrodesis of a severe foot deformity. The patient who can only sit in a wheelchair also needs to maintain this function, which can be destroyed by an uncorrected hip dislocation or scoliosis.

Plastic surgery for drooling
Other than orthopaedic and ophthalmic surgery, plastic surgery has a rôle in cerebral palsy in the treatment of drooling (excessive salivation). I mention this here because parents expect the orthopaedic surgeon to have knowledge of surgical treatment in general.

Drooling is common in babies and young children. When it persists into mid-childhood and beyond, it becomes distressing for parents and sometimes the aware child. Approximately 10 per cent of the cerebral-palsied population have persistent drooling (Koheil *et al.* 1985). Excessive salivation that requires the constant use of a bib is a hindrance to social integration. Head control is important in achieving a good result from the procedures designed to reduce salivation.

Recently biofeedback methods have been reported as promising in relieving drooling. 11 of 12 patients treated with biofeedback techniques were improved (Koheil *et al.* 1985). Tympanic neurectomy and chorda tympanectomy were proposed as a method of alleviating the condition. However, Pariser *et al.* (1978) found an unacceptable recurrence of the drooling with these procedures.

Parotid duct relocation to the tonsillar fossa, originally described by Wilke (1967), has had reasonably good results. Messingill (1978) observed decreased salivation in six of eight patients who had the parotid duct relocation. Tongue function during swallowing, as visualized by cinefluoragraphy, was helpful in prognosis when correlated with the postoperative results. The age when the procedure was performed varied from six to 22 years (mean 12.6 years).

Better results seem to be achieved with parotid duct transplantation and submandibular salivary gland excision (Chait and Kessler 1979, Morgan *et al.* 1981).

Preparation of the child and parents for surgery
The basis of all human relationships is trust. Above all, the child and parents must feel secure with the surgeon. Distrust and anxiety will complicate the postoperative course and can compromise the result by placing the surgeon on the defensive. Defensive attitudes can cause errors in judgement. One does not go to a surgeon (or any physician for that matter) in order to dictate the procedure or method of management. If the surgeon discerns distrust and anxiety, it is better not to do the surgery—or at least defer it until more conducive attitudes prevail.

If possible, it is best for the child to become familiar with the physical therapist for three to six months prior to surgery. The therapist will need the full co-operation of the child in the period of postoperative rehabilitation. The therapist can also assist the surgeon in a preoperative analysis of the many-faceted aspects of the motor disorder: the gait pattern, ranges of motion of joints, the behaviour of the child and the attitude of the parents. The therapist can supplement the physician's task by explaining the reasons for surgery to the child and parents. Ideally the therapist would be familiar with the general surgical plan, the operative procedures and the postoperative rehabilitation plan.

Preoperative preparation of the child takes time, but is rewarding in decreasing postoperative psychological complications and a longer than usual hospital stay (Ferguson 1979, Wolfer and Visintainer 1979). At Children's Hospital at Stanford we have had a special preoperative program with illustrated material, video and hospital play for the past 10 years. Barring physiological complications (*e.g.* postoperative infection), postoperative recovery has been smooth with very little persistent pain or spasm beyond the first 48 hours after surgery.

If we always practised what we preached, in adequately preparing children for surgery, they ought to be admitted to the hospital two or three days in advance. In this way the child would be able to integrate the radical change in his/her life, especially in the modern and highly complex hospital organization (Sylvester 1977). Due to steady progress in the application of biomedical science to the practice of surgery, hospital stays have steadily dropped in paediatric orthopaedic surgery. By 1984 our average hospital stay had decreased to a mean of 4.6 days.

The limited ability of the child to adjust to the myriad of personnel and procedures within eight to 10 hours before a major operation must be considered.

Because professional personnel are always 'so busy', there is considerable merit in Sylvester's (1977) suggestion that the patient should have a 'best friend' in the hospital. At Guy's Hospital in London, a 'best-friend' type person was employed (Parks 1977). This non-medical person was able to establish a supportive relationship with the child and parents, interpret and advise on hospital procedures, and say what was likely to happen next. We cannot forget that surgery is unique; instantly it sets in motion an irreversible biological change, and in cerebral palsy, a sudden structural change as well.

The surgeon can help prepare the child for surgery by talking directly to him or her and answering all questions by both parent and child. The child must be told: (i) that it is going to hurt, but medicines will be given to relieve the discomfort which usually lasts about 48 hours; (ii) where the incisions will be made in the skin; (iii) that a plaster will be applied, and what part of the limb will be enclosed; and (iv) how long the plaster will be on the limb, when walking will be permitted, whether crutches or a wheelchair will be necessary and the duration of non-weightbearing if this is required.

Drug therapy

> *The desire to take drugs is one of the distinguishing features between man and other animals* (Meyer Perlstein).

Postoperative analgesia must be assured, particularly during the first 48 hours. All too often inadequate dosages of narcotics are given. Muscle relaxants are no substitute for effective narcotics to relieve pain. We prefer administering narcotics intravenously through the intravenous line inserted by the anaesthesiologist at the time of surgery. Narcotics can be titrated according to the response. Small doses of intravenous narcotics are effective, but need repeating more frequently than if injected subcutaneously or intramuscularly. Table 6.IV is a guide for postoperative analgesia in children.

The late Dr Meyer Perlstein, when called upon to discuss drug therapy papers read at the annual meeting of the American Academy for Cerebral Palsy and Developmental Medicine, invariably said that alcohol was the best relaxing agent. Another Perlsteinism was: 'This study proves that most drug studies in cerebral palsy are not only not double-blind but are also myopic'.

Over the years many drugs have been promoted for muscle relaxation in cerebral palsy and then discarded because they were eventually found ineffective, primarily by the patient. Dantrolene sodium (Dantrium) was first released for use in 1974. After a flurry of high hopes that this medication would relieve spasticity or increase muscle tone in dystonic and tension athetosis, its use has gradually diminished. Our experience and study with Dantrolene in cerebral palsy was reported by Ford *et al.* (1976). Even though we found some objective improvement in the gait of hemiplegic and diplegic children, no child in the original study has continued its use: partly because of the resultant mental dullness, and the need to monitor liver function with sGOT blood-levels every three to four months. I have occasionally prescribed Dantrolene sodium postoperatively in children who had a

TABLE 6.IV

Postoperative analgesia for children*

Meperidine-Demerol	0.25 to 0.5mg per kg. IV
	Give slowly over two to three minutes
	After initial dose, attempt to leave the child without stimulation in order to monitor effect on state of consciousness and respirations
	If child still very agitated and crying after 10 minutes have elapsed from the initial dose, repeat 0.25mg per kg IV and wait another 10 minutes without stimulation
	Dose can be repeated to a maximum of 1mg per kg per hour
Morphine	0.025mg to 0.05mg per kg IV
	Titration of administration the same as with Demerol
Diazepam (Valium)	Oral administration preferred. Poorly absorbed intramuscularly
	Oral dose 0.1 to 0.2mg per kg
	Intravenous dose 0.05 to 0.1mg per kg **very slowly**—duration of IV dose: five to 10 minutes
	Danger: respiratory depression with rapid IV administration especially if in combination with a narcotic
	Oral dose can be repeated if child is very agitated and has spasm
	Make sure you have given adequate narcotic if the child is in pain.
Narcan	For overdose of narcotic and respiratory depression
	First stimulate patient. If no improvement, start assisted ventilation with a bag and mask and 100% oxygen
	When ventilation is assisted, give Narcan IV in dosage of 0.005 to 0.01mg per kg

*Prepared by Michael Flynn MD, former assistant professor of anesthesiology, Department of Anesthesia, Stanford University School of Medicine, Stanford, California.

severe muscle spasticity unrelieved by diazepam (Valium) and adequate narcotics. It must be taken orally, in an initial dose of 0.5mg per kg bodyweight for each dose four times a day. The dose can be increased to 3mg per kg bodyweight for each dose.

Diazepam (Valium) continues to be the most popular muscle relaxant, although there have been no objective assessment methods to demonstrate reduction of muscle spasticity (Hamilton 1984). Its action is central, and it does lessen anxiety and the startle response. Patients with total body involved spasticity and/or athetosis seem to gain relief from regular administration of diazepam. Its effect is cumulative, so there is still an effect 24 to 36 hours after withdrawal of the medication. Some patients have discontinued its use because it appeared to interfere with their ability to learn new material in school.

Baclofen (Lioresal) is another muscle relaxant which appears effective in spasticity due to a lesion of the spinal cord (*e.g.* traumatic paraplegia, multiple sclerosis); but it is not equally effective in spastic paralysis of cerebral origin, and its use in cerebral palsy has not been established (Barnhart 1985).

Adult living and parent counseling
It seems strange that an orthopaedic surgeon would even attempt to supplement

the counseling rôle which may be the turf of the paediatrician, physiatrist or social worker. Nevertheless I have found that parents and patients consider the orthopaedic surgeon to be a physician and not a technician just following orders. Those surgeons who perform more than an occasional surgery in cerebral palsy have found themselves to be inextricably bound with the patient and the family. He who cuts also counsels. The surgeon wields a powerful therapeutic tool which the patient almost never forgets. The surgeon needs some knowledge gained from experience in dealing with children who have long-term orthopaedic impairments.

Maladjustment and psychological problems
What happens to children with cerebral palsy when they become adults? Are there social and psychological as well as medical problems that evolve? In order to counsel parents on the management of cerebral palsy, one needs to know what lies beyond childhood—beyond the curly-headed smiling child in braces on posters and fund-raising brochures. The focus must be on the longer lifespan:adulthood. In the goal-oriented approach, the direction is always towards optimum independent adult living and community integration, and away from the disease. As I have indicated, we can prevent structural changes and late disability with appropriate orthopaedic surgery, combined with the talents of the physical and occupational therapist. We need to look ahead with the parents, and also prevent maladjustment and psychiatric problems in late adolescence and early adulthood. In the few studies that are available, the family is the key ingredient upon which one has to rely. No substitute for the nuclear family has been found (Davis 1976).

Maladjustment and psychiatric problems were reviewed by Thomas *et al.* (1985). We know that studies of handicapped children suggest a much higher incidence of psychiatric disorders than expected in normal children (Heller *et al.* 1985). Not surprisingly, those with marked handicaps are more likely to have psychological problems. Girls had more anxiety and depression than boys in one study quoted by Thomas *et al.* (1985). My own observations on children with cerebral palsy followed to young adulthood (age 21 to 30 years) suggest that serious emotional breakdown is more likely after age 18 years.

In the patients I have known, there was no relationship with the severity of the handicap and psychological breakdown. Spastic diplegic adolescents and young adults seem more vulnerable; here too the majority were young women. Most had stable families (often they were the only child) who always wanted to do the right and best thing (be it physical therapy, special education or surgery) for their daughter, in the hope that they would somehow become normal. The constant overdirection of the child by parents, physicians and therapists may have set the stage for the emotional crisis.

Reality strikes when you realize that childhood is over. Overachieving in school, in the attempt to prove that innate intellectual defects can be overcome, can create anxiety which is more decorticating than any of the cerebral damage. A belief in 'The Little Engine That Could' fairy-tale syndrome might be destructive: 'I think I can, I think I can, I think I can' (Bettelheim 1977).

Parents then need to know what can happen by adopting the disease-oriented approach. It may take years to judge its emotional cost. A recent follow-up of one of my 27-year-old spastic diplegic patients, a young lady who had completed college and had weathered a serious psychiatric breakdown, possibly said it best: 'I was pissed off at everybody'. Another young lady who also had spastic diplegia, and had eventually recovered from a severe anxiety neurosis, said to me: 'If only people would look at the person behind the handicap'.

Awareness of psychiatric problems, their prevention and psychiatric consultation, should be obvious to the physicians who assume primary responsibility for the care of the child with cerebral palsy (Freeman 1970). The orthopaedic surgeon often must assume the primary rôle as it is forced upon him/her by default and parental expectations.

Awareness of sexual functions

Not to be ignored are sexual problems of the handicapped (Thomas *et al.* 1985). The sexual knowledge of the handicapped is said to be very poor. Sex education and counseling services have been established and should be recommended. Personal accounts of sexual concerns and encounters by the physically handicapped have been published (Bullard and Knight 1981). In sexual practices, other perspectives beyond mere knowledge need to be developed by the handicapped person. How these attitudes and philosophies are inculcated as matters of personal responsibility is beyond the scope of this book.

Outcome studies

Outcome studies of cerebral-palsied children who have reached adulthood may be of some general assistance in counseling parents, even though each child's problems, environment and the times in which they live are particular. O'Reilly (1975) published a study of 336 adult patients. In his patient population, 28 per cent who had normal mentality were sufficient in self-care; one-third were retarded and helpless. The outlook for employment was best in those who had spastic paralysis and had attended regular school. In the whole group, 35.4 per cent had a chance of having an occupation. Institutional care was necessary for 11 per cent of those severely involved; 17 per cent had died. 39 per cent of the patients had no organized activity, were unable to obtain employment, or were sitting at home with nothing to do. O'Reilly called for solutions to the problems of this latter group.

Soboloff (1981) reported a follow-up study of 248 cerebral-palsied adults over the age of 20 years (range 20 to 50 years). Of this population, 48 per cent were self-sufficient community walkers; 30 per cent had part-time care and used the wheelchair except for household walking; 22 per cent were helpless and needed total care. Full-time employment was documented in 31 per cent and, as reported in other studies, the majority had spastic diplegia or hemiplegia. About one-third were homebound or institutionalized. 24 (8 per cent) had married—only three to another person with cerebral palsy. The causes of some of the 15 deaths are tragic but possibly instructive: three respiratory arrests, two cardiac arrests, two suicides, one murdered by his mother who then killed herself, one choked on a hot dog, one fell down a staircase and another off a ramp (Table 6.V).

TABLE 6.V

Long-term follow-up of cerebral-palsied children
(Soboloff 1981)

Age (years)	20–30 =	140
	30–40 =	62
	40–50 =	37
	50+ =	9
	Total = 248	

Independence
Self-sufficient; community walkers = 119
Part-time care; wheelchair; household walkers = 74
Helpless; total care = 55
Total = 248

Employment
Fully employed = 76*
Sheltered workshop = 22
Unemployed = 96
In college = 37
In high school = 27
Total = 248

Living circumstances
Homebound = 41
Institutionalized = 33
Total = 74

Marriage and family
Married and had children = 24
Married non-handicapped = 21
Married to a cerebral-palsied person = 3

*61 had spastic diplegia or hemiplegia.

My 1980 study shows that outcome varies according to time and place. We personally contacted 108 patients who we had followed and were age 18 years or older. Only 16 per cent were not working or in a regular school. And our study of 119 cases with spastic diplegia confirms that the specific type of cerebral palsy is an important factor in independent living (Miranda 1979) (Table 6.VI). All the patients were in a school program. 37 per cent were in a special school and were being prepared for normal integrated school; the mean age of transfer to the regular school was 7.4 years. Only a small number (21) had achieved adulthood; however, their success in achieving independence seems evident from the record of full employment or university education.

The family
The vital rôle of families in health status has received scant attention in the medical literature (Somers 1979, Stein and Jessof 1984). The primary rôle of the family in developing countries was emphasized by Bose (1980) in a discussion about the management of cerebral palsy in Singapore. A recent study by Agosta and Bradley (1985) focuses on the significance of the family and the care of persons with developmental disabilities. The contribution of the family was confirmed in my

TABLE 6.VI

School and work status of 119 children wtih spastic diplegia and follow-up of those age 21 years or older

Schooling	N	%
Regular	75	63
Special school	44	37
Older than age 21 years	21	25
Working and independent	16	
Attending university	5	

Occupations: bookkeeper; auto repair; handicapped children's aid; soap company salesman; secretary; playground director; computer programmer; stockroom clerk; recreation park director (2); special education teacher; insurance underwriter; processing technician; mailroom clerk; sheltered workshop; pizza cook.

TABLE 6.VII

Living environment of severely retarded physically handicapped children and adolescents in La Esperanza Development Centers. San Mateo County, California 1977 and 1981 (from Bleck *et al*. 1981)

1977	%	N	Age range	Mean (years)	Mothers	%
Home	66	71	3–19	9.6	At home, no other job	77
Foster home	16				Work full-time outside	16
Custodial care	18					
North Center 1981						
Home	77	43	4–22	11	At home, no other job	46
Foster home	2				Work full-time outside	48
Custodial care	8					
South Center 1981						
Home	91	46	4–33	13	At home, no other job	64
Foster home	0				Work full-time outside	25
Custodial care	9					

study of 106 cerebral-palsied children under age 18 years: 90 per cent were living at home, 2 per cent were in a foster home, and 8 per cent were in a nursing home.

In 1977 we studied 71 severely mentally and physically handicapped children; and four years later we added another 89 such children who were in special day-care development centres in San Mateo County, California. These studies confirmed the importance of the family, because most children were living at home with their biological parents. The rôle of the mother in caring for the child was particularly significant (Bleck *et al*. 1981) (Table 6.VII). In the 1977 study, mothers who worked outside the home comprised only 16.3 per cent in contrast to the estimate of over 50 per cent of the mothers who work at outside jobs in the United States. The 1981 study of two separate centres revealed that fewer women remained at home in one geographic area (South County) than in 1977, and many more were working outside the home in the North County region. These differences may be due to economic variations in the county, and possibly the effects of the severe inflation from 1977 to 1981. The contribution of these care-giving mothers to the society, and the resultant reduction in public hospital costs, has not become an issue of public knowledge or concern: though perhaps there is a budding awareness of the value of mothers who care for children at home, and a new USA voluntary organization has arisen called 'Mothers at Home'.

The family set-up is changed irreversibly when a handicapped child enters its circle. Life does become more complex. Physicians and paramedics who care for these children and their families might also remember the rôle of the father, and not make life more difficult for them by needless treatments and home program.

Although some physicians might feel that life would be easier without parents and families, the fact is that they exist. We need to appreciate them and listen (Bax 1985). One study has produced convincing evidence that parental estimates of a child's developmental level (when applied to a child who was already defined as developmentally delayed) was quite accurate when compared with formal developmental tests (Coplan 1982).

Summary of counseling points for physicians
Mercer Rang (1982) has encapsulated the best guidelines for counseling parents who have children with chronic handicapping conditions. I can do not better than to quote directly from his booklet (Rang 1982, pp.71–72):

Problems of the chronically handicapped
The chief problem is that their difficulties never go away.
    The physical difficulties impede emotional development.
    The problems remain a life-time preoccupation of the entire family.

CRISIS TIMES:
    1. Prediagnosis—worry that the child is not normal.
    2. On diagnosis—often late: parents blame themselves or their doctor.
    —hard to explain the disease to the parents
    —hard for the parents to understand and accept
    —they need ongoing support
    —'treatment' is not easy and is not curative
    —worry often increases after a few weeks when the full impact sinks in.
    3. School entry—intellectual impairment may have to be faced.
    4. Adolescence—lack of independence must be faced.
    5. Parents' middle age—arrangements for future care must be made.

PARENTS:
Parents usually feel that they lack information; they misunderstand and misquote. Their lives are disrupted—housing, work and finances. Even the apparently successful ones are stressed. They may go through a grief reaction: at each stage the doctor has a special rôle.
    Denial—hide disability; MD suggests investigation.
    Disbelief—shop around for cure; MD puts cranks into perspective.

Anger—quarrel with people who try to help; MD is patient.

Apathy—leave it all to others; MD plans for them.

Acceptance—the sensible attitude; MD's reward.

Helping others—organizing groups, petitions, building residences; MD co-operates.

HANDICAPPED TEENAGERS AND YOUNG ADULTS:

face many problems:

    —at this age they comprehend their future.

    —they recognize their own social insecurity and lack interpersonal skills.

    —the change from being protected to being a social reject.

PHYSICIANS:

have difficulty relating to the chronically handicapped but can follow many helpful approaches:

—thorough assessment on suspicion and without delay

—explanations should be slow, complete and repeated several times

—group therapy important

—establish a management plan—avoid 'try this, try that' approach

—avoid pinning hopes on tomorrow being better than today

—emphasize care rather than cure

—examine repeatedly, looking for an opportunity to offer medical help

—turn pity into action by:

1. suggesting books to read
2. advice on groups to join
3. where to go for treatment
4. selection of schools
5. suggesting helpful toys
6. organizing recreation
7. suggesting holiday relief
8. suggesting baby-sitting.

REFERENCES

Accardo, P. J. (1982) 'Freud on diplegia—commentary and translation.' *American Journal Diseases of Children*, **136**, 452–456.

Agosta, J. M., Bradley, V. J. (1985) *Family Care for Persons with Developmental Disabilities: A Growing Commitment.* 120 Milk Street (8th Floor) Boston, MA 02109: Human Services Research Institute.

American Academy of Pediatrics (1982) 'Policy statement: the Doman-Delacato treatment of neurologically handicapped children.' *Pediatrics*, **5**, 810–811.

American Association of Occupational Therapists (1981) 'The role of occupational therapy as an education-related service: official position paper.' *American Journal of Occupational Therapy*, **35**, 811.

Amiel-Tison, C. (1985) 'Neurological assessment from birth to 7 years of age.' *In:* Harel, S., Anastasiow, N. J. (Eds.) *The At-Risk Infant.* Baltimore and London: Paul H. Brookes. pp. 239–251.

Anastasiow, N. J. (1985) 'Parent training as adult development.' *In:* Harel, S., Anastasiow, N. J. (Eds.) *The At-Risk Infant.* Baltimore and London: Paul H. Brookes. pp. 5–12.

Arnoff, G. (1973) 'There's no play like snow play.' *Canadian Journal of Occupational Therapy*, **40**, 79–82.

Ayres, A. J. (1971) 'Characteristics of types of sensory integrative dysfunction.' *American Journal of Occupation Therapy*, **7**, 329–334.

—— (1972) 'Improving academic scores through sensory integration.' *Journal of Learning Disabilities*, .**5**, 336–343.

—— (1977) 'Effect of sensory integrative therapy on the coordination of children with choreoathetoid movements.' *American Journal of Occupational Therapy*, **31**, 291–293.

—— (1978) 'Learning disabilities and the vestibular system.' *American Journal of Learning Disabilities*, **2**, 18–29.

Bachman, W. H. (1972) 'Variables affecting post-school economic adaptation of orthopaedically handicapped and other health impaired students.' *Rehabilitation Literatures*, **33**, 98–114.

Barber, E. (1978) 'Modifications of a MacLaren Buggy Major for orthopaedic seat inserts.' *Orthotics and Prosthetics*, **32**, 6–9.

Barnhart, E. R. (Ed.) (1985) *Physicians's Desk Reference.* Oradell, N. J. pharmaceutical company literature, Lioresal, Geigy, p. 959; Valium, Roche, pp. 1721–1723.

Bauman, S. (1981) 'Physical aspects of the self. A review of some aspects of body image development in childhood.' *Psychiatric Clinics of North America*, **4**, 455–470.

Bax, M. (1983) 'Abuse and cerebral palsy.' *Developmental Medicine and Child Neurology*, **25**, 141–142.

—— (1985) 'Meeting the parents' needs.' *Developmental Medicine and Child Neurology*, **27**, 139–140.

Beals, R. K. (1966) 'Spastic paraplegia and diplegia: an evaluation of non-surgical and surgical factors influencing prognosis for ambulation.' *Journal of Bone and Joint Surgery*, **48A**, 827–846.

Benedetti, A., Colombo, F. (1981) 'Spinal surgery for spasticity.' *Neurochirurgia*, **24**, 195–198.

—— —— Alexander, A., Pellegri, A. (1982) 'Posterior rhizotomies for spasticity in children affected by cerebral palsy.' *Journal of Neurosurgical Science*, **26**, 179–184.

Bensman, A. S., Szegho, M. (1978) 'Cerebellar electrical stimulation: a critique.' *Archives of Physical Medicine and Rehabilitation*, **59**, 485–487.

Bettelheim, B. (1977) *The Uses of Enchantment.* New York: Vintage Books.

Bleck, E. E. (1971) 'The shoeing of children: sham or science?' *Developmental Medicine and Child Neurology*, **13**, 188–195.

—— (1975) 'Locomotor prognosis in cerebral palsy.' *Developmental Medicine and Child Neurology*, **17**, 18–25.

—— (1977a) 'Rehabilitation engineering for severely handicapped children.' *In:* Ahstrom, J. P. Jr. (Ed.) *Current Management in Orthopaedic Surgery.* St. Louis: C. V. Mosby.

—— (1977b) 'Severe orthopaedic disability in childhood: solutions provided by rehabilitation engineering.' *Orthopaedic Clinics of North America*, **9**, 509–527.

—— (1978) 'Integrating the care of multiply handicapped children.' *Developmental Medicine and Child Neurology*, **20**, 10–13.

—— (1982) 'Cerebral palsy'. *In:* Bleck, E. E., Nagel, D. A. *Physically Handicapped Children: A Medical Atlas for Teachers.* Orlando, Florida: Grune & Stratton.

—— (1984) 'Where have all the CP children gone? The needs of adults.' *Developmental Medicine and Child Neurology*, **26**, 674–676.

—— (1985) 'L'enfant paralyse et son appareillage—concepts de base.' (Translation by Dimeglio, A.) *In: L'Enfant Paralyse. Reéducation et Appareillage.* Paris: Masson. pp. 180–190

—— Headley, L. (1961) 'Treatment and parent counseling for the pre-school child with cerebral palsy.' *Pediatrics*, **27**, 1025–1032.

—— Berzins, U. J. (1977) 'Conservative management of pes valgus with plantar flexed talus flexible.' *Clinical Orthopaedics and Related Research*, **122**, 85–94.

—— Wolf, K. McK., Schafheitle, L. (1981) 'The cost of mothering.' (*Unpublished study.*)

Bliss, C. K. (1965) *Semantography/Blissymbolics.* Sydney: Sematography Publications.

Bobath, B. (1954) 'A study of abnormal postural reflex activity in patients with lesions of the central nervous system.' *Physiotherapy*, **40**, 9–12.

—— (1967) 'The very early treatment of cerebral palsy.' *Developmental Medicine and Child Neurology*, **9**, 373–390.

Bobath, K. (1966) *The Motor Deficit in Patients with Cerebral Palsy. Clinics in Developmental Medicine No. 23.* London: S.I.M.P. with Heinemann Medical; Philadelphia: J. B. Lippincott.

—— (1980) *A Neurophysiological Basis for the Treatment of Cerebral Palsy. Clinics in Developmental Medicine No. 75.* London: S.I.M.P. with Heinemann Medical; Philadelphia: J. B. Lippincott.

—— Bobath, B. (1958) 'An assessment of motor handicap of children with cerebral palsy and their response to treatment.' *Occupational Therapy Journal*, **27**, 1–16.

—— —— (1984) 'The neuro-developmental treatment.' *In:* Scrutton, D. (Ed.) *Management of the Motor Disorders in Children with Cerebral Palsy. Clinics in Developmental Medicine No. 90.* London: S.I.M.P. with Blackwell Scientific; Philadelphia: J. B. Lippincott.

Bolkert, R. (1979) 'Medial uprights for valgus feet, spastic.' *Orthotics and Prosthetics*, **33**, 54–62.

Bosc, K. (1980) 'Management of cerebral palsy in a developing country.' *Orthopaedic Transactions*, **4**, 75.

Bourgeois, O., Chaigne, M. O., Cherpin, J., Minaire, P., Weber, D. (1977) 'Diminues physiques et transports collectifs.' *Institute de Recherche des Transports, Centre d'Evaluation et de Recherche des Nuisances, Bron, France.*

Bragg, J. H., Houser, C., Shumaker, J. (1975) 'Behavior modification: effects on reverse tailor sitting in children with cerebral palsy.' *Physical Therapy*, **55**, 860–868.

Broggi, G., Angelini, L., Giorgi, C. (1980) 'Neurological and psychological side effects after stereotactic thalamotomy in patients with cerebral palsy.' *Neurosurgery*, **7**, 127–134.

—— —— Bono, R., Giorgi, C., Nardocci, N., Franzini, A. (1983) 'Long term results of stereotactic thalamotomy for cerebral palsy.' *Neurosurgery*, **12**, 195–202.

Bronowski, J. (1978) *Magic, Science and Civilization.* New York: Columbia University Press.

Brunnstrom, S. (1962) *Clinical Kinesiology, 3rd edn.* Philadelphia: F. A. Davis.

Bullard, D. C., Knight, S. E. (Eds.) (1981) *Sexuality and Physical Disability.* St. Louis: C. V. Mosby.

Burnett, C. N., Johnson, E. W. (1971) 'Development of gait in childhood. Parts I and II.' *Developmental Medicine and Child Neurology*, **13**, 196–206; 297–315.

Campbell, J., Ball, J. (1978) 'Energetics of walking in cerebral palsy.' *Orthopedic Clinics of North America*, **9**, 374–377.

Campion, M. R. (1985) *Hydrotherapy in Pediatrics.* London: Heinemann.

Campos da Paz, Jr., A. (1980) 'Management of cerebral palsy in Brazil.' *Lecture, Children's Hospital at Stanford, Palo Alto, California.*

—— Nomura, A. N., Braga, L. W., Burnett, S. M. (1984) 'Speculations on cerebral palsy.' *Journal of Bone and Joint Surgery*, **2**, 283. (*Abstract.*)

Carlsen, P. N. (1975) 'Comparison of two occupational therapy approaches for treating the young cerebral-palsied child.' *American Journal of Occupational Therapy*, **29**, 267–272.

Carlson, J. M., Winter, R. (1978) 'The Gilette sitting support orthosis.' *Orthotics and Prosthetics*, **4**, 35–45.

Carrington, E. (1978) 'A seating position for a cerebral-palsied child.' *American Journal of Occupational Therapy*, **32**, 179–181.

Cerny, K. (1978) 'Energetics of walking and wheelchair propulsion in paraplegic patients.' *Orthopedic Clinics of North America*, **9**, 370–372.

Chait, L. A., Kessler, E. (1979) 'An antidrooling operation in cerebral palsy.' *South African Medical Journal*, **56**, 676–678.

Cherpin, J., Minaire, P., Flores, J. L., Weber, D. (1985) 'Study of a village population in France.' (*In preparation.*)

—— Weber, D. (1985) 'Approche fonctionelle de la population francaise. Phase exploratoire et construction du protocole experimental. Rapport final.' *Institute de Recherche des Transports.* Paris, France.

Cohen, M. J., Brick, H. G., Taft, L. T. (1970) 'Some considerations for evaluating the Doman-Delacato "patterning" method.' *Pediatrics*, **45**, 302–314.

Cohen, P., Mustacchi, P. (1966) 'Survival in cerebral palsy.' *Journal of the American Medical Association*, **195**, 642–644.

—— Kohn, J. G. (1979) 'Follow-up study of patients with cerebral palsy.' *Western Journal of Medicine*, **130**, 6–11.

Committee on Children with Disabilities, American Academy of Pediatrics (1985) 'School age children with motor disabilities.' *Pediatrics*, **76**, 648–649.

Conrad, L., Bleck, E. E. (1980) 'Augmented auditory feedback in the treatment of equinus gait in children.' *Developmental Medicine and Child Neurology*, **22**, 713–718.

—— Benick, R., Carnehl, J. H., Hohne, J., Meinck, H. M. (1983) Pathophysiological aspects of human locomotion.' *Advances in Neurology*, **39**, 717–726.

Cooper, I. S., Riklan, M., Amin, I., Waltz, J. M., Cullinan, T. (1976) 'Chronic cerebellar stimulation in cerebral palsy.' *Neurology*, **26**, 744–753.

Cooper, R. R. (1972) 'Alterations during immobilization and degeneration of skeletal muscle in cats.' *Journal of Bone and Joint Surgery*, **54A**, 919–953.

205

Coplan, J. (1982) 'Parental estimate of child's developmental level in a high-risk population.' *American Journal Diseases of Children*, **136**, 101–104.

Cotton, E. (1974) 'Improvement in motor function with the use of conductive education.' *Developmental Medicine and Child Neurology*, **16**, 637–643.

—— (1977) 'A bedroom routine for the cerebral palsied child.' *Study Group on Integrating Multiply Handicapped Children, St. Mary's College, Durham, England*. London: The Spastics Society Medical Education and Information Unit.

Craig, C. L., Sosnoff, F., Zimbler, S. (1984) 'Seating in cerebral palsy—a possible advance.' *Orthopaedic Transactions*, **8**, 456. (*Abstract.*)

Craig, J. J., Mathias, A. (1977) 'Forest Town boot.' *Physical Therapy*, **57**, 918–920.

Cristarella, M. C. (1975) 'Comparison of straddling and sitting apparatus for the spastic cerebral palsied child.' *American Journal of Occupational Therapy*, **29**, 273–276.

Davis, K. (1976) 'The changing family in industrial societies.' Reprint from Jackson, R. C., Morton, J. (Eds.) *Family Health Care: Health Promotion and Illness Care*. Berkeley, California: School of Public Health, University of California.

Davis, R., Barolat-Romana, G., Engle, H. (1980) 'Chronic cerebellar stimulation for cerebral palsy—5 year study.' *Acta Neurochirurgica*, Supplement 30, 317–322.

Denhoff, E. (1981) 'Current status of infant stimulation or enrichment programs for children with developmental disabilities.' *Pediatrics* **67**, 32–37.

Doman, R. J., Spitz, E. B., Zucman, E., Delacato, C., Doman, G. (1960) 'Children with severe brain injuries—results of treatment.' *Journal of the American Medical Association*, **174**, 257–262.

Duncan, W. R. (1960) 'Tonic reflexes of the foot.' *Journal of Bone and Joint Surgery*, **42A**, 859–868.

—— Mott, D. H. (1983) 'Foot reflexes and use of the "inhibitive cast".' *Foot and Ankle*, **4**, 145–148.

Eiser, C., Patterson, D. (1983) '"Slugs and snails and puppy-dog tails"—children's ideas about the inside of their bodies.' *Child Care Health Development*, **4**, 233–240.

Ellenberg, J. H., Nelson, K. B. (1981) 'Early recognition of infants at high risk for cerebral palsy: examination at four months.' *Developmental Medicine and Child Neurology*, **23**, 705–716.

Fay, T. (1958) 'Neuromuscular reflex therapy for spastic disorders.' *Journal of Florida Medical Association*, **44**, 1234–1240.

—— (1977) 'The neurophysical aspects of therapy in cerebral palsy.' *In:* Payton, O. D., Hirt, S., Newton, R. A. (Eds.) *Neurophysiological Approaches to Therapeutic Exercise*. Philadelphia: F. A. Davis. pp. 237–246.

Feagans, L. (1983) 'A current view of learning disabilities.' *Journal of Pediatrics*, **102**, 487–493.

Feldkamp, M. (1979) 'Motor goals of therapeutic horseback riding for cerebral palsied children.' *Rehabilitation*, **18**, 56–61.

Ferguson, B. F. (1979) 'Preparing young children for hospitalization: a comparison of two methods.' *Pediatrics*, **64**, 656–664.

Ferry, P. C. (1981) 'On growing new neurons. Are early intervention programs effective?' *Pediatrics*, **67**, 38–44.

Fisher, S. V., Patterson, R. P. (1981) 'Energy cost of ambulation with crutches.' *Archives of Physical Medicine and Rehabilitation*, **62**, 250–256.

Ford, L. F., Bleck, E. E., Aptekar, R. G., Collins, F. J., Stevick, D. (1976) 'Efficacy of dantrolene sodium in the treatment of spastic cerebral palsy.' *Developmental Medicine and Child Neurology*, **18**, 770–783.

Freeman, R. D. (1970) 'Psychiatric problems in adolescents with cerebral palsy.' *Developmental Medicine and Child Neurology*, **12**, 64–70.

Freud, S. (1893) 'Les diplégies cérébrales infantiles.' *Revue Neurologigue*, **1**, 177–183.

Fulford, G. E., Cairns, T. P., Sloan, Y. (1982) 'Sitting problems of children with cerebral palsy.' *Developmental Medicine and Child Neurology*, **24**, 48–53.

Garrett, A. L., Lister, M., Drennan, J. (1966) 'New concept in bracing for cerebral palsy.' *Physical Therapy*, **46**, 728–733.

Gillette, H. (1969) *Systems of Therapy in Cerebral Palsy*. Springfield, Ill.: C. C. Thomas.

Golden, G. S. (1980) 'Nonstandard therapies in the developmental disabilities.' *American Journal of Diseases of Children*, **134**, 487–491.

Goldkamp, O. (1984) 'Treatment effectiveness in cerebral palsy.' *Archives of Physical Medicine and Rehabilitation*, **65**, 232–234.

Goldner, J. L. (1985) *Personal communication*.

Gollnitz, G., Schulz-Wulf, G. (1973) 'Rhythmisch-pscyhomotrische Musiktherapie. Eine gezielter Behgandîung entwicklungsgeschadigeter Kinder und Jungendlicher.' *Sammlung Zwangloser Abhandlungen auz dem Gebiete der Psychiatrie und Neurologie*, **44**, 1–112.

206

Gornall, P., Hitchcock, E., Kirkland, I. S. (1975) 'Stereotaxic neurosurgery in the management of cerebral palsy.' *Developmental Medicine and Child Neurology*, **17**, 279–286.

Griffin, P. P., Wheelhouse, W. W., Shiavi, R., Bass, W. (1977) 'Habitual toe-walkers.' *Journal of Bone and Joint Surgery*, **59A**, 97–101.

Hagbarth, K. E., Eklund, G. (1977) 'The muscle vibrators—a useful tool in neurological therapeutic work.' *In:* Payton, O. D., Hirt, S., Newton, R. A. (Eds.) *Scientific Basis for Neurophysiologic Approaches to Therapeutic Exercise.* Philadelphia: F. A. Davis. pp. 133–145.

Hamilton, M. S. (1984) 'Centrally acting muscle relaxants.' *Drug Information News Letter.* Stanford, California: Stanford University Hospital.

Hanks, S. B., Macfarlane, D. W. (1969) 'Device for heel-cord stretching and gait training.' *Physical Therapy*, **49**, 380–381.

Hare, N. (1977) 'Abduction pants.' *Physiotherapy*, **63**, 227.

Hari, M., Tillemans, T. (1984) 'Conductive education.' *In:* Scrutton, D. (Ed.) *Management of the Motor Disorders of Children with Cerebral Palsy. Clinics in Developmental Medicine No. 90.* London: S.I.M.P. with Blackwell Scientific; Philadelphia: J. B. Lippincott.

Harris, S., Hinderer, K., Staheli, L., Chew, D., McLaughlin, J. F. (1985) 'Effects of "tone-reducing" and standard short leg casts: a single subject study design.' *Scientific program, American Academy for Cerebral Palsy and Developmental Medicine, Seattle.*

Harrison, A. (1977) 'Augmented feedback training of motor control in cerebral palsy.' *Developmental Medicine and Child Neurology*, **19**, 75–78.

Hassakis, P. C. (1974) 'Outcomes of cerebral palsy patients.' *Annual Meeting of the American Academy for Cerebral Palsy, Denver, Colorado.*

Hayes, N. K., Burns, Y. R. (1970) 'Discussion on use of weight-bearing plasters in reduction of hypertonicity.' *Australian Journal of Physiotherapy*, **16**, 108–117.

Helander, E., Mendis, P., Nelson, G. (1983) *Training Disabled People in the Community.* Geneva: World Health Organization.

Heller, A., Rafman, S., Zvagulis, I., Pless, I. V. (1985) 'Birth defects and psychosocial adjustment.' *American Journal of Diseases of Children*, **139**, 257–263.

Hengst, C. (1976) 'Sport therapy and rehabilitation—especially riding therapy.' (Sport als Mittel der Therapie and Rehabilitation insbesondere Reittherapie'). *Zeitschrift für Orthopedie,* **114**, 690–691.

Herbison, B. J., Jaweed, M. M., Ditunno, J. F. (1978) 'Muscle fiber atrophy after cast immobilization in the rat.' *Archives of Physical Medicine and Rehabilitation*, **59**, 301–305.

Hoffer, M. M., Feiwell, E., Perry, J., Bonnett, C. (1973) 'Functional ambulation in patients with myelomeningocele.' *Journal of Bone and Joint Surgery*, **55A**, 137–148.

—— Koffman, M. (1980) 'Cerebral palsy: the first three years.' *Clinical Orthopaedics and Related Research*, **151**, 222–227.

Hollis, L. I. (1974) 'Skinnerian occupational therapy.' *American Journal of Occupational Therapy*, **28**, 208–213.

Holm, V. A. (1983) 'A western version of the Doman-Delacato treatment of patterning for developmental disabilities.' *Western Journal of Medicine*, **139**, 553–556.

—— Harthun-Smith, L., Tada, W. L. (1983) 'Infant walkers and cerebral palsy.' *American Journal of Diseases of Children*, **137**, 1189–1190.

Holte, R. N. (1980) *Final Report: A Modular System for Seating the Multiply Handicapped Child.* Project 6607-1181-51, National Health Research and Development Program, Ottawa, Canada: Health and Welfare.

Ingram, T. T. S., Jameson, S., Errington, J., Mitchell, R. G. (1964) *Living with Cerebral Palsy. Clinics in Developmental Medicine No. 14.* London: Spastics Society Medical Education and Information Unit with Heinemann Medical.

Ivan, L. P., Ventureyra, E. C., Wiley, J., Doyle, D., Pressman, E., Knights, R., Guzman, C., Uttley, D. (1981) 'Chronic cerebellar stimulation in cerebral palsy.' *Surgical Neurology*, **15**, 81–84.

Jesien, G. (1984) 'Home-based early intervention: a description of the Portage Project model.' *In:* Scrutton, D. (Ed.) *Management of Motor Disorders of Children with Cerebral Palsy. Clinics in Developmental Medicine No. 90,* London: S.I.M.P. with Blackwell Scientific; Philadelphia: J. B. Lippincott. pp. 36–48.

Jones, R. B. (1975) 'The Vojta method of treatment of cerebral palsy.' *Physiotherapy*, **61**, 112–113.

Kabat, H. (1977) 'Studies on neuromuscular dysfunction.' *In:* Payton, O. D., Hirt, S., Newton, R. A. (Eds.) *Scientific Basis for Neurophysiologic Approaches to Therapeutic Exercise.* Philadelphia: F. A. Davis. pp. 219–235.

—— Knott, M. (1953) 'Proprioceptive facilitation techniques for treatment of paralysis.' *Physical*

Therapy Review, **33**, 53–64.
Kanda, T., Yuge, M., Yamori, Y., Suzuki, J., Fukase, H. (1984) 'Early physiotherapy in the treatment of spastic diplegia.' *Developmental Medicine and Child Neurology*, **26**, 438–444.
Kanter, R. M., Clark, D. C., Allen, L. C., Chase, M. A. (1976) 'Effects of vestibular stimulation on nystagmus response and motor performance in the developmentally disabled infant.' *Physical Therapy*, **156**, 414–421.
Kassover, M., Tauber, C., Oau, J., Johnson, S., Pugh, J. (1984) 'Auditory feedback in spastic diplegia: gait analysis.' *Transactions of Orthopaedic Research Society, 30th annual meeting, Atlanta, Georgia.*
Kavanagh, C. A., Banco, L. (1982) 'The infant walker: a previously unrecognized health hazard.' *American Journal of Diseases of Children*, **135**, 205–206.
Koheil, R., Sochaniwskyj, A., Bablich, K., Kenny, D., Milner, M. (1985) 'Biofeedback techniques and behaviour modification in the conservative remediation of drooling in children with cerebral palsy.' *Scientific program American Academy for Cerebral Palsy and Developmental Medicine, Seattle.*
Kohn, J. (1982) 'Multiply handicapped child.' *In:* Bleck, E. E., Nagel, D. A. (Eds.) *Physically Handicapped Children: A Medical Atlas for Teachers. 2nd edn.* Orlando, Florida: Grune & Stratton.
—— Enders, S., Preston, J., Motloch, W. O. (1983) 'Provision of assistive equipment for handicapped persons.' *Archives of Physical Medicine and Rehabilitation*, **64**, 378–381.
Köng, E. (1966) 'Very early treatment of cerebral palsy.' *Developmental Medicine and Child Neurology*, **8**, 198–202.
Kvashnik, B. L., Pelevin, V. V., Deniskina, L. N. (1978) 'Opyt griaxelech eniia na lechebnom pliazhe sanatoriia.' *Voprosy Kurotologii, Fizioterapii Lechebnoi Fizicheskoi Kultury (Moskova)*, **4**, 82.
LeBlanc, M. (1982) 'Systems and devices for nonoral communication.' *In:* Bleck, E. E., Nagel, D. A. (Eds.) *Physically Handicapped Children: A Medical Atlas for Teachers.* Orlando, Florida: Grune & Stratton. pp. 159–169.
Lee, C. L. (1982) 'Role of lower extremity bracing in cerebral palsy.' *Developmental Medicine and Child Neurology*, **24**, 250–251. (*Abstract.*)
—— Bleck, E. E. (1980) 'Surgical correction of equinus deformity in cerebral palsy.' *Developmental Medicine and Child Neurology*, **22**, 287–292.
Letts, R. M., Fulford, R., Eng, B., Hobson, D. A. (1976) 'Mobility aids for the paraplegic child.' *Journal of Bone and Joint Surgery*, **58A**, 38–41.
Letts, M., Stevens, L., Coleman, J., Kettner, R. (1983) 'Puppetry and doll play as an adjunct to pediatric orthopaedics.' *Journal of Pediatric Orthopaedics*, **3**, 605–609.
Levine, M. S., Kliebhan, L. (1981) 'Communication between physician and physical and occupational therapists: a neurodevelopmentally based prescription.' *Pediatrics*, **68**, 208–214.
Maloney, F. P., Mirrett, P., Brooks, C., Johannes, K. (1978) 'Use of the goal attainment scale in the treatment and ongoing evaluation of neurologically handicapped children.' *American Journal of Occupational Therapy*, **32**, 505–510.
Martin, J. E., Epstein, L. H. (1976) 'Evaluating treatment effectiveness in cerebral palsy.' *Physical Therapy*, **56**, 285–294.
McCollough, N. C. III (1985) *Critical Needs of the Child with Long Term Orthopaedic Impairment, Conference Report, October 18–20, 1984.* Washington, D.C.: American Academy of Orthopaedic Surgeons.
McLellan, L. (1984) 'Therapeutic possibilities in cerebral palsy: a neurologist's view.' *In:* Scrutton, D. (Ed.) *Management of the Motors Disorders of Children with Cerebral Palsy. Clinics in Developmental Medicine No. 90.* London: S.I.M.P. with Blackwell Scientific; Philadelphia: J. B. Lippincott.
McNaughton, S. (1977) 'Blissymbolics and technology.' *Proceedings of the Workshop on Communication Aids for the Handicapped.* Ottawa, Canada: Peter Nelson, National Research Council.
—— (1982) 'Augmentative communication system: Blissymbolics.' *In:* Bleck, E. E., Nagel, D. A. (Eds.) *Physically Handicapped Children: A Medical Atlas for Teachers. 2nd edn.* Orlando, Florida: Grune & Stratton. pp. 146–154.
Messingill, R. (1978) 'Follow-up investigation of patients who have had parotid duct transplantation surgery to control drooling.' *Annals of Plastic Surgery*, **2**, 205–208.
Messner, D. (1976) 'The mountain does it for me.' *16 mm film, Denver, Colorado: Children's Hospital Medical Center.*
Michaelis, R., Haas, G., Buchwald-Saal, M. (1985) 'Neurological development and assessment in infants at risk.' *In:* Harel, S., Anastasiow, N. J. (Eds.) *The At-Risk Infant.* Baltimore and London: Paul H. Brookes. pp. 269–273.
Milani-Comparetti, A. (1979) 'Priorities in rehabilitation: a progress report on a community program.'

Presented as the 1979 Mary Elaine Meyer O'Neal Award Lectureship in Developmental Pediatrics, Omaha, Nebraska.

Miller, T. G., Goldberg, K. (1975) 'Sensorimotor integration: an interdisciplinary approach.' *Physical Therapy*, **55**, 501–504.

Miranda, S. (1979) 'Outcomes of spastic diplegia.' *Unpublished study. Palo Alto, California: Children's Hospital at Stanford.*

Montgomery, P., Richter, E. (1977) 'Effect of sensory integrative therapy on the neuromotor development of retarded children.' *Physical Therapy*, **57**, 799–806.

Morgan, R. F., Hansen, F. C., Wells, J. H., Hoopes, J. E. (1981) 'The treatment of drooling in the child with cerebral palsy.' *Maryland State Medical Journal*, **30**, (6), 79–80.

Motloch, W. M. (1977) 'Seating and positioning for the physically impaired.' *Orthotics and Prosthetics*, **31**, 11–21.

Mott, D. H., Yates, L. (1981) 'An appraisal of inhibitive casting as an adjunct to the total management of the child with cerebral palsy.' *Proceedings of the American Academy for Cerebral Palsy and Developmental Medicine Annual Meeting, Detroit.*

Mothers at Home (1984) 9673 Lee Highway, Fairfax, Virginia 22031.

Nelson, K. B., Ellenberg, J. H. (1981) 'Apgar scores as predictors of chronic neurologic disability.' *Pediatrics*, **68**, 36–44.

—— —— (1982) Children who "outgrew" cerebral palsy.' *Pediatrics*, **69**, 529–536.

—— —— (1984) 'Obstetric complications as risk factors for cerebral palsy or seizure disorders.' *Journal of the American Medical Association*, **251**, 1843–1848.

Norlin, R., Thaczok, A. (1985) 'One-session surgery for correction of lower extremity deformities in children with cerebral palsy.' *Journal of Pediatric Orthopaedics*, **5**, 208–211.

Nwaobi, O. M., Brubaker, C. E., Cuskick, B., Sussman, M. D. (1983) 'Electromyographic investigation of extensor activity in cerebral palsied children in different seating positions.' *Developmental Medicine and Child Neurology*, **25**, 175–183.

Ohye, C., Miyazaki, M., Hirai, T., Shibazaki, T., Nagaseki, Y. (1983) 'Sterotactic selective thalamotomy for the treatment of tremor type of cerebral palsy in adolescence.' *Child's Brain*, **10**, 157–167.

O'Reilly, E. D. (1975) 'Care of the cerebral palsied: outcomes of the past and needs for the future.' *Developmental Medicine and Child Neurology*, **17**, 141–149.

Paine, R. S. (1962) 'On the treatment of cerebral palsy: the outcome of 177 patients, 74 totally untreated.' *Pediatrics*, **29**, 605–616.

Parette, H. P. Jr., Hourcade, J. J. (1983) 'Early intervention: a conflict of therapist and educator.' *Perceptual and Motor Skills*, **57**, 1056–1058.

—— —— (1984) 'How effective are physiotherapeutic programmes with young mentally retarded children who have cerebral palsy?' *Journal of Mental Deficiency Research*, **28**, 167–175.

Pariser, S. C., Blitzer, A., Binder, W. J., Friedman, W. F., Marovitz, W. F. (1978) 'Evaluation of tympanic neurectomy and chorda tympanectomy surgery.' *Otolaryngology*, **86**, 308–321.

Parks, L. (1977) 'The need for "someone with nothing to do".' *Study Group on Integrating the Care of Multiply Handicapped Children, St. Mary's College, Durham, England. The Spastics Society Medical Education and Information Unit.*

Parmelee, A. H., Cohen, S. E. (1985) 'Neonatal follow-up for infants at risk.' *In:* Harel, S., Anastasiow, N. J. (Eds.) *The At-Risk Infant.* Baltimore and London: Paul H. Brookes. pp. 269–273.

Peacock, W. J., Arens, L. J. (1982) 'Selective posterior rhizotomy for relief of spasticity in cerebral palsy.' *South African Medical Journal*, **62**, 119–124.

Perry, J. (1974) *Personal communication.*

—— Jones, M. H., Thomas, L. (1981) 'Functional evaluation of Rolfing in cerebral palsy.' *Developmental Medicine and Child Neurology*, **23**, 719–729.

Polatajko, H. J. (1985) 'A critical look at vestibular dysfunction in learning-disabled children.' *Developmental Medicine and Child Neurology*, **27**, 283–292.

Rang, M. (1982) *The Easter Seal Guide to Children's Orthopaedics.* Ontario, Canada: The Easter Seal Society.

Ring, N. D., Nelham, R. L., Pearson, D. A. (1978) 'Molded supportive seating for the disabled.' *Prosthetics and Orthotics International*, **2**, 30–34.

Robertson, L. T., Meek, M., Smith, W. L. (1980) 'Speech changes in cerebral palsied patients after cerebellar stimulation.' *Developmental Medicine and Child Neurology*, **22**, 608–617.

Rood, M. S. (1954) 'Neurophysiologic reactions as a basis for physical therapy.' *Physical Therapy Review*, **34**, 444–449.

Root, L. (1977) 'The total body involved cerebral palsy patient.' *Instructional course lectures, Annual Meeting, American Academy of Orthopaedic Surgeons*, Las Vegas, Nevada.

Rose, J., Mederios, J. M., Parker, R. (1985) 'Energy cost index as an estimate of energy expenditure of cerebral-palsied children during assisted ambulation.' *Developmental Medicine and Child Neurology*, **27**, 485–490.

Rosemeyer, B., Stürz, H. (1977) 'Musculus quadriceps femoris bei Immobilization und remobilisation.' *Zeitschrift für Orthopädie*, **115**, 182–188.

Rosenthal, R. K. (1984) 'The use of orthotics in foot and ankle problems in cerebral palsy.' *Foot and Ankle*, **4**, 195–200.

—— Deutsch, S. D., Miller, W., Schumann, W., Hall, J. E. (1975) 'A fixed ankle below-the-knee orthosis for the management of genu recurvatum in spastic cerebral palsy.' *Journal of Bone and Joint Surgery*, **57A**, 545–549.

Russell, G., Sharp, E., Iles, G. (1976) 'Clinical biofeedback applications in pediatric rehabilitation.' *Inter-Clinics Information Bulletin*, **15**, 1–6.

Samilson, R. L., Hoffer, M. M. (1975) 'Problems and complications in orthopaedic management of cerebral palsy.' *In:* Samilson, R. L. (Ed.) *Orthopaedic Aspects of Cerebral Palsy. Clinics in Developmental Medicine, Nos. 52/53.* London: S.I.M.P. with Heinemann Medical; Philadelphia: J. B. Lippincott. pp. 258–274.

Sherzer, A. L. Mike, V., Ilson, J. (1976) 'Physical therapy as a determinant of change in the cerebral palsied infant.' *Pediatrics*, **58**, 47–51.

Schlesinger, E. R., Allaway, N. C., Peitin, S. (1959) 'Survivorship in cerebral palsy.' *American Journal of Public Health*, **49**, 343–354.

Schowalter, J. E. (1977) 'The modification of behavior modification.' *Pediatrics*, **59**, 130–131.

Schutt, B. (1981) 'Kindliche Huftluxation und Neuro-Physiotherapie nach Vojta.' *Fortschritte der Medizin*, **99**, 1410–1412.

Scrutton, D. (1984) 'Aim-oriented management.' *In:* Scrutton, D. (Ed.) *The Management of Motors Disorders of Children with Cerebral Palsy. Clinics in Developmental Medicine No. 90*, London: S.I.M.P. with Blackwell Scientific; Philadelphia: J. B. Lippincott.

Seeger, B. R., Caudry, D. J., Scholes, J. R. (1981) 'Biofeedback therapy to achieve symmetrical gait in hemiplegic cerebral palsied children.' *Archives of Physical Medicine and Rehabilitation*, **62**, 364–368.

—— —— (1983) 'Biofeedback therapy to achieve symmetrical gait in children with hemiplegic cerebral palsy: long-term efficacy.' *Archives of Physical Medicine and Rehabilitation*, **64**, 160–162.

—— —— O'Mara, N. A. (1984) 'Hand function in cerebral palsy: the effect of hip-flexion angle.' *Developmental Medicine and Child Neurology*, **26**, 601–606.

Sellick, K. J., Over, R. (1980) 'Effects of vestibular stimulation on motor development of cerebral-palsied children.' *Developmental Medicine and Child Neurology*, **22**, 476–483.

Sharrard, W. J. W. (1976) 'Indications for bracing in cerebral palsy.' *In:* Murdoch, G. (Ed.) *The Advance in Orthotics.* London: Edward Arnold. pp. 453–461.

Skinner, B. F. (1971) *Beyond Freedom and Dignity.* New York: Knopf.

Slominski, A. H. (1984) 'Winthrop Phelps and the Children's Rehabilitation Institute.' *In:* Scrutton, D. (Ed.) *Management of the Motor Disorders of Children with Cerebral Palsy. Clinics in Developmental Medicine No. 90.* London: S.I.M.P. with Blackwell Scientific; Philadelphia: J. B. Lippincott. pp. 59–74.

Soboloff, H. R. (1981) 'Long term follow-up of handicapped children.' *Paper read at the Eighth World Congress of Social Psychiatry, Zagreb, Yugoslavia.*

Somers, A. R. (1979) 'Marital status, health, and the use of health services.' *Journal of the American Medical Association*, **241**, 1818–1822.

Sparrow, S., Zigler, E. (1978) 'Evaluation of patterning treatment for retarded children.' *Pediatrics*, **62**, 137–150.

Stamp, W. G. (1973) 'Bracing in cerebral palsy.' *Instructional Course Lectures, American Academy of Orthopaedic Surgeons*, **18**, 286–306.

Staros, A., LeBlanc, M. (1975) 'Orthotic components and systems.' *In:* American Academy of Orthopaedic Surgeons (Eds.) *Atlas of Orthotics—Biomechanical Principles and Applications.* St. Louis: C. V. Mosby.

Stein, R. E. K., Jessof, D. J. (1984) 'Relationship between health status and psychological adjustment among children with chronic conditions.' *Pediatrics*, **73**, 169–174.

Sussman, M. D. (1983) 'Casting as an adjunct to neurodevelopmental therapy in cerebral palsy.' *Developmental Medicine and Child Neurology*, **25**, 804–805.

—— Cusick, B. (1979) 'Preliminary report: the role of short-leg, tone-reducing casts as an adjunct to

210

physical therapy of patients with cerebral palsy.' *Johns Hopkins Medical Journal*, **145**, 112–114.

—— —— (1981) 'Early mobilization of patients with cerebral palsy following muscle release surgery.' *Orthopaedic Transactions*, **5**, 193.

Sutherland, D. H., Olshen, R., Cooper, L., Woo, S. K. (1980) 'The development of mature gait.' *Journal of Bone and Joint Surgery*, **62A**, 336–353.

Sylvester, E. (1977) 'Psychological problems in pediatric orthopaedic patients.' *Lecture at Children's Hospital at Stanford, Palo Alto, California.*

Sziklai, I., Grof, J. (1981) 'Effect of immobilization by plaster on the level of various energy metabolites in skeletal muscle.' *Acta Physiologica Academiae Scientiarum Hungaricae*, **58**, 47–51.

Taft, L. T. (1972) 'Are we handicapping the handicapped?' *Developmental Medicine and Child Neurology*, **14**, 703–704.

Tabary, J. C., Tabary, C., Tardieu, C., Tardieu, G., Goldspink, G. (1972) 'Physiological and structural changes in the cat's soleus muscle due to immobilization at different lengths by plaster casts.' *Journal of Physiology*, **224**, 231–244.

Tauffkirchen, E. (1978) 'Hippotherapy—a supplementary treatment for motion disturbance caused by cerebral palsy' ('Reittherapie-eine erweiterte behandlung bei zerebralen Bewegenungsstorungen'). *Pädiatrie und Pädologie*, **13**, 405–411.

Taylor, S., Kling, T. F. (1984) 'An improved system of orthotic management in neuromuscular disease.' *Orthopaedic Transactions*, **8**, 105.

Terver, S., Levai, J. P., Bleck, E. E. (1981) 'Motricité cérébrale readaption neurologie du developpement.' *Motricité Cérébrale*, **2**, 55–68.

Thomas, A., Bax, M., Coombes, K., Goldson, E., Smyth, D., Whitmore, K. (1985) 'The health and social needs of physically handicapped young adults: are they being met by statutory services?' *Developmental Medicine and Child Neurology.* Supplement No. 50.

Thompson, S. (1977) 'Results of questionnaire on therapy.' Regional Course, *American Academy for Cerebral Palsy and Developmental Medicine*, New Orleans.

Tizard, J. P. (1980) 'Cerebral palsies: treatment and prevention. The Croonian Lecture 1978.' *Journal of the Royal College of Physicians, London*, **14**, 72–77.

Trefler, E., Hanks, S., Huggins, P., Chiarizzo, S., Hobson, D. A. (1978) 'A modular seating system for cerebral palsied children.' *Developmental Medicine and Child Neurology*, **20**, 199–204.

Van der Velde, C. D. (1985) 'Body images of one's self and of others: developmental and clinical significance.' *American Journal of Psychiatry*, **142**, 527–537.

Vasin, N. I., Nodvornik, P., Lesnov, N., Kadin, A. L., Shramka, M. (1979) 'Stereotaxic combined dentate-thalamotomy in the treatment of spastic-hyperkinetic forms of subcortical dyskinesias.' *Zhurnal Voprosy Neirokhirurgii Imeni N.N. Burdenko (Moskova)*, **6**, 23–28.

Von Wendt, L., Ekenberg, L., Dagis, D., Janlert, U. (1984) 'A parent-centered approach to physiotherapy for their handicapped children.' *Developmental Medicine and Child Neurology*, **26**, 445–448.

Vojta, V. (1981) *Die zerebralen Bewegunstrorungen im Säuglingsalter, Früdiagnose und Frütherapie*, 3rd edn. Stuttgart: F. Enke. pp 183–189.

—— (1984) 'The basic elements of treatment according to Vojta.' *In:* Scrutton, D. (Ed.) *The Management of the Motor Disorders of Children with Cerebral Palsy. Clinics in Developmental Medicine No. 90.* London: S.I.M.P. with Blackwell Scientific; Philadelphia: J. B. Lippincott. pp. 75–85.

Waltz, J. M., Davis, J. A. (1983) 'Cervical cord stimulation in the treatment of athetosis and dystonia.' *Advances in Neurology*, **37**, 225–237.

Watt, J., Sims, D., Harckham, F., Schmidt, L., McMillan, A., Hamilton, J. (1984) 'A prospective study of inhibitive casting as an adjunct to physiotherapy in the cerebral palsied child.' *Orthopaedic Transactions*, **8**, 110.

Weber, S. (1983) 'Indication for exercise therapy in infancy in prevention of childhood cerebral palsy' ('Indikation zur krankengymnastischen Behandlung im Säuglingsalter zur Prophylaze infantiler Zerebralparesen'). *Klinische Pädiatrie*, **195**, 347–350.

Westin, G. W., Dye, S. (1983) 'Conservative management of cerebral palsy in the growing child.' *Foot and Ankle*, **4**, 160–163.

White, R. (1984) 'Sensory-integrative therapy for the cerebral-palsied child.' *In:* Scrutton, D. (Ed.) *Management of the Motor Disorders of Children with Cerebral Palsy. Clinics in Developmental Medicine No. 90.* London: S.I.M.P. with Blackwell Scientific; Philadelphia: J. B. Lippincott. pp. 86–95.

Whittaker, C. K. (1980) 'Cerebellar stimulation in cerebral palsy.' *Journal of Neurosurgery*, **52**, 648–653.

211

Wilke, T. F. (1967) 'The problem of drooling in cerebral palsy: a surgical approach.' *Canadian Journal of Surgery*, **10**, 60–67.

Williams, I. (1977) 'The consequences of orthopaedic surgery in the adolescent cerebral palsied: medical education and parental attitudes.' *Paper read at the Study Group on Integrating the Care of Multiply Handicapped Children, St. Mary's College, Durham, England.* London: The Spastics Society Medical Education and Information Unit.

Wolfer, J. A., Visintainer, M. A. (1979) 'Prehospital psychological preparation for tonsillectomy patients: effects on children's and parents' adjustment.' *Pediatrics*, **64**, 646–655.

Woolridge, C. P., McLaurin, C. (1976) 'Biofeedback-background and applications to physical rehabilitation.' *Bulletin of Prosthetic Research*, Spring, 25–37.

World Health (1984) May, 4, 5, 20, 25.

Wright, T., Nicholson, J. (1973) 'Physiotherapy for the spastic child: an evaluation.' *Developmental Medicine and Child Neurology*, **15**, 146–163.

Yates, H., Mott, D. H. (1977) 'Inhibitive casting.' *Paper read at the First William C. Duncan Seminar on Cerebral Palsy.* Seattle: Children's Orthopaedic Hospital and Medical Center and the University of Washington.

Zachazewski, J. E., Eberle, E. D., Jefferies, M. (1982) 'Effect of tone-inhibiting casts and orthoses on gait. A case report.' *Physical Therapy*, **62**, 453–455.

7
SPASTIC HEMIPLEGIA

Characteristics and natural history

The typical posture of the child with spastic hemiplegia consists of equinus of the foot and ankle, flexion of the elbow, wrist and fingers, and an adducted thumb (Fig. 7.1). Variations of this pattern will be found whether the spastic paralysis is barely discernible or severe. In mild forms of hemiplegia, the upper-limb involvement is not noticed until the child runs and 'stresses' the central nervous system. Varus of the foot is usual; pes valgus does occur, but not nearly as often as in spastic diplegia.

Most of these children begin independent walking between the ages of 18 and 21 months, gain independence in activities of daily living, are able to talk, can participate in peer group activities and attend regular school. Their greatest handicap can be mental retardation, behavioural problems, and late-onset convulsive disorder (Perlstein and Hood 1956, Jones 1976).

General management

Physical and occupational therapy

Because children who have spastic hemiplegia have an intact unilateral sensory and motor system, the management of their motor problems to achieve function for independent living is not difficult. They need only short-term supervision, if any, by a physical or occupational therapist. The therapist can be of great help in analyzing the functional capacity of the hand, the sensibility, the active and passive ranges of motion of the fingers and wrist, and the strength of the controlling muscles. The therapist can also suggest ways to practise and to use adaptive devices for efficiency in bimanual skills.

Orthotics

Orthotic use is minimal, and usually consists of the plastic ankle-foot orthosis at an early age in an attempt to control ankle equinus and prevent contractures— although we have little evidence that this occurs (see Chapter 6).

Upper-limb orthoses are temporary expedients, and do not seem to be effective in encouraging function or in correcting contractures. Most of us have used the opponens-type splint to keep the thumb out of the palm in young children while their nervous system is maturing. Similar use has been made of plastic volar wrist-extension splints. Both are used only part of the day, because they seem to interfere with the child's hand function and attempts to adapt. Moberg (1984) makes the good point that the usual volar hand and finger splint covers the area where tactile gnosis is important in order to grasp. He suggests that this part of the splint be replaced with soft non-elastic straps.

Although night splinting of the hand and fingers is often recommended to prevent contractures, there are no data to confirm their efficacy. The hand and

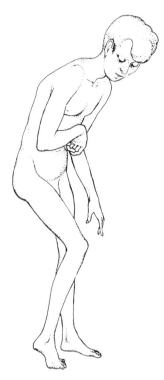

Fig. 7.1. Typical posture, spastic hemiplegia.

wrist are usually relaxed during sleep. Splinting, however, is 'something to do' and cannot be entirely condemned if it satisfies the needs and perceptions of the parents, physician and therapist in the management of the very young hemiplegic child.

Management
Surgical management of the lower limb is mainly for equinus due to contractures of the triceps surae, and to prevent fixed varus deformities when dynamic inversion of the foot occurs during gait. Surgery of the hand and upper limb is highly selective. While surgery can improve upper-limb function and appearance, it never restores hand function to normal—mainly because of the almost universal defect in stereognostic sensation in the involved limb. Surgery is a mere incident in their lives.

The major thrust of the management program is educational and behavioral, to allow as normal a maturation as possible so that independent function and community integration can be achieved.

Upper-limb surgery
Evaluation of the hand for surgery
The following factors need to be considered and examinations conducted in the assessment of the hand and upper limb:

214

1. TYPE OF MOTOR DISORDER: SPASTIC OR ATHETOID?

Dystonic posturing of the hand and upper limb is often confused with that of spastic paralysis especially in patients with hemidystonia.

Dystonia is differentiated from spasticity when relaxation of the patient restores the hand to a normal posture, when there are no contractures or increased stretch reflexes and when the deep tendon reflexes are either normal or hypoactive (Fig. 1.3).

Tendon lengthenings or transfers in dystonic hands either fail to relieve the flexed posture of the wrist or fingers, or cause a reversal to an extension posture.

2. BEHAVIORAL STATUS AND INTELLECTUAL FUNCTION

The patient must have sufficient intellectual function and emotional stability to comprehend the goals of surgery and to co-operate in the optimum restoration of hand function postoperatively (Zancolli and Zancolli 1981).

3. HAND SENSATION

Most patients with hemiplegia have deficient stereognosis (tactile gnosis). The tests for shape recognition are done with the eyes occluded and using the normal hand as a control (Fig. 2.28).

For patients who can articulate or indicate the difference between one and two points, Moberg's two-point discrimination test with a paper-clip may be more useful (Fig. 2.29), especially in those patients who have a bilateral motor involvement. Moberg points out that this test must be carefully performed by stabilizing the patient's and the examiner's fingers, so that the skin does not blanch from the pressure applied through the tips of the clip. The pressure should not exceed 10g (Moberg 1976, 1984).

We have tried the Moberg paper-clip test and compared it to shape recognition in our patients with cerebral palsy. Our preliminary results indicate that it is probably as accurate as shape recognition and simpler to perform.

Thus far it appears that those with spastic diplegia have normal two-point discrimination and normal shape recognition.

Moberg emphasizes the importance of tactile gnosis as the highest quality of sensibility; it puts 'eyes' on the fingertips. Without it, visual feedback is necessary and this can provide control of only one hand at a time.

Sensory tests involving pins, touching or testing temperatures have no relevance in the evaluation for hand surgery. More sophisticated sensory tests of finger and thumb pulp have been described. The 'pulp-writing' test was found to be more indicative of higher functions than the two-point discrimination test after sensory-nerve reconstructive surgery (Hirasawa *et al.* 1985). In this test, the patient's eyes are closed and the examiner writes letters with a blunt rod on the pulp of the patient's finger. The patient then draws his impressions of the letters on a prepared outline of the thumb pulp. This test might give more information about sensibility and prognosis in cerebral-palsied hands than other tests. The results would depend very much on the intelligence and age of the patient.

Goldner and Felic (1966) long ago recognized the importance of good

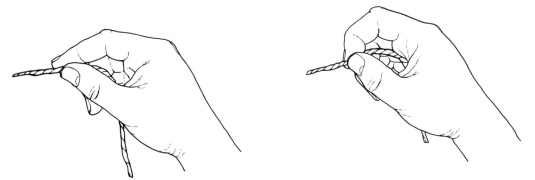

Fig. 7.2. Pinch. *Left:* thumb and index extended. *Right:* thumb and index flexed. These represent terminal positions for digits when executing this pattern of movement.

sensation in the prognosis for function in cerebral-palsied hands. If tactile gnostic sensation is deficient, patients and parents need to be informed: and while this deficiency is not an absolute contra-indication to surgery, it does compromise the result. No 'therapy' has been discovered to restore defective sensation even by 'early intervention'.

4. HAND FUNCTION IN ACTIVITIES OF DAILY LIVING
How the patient manages such actions as turning on a light-switch and faucets, dressing, toileting, bathing and grooming should be part of the examination.

Moberg (1962) suggests various tasks to test precision grip: (i) screw on a bolt, (ii) wind a wrist-watch, (iii) sew with a needle, (iv) knot a piece of string, (v) lift a teacup with the thumb and forefinger, and (vi) button and unbutton. Gross grip can be functionally assessed by the ability to (i) work with a heavy handled object like a wheelbarrow, (ii) use a spade, (iii) manipulate a doorknob, (iv) hold a bottle and (v) carry a basket.

Elliott and Connolly's (1984) classification of manipulative hand movements as intrinsic movement patterns of the digits might be a better method of analysis. These intrinsic movements have been subdivided into simultaneous patterns as simple synergies of pinch, dynamic tripod (*e.g.* holding a pencil) and squeeze; the reciprocal synergies of thumb function are twiddle, rock, radial roll, index roll and full roll. Sequential patterns are those in which movement is step-like: rotary step (*e.g.* moving a circular object with the fingertips), interdigital step (*e.g.* a pen or chopstick is turned from one end to the other), and linear step (where the fingers are repositioned along the linear axis of an object, as in playing a violin). The palmar slide is the action of the thumb against the index finger, while the other fingers grasp an object (*e.g.* when uncapping a fountain pen) (Figs. 7.2 to 7.13, reproduced by permission from Elliott and Connolly 1984).

5. VOLUNTARY GRASP AND RELEASE PATTERNS
Voluntary grasp and release patterns have been classified into three types (Zancolli *et al.* 1983): *(Continued on page 221)*

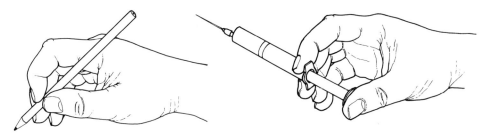

Fig. 7.3. Dynamic tripod: small, simultaneous flexion and extension movements of the thumb, index finger and digit 3 manipulate pen.

Fig. 7.4. Squeeze: precise configuration of fingers is determined by shape of syringe. Simultaneous flexion of thumb, index and digit 3 will drive plunger into barrel.

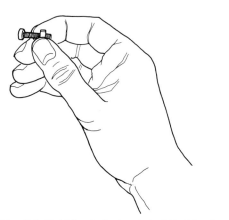
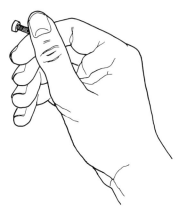

Fig. 7.5. Twiddle. *Left:* thumb in full abduction. *Right:* thumb in partial adduction, with concurrent index flexion. Extent of thumb adduction is quite variable, depending on extent of movement required in alternating between postures illustrated.

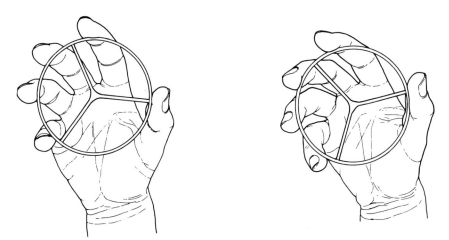

Fig. 7.6. Rock: illustrated in ventral view with a petri dish. *Left:* thumb in partial abduction. *Right:* thumb in partial adduction.

217

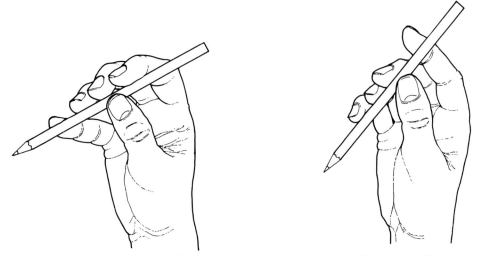

Fig. 7.7. Rock: illustrated with pencil held transversely in radial-ulnar axis. Movements of thumb and digit 3 are much reduced compared with movements of other digits. *Left:* ulnar digits relatively extended. *Right:* ulnar digits relatively flexed.

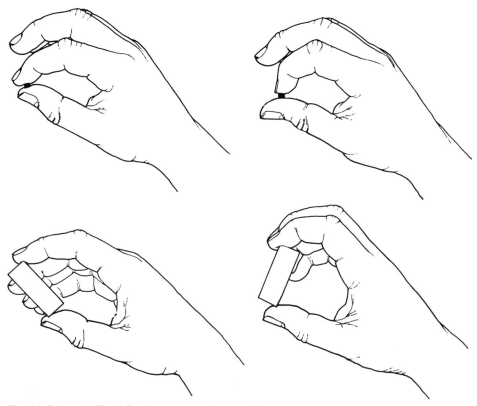

Fig. 7.8. Index roll. *Top left:* slight reciprocal flexion of thumb and extension of index, and *top right:* the reverse. Full roll *(bottom left and right)* as for index roll, but with involvement of additional digits. The object rocks about the radio-ulnar axis as a result of movement between the positions illustrated.

218

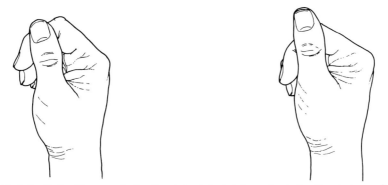

Fig. 7.9. Radial roll. In this example the thumb is abducted throughout; in other instances it may be partially adducted, consequently operating radial index more distally. *Left:* index less flexed. *Right:* index more flexed.

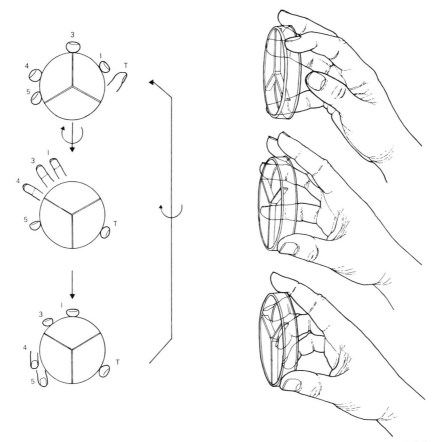

Fig. 7.10. Rotary step. A schematic representation of positions in which the digits are placed *(left)* and successive postures of the hand *(right)*. Sequence *(right, top to bottom)* shows successive phases in clockwise rotation totalling approximately 120° of object rotation. This occurs between transitions *top* to *center* and *bottom* to *top*, as indicated by the rotary arrows.

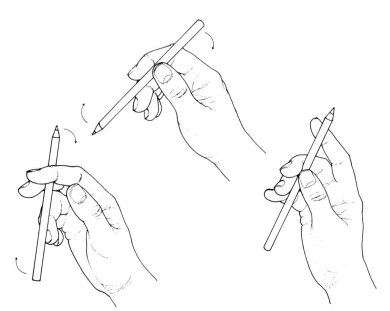

Fig. 7.11. Interdigital step: from *center* to *left* the object is rotated by extension of ulnar digits, especially digit 3. Flexed thumb passes under rotating object to assume its position shown *left*. From *left* to *right*, thumb and ulnar digits flex to grasp object and index extends and may lose contact with it. From *right* to *center*, index flexes to preserve position of object against thumb, while ulnar digits flex to reposition below object in readiness for next cycle.

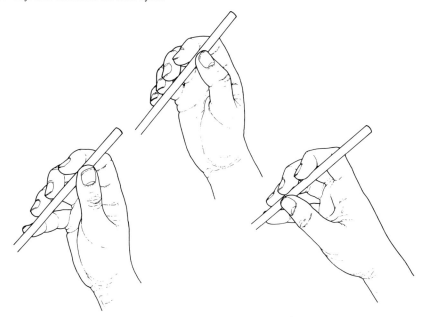

Fig. 7.12. Linear step: from *center* to *left*, ulnar digits extend inter-phalangeally, but flex at carpo-metacarpal joints, sliding along object. From *left* to *right*, thumb abducts to oppose ulnar digits. From *right* to *center*, index flexes to restore initial posture.

220

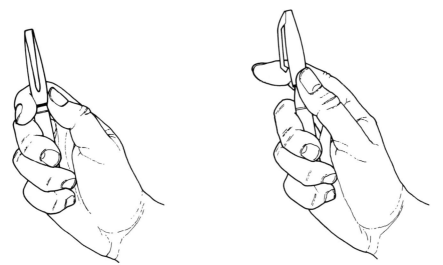

Fig. 7.13. Palmar slide: the movement, illustrated in change from *left* to *right*, involves extension of thumb and radial deviation of index, with some extension.

Pattern I: the fingers actively extend with the wrist in less than 20° of flexion. Surgery is indicated.

Pattern II: the wrist and fingers are constantly in flexion. Active finger extension occurs only when the wrist is flexed more than 20°. This pattern has been divided into two groups:

Pattern IIa: when the wrist and fingers are flexed, active extension of the wrist is possible because the wrist extensors exert good voluntary control.

Pattern IIb: when the fingers are flexed, wrist extension is not possible because the wrist extensors are weak or lack voluntary control. In these patients the hand can open only by wrist flexion, which creates a tenodesis effect on the finger extensors. Surgery can improve function.

Pattern III: this is a severe flexion deformity of the hand, without finger extension even with maximum wrist flexion, and with no active wrist extension with the fingers flexed. Passive extension of the fingers and thumb is possible when the wrist is flexed. Function will not improve much with surgery, but appearance may be greatly improved.

In an earlier publication Zancolli and Zancolli (1981) gave a more refined classification of cerebral palsy hand dysfunction and deformity (Table 7.I).

In the examination, the effect of wrist on finger extension should be observed. Very often finger extension occurs not by active extension, but by the tenodesis effect of the extensor digitorum communis as the wrist drops into flexion. In these cases wrist stabilization or an extension contracture of the wrist will preclude opening the hand for release from the grasp.

Goldner's original classification (1975) is useful and straightforward:

1. Minimal involvement. The patient's hand has pinch, grasp and release, but lacks dexterity and speed. No surgery is indicated.

221

TABLE 7.I
Classification of cerebral palsy hand dysfunction and deformity (from Zancolli and Zancolli 1981)

I Extrinsic Type
General fully developed pattern:
Upper limb with internal rotation of the shoulder, flexion of the elbow, pronation of the forearm, flexion of the wrist and fingers, adduction or adduction/flexion of the thumb, 'swan-neck' deformities of the fingers (occasionally)
Group 1 – minimal spasticity in the flexor carpi ulnaris
– active finger extension with *less than* 20° wrist flexion
Group 2 – finger extension with *more than* 20° wrist flexion
subgroup 2a – active wrist extension with fingers flexed; therefore, most of the spasticity is in the finger-flexor muscles
subgroup 2b – no active wrist extension with the fingers flexed; therefore, no voluntary control of wrist-extensor muscles
Group 3 – wrist or finger extension impossible even with maximal flexion of the wrist
(In all 3 groups—thumb-in-palm).

II Intrinsic Type
Intrinsic-plus deformity; usually occurs in mixed type of paralysis—spastic and athetoid.

Surgical decisions based upon the classification:
Groups 1 and 2-surgery indicated for functional pinch, grasp and release (N.B. will always prefer uninvolved hand)
Group 3-surgery for appearance, hygiene and comfort.

---

2. Thumb-in-palm, wrist flexed moderately; to extend the fingers the wrist must be dropped into full flexion (tenodesis effect on the finger extensors) (Fig. 7.14).

3. Thumb-in-palm, wrist and fingers completely flexed; the patient is unable to extend the fingers (Fig. 7.15). Surgery is indicated to improve appearance and hand hygiene.

To the above classification I would add the following observations to assist in decision-making for surgery:

1. Voluntary control.

2. No voluntary control; mirror movements by the opposite hand are the controlling mechanism. Mirror movements are probably normal up to the age of six or seven years in some children. These can be ascertained by asking the child to place his hands on the table-top and perform alternating movements (*e.g.* finger tapping or rapid pronation and supination) with one hand alone, and then the other hand.

3. No voluntary or mirror movement control.

Surgery may be indicated in the first two patterns. In the third, restoration of any function cannot be promised; surgery is indicated for appearance, hygiene and comfort.

Although the above patterns are useful to organize thinking and examining, they are only general guides and cannot be slavishly applied in decisions for specific surgery. Only examination, repeat examination and repeat examination of the patient's hand and upper limb will allow a reasonably correct plan for surgical treatment.

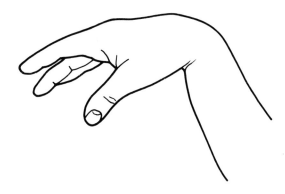

Fig. 7.14. Spastic hand pattern II. To open the fingers, wrist must flex, exerting a tenodesis effect on the finger extensor tendons.

Electromyographic evaluation

Electromyography of the spastic muscle to be lengthened or transferred has been used as an additional method of analysis for many years. Samilson and Morris (1964) found continuous activity of spastic muscles, and thought that some of their postoperative tendon transfers or lengthenings resulted in restoration of some normally timed electrical activity.

Feldkamp and Guth (1980) also used electromyographic analysis of spastic hand function preoperatively. However, it is not clear how their studies or those of Samilson and Morris aided in decision-making for surgery.

Hoffer *et al.* (1979) did use the electromyographic information preoperatively. They transferred the tendons of muscles only when these muscles showed isolated electrical activity in grasp in those with weak grasp, and only muscles that had isolated activity in release in hands with a poor release. Hoffer *et al.* (1983) made the case for dynamic electromyography in surgery for adduction contractures of the thumb. If selective control of the adductor pollicis was found in electromyograms, and they had a key pinch, only partial adductor pollicis myotomy was performed. If they found neither selective control nor key pinch, then they performed a total myotomy of the adductor pollicis muscle.

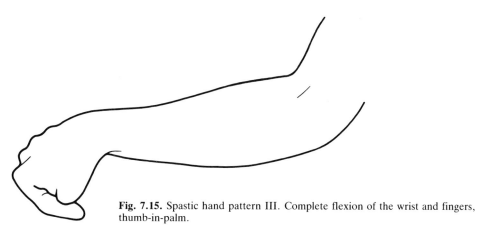

Fig. 7.15. Spastic hand pattern III. Complete flexion of the wrist and fingers, thumb-in-palm.

Mowery *et al.* (1985) used preoperative and postoperative electromyograms of muscles in which tendon transfer was planned in 12 patients with cerebral palsy. Postoperative electromyograms in four of 16 muscles tested showed changes in their preoperative electrical activity: three continuously firing muscles became phasic, and only one muscle changed phase to match that of its recipient.

The reports of Hoffer *et al.* (1979, 1983) seem to be alone in suggesting that electromyographic studies are useful for deciding on appropriate upper-limb surgery. The technology is still relatively new, and with increasing appropriate and skilled use will be found helpful as another laboratory tool to refine surgery of the spastic hand.

Myoneural blocks
Infiltration of the muscle bellies of the flexor muscles of the wrist and fingers with lidocaine (either 0.5 or 1 per cent*) is useful to determine whether the spastic flexor muscles of the wrist or fingers are preventing voluntary extension of the wrist or fingers (Goldner 1983, Moberg 1985). In contrast to a local anesthetic block of the median nerve, a myoneural block obviates the loss of finger sensation which occurs over a fairly large area of the palm and fingers. This loss of sensation might alter the functional evaluation considerably, because Moberg's study (1976) indicates the important rôle of cutaneous sensory endings in providing feedback of joint-position sense: 'There is no "muscle sense" in man' (p. 34).

Infiltration of the biceps muscle with the local anesthetic may help to decide the effect of muscle release in flexion deformities of the elbow. In two patients who had severe, painful and disabling contraction of the elbow flexor muscles in hemidystonia, I infiltrated the biceps brachii with 45 per cent alcohol. This gave me, the patient and the family two to four weeks to decide on the effects of denervating the biceps brachii in order to reduce the severe elbow-flexion posture. I would not recommend infiltration of the forearm musculature with alcohol. Its effects can be very destructive on the adjacent peripheral nerves, and the resultant paralysis might last a distressing three to four months.

Prerequisites for surgery
Judging from the reports of the number of patients with cerebral palsy who had hand surgery compared with the whole of the cerebral palsy population, the indications when applied for surgery have restricted the number of patients operated on (Goldner 1955, Chait *et al.* 1980, Zancolli and Zancolli 1981, Hoffer *et al.* 1983, Mowery *et al.* 1985).

1. SPASTIC PARALYSIS
Although a satisfactory surgical result may be possible when the spastic hand has a minor degree of athetosis (*e.g.* chorea), the best results are achieved only in those with spastic paralysis, and most of these have hemiplegia. In one study of results of

---

*The dose of lidocaine should not exceed 4.5mg/kg in children over 10 years and in adults; in children under age 10, the dosage should be adjusted downward according to the usual pediatric drug dose rules (*e.g.* Clark's).

87 spastic hands, only two had quadriplegia; all the others had hemiplegia (Zancolli and Zancolli 1981).

As I have urged in previous sections, spastic hands must be differentiated from those with dystonic posturing. This error in diagnosis seems to be prevalent. The dystonic hand will be completely relaxed during sleep, with sedation and voluntarily. There are no contractures and no increased stretch reflexes. The deep-tendon reflexes are normal or hypotonic. If tendon transfers are done in a dystonic hand, the reverse and equally disabling dynamic posture can result.

2. AGE OF THE PATIENT

Most experienced surgeons in this field recommend deferring surgery until age five years or older. By this time the child can co-operate in the preoperative analysis and the postoperative regimen. An exception to this advice is that of Goldner (1983). He will lengthen a wrist tendon (usually the flexor carpi ulnaris) in a three-year-old if it is deforming and contracted. This procedure is always followed by prolonged splinting.

Lipp and Jones (1984) strongly recommended that this procedure could and should be done at age three years, based upon their results of transfer of the flexor carpi ulnaris to correct the flexion-pronation deformity of the wrist.

3. SENSATION

Although stereognosis is absent in the majority of patients with spastic hemiplegia, this is not a contra-indication to surgery. If this sensation of tactile gnosis is normal, then the result will be better.

4. MENTAL STATUS

The mental status obviously will affect the result. Severely retarded children and adults will not obtain the desired functional result. Of more importance is their behaviour. Emotional instability with increased spasticity in response to stimuli will compromise the function (Zancolli et al. 1983).

5. VOLUNTARY CONTROL

This is most important for function after reconstructive surgery. Some ability to extend the fingers with active wrist flexion assures a better result. The best candidates for surgery are those who have either patterns I or II (Zancolli et al. 1983) or Goldner group 2 (1975).

Goals of surgery

The goals are to improve the function and appearance of the hand. The patient and the parents must be told that the hand will never be normal—it will be a helping hand. It is wise to not only state this fact, but also put it in writing (Goldner 1983). However, with the proper selection of the patient for surgery and the proper selection of the specific procedures, the surgical results are much better than the conservative methods of splinting, stretching or special therapies.

When discussing the proposed plan of surgery with the parents and child, the

TABLE 7.II

Functional classification (from Mowery *et al.* 1985)

Excellent	Good use of hand, effective grasp and release, voluntary control.
Good	Helper hand, effective grasp and release, some voluntary control.
Fair	Helper hand, no effective use, moderate grasp and release, fair control.
Poor	Paperweight, absent grasp and release.

surgeon should reiterate that additional surgery may be necessary to accomplish the goal. This will be true even though most of us now try to do multiple surgical procedures at one stage. The preoperative analysis and planning, while very good, is not perfect.

Appearance of the hand will usually be improved with surgery. Appearance often outweighs the functional result; after all, the hand is a highly visible part of the human anatomy. In the analysis of results, authors often comment on the improved appearance as an important parameter of the outcome (Chait *et al.* 1980, Zancolli and Zancolli 1981, Mowery *et al.* 1985).

Improvement of appearance is often termed 'cosmetic'. However, to deny the human need of looking one's best is to deprive the person with spastic hemiplegia and a deformed hand the opportunity to overcome just one obstacle for achievement. While it is true that we should strive to look at the person behind the handicap, it is also true that this is a process which takes time and understanding by others. Rather than hide the deformed hand in the pocket or explain it in detail to the other person, it seems that a more normal hand will help to improve initial relationships and increase chances in a job interview. So surgery to improve the appearance of the hand can be a most important functional as well as psychological goal.

I have observed that my hemiplegic patients over age 18 years want their hands to be 'fixed' without any regard for function. They readily accept arthrodesis of the wrist, finger flexor tendon lengthenings and thumb reconstructive surgery. With the American people spending billions of dollars a year on grooming aids and cosmetics, is it irrational and unwarranted to want the best possible appearance?*

Surgical procedures for the upper limb
It must be realized that no single procedure offers the complete reconstruction of the spastic hand and wrist. The procedures described are reliable, but must be combined according to the preoperative analysis; multiple procedures at one stage are usually necessary to achieve the desired result. House *et al.* (1981) give an example of the need for multiple procedures; they performed 165 different procedures for the thumb-in-palm deformity in 56 patients.

The best way of assessing the results is to use a preoperative and postoperative functional classification (Table 7.II). In the paper by Mowery *et al.* (1985), the

*Retail sales of toiletries USA 1982: $17,768 billion; source: US Bureau of the Census (1984) *Statistical Abstracts of the United States (104th edn.)* Washington DC: Government Printing Office.

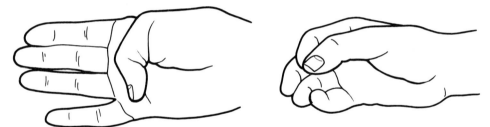

Fig. 7.16. *Left:* thumb-in-palm deformity due to spastic adductor pollicis and flexor pollicis longus. *Right:* normal pinch.

functional grade after hand surgery improved by at least one level in all patients. Of the 12 patients reported, results were evenly divided into excellent, good and fair.

A more elaborate and precise method of evaluation of the results of surgery was published by Swanson (1982) and Zancolli *et al.* (1983).

Thumb deformities
Whether the thumb is only adducted (either a dynamic or a fixed deformity) due to contracture, or is a thumb-in-palm deformity, the objective is to get the thumb out of the palm and to restore pinch. True opposition by pulp pinch cannot be achieved in most. This is not a functional pinch. A 'key' pinch will suffice (Figs. 7.16, 7.17).

Based upon my observations of children with cerebral palsy in Asian countries, the adduction contracture of the thumb might be useful to manipulate chopsticks. The adducted thumb normally stabilizes one of the sticks against the ring finger.

SPASTIC DYNAMIC ADDUCTION
This deformity is due to spasticity of the adductor pollicis muscle, with the metacarpal and interphalangeal joints maintained in extension. If the deformity is only dynamic, passive abduction of the thumb is possible, and the adducted position interferes with the release of the side pinch to the index finger. In this case, a simple release of the adductor insertion through an ulnar incision over the metacarpal-phalangeal joint is sufficient. Goldner (1983) sutures this insertion to the annular ligament of the metacarpal-phalangeal joint as a controlled lengthen-

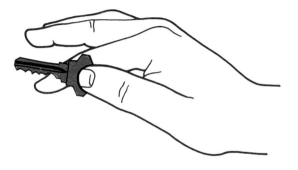

Fig. 7.17. Key pinch: the thumb pulp opposes the radial side of the index finger.

ing, if arthrodesis of this joint is not necessary. If arthrodesis is required, then the adductor pollicis insertion is sutured more proximally. Hoffer *et al.* (1983) advise more selectivity in tenotomy of the adductor pollicis based upon the dynamic electromyograph. If the adductor muscle demonstrates selective control during grasp and release, then only myotomy of the transverse fibers is needed. If there is non-selective control (a patterned type of contraction with continuous firing of the muscle), a complete myotomy of the adductor pollicis muscle was recommended. These procedures were done through a z-plasty incision in the web space. The thumb procedures were always combined with tendon transfers at the wrist or fingers, and in some with a capsulodesis of the first metacarpal-phalangeal joint.

ADDUCTION CONTRACTURE

When a severe adduction contracture of the thumb occurs (which is very rare in children), then a release of the origin of the adductor pollicis is necessary. This procedure, introduced by Matev (1963), uses a palmar incision. Goldner (1983) found the palmar approach unnecessary; the origin release from the third and second metacarpals can be done through a dorsal incision. The first dorsal interosseus muscle aggravates these severe adduction deformities, and can be released from the first and second metacarpals (Goldner 1955, 1975, 1983; Silver *et al.* 1976; House 1981).

SKIN WEB-SPACE CONTRACTURE

A z-plasty of the web space is almost never required in children with cerebral palsy. Goldner (1983) advised that the flap of skin on the thumb side of the incision be made larger so that with undermining the dorsal skin advancement of both flaps and a loose closure can be accomplished.

The various techniques of z-plasty of the thumb web space have been described in detail by Meyer et al. (1981).

If in severe skin contractures the web-space skin cannot be completely closed even with z-plasty, then a full-thickness skin graft from the elbow flexor crease is a solution (Goldner 1983).

THUMB-IN-PALM

This is the commonest thumb deformity; as well as the adduction spasticity and eventual contracture there is a flexion spasticity and contracture of the flexor pollicis longus, and at times also the flexor pollicis brevis and the abductor pollicis brevis (Goldner 1983). Several procedures are required to alleviate the untenable position of the thumb so that grasp can occur, and if possible to restore lateral or key pinch:

1. Release of the adductor pollicis (depending upon the degree of the dynamic deformity) and contracture and release of the first dorsal interosseus.

2. Release of the flexor pollicis brevis and abductor pollicis brevis insertions from the thumb sesamoid bones and resuturing of the insertions proximally after arthrodesis of the metacarpal-phalangeal joint (Goldner 1983).

3. Arthrodesis of the metacarpal-phalangeal joint if unstable (excessive

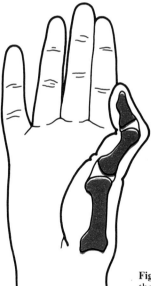

Fig. 7.18. Common posture of the thumb with instability in extension at the metacarpal-phalangeal joint.

motion) in both flexion and extension, or capsulodesis of the joint if hyperextendable (Zancolli *et al.* 1983) (Fig. 7.18).

4. Lengthening of the flexor pollicis longus and reinforcement if it has weak muscle power (Goldner 1983), or transfer of this tendon to the radial side of the proximal phalanx with arthrodesis of the interphalangeal joint of the thumb in 15° of flexion (Smith 1982).

5. Rerouting of the extensor pollicis longus (Goldner 1983, Manske 1984).

6. Reinforcement of the abductor and extensor pollicis longus.

7. Shortening by plication of the tendon of the abductor pollicis longus.

ARTHRODESIS OF THE METACARPAL-PHALANGEAL JOINT

This procedure can be done in children who have open epiphyses (Goldner 1975, 1983; Zancolli *et al.* 1983). Through a midlateral ulnar incision over the joint, the lateral band is retracted dorsally, the ulnar collateral ligament and capsule cut, the joint opened and the articular cartilage on both surfaces removed. In children it is safer to 'nibble' away the cartilage with a rongeur. The joint surfaces are coapted manually in 5° of flexion. Using a motorized drill, a single smooth pin is drilled through the center of the proximal phalanx in line with the center of the nail. Then with the joint flexed 5°, the pin is drilled in retrograde manner into the first metacarpal. The phalanx is rotated so that the palmar thumb-pad coincides with the radial aspect of the index finger. Smooth pins are inserted at a 45° angle across the joint to secure the arthrodesis. Small bone chips can be added to any gaps in the arthrodesis site (Fig. 7.19).

The ends of the pins are clipped off beneath the skin and removed when the arthrodesis is solid (eight to 12 weeks). A plaster holds the thumb and wrist in position while healing occurs.

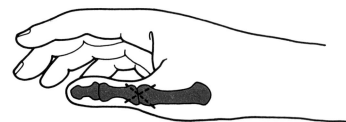

Fig. 7.19. Arthrodesis of the metacarpal-phalangeal joint of the thumb with crossed fixation pins.

In skeletally mature patients I prefer a small (³⁄₃₂in) screw for fixation. After the joint surfaces are denuded, the joint is manually compressed and held in the proper position. A small hole of the same diameter as the screw is bored with an air-powered dental burr in the distal end of the dorsal surface of the metacarpal neck. This hole is then drilled obliquely into the center of the proximal phalanx. With the burr, the entry hole in the metacarpal is enlarged so that the screw-head can be countersunk slightly. The screw is then inserted and the joint surfaces compressed (Fig. 7.20). With this rigid fixation, it is possible to remove the postoperative plaster in three to four weeks so that early motion of the hand and wrist can commence. If the screw-hole in the metacarpal breaks during the procedure, all is not lost. The joint can always be secured with multiple crossed pins (in adults I prefer threaded pins or wires).

CAPSULODESIS OF THE METACARPAL-PHALANGEAL JOINT
This operation has been recommended if the metacarpal-phalangeal joint is unstable in hyperextension but not flexion (Filler *et al.* 1976, Zancolli 1979, Zancolli *et al.* 1983). It consists of detachment of the volar capsule of the metacarpal-phalangeal joint from the first metacarpal and advancement of the capsular attachment proximally into a groove in the metacarpal shaft. Fixation is with a pullout suture, threaded first through the capsule and then through two drill holes directed dorsally in the neck of the metacarpal, and tied over a button on the dorsum of the first metacarpal (Fig. 7.21). 30° of flexion are recommended by advocates of the procedure. Plaster immobilization is six weeks postoperatively.

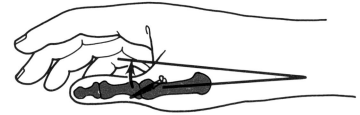

Fig. 7.20. Arthrodesis of the metacarpal-phalangeal joint of the thumb with small screw fixation. The joint is flexed 5° to 10° for optimum function.

230

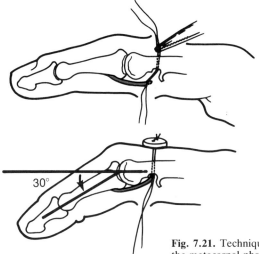

Fig. 7.21. Technique for volar capsule advancement to stabilize the metacarpal-phalangeal joint of the thumb.

LENGTHENING AND REINFORCEMENT OF THE FLEXOR POLLICIS LONGUS

This should be done if the distal phalanx of the thumb is persistently flexed. Contracture of the flexor pollicis longus contributes to the thumb-in-palm. A weak muscle decreases endurance of grasp and pinch (Goldner 1983). Lengthening is not indicated if there is no flexion contracture found on 30° of wrist extension and passive hyperextension of the thumb. Reinforcement would not be indicated if the extensor muscles are half normal strength or better, or if reinforcement of the extensor and abductor pollicis longus is not done. The indications to reinforce the flexor pollicis longus muscle are probably uncommon.

Lengthening and reinforcement can be done through an incision over the volar radial surface of the wrist and forearm. To determine the amount of lengthening, the wrist is placed in 15° extension with the thumb held in full abduction and the proximal phalanx held in neutral extension. The resultant amount of flexion at the distal joint is measured, and the flexor pollicis longus tendon is lengthened 0.5mm per degree (Goldner 1983). The lengthening is done above the transverse carpal ligament so that the suture line will not impinge on this ligament.

Reinforcement is with the brachioradialis (which must be extensively mobilized) or a flexor digitorum superficialis tendon. The pronator teres is said to be usable as well (Goldner 1983). If the flexor superficialis is selected, it is adjusted to one-half its resting length for the suture to the flexor pollicis longus tendon.

Smith (1982) described the transfer of the flexor pollicis longus tendon to the radial side of the proximal phalanx of the thumb combined with arthrodesis or tenodesis of the distal phalanx in 15° of flexion. Smith reported improvement in grasp in seven patients but pinch and the ability to manipulate small objects was not improved. The ability to manipulate small objects is not the usual result in most surgery of the hand in cerebral palsy. The motor control and sensation originating in the brain is deficient.

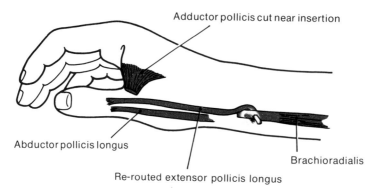

Adductor pollicis cut near insertion

Abductor pollicis longus

Brachioradialis

Re-routed extensor pollicis longus

Fig. 7.22. Technique for reinforcement of thumb abduction by transfer of the brachioradialis to the rerouted extensor pollicis longus. The abductor pollicis longus can be shortened and advanced.

REROUTING OF THE EXTENSOR POLLICIS LONGUS TENDON

This procedure is almost always performed in conjunction with other techniques for correction of the thumb-in-palm. Through a lazy-s incision from the metacarpal-phalangeal joint of the thumb to about 4cm proximal to the wrist, the extensor pollicis longus tendon is dissected from its dorsal hood insertion to its musculo-tendinous junction. The tendon is lifted out of its fibro-osseus tunnel in the radial styloid and shifted to the radial side of the wrist. It is held in its new location by fashioning a flap of subcutaneous fascia and fat to make a tunnel 3 to 4cm long (Figs. 7.22, 7.23).

Manske (1984) observed in spastic thumb deformities that the distal phalanx extended during finger extension (indicating in-phase muscle function of the extensor pollicis longus) and also that the extensor pollicis longus acted as a thumb adductor (noted as well by other surgeons). His procedure in 17 patients was to detach the extensor pollicis longus at the extensor hood, withdrawing the tendon into the forearm, rerouting it through the first extensor compartment and suturing it to the first metacarpal-phalangeal joint capsule and extensor hood. The

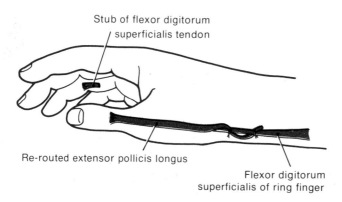

Stub of flexor digitorum superficialis tendon

Re-routed extensor pollicis longus

Flexor digitorum superficialis of ring finger

Fig. 7.23. Technique for reinforcement of thumb abduction by transfer of the flexor digitorum superficialis to the rerouted extensor pollicis longus.

232

procedure was done in conjunction with the usual myotomies of the spastic intrinsic thumb muscles. His results were good after an average follow-up of 28 months.

Two muscle-tendon units can be used: the flexor digitorum superficialis of the long or ring finger or the brachioradialis. The superficialis tendon is cut at the proximal phalanx of the finger, pulled out through a separate incision 8 to 10cm above the wrist and rerouted subcutaneousiy to the extensor pollicis longus. The brachio-radialis is detached at its insertion on the radius, and the muscle mobilized to the junction of the upper and middle thirds of its belly.

The tendons of either are woven into the extensor pollicis longus tendon after the thumb has been repositioned. To determine the proper tension of the transferred tendon, a temporary anchoring suture is used so that the thumb can move passively to the index finger with the wrist in the neutral position, and to allow passive extension of the thumb about 2.5cm from the index finger. It is not necessary to detach the extensor pollicis tendon from its muscle belly, because keeping it in continuity will help prevent volar displacement of the rerouted tendon (Goldner 1983).

ARTHRODESIS OF THE DISTAL INTERPHALANGEAL JOINT OF THE THUMB
Arthrodesis of this joint is indicated if it is hypermobile in extension, flexion, radial or ulnar deviation. It is not indicated if the distal phalangeal flexion and extension are controlled by the muscle-tendon unit (Goldner 1983).

The operative technique consists of removing the articular surfaces of the joint, and securing it in $5°$ to $10°$ of flexion with threaded pins cut off beneath the skin.

Wrist- and finger-flexion deformities

A spastic wrist-flexion deformity is often due to a combination of both wrist- and finger-flexor spasticity. Only a careful and repeat examination allows discernment if one or the other or both predominate. The possibility that the flexor muscle spasticity prevents active extension of the wrist can be determined by infiltration of the flexor muscle bellies in the proximal forearm with 0.5 or 1 per cent lidocaine.

Tendon lengthening

To avoid overlengthening of the finger-flexor tendons, a controlled lengthening is used to retain the 'normal' tension so that when the hand is relaxed and the wrist in neutral position, the fingers assume their normal flexed position (as it is with your own hand when relaxed on a desk-top with the forearm supinated). When lengthening a contracted wrist-flexor muscle-tendon unit, enough elongation of the tendon should permit about $20°$ of wrist extension.

One way to estimate the amount of z-lengthening of a tendon, to restore its resting length and preserve the proper tension for function, is to lengthen it approximately one-half of the contracted resting state of the muscle. One way to do this is to incise and split the tendon longitudinally for a distance of double the estimated amount of lengthening needed (in general plan to lengthen 0.5mm for every degree of flexion contracture; *e.g.* 40° of contracture = 20mm of lengthening). A 2cm lengthening would require a 4cm split in the tendon; a suture is placed in the distal end of one of the splits in the tendon, which is then cut distal to the suture. Next, this distal end is brought proximally 2cm and sutured to the adjacent intact split tendon, which is then cut proximally. The two slips of tendon are sutured side by side. Handling dangling tendon ends is avoided by this method (Goldner 1983). The suture should be temporary until the proper resting position of the fingers is observed. It is safer to underlengthen, since overlengthening results in too much loss of muscle strength.

In young children, Goldner advised lengthening of the flexor carpi radialis ('the heel cord of the hand') when it appears to be the major deforming force. In other cases it may be the flexor carpi ulnaris. Zancolli and Zancolli (1981) found tenotomy to be a satisfactory solution only in cases of mild flexion deformities.

I have found few children whom I thought were candidates for wrist-flexor tendon lengthening. In any case, overlengthening and lengthening of both wrist-flexor tendons should be avoided.

Lengthening of the finger-flexor tendons is performed in the forearm. When necessary to overcome severe flexion of the digits when the wrist is dorsiflexed to neutral, the flexor digitorum superficialis tendons can be lengthened by the z-method described above. Simultaneous lengthening of the flexor digitorum profundus tendons is not advised.

Another procedure to relieve the flexion deformities of the fingers was proposed by Braun *et al.* (1974). The profundus tendons are sectioned above the wrist, and their proximal ends are sutured to the distal ends of the cut superficialis tendons. The procedure (as in lengthening of both superficialis and profundus tendons) can result in pronounced weakness of finger flexion and the subsequent development of an intrinsic-plus deformity, with the fingers practically fixed in extension. Braun had this kind of result initially, and in subsequent patients recommended postoperative splinting of the fingers in 45° of flexion.

Other methods to lengthen spastic and contracted finger and wrist flexors are variations of release of the flexor muscle origins at the elbow. The variations depend upon the range of finger extension possible when the wrist is flexed:

1. If finger extension is possible with the wrist flexed less than 50°, Zancolli and Zancolli (1981) recommended section of the aponeurosis of the origin of the flexor muscles at the medial epicondyle of the humerus.

2. If finger extension is possible only with the wrist flexed more than 50°, then the entire flexor origin is detached from the humerus (Zancolli and Zancolli 1981). This 'flexor slide' operation, in which the origins are detached and allowed to slide distally, was reported by Inglis and Cooper (1966). It was reviewed as the operation first described by Max Page in 1923 in a report by White (1972), who had 11 failures with this operation in 21 patients. To ensure a complete relief of the flexion contracture of the wrist and fingers, Hadad (1977) added the release of the origins of the flexor digitorum profundus muscles. But it seems as if this extensive and non-selective release of the flexor-muscle origins results in loss

of flexion power, while with a more limited release, the problem is a failure of correction. Selective lengthening and/or transfer of tendons is probably a better solution.

Summary of surgical treatment of wrist- and finger-flexion deformities
Although it is impossible to offer a recipe for what is to be done, the trinity of Zancolli, Goldner and Swanson (Zancolli *et al.* 1983) did attempt to give some recommendations which depend upon which of the three hand patterns occur:

Pattern I. Mild flexion spasticity, especially of the flexor carpi ulnaris and the finger flexors. Perform tenotomy of the flexor carpi ulnaris and musculoaponeurotic release of the flexor origins.

Pattern II. If wrist extensors are weak or absent, transfer the flexor carpi ulnaris to the extensor carpi radialis brevis.

If finger extension is possible with less than 50° of wrist flexion, perform musculoaponeurotic release of the origins of the flexor muscles.

If finger extension is possible only with more than 50° of wrist flexion, do the more extensive release of the flexor muscle origin with a pronator teres release if desired.

Pattern III. Severe flexion of the fingers and inability to extend with full wrist flexion. Do multiple tendon lengthenings in the forearm.

In all patterns, the adducted thumb or the thumb-in-palm is treated as described in the preceding section.

Postoperative care of tendon lengthenings and transfers
Four weeks of immobilization in dressings and splints are usually followed by six to eight weeks of intermittent daytime splinting and all-night splinting with the wrist in neutral position and the fingers extended. During these latter eight weeks the splint can be removed three to four times a day, for periods of up to an hour, for guided functional activities and restoration of motion. Flexible action splints can be used, but excessive pulling by the elastic should not be so great as to elicit a stretch reflex, cause hyperextension of the wrist or preclude flexion of the fingers. This protection is necessary while the collagen fibers mature and recontracture is a risk.

This postoperative regimen undoubtedly varies with the experience of the surgeon, the type of motor disorder and the co-operation of the patient and parents. Therefore my recommendations are only a general guide for a postoperative plan. Some patients may need months of postoperative splinting. All need functional hand activities to obtain the best postoperative result (washing dishes, for instance, can be good home occupational therapy). Bimanual activities should be chosen.

Wrist arthrodesis
Wrist arthrodesis is rarely indicated. I have only performed it when the goal is mainly a normal appearance and a paperweight (stabilizing) function if feasible, and when there is deformity of the carpal bones due to the longstanding flexion contracture of the wrist and fingers.

Arthrodesis should *not* be done if:
(1) The fingers can extend only by flexing the wrist
(2) The fingers can flex only by extending the wrist
(3) Tendon transfers are feasible to improve the wrist position.

Wrist arthrodesis is a satisfactory solution for a severe wrist flexion deformity if:
(1) There is general poor muscle control and strength that precludes active flexion and extension
(2) There is a severe fixed deformity that precludes correction by tendon lengthenings and transfer
(3) Tendon transfers have been done and the wrist position is either not corrected or hyperextended.

OPERATIVE TECHNIQUE
A dorsal longitudinal incision exposes the extensor tendons, which are then retracted. The dorsal capsule of the joint is opened and the navicular and lunate bones excised; the articular surfaces of the carpal bones and distal radius are denuded of cartilage. The denuded articular surface of the capitate is fixed to the saucer-like depression in the denuded articular surface of the radius. A Steinman pin is introduced at the distal end of the third metacarpal in the web space between the third and fourth metacarpal heads. The pin is driven straight through the base of the third metacarpal, across the carpal bones, through the capitate and into the center of the distal radial epiphysis into the shaft of the radius. Iliac bone grafts are added. A plaster cast is used until fusion is solid.

POSITION OF THE WRIST IN ARTHRODESIS
The best position is with the wrist extended to the point where the first metacarpal is in alignment with the shaft of the radius (Figs. 7.19, 7.20). The contracted wrist- and finger-flexor tendons are lengthened the proper amount. To prevent an intrinsic-plus hand with no finger flexion, overlengthening of the flexor digitorum profundus should be avoided. The thumb-in-palm deformity can be managed with the procedures previously described.

Finger-hyperextension deformity ('swan-neck')
The 'swan-neck' deformity of the fingers is a hyperextension of the proximal interphalangeal joints and flexion of the distal interphalangeal joint. It is caused by a persistent flexed posture of the wrist; spasticity of the intrinsic muscles is secondary. The flexion of the wrist results in pulling of the extensor tendons across the dorsum of the proximal interphalangeal joints with stretching of the volar capsules.

Surgical treatment is indicated only when the fingers lock in extension and cannot be actively flexed. The wrist-flexion deformity must also be corrected in all cases.

Two surgical procedures to correct the deformity have been described. I prefer

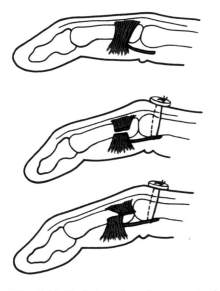

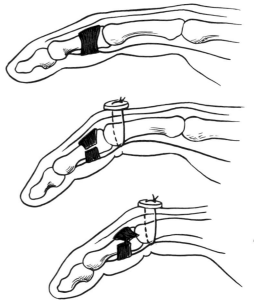

Fig. 7.24. Technique for advancement of volar capsule of proximal interphalangeal joint and retinacular overlap to correct hyper extension locking of proximal joint ('swan-neck' deformity). This can be combined with flexor superficialis tenodesis (Fig. 7.25).

Fig. 7.25. Technique for tenodesis of flexor digitorum superficialis to correct hyperextension deformity of proximal interphalangeal joint. This can be combined with volar capsular advancement (Fig. 7.24).

to combine both, because I observed unwelcome recurrences of the deformity in some patients who have generalized increased ligamentous laxity.

VOLAR CAPSULODESIS

Radial and ulnar midlateral incisions over the proximal interphalangeal joint expose the retinacula which are incised (Goldner 1975, 1983). The volar joint capsule is detached from the distal end of the proximal phalanx and pulled proximally to flex the joint 45°. The capsule is anchored to its new attachment with sutures passed through the bone and tied to a dorsal button. The retinacula are sutured by overlapping the dorsal leaf distally and the volar leaf proximally (Fig. 7.24).

FLEXOR SUPERFICIALIS TENODESIS

The flexor tendons are exposed through a midlateral incision over the proximal joint, and the sheath is then opened; the tendons are retracted volar-ward (Swanson *et al.* 1960). The volar aspect of the proximal phalanx is stripped of its periosteum. The superficialis tendon is then sutured to the distal end of the proximal phalanx through two drill holes directly dorsally in the distal end of the phalanx. The suture is tied over a button on the dorsum of the finger (Fig. 7.25). The proximal phalanx should be flexed about 45°.

In both reconstructions, a fine smooth pin driven from the proximal end of the middle phalanx through to the distal end of the proximal phalanx prevents disruption of the capsule and tendon while healing occurs. The pin can be removed in three to four weeks.

The postoperative immobilization consists of a plaster with the wrist in neutral position and the fingers flexed for six weeks.

Pronation deformity of the forearm

Pronation spasticity and early contracture are common. Posterior subluxation of the radial head occurs early in life, and often accounts for a fixed deformity that limits elbow extension. Posterior dislocation of the radial head occurs as the child matures. Pletcher *et al.* (1976) found this deformity in 2.4 per cent of 384 elbows, in 184 patients with cerebral palsy.

Aitken (1952) described these identical changes in the elbow in a study of children with Erb's obstetrical paralysis. He described subtle early signs of posterior subluxation of the radial head and increased posterior bowing of the ulna. Dislocation of the radial head occurred between the ages of five and eight years. The mechanism of the gradual displacement of the radial head was thought to be due to the pull of the pronator teres when forced supination was imposed by treatment, and contracture of the interosseus membrane was the deforming force on the ulna.

Although Keats (1974) reported success with bilateral radial head excision in a seven-year-old child with cerebral palsy, I had poor results long ago in two children who had closed epiphyses (I would not excise the radial head in a growing child). Aitken (1952) also reported poor results with excision.

Indications for surgery

Prevention of subluxation of the radial head seems possible if the pronation contracture is relieved early enough, probably before the age of three years. In older children who have a pronation contracture and some evidence of active voluntary supination, pronator teres tenotomy has improved active supination. In children who have spastic hemiplegia, the ability to supinate is crucial for participation in ball-games. It is not too easy to catch a ball when one hand is supinated and the other pronated.

Pronator teres tenotomy can be performed alone or in combination with a flexor carpi ulnaris transfer to the distal radius (Green and Banks 1962). I have not found it necessary to do the flexor carpi ulnaris transfer merely to improve active supination. Sakellarides *et al.* (1981) had disappointing results with this procedure, and had much better results when he performed a transfer of the pronator teres insertion.

In my own experience, simple tenotomy of the pronator teres is sufficient. House (1975) was of the same opinion. Good results have also been reported with more complex procedures, such as transfer of the pronator teres posteriorly to the anterolateral border of the radius (Sakellarides *et al.* 1981) or to the extensor carpi radialis brevis (Colton *et al.* 1976, Patella and Martucci 1980).

The operative technique of pronator teres tenotomy is simple. A straight incision is made over the insertion of the tendon on the volar aspect of the proximal shaft of the radius. The tendon is detached from its insertion and excised up to its muscle. Immobilization of the forearm in supination for three weeks, followed by active supination exercises, has been sufficient. Supination function activities such as opening doorknobs, jar tops and catching a large ball appear effective in achieving the desired result.

Complete active supination is rarely achieved. No active supination is ever achieved in those patients who have no evidence of active voluntary control of supination, which is highly dependent upon the activity of the biceps brachii muscle. In the report of the procedure by Sakellarides *et al.* (1981), 82 per cent were judged to have good or excellent results, with an average gain of 46° of active supination.

Elbow-flexion deformity
Indications for surgery
If elbow extension lacks only 30° to 40°, the problem is probably not worth treating. The most frequent need to correct the flexed elbow is in spastic hemiplegia, although Mital (1979) did surgery on spastic quadriplegics to gain elbow extension in order to facilitate walking with crutches in six patients; all became independent in walking with crutch support.

Despite the original pessimism of Samilson and Hoffer (1975) on the results of surgery for the spastic elbow flexion contracture, more recent reports have recommended the procedure. Goldner *et al.* (1977) reported 32 cases followed from one to 22 years; the flexion contracture recurred in only three patients, and four had a slow recovery of flexion strength. Mital (1979) performed a surgical release in 32 elbows (26 patients), with good results on follow-up of 25 patients.

To ascertain the effect of surgically decreasing the spastic elbow flexion, Goldner's (1983) recommendation to infiltrate the biceps and brachialis muscles with lidocaine has merit.

Operative techniques
Mital (1979) used a lazy-s incision, beginning on the anterolateral aspect of the distal third of the arm and crossing the elbow crease to end on the anteromedial aspect of the forearm. The lacertus fibrosis was excised, the biceps tendon z-lengthened and the brachialis aponeurosis incised transversely in two or three locations so that the muscle could be stretched on extension of the elbow. Anterior capsulotomy was rarely done, but it is obviously necessary in severe contractures. The anatomy of the nerves and vessels needs to be remembered in the dissection.

Goldner (1983) uses a curved incision anterior to the medial epicondyle of the humerus. The ulnar nerve is isolated and the origins of the flexor carpi ulnaris, radialis brevis and pronator teres are detached from the proximal ulna. The lacertus fibrosis is incised and the biceps tendon and the brachialis are z-lengthened at their insertions. If more extension is needed, the anterior capsule is incised. The ulnar nerve is mobilized and transferred anteriorly. If the brachioradialis is very spastic and contracted, it too is released from its origin on the humerus.

Postoperative care

It seems wise to use splinting in just enough extension to obviate excessive stretch on the nerves and vessels and with heavily padded dressings. Intermittent supervised flexion and extension exercise with extension splinting can be started within a week. The day-splinting continues for three weeks, and night-splinting in extension for three months. Because the elbow joint is extremely prone to arthrofibrosis and stiffness, postoperative care and encouragement of early motion is important to achieving a good result. My experience in elbow-joint arthrotomy and capulotomy, in cases other than cerebral palsy, has shown me the value of continuous passive motion (CPM) machines for the first seven to 14 days postoperatively.

Complications of elbow flexor release (other than what might be expected from overstretching of the nerves and vessels, hematoma and infection) can include a fixed elbow extension posture and contracture. This position of constant elbow extension is much worse than a flexion contracture. I have seen it in only one patient, who had tension athetosis that had been confused with spasticity. Only awareness of the peculiarities of the motor disorders in cerebral palsy pre-operatively can prevent this kind of distressing result.

Elbow flexion posturing in hemidystonia is not accompanied by any contracture or skeletal change. In some patients, the hyperflexed posture of the elbow during waking hours is quite uncomfortable (it disappears during sleep). Such patients ask for relief.

To assess the effect of surgery in this kind of problem, I infiltrate the biceps muscle with 1 per cent lidocaine solution. If this provides significant relaxation of the hyperflexed posture, a neurectomy of the musculocutaneous nerve has effected sustained relief in two patients followed-up for 11 and 12 years. The brachialis muscle continued to function for active flexion of the elbow; the dystonic flexion posture was reduced to tolerance and comfort.

Internal rotation contracture of the shoulder

Very rarely, a spastic contracture of the pectoralis major and subscapularis preclude the neutral or slightly externally rotated position of the shoulder and thus interferes with function of the hand. This dysfunctional position may be more common in athetosis or mixed types of cerebral palsy (Goldner 1983). A logical solution is lengthening of the pectoralis major tendon and subscapularis myotomy (Goldner 1983). I have performed shoulder surgery in a six-year-old with spastic quadriplegia and satisfactory hand function. He had a severe forward cupping of the shoulders as well as restriction of external rotation. Shoulder position was improved by bilateral pectoralis major lengthening, subscapularis myotomy and especially pectoralis minor tenotomy.

Surgery of the lower limb

Equinus deformity

> *'A little equinus is better than calcaneus.'*

In all the spastic types of cerebral palsy, the equinus position of the foot receives the most attention. It is the most visible of the abnormal postures. Consequently, treatment efforts are often directed zealously to correcting it, either with passive stretching by the parents and the physical therapist, or with plaster immobilization, or with a variety of surgical techniques. Conservative methods of management with plaster, myoneural blocks and orthotics are discussed in Chapter 6.

In hemiplegia, even minor degrees of equinus are noticeable because of the obvious comparison with the normal side. Although the description of the surgical management of equinus is described in this chapter on hemiplegia, the same procedures are applicable to equinus in spastic diplegia and the total body involved. The rôle of the spastic hamstring muscles in dynamic equinus sometimes found in spastic diplegia can be found in Chapter 8.

Indications for surgery
Is the plantar-flexed position of the ankle and foot detrimental to achieving functional walking? We know that patients with cerebral palsy will walk despite equinus if their neurological status permits. We also know that the lack of normal equilibrium reactions cannot be compensated for by the plantigrade foot. Patients who only have ataxia do not usually have equinus, yet their ability to balance can be so poor that a four-post walker is necessary. Normal people run (as opposed to jog) in equinus. Ballet artistes seem to have perfect postural control on tiptoe. Most women who wear high-heeled shoes walk in equinus all day. So what is so bad about having an equinus deformity throughout life?

Weight-bearing in equinus does result in all the bodyweight concentrated on the metatarsal head region of the foot. Eventually painful callosities occur, and walking is compromised because of foot discomfort and pain. The equinus position of the ankle is unstable, because in this position the talus is not securely locked in the ankle mortice; as a result the ankle joint is prone to inversion sprains and strains.

In hemiplegia, unilateral equinus creates a relative lengthening of the limb, a pelvic obliquity and compensatory postural lumbar scoliosis. The result is a limp. Furthermore, persistent equinus necessitates a greater degree of knee and hip flexion during the swing phase of gait in order for the foot to clear the ground; or if the quadriceps is spastic, the constant extension of the knee causes the patient to circumduct the limb in order for the foot to clear in swing phase. A slight degree of equinus (5°) can compensate for shortness of the limb which occurs frequently in hemiplegia (usually no more than 1.5cm).

Examination for contracture
Surgery is indicated for a contracture of the triceps surae. If the foot can be dorsiflexed to the neutral (zero) position when measured with the plantar aspect of the heel and *the foot inverted* (to lock the talonavicular joint and prevent false dorsiflexion at the midtarsal joint) and with the knee extended, surgery is not indicated in most patients.

To differentiate a contracture from spasticity alone demands a very slow and careful dorsiflexion of the ankle, first with the knee flexed and then extended. Truscelli *et al.* (1979) separated the contracture from the spasticity by creating ischemia of the limb with a pneumatic torniquet inflated to 200mm Hg pressure for 20 minutes; then they determined the true shortening of the muscle with the usual measurements of the range of passive dorsiflexion of the ankle.

The examination should also include the ability of the patient to dorsiflex the ankle voluntarily with the knee extended. Often this is not possible, and dorsiflexion will occur only with simultaneous hip and knee flexion against resistance. This is a reflex motion found in upper motor-neuron disorders. It accounts for the observation that patients who have only this flexor withdrawal reflex (or 'confusion' reflex) will usually walk with a steppage gait in order for the foot to clear the floor on swing phase.

Function of the gastrocnemius and soleus muscle
Electromyographic gait studies have demonstrated that the gastrocnemius and soleus muscles become active at heel strike and continue their activity through the mid-stance phase of gait. The function of the calf muscles is to reduce forward acceleration of the tibia during the stance phase. The muscle does not 'push off' at toe contact. Instead, the terminus of the stance phase is mechanical when the foot action consists of a passive 'roll-off' motion (Perry *et al.* 1974). Sutherland *et al.* (1980), in a study of the function of the ankle plantar flexors, emphasized the importance of these muscles to resist, arrest and reverse dorsiflexion. Other than the resistance of dorsiflexion, the ankle plantar flexors adjust the limb length and restrain the drop of the body's center of gravity; this action minimizes the vertical oscillations of the center of gravity during gait, and energy is conserved.

Constant contraction of the calf muscles (as occurs in spastic paralysis, and especially with a fixed equinus due to contracture) eliminates the 'roll-off'; the patient vaults over his foot, raises the vertical oscillation of the center of gravity and thus expends more energy. A paralysis of these muscles induced by a local anesthetic block of the tibial nerve demonstrated drastic changes in the gait variables: ankle dorsiflexion increased during stance, and the opposite heel did not leave the floor until weight was transferred to the opposite foot. The result was to shorten the step length, reduce the gait velocity, increase the vertical and forward velocities of the center of gravity (center of mass) and increase the energy expenditure (Sutherland *et al.* 1980). These accurate measurements on the effect of weakening the calf muscles should be a sufficiently strong reason to avoid a surgical procedure which would overcorrect the contracture. A calcaneus deformity is functionally worse than a moderate degree of equinus.

Mechanism of the contracture
In a normal person the ankle plantar flexors have 17 times the potential torque of the ankle dorsiflexors, and yet there is no calf-muscle contracture (Perry 1985). This is because when normal people walk, passive dorsiflexion of the ankle occurs in stance phase so that periodic elongation of the calf muscles prevents excessive shortening. The dorsiflexors lift the foot in the swing phase and decelerate plantar flexion during at-heel strike until the foot is flat; their strength requirements are much less than those of the plantar flexors.

242

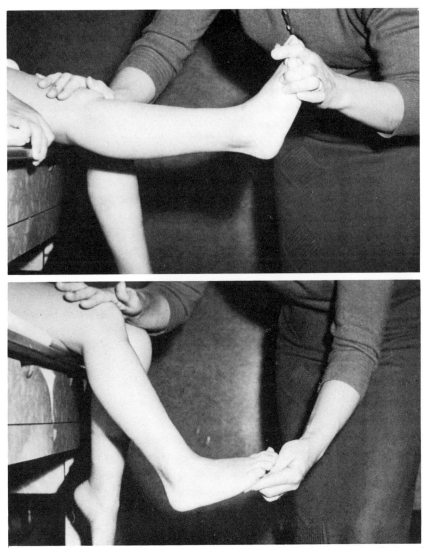

Fig. 7.26. *Top:* with knee extended and foot in varus, limited passive dorsiflexion of the ankle demonstrates contracture of gastrocnemius-soleus muscles. *Bottom:* with knee flexed, passive dorsiflexion of ankle is easily accomplished. This indicates more contracture in gastrocnemius muscle.

In spastic paralysis, constant contraction of the calf muscles and insufficient central control of ankle dorsiflexion fails to preserve the elasticity of the calf muscles (Fig. 7.26). As skeletal growth occurs, the muscle length fails to keep up with the bone length. At the microscopic level, Tardieu *et al.* (1977) found in cats that the sarcomere length of the calf muscle fibers were the same, regardless of the angle of dorsiflexion of the ankle. This mechanism was thought to explain why muscles adapt to skeletal growth, and in some cases of cerebral palsy this

243

mechanism was absent with a resultant contracture. Another explanation came from the experimental data of Huet de la Tour *et al.* (1979), where a reduction of sarcomeres in the muscle fiber as well as a loss of its extensibility after prolonged and sustained contractions was observed in experimental tetany resembling spastic paralysis.

In a unique experiment which studied the growth of the gastrocnemius muscle in hereditary spastic mice, Ziv *et al.* (1984) confirmed the view that muscle growth was not interstitial but was appositional at the musculotendinous junction. The cells here added sarcomeres to the end of the muscle fiber. In these spastic mice, growth of the muscle was definitely reduced and contractures ensued. The authors concluded that the contracture of the muscle in children is due to the failure of its growth, which in turn is the result of a spastic muscle's inability to stretch to its full length.

The velocity of muscle growth is greatest from birth to age four years, when muscles double in length; from then until skeletal maturity they double in length again (Rang *et al.* 1986). This phenomenon of early rapid growth explains the observation that recurrence of contracture after Achilles tendon lengthening is more common when done in early childhood. Lee and Bleck (1980) had a 75 per cent recurrence rate in children at age two years, 25 per cent at four years, 14 per cent at seven years and none (N = 31) at eight years and older.

The experiment in which springs were attached to the wings of chickens, so that constant stretch was applied to the wing muscles, did demonstrate an increase in length of the muscles (Barnett *et al.* 1980). Perhaps this provides a rationale for keeping a child's ankle constantly dorsiflexed in plasters ('inhibitive' or ordinary) orthotics (TRAFOS—'tone-reducing ankle foot orthoses' or ordinary AFOS) to prevent spastic equinus contracture. However, muscle atrophy due to disuse will also occur. And would it be practical for everyday living and functioning?

Unlike in children, adult muscle contractures are accompanied by loss of sarcomeres; there is no growth, and therefore few recurrences after lengthenings.

Surgical procedures
What surgical procedure do you perform to correct an equinus deformity? Many have been proposed: neurectomy of the gastrocnemius and/or soleus muscles, gastrocnemius lengthening, gastrocnemius origin recession, Achilles tendon lengthening and Achilles tendon translocation. All are designed to reduce the increased stretch reflex and to lengthen the muscle. All weaken the muscle. Which one strikes the best compromise between relieving the contracture and preserving the strength?

This dilemma is physiologically based. The excursion of muscles is determined by the length of their fibers (the number of sarcomeres); the strength is determined by the number of fibers. Achilles tendon lengthening reduces the excursion of the gastrocnemius-soleus muscle, but this excursion to dorsiflex the ankle actively remains in the same range as before; only passive dorsiflexion is increased. Lengthening weakens the muscle. We have no solution except to try to avoid too much lengthening of the tendon.

Denervation of the muscle by neurectomy no longer seems popular. Neurectomy paralyzes the muscle but does not lengthen it. Silver and Simon (1959) have reported success with neurectomy of the gastrocnemius when combined with the recession of its orgins (Silfverskiöld 1923–24, Silver 1977).

Vulpius is credited with the operation designed to lengthen the gastrocnemius only and thereby spare the soleus muscle (Vulpius and Stoffel 1913, Vulpius 1920). This operation consists of an inverted v incision in the gastrocnemius tendinous aponeurosis and forcing the ankle into dorsiflexion, followed by plaster immobilization. This procedure was modified by Strayer (1950, 1958) and then by Baker (1954, 1956). In the Strayer procedure the gastrocnemius aponeurosis is sectioned transversely, the muscle bellies dissected free of the underlying soleus muscle, the foot dorsiflexed and a plaster applied. Baker's modification was a tongue-in-groove incision in the aponeurosis and section of the median raphe of the soleus muscle, foot dorsiflexion and plaster immobilization.

The basis for the Vulpius, Strayer and Baker procedures was the positive Silfverskiold test, in which ankle dorsiflexion was greater with the knee flexed than extended (Fig. 26). However, Perry *et al.* (1974) clearly demonstrated with electromyograms that the test is unreliable. Usually when the ankle was dorsiflexed 90°, electrical activity was recorded in *both* the gastrocnemius and soleus muscles. Indeed, in two patients with a positive Silfverskiold test, the gait electromyograms showed premature contraction of the soleus and the gastrocnemius muscles on swing phase. In 95 per cent of the patients with spastic equinus, both muscles are firing abnormally (Perry 1985).

The Strayer-Baker type of gastrocnemius lengthening (termed 'recession' by Strayer 1950) has lost its popularity with many surgeons. Its goal was to relieve the contracture and preserve strength. Bassett and Baker (1966) had only a 4 per cent recurrence rate after this procedure, but the length of follow-up was not specified. Unfortunately the recurrence rate on longer follow-up was unacceptably high. In a study of 51 such procedures by Lee and Bleck (1980), followed for at least two years, unacceptable equinus recurred in 29 per cent. Schwartz *et al.* (1977), in a 20-year follow-up study, found recurrent equinus in 41 per cent after the Strayer-Baker method. The significance of this report was that it came from the same institution which described the procedure originally.

Craig and Van Voren (1976) measured the proximal migration of the gastrocnemius muscle bellies after gastrocnemius muscle lengthening and Achilles tendon lengthening with metallic markers and radiographic examinations. The postoperative radiographs showed a proximal shift of just 0.8cm of the gastrocnemius muscle after the Achilles lengthening, and a 4.7cm shift after the Strayer gastrocnemius lengthening. Based upon this data they recommended both operations at the same time. Equinus recurred in 9 per cent of cases.

I have done the classic Strayer lengthening in only four patients in the past 10 years. My criterion for performing this operation is spastic equinus with a definite contracture of what seems to be the gastrocnemius manifested on examination. With the foot in varus and the knee flexed 90°, ankle dorsiflexion to 5° or 10° was easy. This situation is rarely encountered; two of my patients had spastic paralysis

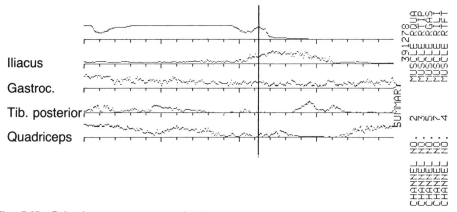

Fig. 7.27. Gait electromyogram: spastic diplegia. Demonstrates continuous contraction of the gastrocnemius during both phases of the gait cycle. It should be active only in stance. Note normal iliacus activity, abnormal action of the posterior tibial in swing phase and prolonged action of quadriceps during stance.

after a head injury and were skeletally mature. A gait electromyogram can be of considerable assistance in making the decision (Fig. 7.27). Sharrard and Bernstein (1972) compared recurrence rates of 23 per cent after coronal lengthening of the Achilles tendon, with 15 per cent after gastrocnemius recession (20 of 53 of these also had a gastrocnemius neurectomy). They found that postoperative bracing did not affect the result or the recurrence rate. They also said that the success rate of the operation should not be related exclusively to the recurrence of equinus, because a small amount of equinus was much more desirable for a functional gait than excessive weakness of the triceps surae produced by too much zeal in preventing recurrence (Fig. 7.28). It is better to perform a second operation to relieve unacceptable equinus than to risk a calcaneus deformity.

Achilles tendon lengthening appears now to be the most acceptable way to correct equinus, providing it is not overdone. The z-lengthening method may cause overcorrection, although it has its adherents (Grabe and Thompson 1979). Gaines and Ford (1984) have attempted (successfully, according to their paper) a study assessing the amount of lengthening needed, among three types of patients with cerebral palsy; they were prospectively selected according to gradings of the spasticity, voluntary control and strength of the muscle. A combination of three grades of spasticity and voluntary control-strength was used to place the ankle either at neutral, 10° or 20° of dorsiflexion, to determine the proper tension under which to suture the Achilles tendon after the z-lengthening. This rather complicated system of preoperative analysis seems to have worked; they had no cases of postoperative calcaneous deformity.

Open versus percutaneous sliding lengthening
Most surgeons today have found the sliding method of lengthening either by the White (1943) or the Hoke (Roberts 1953, Goldner 1954) more controlled and very

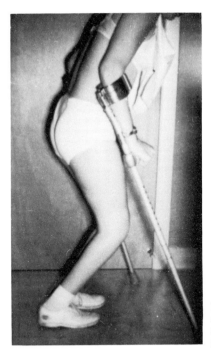

Fig. 7.28. Crouch posture and gait, due to overlengthening of the Achilles tendon and resultant loss of muscle strength of the gastrocnemius-soleus which normally prevents forward acceleration of the tibia.

satisfactory. Many surgeons seem to prefer the percutaneous method to the open method of Achilles tendon lengthening (Coleman 1983, Lake *et al*. 1985). Whether the tendon is exposed and lengthened or cut in the proper places by the blind percutaneous technique, the principle is the same (White 1943, Crenshaw 1963).

White observed that the Achilles tendon rotated 90° on its longitudinal axis between its origin and insertion; the rotation from the posterior aspect was from medial to lateral. Cummins and colleagues, in a study of 100 tendons, found 52 per cent that rotated the least where the soleus comprised one-third of the posterior surface and the gastrocnemius two-thirds; in 35 per cent the soleus and gastrocnemius each comprised half the posterior surface; in 13 per cent with extreme rotation of the tendon, the soleus was two-thirds and the gastrocnemius one-third of the posterior surface (Crenshaw 1963).

The White technique is to cut the anterior two-thirds of the tendon distally near the insertion and the medial two-thirds 5 to 7cm proximal to the distal cut. Because of the variations in the twist of the tendon and the ankle dorsiflexion force necessary to produce the lengthening with the White percutaneous method ('The foot was dorsiflexed forcefully until a snap was heard'—Lake *et al*. 1985), I prefer the Hoke open method where I can see the tendon slide and cut a tiny fiber or two when necessary to facilitate sliding without undue force. Tibiae have been fractured due to excessive force in dorsiflexing the foot when the percutaneous method was tried, particularly in patients with thin osteoporotic bones (Samilson 1966). Rang *et al*. (1986) make the point that with the percutaneous method, the opportunity to lengthen the toe flexor tendons is lost; in the open method, these can be easily lengthened if acute flexion of the great and/or lesser toes is evident after Achilles tendon lengthening and when the ankle is dorsiflexed to neutral.

The successful results of sliding Achilles tendon lengthenings have been reported by Banks and Green (1958), Banks (1977), Lee and Bleck (1980) and Banks (1983), with recurrence rates between 2 and 9 per cent. Our regimen (Lee and Bleck 1980) differed from that of Banks and Green in that we did not use physical therapy and definite exercises, daytime orthosis or night splints postoperatively. The difference in the recurrence rate of 2 per cent does not appear significant. Our experience shows that an elaborate postoperative regime of splints and exercises is usually superfluous (the children aged five years and older wore only tennis shoes after plaster removal, and there was only one recurrence). Two cases developed postoperative calcaneus (4 per cent). In the 15 lengthenings age four years or younger the recurrence rate was 33 per cent. Given the greater velocity of growth which doubles the length of the limb up to age four years, I doubt that exercises, physical therapy, night splints and orthoses would have made much difference to this recurrence rate.

A different procedure to alleviate equinus is a translocation of the Achilles tendon (Throop *et al*. 1975). The Achilles tendon was moved to a more anterior insertion on the calcaneus. The rationale for this procedure in 79 cases was to preserve the strength of the triceps surae muscle; they estimated that the plantar flexion strength was reduced by 50 per cent. Their correction rate was 89.9 per cent. These results do not seem to be appreciably different from those reported with sliding Achilles tendon lengthening. The translocation procedure is more complicated than lengthening, and although the authors reported no increased morbidity with this procedure, Achilles tendon lengthening seems simpler. Why not do the least complex procedure if the results are similar?

Westin and Dye (1983) have persisted in the conservative management of spastic equinus, using plasters over a period of 27 years. In a retrospective review of 194 patients, 61 per cent had plaster alone, 23 per cent had both plaster and surgery, and 16 per cent were not treated but only observed. They concluded that their decreasing incidence of surgery for equinus (from 33 operations in 1952 to 1961, to 19 operations from 1970 to 1979) is a reflection of their recognition that a major cause of the equinus is hamstring muscle spasticity rather than spasticity primarily of the gastrocnemius-soleus muscles. This observation has validity, particularly when considering the surgical treatment of equinus in young children with spastic diplegia.

The prolonged plaster immobilization for equinus has some theoretical merit, based upon the observations of appositional muscle growth in spastic mice. The muscle grows along with the bone as long as it is kept stretched to is resting length (Rang *et al*. 1986).

Hoke Achilles tendon lengthening operative technique
Through a longitudinal posterior medial incision (5 to 7cm), the posterior portion of the Achilles tendon is exposed and (if possible) its sheath preserved. Three cuts

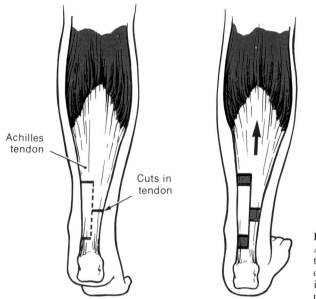

Achilles
tendon

Cuts in
tendon

Fig. 7.29. Technique of Hoke Achilles tendon lengthening. The tendon cuts are allowed to slide only to the point where the ankle is dorsiflexed to neutral and no more.

are made in the tendon: (i) one half medially and distally; (ii) half medially and proximally; and (iii) one half is cut laterally between the two medial cuts. The ankle is dorsiflexed just to the neutral (zero) position with the foot in varus; the tendon ends slide apart, leaving a lateral splice in between. No tendon sutures are necessary (Fig. 7.29). Dorsiflexion of the foot should be possible without force—the pressure of two fingers is all that is necessary. If the tendon does not slide apart easily, a few additional fibers may be cut.

In mild contractures (< 10° of equinus), a transverse incision can be used; the resultant incisional scar is barely visible. I have also used two separate transverse incisions 3 to 4cm apart in more severe contractures, but it is necessary to undermine the skin in order to see the tendon.

In the application of the postoperative plaster it is vital that the foot is not forced into more than neutral dorsiflexion; otherwise the tendon will be overlengthened and strength impossible to restore. Generally I use a long-leg plaster for six weeks, though I may reduce the plaster to a short leg (below-the-knee) in three weeks, if it is convenient for the patient. Patients are allowed to walk the first day postoperatively with weight-bearing to tolerance. Most children do so within two days. Crutches and walkers are necessary only if the child needs them for postural stability.

After plaster removal, ordinary low quarter shoes or tennis shoes are adequate (Lee and Bleck 1980). In the rare cases which require repeat surgery, I use plastic ankle-foot orthoses for six months.

A similar early weight-bearing program in short-leg plasters after one to two days postoperatively has been successfully used by Sirna and Sussman (1985). They applied Buck's traction immediately after surgery to overcome the flexed knee posture.

White technique of sliding Achilles tendon lengthening
This was used by Banks and Green (1958). Half the tendon is cut proximally in its posterior-lateral segment, and half distally in its anterior-medial segment. The ankle is dorsiflexed to neutral and plaster immobilization is used as with the Hoke method described above.

Percutaneous sliding Achilles tendon lengthening
Through a skin stab wound, the surgeon makes three cuts in the tendon: a distal and proximal cut laterally, and a medial cut between these two (Coleman 1983). Lake *et al.* (1985) performed percutaneous lengthening with two stab wounds 3cm apart: one half of the medial side distally and one half the lateral side proximally. Immobilization of the dorsiflexed ankle in plaster and immediate ambulation were implemented.

I have continued to use the open Hoke method because it has been reliable. Even in a teaching institution it has produced overcorrection in only two lengthenings in some 175 cases in the past 14 years, it has few complications and gives satisfactory results. In a teaching program it might be better to see first what you are doing to the tendon, before adopting the blind percutaneous approach. Experience is a good teacher.

Gastrocnemius-lengthening operative technique
A 5 to 7cm longitudinal incision is made at the junction of the proximal and middle thirds of the calf, where the muscle bellies of the gastrocnemius join to form the broad gastrocnemius aponeurosis overlying the soleus muscle (Strayer 1950, Baker 1956). The sural vein and nerve are retracted. One end of the gastrocnemius aponeurosis is identified and separated from the underlying soleus. The aponeurosis is cut transversely (a 1 to 2cm segment can be removed). The muscle bellies of the gastrocnemius are easily separated from the soleus. The knee is then extended and the ankle dorsiflexed. A long-leg walking plaster is used for six weeks postoperatively.

The Baker modification of the Strayer procedure is a proximally directed 'tongue' cut in the aponeurosis. The base of the 'tongue' is distal. When the ankle is dorsiflexed with the knee extended, the 'tongue' slides distally to effect the lengthening. Most often the median fibrous raphe of the soleus was cut and when insufficient lengthening occurred, the surgeon stripped the soleus muscle fibers from the emerging Achilles tendon. This extensive muscle-stripping possibly caused more scar tissue formation and accounted for the high recurrence rate of contracture reported.

Postoperative calcaneus deformities after surgical procedures to overcome equinus are usually due to overlengthening of the gastrocnemius-soleus muscles. Although this complication is rare (about 1 per cent of cases in my experience) there are multiple factors that may produce the unwanted result in the best of surgical hands. I have observed postoperative calcaneus most often after surgical correction of severe pes valgus, with either extra-articular subtalar or triple arthrodesis in total body involved patients. In pes valgus it is practically always necessary to lengthen the Achilles tendon and allow it to slide so that the foot can be manipulated into the corrected position. These partly ambulatory patients usually have severe spasticity, so that when the plantar flexor muscles are weakened the antagonist dorsiflexor muscles become predominant.

Operative shortening of the Achilles tendon has not been successful in correcting this distressing postoperative complication. If the anterior tibial muscle is spastic, it may be transferred through the interosseus membrane to the os calcis at the insertion of the Achilles tendon. To avoid further deformity due to the resulting imbalanced spasticity of the peroneal muscles, subtalar arthrodesis or triple arthrodesis of the foot might be considered (depending on age). If arthrodesis has been done, then lengthening of the anterior tibial tendon will at least reduce the force of ankle dorsiflexion.

The most satisfactory solution, with or without anterior tibial tendon transfer, has been to stop all ankle motion with a rigid plastic ankle-foot orthosis which holds the foot in slight equinus. Foot-ankle function can be restored with the addition of a rocker-sole and a cushion heel to the shoe. The principle applied is the same one used in lower limb prosthetics with the SACH (solid ankle cushion heel) foot.

Dynamic equinus deformity in hemidystonia
I have performed neurectomy of both gastrocnemius muscle heads in three patients who had severe and disabling dystonic equinus deformity. When relaxed, all patients had a full range of passive dorsiflexion of the ankle well above the neutral position. All were over 13 years of age and had had long and extensive trials of various physical therapy methods, muscle-relaxing drugs and restrictive ankle orthoses. The preoperative assessment in all was with 45 per cent alcohol myoneural blocks of the gastrocnemius muscle heads. These blocks resulted in improvement of the equinus for a period of two to six weeks. Most importantly, no 'athetoid shift' to the opposite dystonic pattern occurred. In all three patients, a neurectomy of the medial and lateral heads of the gastrocnemius was performed through a transverse incision just distal to the popliteal crease. A long-leg walking plaster was used for three weeks postoperatively to ensure wound healing.

Follow-up observation for eight years confirmed no recurrence of the severe disabling dynamic equinus posturing of the foot. In these patients the weakening of the gastrocnemius did not relieve all the equinus posturing or convert the gait into the normal heel-toe pattern, but it did allow the use of a plastic ankle-foot orthosis. The gait, while not normal, was at least more functional. Calcaneus deformities have not occurred.

Spastic pes varus

> *'Thou shalt not varus'* (old orthopaedic adage).

The etiology of varus deformity of the foot in cerebral palsy is not complex. It is

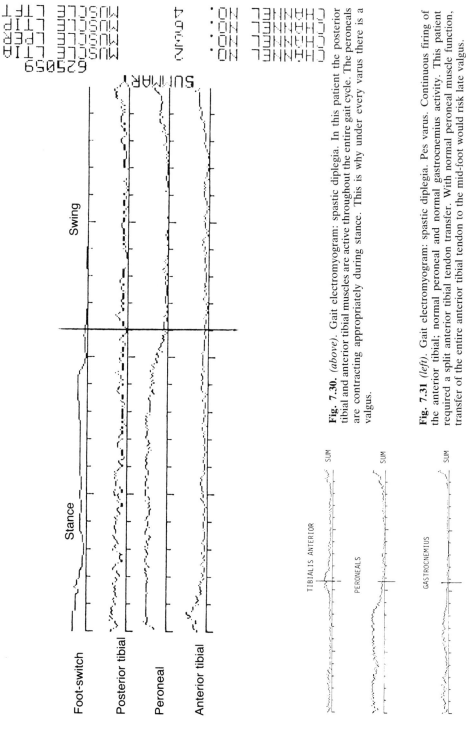

Fig. 7.30. (*above*). Gait electromyogram: spastic diplegia. In this patient the posterior tibial and anterior tibial muscles are active throughout the entire gait cycle. The peroneals are contracting appropriately during stance. This is why under every varus there is a valgus.

Fig. 7.31 (*left*). Gait electromyogram: spastic diplegia. Pes varus. Continuous firing of the anterior tibial; normal peroneal and normal gastrocnemius activity. This patient required a split anterior tibial tendon transfer. With normal peroneal muscle function, transfer of the entire anterior tibial tendon to the mid-foot would risk late valgus.

due to spastic muscle imbalance where the force of the spastic foot invertor muscles exceeds that of the spastic evertors. In this respect the cause of the varus deformity is different from flaccid paralysis, where the imbalance is due to weakness or absence of the evertor muscles. Our electromyographic gait analyses of cases of spastic varus deformities, in which we recorded the simultaneous electrical activity of the posterior tibial, anterior tibial and peroneal muscles, clearly indicated that all these muscles fired during gait—albeit often out of phrase (Fig. 7.30). This is why underneath every varus there is a valgus. If the invertor spasticity is decreased too much, the evertor spasticity predominates and the foot which was formerly in varus ends up in valgus.

Only two muscles account for the varus deformity: the posterior tibial, which causes hind-foot varus, and the anterior tibial which causes mid-foot varus. Either or both may be responsible. Judging from the literature, most surgeons in recent years have concentrated on the posterior tibial muscle.

Spasticity and contracture of the gastrocnemius-soleus accounts for some varus, but this is in the ankle and positional due to the obliquity of the ankle axis of dorsi-plantar flexion (Inman 1976). This axis is in the line constructed through the tips of the ankle malleoli, and slopes downward obliquely from lateral to medial. Because of the oblique axis of the ankle joint, the foot is directed medially on plantar flexion and laterally on dorsiflexion. However, this anatomical construction does not cause inversion at the subtalar joint or the mid-tarsal joints of the foot. If we recognize these aspects of varus, then the surgeon will not be disappointed by the failure of Achilles tendon lengthening to correct a dynamic pes varus.

Indications for surgery
Surgical treatment is generally indicated in a child more than four years old, when the deforming force of the spastic muscle persists and cannot be controlled with an orthosis. If surgery is delayed, skeletal changes in the direction of the dynamic deformity will result. Early surgery on the tendons is indicated to prevent late fixed bony deformities that can be corrected only with surgery of the bones and joints, and the attendant loss of foot mobility and greater morbidity.

A varus foot is an uncomfortable foot. Walking on the outer border of the foot eventually causes a painful callous over the base of the fifth metatarsal. When severe, shoes or sandals can no longer be worn and recurrent ankle sprains occur. Participation in sport becomes almost impossible, and ski boots do not fit.

The *selection* of the patient for surgery of the posterior tibial tendon is based upon the clinical examination of gait observation of the foot position during the stance phase, and the passive correction of the foot to the neutral position. Soft-tissue surgery alone will not correct a fixed skeletal deformity.

The gait electromyogram is useful in making a decision (Hoffer 1976, Perry and Hoffer 1977, Adler *et al.* 1985). Continuous activity of the posterior tibial muscle indicates lengthening; if this muscle has activity in swing phase, then transfer is selected (Fig. 7.30). If the anterior tibial shows continuous and out-of-phase activity, a split anterior tibial tendon transfer should be considered (Fig. 7.31). As mentioned previously, most of our patients had either normal, prolonged or dysphasic activity in the peroneals in pes varus.

The choice of surgical procedure to correct pes varus is very wide (Fig. 7.32). It seems inconceivable that any more operations could be devised for the poor spastic posterior tibial muscle and its tendon. According to reports, and the excellent results on follow-up examinations, the surgeon can lengthen the tendon, cut it at its musculo-tendinous junction in the calf, transfer it anteriorly through the interosseus membrane, reroute it anterior to the medial malleolus, and now in the late 1980s split it in two and transfer its lateral half to the peroneus brevis tendon.

Supramalleolar lengthening of the posterior tibial tendon remains my choice for correction of varus of the hind-foot (Fig. 7.32b). It has been the preference of Banks and Panagakos (1966), Tachdjian (1972) and Coleman (1983). In 21 patients, Root and Kirz (1982) reported poor results in nine and good in 12. The only poor results I have had were in those patients in whom the hind-foot varus was corrected but mid-foot varus persisted due to the concomitant spasticity of the anterior tibial muscle; these required a transfer of the anterior tibial tendon. Spastic metatarsus adductus cannot be alleviated with either posterior tibial or anterior tibial tendon procedures. This should be obvious, but sometimes we tend to overgeneralize in the definition of pes varus.

Intramuscular tenotomy of the posterior tibial tendon in the middle third of the calf was described by Ruda and Frost (1971) (Fig. 7.32b). No plaster immobilization was used; the patients walked soon after surgery. Nather *et al.* (1984), in experimental intramuscular lengthenings in rabbits, confirmed that without plaster

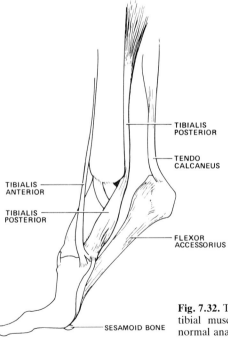

TIBIALIS POSTERIOR

TENDO CALCANEUS

TIBIALIS ANTERIOR

TIBIALIS POSTERIOR

FLEXOR ACCESSORIUS

SESAMOID BONE

Fig. 7.32. The variety of operative procedures on the posterior tibial muscle-tendon to alleviate spastic pes varus. *Left: normal anatomy. (Figure continues opposite.)*

254

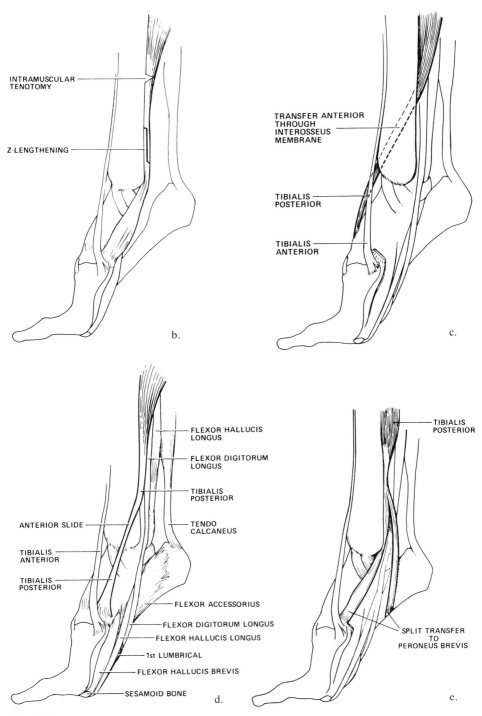

INTRAMUSCULAR
TENOTOMY

Z-LENGTHENING

b.

TRANSFER ANTERIOR
THROUGH
INTEROSSEUS
MEMBRANE

TIBIALIS
POSTERIOR

TIBIALIS
ANTERIOR

c.

FLEXOR HALLUCIS
LONGUS

FLEXOR DIGITORUM
LONGUS

TIBIALIS
POSTERIOR

TENDO
CALCANEUS

ANTERIOR SLIDE

TIBIALIS
ANTERIOR

TIBIALIS
POSTERIOR

FLEXOR ACCESSORIUS

FLEXOR DIGITORUM LONGUS

FLEXOR HALLUCIS LONGUS

1st LUMBRICAL

FLEXOR HALLUCIS BREVIS

SESAMOID BONE

d.

TIBIALIS
POSTERIOR

SPLIT TRANSFER
TO
PERONEUS BREVIS

e.

Fig. 7.32b-e.

255

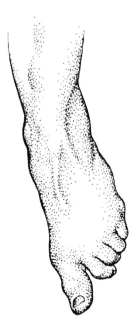

Fig. 7.33. Postoperative pes valgus after transfer of the posterior tibial tendon through the interosseus membrane to the dorsum of the foot. Solution: cut the posterior tibial tendon and subtalar extra-articular arthrodesis.

immobilization this type of lengthening did not change while healing occurred. The gap in the tendon remained the same. In the 29 cases of Ruda and Frost there were no failures and only two recurrences. This operation was recommended in children younger than age six years.

Tenotomy of the posterior tibial tendon at its insertion on the navicular bone is not recommended because of the great risk of a late valgus deformity. Collapse of the longitudinal arch in disruptions of the posterior tibial tendon at its insertion in adults has been reported (Kettlekamp and Alexander 1969, Goldner *et al.* 1974, Jahss 1980, Mann and Specht 1982, Johnson 1983, Funk *et al.* 1986). Overlengthening of the posterior tibial tendon can theoretically result in the same reverse deformity.

Transfer of the posterior tibial tendon to the dorsum of the foot through the interosseous membrane has had its adherents and detractors (Fig. 7.32c). Bisla *et al.* (1976) reported good results in 13 of 19 cases; Turner and Cooper (1972) had poor results in 10 of 14 patients, in whom reversal from varus to valgus occurred. Banks (1975) had only moderate success. Schneider and Balon (1977) reported poor results; within one year 68 per cent of the feet were either in valgus or calcaneus. Root and Kirz (1982) performed 67 transfers in 59 patients, and had better results: 22 excellent, 25 good and 12 poor (18 per cent). These 12 developed valgus, which was not deemed severe enough to merit further corrective surgery.

Miller *et al.* (1982) transferred the posterior tibial tendon through the interosseus membrane to the dorsal-lateral aspect of the foot in seven patients (nine feet) who had cerebrospastic paralysis (two were post-head injury). They had a 56 per cent failure rate, with four overcorrections to valgus and one undercorrection

(Fig. 7.33). These orthopaedists recommended that a posterior tibial tendon transfer anteriorly should be done in cerebral palsy only if confirmation of its swing-phase activity is found on gait electromyography.

Transfer of the posterior tibial tendon anteriorly through the interosseous membrane was originally used successfully in cases of flaccid and spastic paralysis of the dorsiflexor muscles of the ankle. Watkins *et al.* (1954) performed the transfer in seven patients with spastic paralysis; the results were excellent in two, good in three and fair in one (one patient was lost to follow-up). In one patient (presumably the fair result) a valgus deformity occurred. These original authors cautioned against transferring the tendon too far laterally in the foot in spastic paralysis. 12 of their 29 patients had a triple arthrodesis combined with the transfer. They did not delineate the motor problem in whom the arthrodesis was used in combination.

In reviewing the literature, one is struck by the recurring reports of transfer of the posterior tibial tendon to the dorsum of the foot. The operation is at least 50 years old (Mayer 1937). Some reports praise the procedure as being the best for a spastic pes varus (Gritzka *et al.* 1972, Bisla *et al.* 1976, Williams 1976), while others reflect disappointment—particularly with the later valgus and calcaneus deformities. The clever answer might be that those who are happy with the results are better surgeons; but I think the key factor influencing the good results is insertion of the tendon to prevent overcorrection. Williams (1976) advised anchoring the tendon to the mid-dorsum of the foot. Often it is necessary to correct the equinus at the same time, and overlengthening of the Achilles tendon would be more deterimental when the spastic posterior tibial tendon is transferred anteriorly under tension; it can then act as a strong dorsiflexion force.

Transposition of the posterior tibial tendon anterior to the medial malleolus was devised by Baker and Hill (1964) (Fig. 7.32d). In this simple procedure, the posterior tibial tendon was removed from its sheath through two incisions proximal and distal to the medial malleolus, and then allowed to slide anteriorly to act as a dorsiflexor of the ankle (Fig. 32). Bisla *et al.* (1976) had poor results with this procedure. In 1985 Lester and Johnson reviewed the 'Baker slide operation' in 28 patients (35 feet) who had an average follow-up of 10.4 years. Achilles tendon lengthening was done with the procedure in 18 feet; 15 feet had a previous Achilles lengthening. Their results were very good in 30 of the 35 feet. Two feet had continued hind-foot varus and three developed a calcaneocavus deformity. These two cases had simultaneous Achilles tendon lengthening. In 10 feet that had only the posterior tibial transposition and no Achilles tendon lengthening, no late calcaneus deformities ensued. With an 85 per cent success rate, this operation will probably have a resurrection. However, Lester and Johnson were quite specific in stating that the operation was for hind-foot varus, which they did not attempt to correct with a split transfer of the anterior tibial tendon.

The nefarious posterior tibial tendon has had yet another procedure devised for it and reported in the past few years. This is the *split posterior tibial tendon transfer*, in which half the tendon is transferred to the peroneus brevis tendon to correct the spastic hind-foot varus (Figs. 7.32e, 7.34). Green *et al.* (1983) had excellent results in all 16 patients who had this operation. They had no valgus or

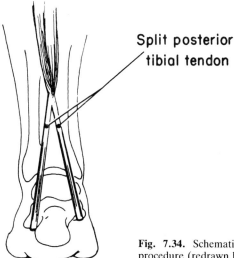

**Split posterior
tibial tendon**

Fig. 7.34. Schematic drawing of the split posterior tibial tendon procedure (redrawn by permission from Kling *et al.* 1985).

calcaneus deformities in a minimum two year follow-up. Kling *et al.* (1985) were also enthusiastic with their results, which were excellent in 35 of 37 feet with spastic equinovarus deformities. Achilles tendon lengthening was usually done in combination with the transfer. It seems probable that we have exhausted all the possibilities with this tendon in cerebral palsy.

Green *et al.* (1983) wrote that simple lengthening of the posterior tibial gave them the best results. They changed to the split posterior tibial transfer because they felt theoretically that lengthening of the Achilles tendon and the posterior tibial would weaken the plantar flexor muscles too much. They also feared that overlengthening of the posterior tibial tendon would result in a late valgus deformity. I agree with Green and his colleagues that simple lengthening has been quite satisfactory in correction of the hind-foot varus. I have been unable to gauge accurately the strength of the plantar flexors in cerebral palsy. Few patients with cerebral palsy can tiptoe, to enable measurement of the standing strength of the ankle plantar flexor muscles. In normal persons this is the recognized manner to test the strength of the calf muscles.

Posterior tibial tendon lengthening
In order to confirm my impression of the efficacy of the posterior tibial tendon lengthening, I reviewed the operative notes and charts of patients who had only this procedure for spastic pes varus, usually in combination with a sliding Achilles tendon lengthening for the equinus (Table 7.III). While admitting the defects of retrospective review, it appears that posterior tibial tendon lengthening has been successful in correcting the deformity. Two of the 47 feet developed late valgus; this was probably due to overlengthening of the tendon. Four feet had a recurrence of the varus but it was in the mid-foot; a split anterior tibial tendon transfer corrected

258

TABLE 7.III

Retrospective review of posterior tibial tendon lengthening with and without transfer of anterior tibial tendon and with transfer of anterior tibial tendon alone for spastic pes varus 1956–1982

Diagnosis	N	Follow-up (mean yrs.)	Recurrence	Late valgus
Posterior tibial tendon lengthening only (supramalleolar-Z type)				
Spastic hemiplegia	23	7.0	2	2
Spastic diplegia	16	7.5	2	
Spastic quadriplegia	4	8.5		
Total patients	43			
Total feet	47	7.5	4 (8%)	2 (4%)
Posterior tibial tendon lengthening with anterior tibial tendon transfer				
Spastic hemiplegia	9	7.0		2*
Spastic diplegia	12	8.0		1*
Spastic quadriplegia	1	10.0		
Total patients (all unilateral)	22	8.0	0	3 (13%)

*Whole tendon transferred to mid-foot in these three patients; all others had split transfers.

Split anterior tendon transfer alone				
Spastic hemiplegia	6	8.0		
Spastic diplegia	2	4.0		
Total patients (all unilateral)	8	6.0	0	0

it nicely. I did not attempt to assess the preoperative or postoperative strength of plantar flexion, being satisfied preoperatively with a passively correctable foot and postoperatively with a foot in neutral position of the heel and forefoot.

Twenty-two of my patients had the posterior tibial tendon lengthening and the anterior tibial tendon transfer at the same time. Three of these developed late valgus; in these three the entire tendon had been transferred to the mid-dorsum of the foot. All others had a split anterior tibial tendon transfer.

Since 1977 we have relied more on the gait electromyograms to help us decide whether to do both the anterior tibial tendon transfer and the posterior tibial tendon lengthening. If there is varus of the hind-foot, and the tendon of the posterior tibial is prominent and under obvious tension on passive eversion of the heel, then I lengthen it. If in the same patient the mid-foot moves into dynamic varus, especially on the maneuver of resistance against flexion of the hip with the knee flexed (flexor withdrawal or 'confusion' reflex), then the split anterior tibial tendon transfer is included.

Only eight patients had a split anterior tibial tendon transfer alone because they did not have hind-foot varus or resistance to passive eversion of the heel. They did have electromyographic confirmation of continuous activity of the anterior tibial muscle during gait (Fig. 7.31). To repeat: clinical examination must always be combined with the laboratory results, *i.e.* the electromyographic gait examination.

Operative technique of posterior tibial tendon lengthening
Through a 3 to 5cm incision directly over the posterior tibial tendon *proximal* to the

medial malleolus, the tendon is z-lengthened. The heel is everted to the neutral position and the split tendon is sutured side-to-side, with just enough tension to prevent it from wrinkling. A short-leg plaster is worn for six weeks. The procedure can be combined with a sliding Achilles tendon lengthening.

Operative technique of the split anterior tibial tendon transfer ('SPLATT')
Three incisions are required. The first is over the dorsal-medial aspect of the first cuneiform bone and the base of the first metatarsal. The lateral half of the anterior tibial tendon is cut at its insertion and the tendon slit in half proximally. The second incision is made just lateral to the tibial crest of the musculotendinous junction of the anterior tibial at about the level of the distal and middle thirds of the leg. The fascial envelope over the muscle is incised and the lateral half of the tendon brought out through this wound. The third longitudinal incision is made over the dorsum of the cuboid, and the tendon passed subcutaneously from the second incision to the cuboid region. Two convergent drill holes, large enough to accommodate the tendon (⁷⁄₆₄ or ⁹⁄₆₄ inches), are drilled in the cuboid. The lateral half of the transferred tendon is passed through these holes and sutured to itself under tension with the foot slightly dorsiflexed and the hind-foot in eversion (Hoffer *et al.* 1974, 1985). A short-leg walking plaster is worn for six weeks. Hoffer and colleagues advise use of an orthosis for six months postoperatively.

I have had difficulty in maintaining the drill hole in the cuboid (the roof breaks) in some cases, especially in young children whose bones are small and cartilaginous. In these instances, the results seem just as good when the tendon is anchored with strong sutures to the peroneus tertius tendon and the thick periosteum of the cuboid. To prepare for this contingency, the periosteum of the cuboid should be carefully preserved when exposing the bone prior to making the drill holes.

Hoffer *et al.* (1985) combined the 'SPLATT' with an intramuscular posterior tibial lengthening when there was a relatively fixed hind-foot varus and continuous firing of the posterior tibial tendon on gait electromyograms. All cases had an Achilles tendon lengthening to correct the equinus. The posterior tibial tendon was lengthened in eight of their 27 feet reported. The split anterior tibial tendon transfer alone was performed when the electromyogram showed continuous activity of the muscle. Their results were quite satisfactory; only two had a recurrent equinus and one had a recurrence of a mild dynamic varus. Given the 10-year follow-up and results like these, who can argue about their approach to the treatment of dynamic pes varus?

Hind-foot varus, not passively correctable: closed wedge osteotomy of the calcaneus
If passive correction of the hind-foot varus deformity is not possible, a closed wedge osteotomy of the calcaneus is an effective procedure. It must be combined with a posterior tibial tendon lengthening and, if required, Achilles tendon lengthening (Silver *et al.* 1967). I have found it useful in a few patients who had fixed varus of the heel after overcorrection of a subtalar extra-articular arthrodesis performed for a pes valgus.

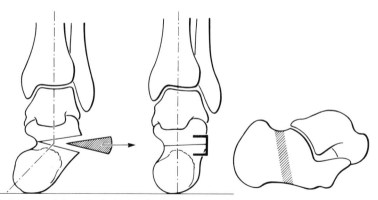

Fig. 7.35. Technique of lateral closing-wedge osteotomy of calcaneus for fixed hind-foot varus deformity.

Through a lateral oblique incision, coursing from a point anterior to the Achilles tendon to a distal point almost parallel to the peroneal tendons, the lateral aspect of the calcaneus is exposed subperiosteally. A laterally based wedge of bone is removed from the calcaneus. Sufficient bone is removed to correct the heel varus to neutral when the wedge is closed. A staple maintains the closure (Fig. 7.35).

Hind-foot and mid-foot varus, not passively correctable: triple arthrodesis
If the varus of the hind- and mid-foot cannot be passively corrected, a triple arthrodesis is the time-tested and best procedure in children over the age of 12 years. The deforming force of the spastic muscles should be relieved by lengthening of the posterior tibial and Achilles tendons. If the peroneal muscles are non-functional, the anterior tibial tendon should be transferred to the mid-dorsum of the foot.

In cerebral palsy, triple arthrodesis is not often performed in pes varus, because early muscle lengthenings and tendon transfers to balance the spastic muscle deforming forces are successful. Horstmann and Eilert (1977) reported triple arthrodesis in only 37 patients from a pool of 899 with cerebral palsy. Only 20 of these had equinovarus deformities, but were more successfully corrected with triple arthrodesis than valgus deformities.

Ireland and Hoffer (1985) found triple arthrodesis a successful procedure in 18 of 20 cerebral-palsied patients whose mean age was 15.5 years. They did report four talonavicular joint non-unions. Non-union of this joint is fairly common. Perhaps this occurs because of inadequate contact between the head of the talus and the navicular articulating surface. Removal of an excessive amount of talar head is to be avoided, and it should be contoured to fit snugly against the navicular surface. Orthopaedic surgeons have been concerned that after a triple arthrodesis a 'ball and socket' ankle might develop after many years and cause intractable ankle pain. I believe I have one patient who does have ankle-joint pain secondary to this phenomenon. The explanation for the ball and socket joint is the function of the subtalar joint which absorbs the torques between the foot and the floor during the

261

stance phase of gait, when the lower limb abruptly changes from internal rotation to external rotation. If these rotational forces cannot be absorbed at the subtalar joint due to arthrodesis, the next proximal joint that may do so is the ankle (Inman 1976). Not every patient who has a triple arthrodesis will develop a 'ball and socket' ankle joint. This inconsistency might be explained by the great individual variations that occur in the axis of the ankle joint. This axis is oblique, and it corresponds almost exactly to a line drawn just through the tips of the malleoli. When a second line is drawn through the midline of the tibia, the ankle axis has a mean of 82.7° (SD + 3.7°; range 74° to 94°) (Inman 1976). It is possible that the more horizontal the axis of the ankle joint, the more rotation is possible; such patients are more likely to develop a late 'ball and socket' ankle after triple arthodesis.

The operative technique of triple arthrodesis is described in so many surgical technique textbooks that the details need not be repeated here. I use the technique which is an adaptation of several methods and preferred by the Campbell Clinic (Edmonson and Crenshaw 1980). The skin incision is on the lateral aspect of the foot and courses obliquely from the talar head to the peroneal tendons in a line that bisects the heel. The three joints are resected in the following order: calcanealcuboid, talonavicular and subtalar. A lamina spreader helps to visualize the subtalar articular surfaces. Excessive valgus position of the foot due to over-generous removal of laterally based wedges from the three joints should be avoided.

I do not use staples or other forms of external fixation. Two Steinman pins, one through the heel across the subtalar joint and one dorsally across the talonavicular joint, permit the application of a heavily padded postoperative plaster. I sandwich the foot and ankle between dorsal and plantar ABD pads that are secured with rolled cast padding before the plaster is applied (Roberts 1953). This padding accommodates the postoperative swelling, and the plaster seldom needs to be split. The long-leg plaster and pins are removed four weeks postoperatively. A short-leg walking plaster is used for an additional four to six weeks.

Continuous suction drainage of the wound up to 48 hours after surgery has continued to be a useful additional detail that has helped prevent wound breakdown.

Pes valgus

Although pes valgus occurs in patients with spastic hemiplegia, it is more common in spastic diplegia. In one study of 230 patients with cerebral palsy and foot deformities, pes varus occurred in 94 per cent of spastic hemiplegics. Pes valgus was more common in quadriplegics and diplegics—64 per cent (Bennet *et al.* 1982).

The management of pes valgus is discussed in Chapter 8.

Pes cavus—cavovarus or calcanealcavus?

Pes cavus is only occasionally seen in spastic hemiplegia. In Wilcox and Weiner's (1985) description of their dome osteotomy for cavus, only two of 22 patients reported had cerebral palsy.

Although pes cavus theoretically is caused by spasticity of the intrinsic muscles

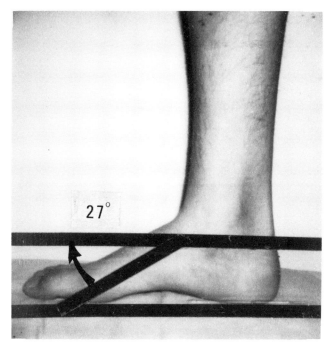

Fig. 7.36. Photograph of foot in weight-bearing; measurement to determine clinically the degree of forefoot equinus (cavus). The angle between a line parallel to the weight-bearing surface of the heel and the shaft of the first metatarsal defines the degree of cavus. If 40° or more, there is definite cavus.

of the foot, in my experience it has followed Achilles tendon lengthening (not once but three times in one patient) due to a confusion of forefoot equinus with ankle equinus. In cavus, the primary problem is excessive plantar flexion of the tarsal and metatarsal bones beyond the range of normal. As in flaccid paralysis, weakening the triceps surae creates excessive dorsiflexion of the calcaneus, and the substitution of the toe flexor muscles for the gastrocnemius-soleus 'pulls' the forefoot to the hind-foot; the deformity is calcanealcavus (Coleman 1983, Dillin and Samilson 1983). The higher the arch of the foot, the more discomfort ensues due to the excessive pressure of weight-bearing on the metatarsal heads and strain on the mid-tarsal joints at the apex of the arch.

Measurement of cavus
It is useful to have some objective method of determining the degree of cavus. One method I use is to measure the angle made by a line through the first metatarsal shaft and the plantar surface of the heel when weight-bearing or when the foot is passively dorsiflexed. On weight-bearing, the foot perceived to be normal has an angle between these two landmarks of 25° in a range of 20° to 40°. Feet with this angle greater than 40° have excessive forefoot equinus and can be termed cavus deformities (Fig. 7.36). This measurement can be used at the time of surgical correction.

Barenfeld *et al.* (1971) measured the degree of forefoot equinus on standing lateral radiographs of normal children's feet. The obtuse angle between the

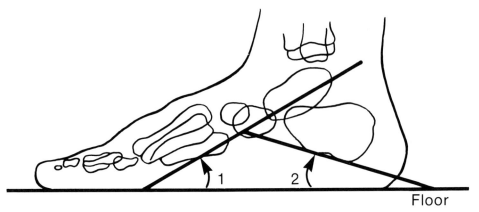

Fig. 7.37. Tracing of weight-bearing radiograph of a child's foot. Angle 1 is the talar plantar flexion angle (normal mean 26.5°, SD 5.3°). Angle 2 is the calcaneal dorsiflexion angle (normal mean 16.8°, SD 5.6°). A calcaneal dorsiflexion angle >25° indicates a calcaneus deformity (Bleck and Berzins 1977).

horizontal plane of the calcaneus and a line along the shaft of the first metatarsal varied from 140° to 160°. If this angle was less than 140°, the foot was defined as cavus. In 75 per cent of the children with pes cavus, the angle was less than 125°.

The extent of the abnormality is defined by radiographic measurements of the dorsiflexion angle of the calcaneus with the horizontal plane when the patient is standing (Fig. 7.37). The normal upper limit with this measurement is about 25°. If this angle is 30° or more, the deformity called 'calcaneus' is certain.

Management of pes calcanealcavus
No conservative management has been successful and orthotic treatment is useless (Coleman 1983). Surgery is indicated in children under the age of 10 years to prevent the severe and often symptomatic deformity in adolescence. In older children and adolescents, it is probably wise to perform the extensive surgery required in this difficult deformity only if the patient has symptoms of foot discomfort.

Calcanealcavus in children between the ages of five and 10 years will require first an extra-articular subtalar arthrodesis to stabilize the hind-foot, followed six weeks later by transfer of the peroneal and posterior tibial tendons to the calcaneus in order to substitute for the weak triceps surae muscle (Coleman 1983). In cerebral palsy, the spastic anterior tibial muscle is usually the major deforming force in causing the imbalance. If so, I transfer it rather than the peroneals or the posterior tibial which are plantar flexors. In all cavus deformities it is necessary to do a plantar fasciotomy and a myotomy of the origin of the flexor digitorum brevis muscles ('plantar release') as well as the preceding operations. Calcanealcavus in children with the spastic type of cerebral palsy over the age of 12 years will require the 'plantar release', a triple arthrodesis, a crescentric osteotomy of the calcaneus (Samilson 1976), and usually a transfer of the deforming spastic anterior tibial muscle-tendon to the calcaneus (Fig. 7.38). The problem with triple arthrodesis in

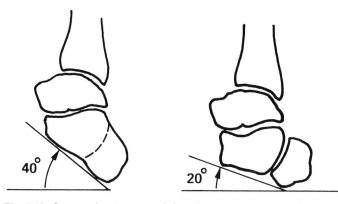

Fig. 7.38. Crescentric osteotomy of the calcaneus to correct a calcaneus deformity.

correcting a severe forefoot equinus is that removal of the talar head and neck is limited by the tibial articular surface of the talus; excessive dorsiflexion of the forefoot by resection of more and more of the talar neck will compromise the integrity of the ankle joint. It is then necessary to do a form of mid-tarsal osteotomy with the dorsally based wedge. In cerebral palsy I have used the metatarsal-cuneiform osteotomy-arthrodesis described by Jahss (1980) for idiopathic pes cavus and that associated with club foot and flaccid paralysis (Bleck 1984). I would recommend that the triple arthrodesis and calcaneal osteotomy be done, and then in the operating room the degree of forefoot equinus can be measured as described. If it does not exceed the clinical measurement of 30°, then additional mid-tarsal or metatarsal-cuneiform dorsally based wedge osteotomies need not be performed (Fig. 7.39).

The 'Akron midtarsal dome osteotomy' (Wilcox and Weiner 1985) is probably

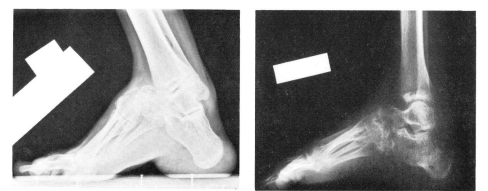

Fig. 7.39. *Top:* severe calcaneus deformity; spastic diplegia. The patient had two Achilles tendon lengthenings and a posterior capsulotomy of the ankle joint in attempts to correct ankle equinus. *Bottom:* postoperative crescentric calcaneal osteotomy and midtarsal osteotomy arthrodesis to correct the severe deformity shown *top*.

best applied in cavovarus deformities. The v-osteotomy of the mid-tarsus in the coronal plane, with the point of the v in the middle cuneiform bone, is yet another method to correct the forefoot equinus (Japas 1968). It is designed to avoid forefoot shortening that can occur when a large dorsally based wedge of bone is removed from the mid-tarsal joints in order to correct the forefoot equinus. Because of my limited experience and technical difficulties with this procedure, I have not used it in cerebral palsy. Nor have I had an occasion to use Swanson's v-type osteotomies at the base of the metatarsals to correct cavus (Swanson *et al.* 1966). Perhaps it would be useful in rigid pes cavus without a hind-foot deformity, *i.e.* neither calcaneus or varus. In cerebral palsy this is hardly ever the case.

Management of pes cavovarus
If pes cavovarus ever occurs in cerebral palsy, the decision to perform only the plantar release can be made by application of Coleman's block test. The child stands on a one-inch block of wood so that the heel rests on it and the foot is diagonally placed to allow the medial half of the forefoot to drop downward on the floor. If the varus of the heel corrects with this maneuver, the deformity is flexible and a plantar release indicated. If it does not correct this way, additional bone surgery will be necessary (Coleman 1983).

Metatarsus adductus
Pathogenesis
The pathogenesis of metatarsus adductus in the spastic paralysis of cerebral palsy appears to be the spastic abductor hallucis muscle. In children the deformity is dynamic and later evolves into a fixed skeletal one (Bleck 1967). I originally noted a unilateral hallux valgus, and bunion in spastic hemiplegia on the side of the paralysis (Fig. 7.40); this seems more prone to occur after Achilles tendon lengthening in some patients who have spasticity of the intrinsic muscles of the foot. These muscles are active during the stance phase of gait, and the abductor hallucis is a major intrinsic muscle of the foot. Probably with weakening of the gastrocnemius-soleus muscle, the intrinsic muscles of the foot act as substitutes during walking and running (Fig. 7.41).

Indications for treatment
The indications for treatment in the young child who has a dynamic metatarsus adductus is the recognition that it will eventually become a fixed deformity. I originally ascertained that the abductor hallucis was a dynamic force in adducting the forefoot by infiltration of its muscle belly with 5 to 10ml of 1 per cent lidocaine. This invasive procedure can be eliminated by comparing an anterior-posterior radiograph of the foot when the child stands with another radiograph taken when the forefoot is manually abducted against the heel (a lead apron and gloves are necessary to protect the physician when this is done). If the radiograph shows passive correction of the metatarsal adduction, abductor hallucis release is indicated. A simple release is not indicated if there is a fixed deformity, particularly

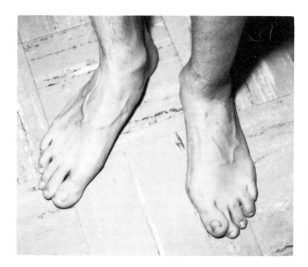

Fig. 7.40. Unilateral hallux valgus on the involved limb in a patient with spastic hemiplegia.

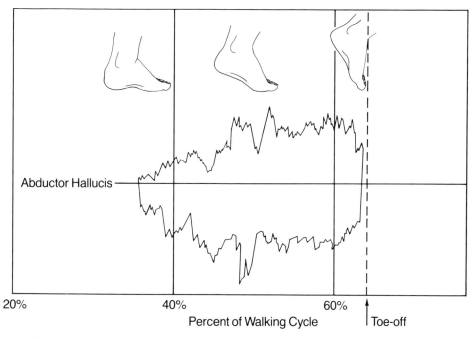

Abductor Hallucis

20% 40% 60%

Percent of Walking Cycle

Toe-off

Fig. 7.41. Gait electromyograms show that the abductor hallucis is a stance-phase muscle.

267

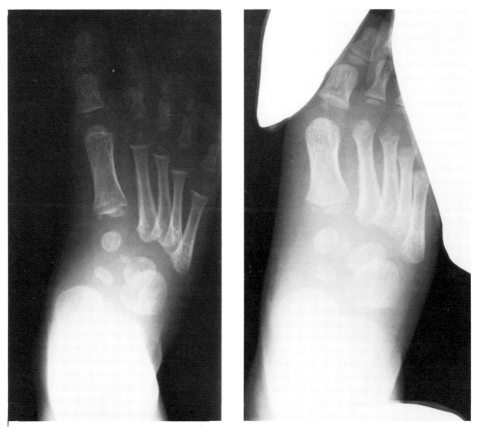

Fig. 7.42. *Left:* metatarsus adductus. *Right:* the adduction of the metatarsals fails to correct with passive abduction of the forefoot. Therefore this is a fixed and not a dynamic deformity. Abductor hallucis tenotomy is not indicated.

of the first metatarsal. In this case it is a fine procedure to produce hallux valgus and a bunion (Fig. 7.42).

If the metatarsals are fixed in adduction and abduction occurs only at the mid-tarsal joints, it is not passively correctable. In these cases more extensive surgery is required. The use of a simple grading system to define the severity of the metatarsus adductus assists in the decision. The heel bisector method visualizes the plantar weight-bearing aspect of the heel as an ellipse, the major axis of which bisects the heel and forms the center line of the foot. In normally aligned feet (85 per cent, according to Bleck 1971) this line falls between the second and third toes. This center line is through the third toe in mild metatarsus adductus, between the third and fourth toes in moderate and between the fourth and fifth toes in severe cases (Bleck 1983) (Fig. 2.40).

In mild and moderate fixed metatarsus adductus, the surgery does not seem worthwhile. In severe cases the tarsal-metatarsal capsulotomies are satisfactory up to the age of three or four years (Heyman *et al.* 1958). After that age, metatarsal osteotomies with laterally based wedges at the proximal ends of these bones correct with greater facility than capsulotomies (Berman and Gartland 1971). In cerebral palsy an abductor hallucis release should also be done.

Coleman (1983) has used the open-wedge medial cuneiform osteotomy with either a homogenous or an autogenous bone graft, and six weeks of fixation with a threaded pin to prevent collapse of the osteotomy in cases of residual metatarsus adductus in congenital club foot. I have not used this method in cerebral palsy, but have tried it in severe metatarsus adductus in children at age six years; I used freeze-dried bone homografts, which failed to incorporate even after eight weeks. Coleman is correct; a threaded pin seems to be necessary. It seems excessive to keep a child non-weightbearing and in plaster for many weeks while awaiting healing. I believe an autogenous graft is preferable to ensure more rapid healing of the osteotomy.

Operative technique—modifications of capsulotomies and osteotomies for metatarsus adductus
The only modification I have made from the description of these operations is to use two longitudinal incisions on the dorsum of the foot: one between the first and second metatarsals and the other over the fourth metatarsal. In performing the osteotomies, a small Kerisan upbiting rongeur is a convenient and gentle way of removing the laterally based wedge of bone. In both the capsulotomies and osteotomies, Kirschner wires are driven from the medial distal and lateral distal sides of the first and fifth metatarsals through their shafts and into the tarsal bones. These hold the corrections reasonably well in padded plasters for four to six weeks while healing occurs. Another method of pin fixation has been described by Tachdjian (1972).

Operative technique—abductor hallucis release
A 2.5cm incision is made over the medial aspect of the first metatarsal, and the tendon of the abductor hallucis is found and grasped with a Kocher hemostat (Fig. 7.43). The tendon is cut distal to the hemostat and the tendon is pulled out of the wound so that a 1cm piece can be excised. With the forefoot held in abduction and the heel in the neutral position, a short-leg walking plaster is applied and worn for six weeks. No special shoes or splints have been necessary after plaster removal.

The results of this procedure have been excellent, providing it is done when there is no fixed deformity (Bleck 1967). In two of my patients who had a fixed adduction of the first metatarsal, hallux valgus developed later.

Hallux valgus and bunion
The pathogenesis of hallux valgus can be a spastic adductor hallucis muscle alone or in combination with excessive adduction of the first metatarsal. In many patients it is secondary to pes valgus, which causes excessive pressure on the medial border of

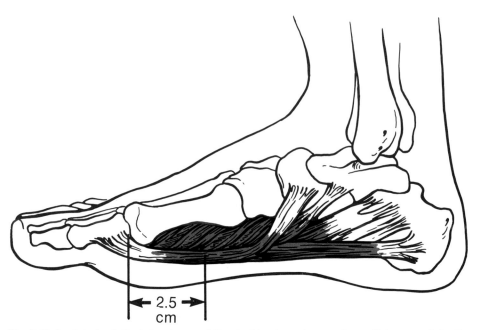

Fig. 7.43. In abductor hallucis tenotomy a 2.5cm incision is made over the medial aspect of the first metatarsal neck and proximal shaft. A 1cm section of the abductor hallucis tendon is resected.

the foot and great toe. The great toe is forced into progressive abduction (Holstein 1980).

The indications for surgery are a painful bunion over the head of the first metatarsal and painful callosities over the medial aspect of the great toe. In some patients a recurrent ingrown great toenail results from the pressure on the medial distal end of the great toe, which is not only in valgus but also rotated internally.

Selection of the surgical procedure. If the hallux valgus is secondary to pes valgus, then the foot deformity must also be corrected in addition to correcting the hallux valgus. In children under the age of 12 years, a subtalar extra-articular arthrodesis is the usual procedure to correct pes valgus (see Chapter 8); in older children and skeletally mature patients, triple arthrodesis is most often selected. Severe hallux valgus can be prevented when it is recognized early in pes valgus in cerebral palsy; in this case a subtalar extra-articular arthrodesis to bring the foot into a neutral weight-bearing position prevents progression of the great toe abduction deformity.

Symptomatic and primary dynamic hallux valgus (without pes valgus and/or adduction of the first metatarsal) can be relieved with a tenotomy of the adductor hallucis through a short linear incision in the first web space.

In children if the hallux valgus is fixed and symptomatic, the correction is possible with adductor hallucis tenotomy, lateral capsulotomy of the metatarsal-phalangeal joint and pin fixation of the great toe to the first metatarsal. Sequist (1977) reported success with this method in 20 of 26 patients. However, in most of our child patients the hallux valgus is secondary to pes equinovalgus which should be corrected first with subtalar arthrodesis.

In adolescents and adults with cerebral palsy I prefer to correct the skeletal deformities in hallux valgus. The adductor hallucis tenotomy is always done. An osteotomy of the first metatarsal to correct its adduction deformity can be done through the neck of the metatarsal as described by Mitchell *et al.* (1958), Carr and Boyd (1968) and Wu (1986). The crescentric osteotomy in the proximal shaft of the first metatarsal used by Mann (1986) may be preferable to the one through the neck. The Mitchell osteotomy is easy to displace dorsally and compromise the result. Although I have not seen avascular necrosis in the head of the first metatarsal with the Mitchell procedure, others have reported it. It probably occurs by interfering with the blood supply of the bone on the lateral aspect of the head and neck if capsulotomies and extensive dissection are done with the osteotomy of the neck.

Excessive removal of the prominence on the medial aspect of the first metatarsal head should be avoided, and the osteotomy should not go beyond the ridge which separates the articular cartilage of the metatarsal from the bone (Mann 1986). If the prominence disappears with the realignment of the first metatarsal osteotomy, there is nothing to remove. Normal feet have a slight medial bulge on the metatarsal head.

If the hallux valgus does not correct at the time of the first metatarsal osteotomy, I prefer to correct this with a closed wedge osteotomy at the base of the proximal phalanx (Goldner 1981). This procedure has preserved motion of the metatarsal-phalangeal joint. Attempts to 'reef' the medial capsule of the joint, to correct the hallux valgus, seem to create undesirable stiffness of the joint.

Because of discouraging results with the Mitchell metatarsal osteotomy and the McBride (1928) adductor hallucis transfer and exostectomy, Renshaw *et al.* (1979) prefer arthrodesis of the metatarsal-phalangeal joint of the great toe and removal of the medial bump (exostosis) on the head of the first metatarsal (McKeever 1952). Arthrodesis is a permanent solution and is probably indicated in those patients who have degenerative arthritis of the joint. The arthrodesis of the joint should be in varying degrees of dorsiflexion depending upon heel height (and presumably the amount of equinus during the stance phase of gait in cerebral palsy); in McKeever's cases the great toe dorsiflexion varied between 15° and 35°. I have not had occasion to fuse the joint.

Goldner (1981) corrected 26 feet in 16 patients with the adductor hallucis tenotomy, proximal shaft metatarsal osteotomy and the osteotomy at the base of the proximal phalanx. In his patients, followed from two to 20 years, none developed a degenerative arthritis of the first metatarsal-phalangeal joint and none needed arthrodesis of the joint.

With careful observation one can appreciate that much of the hallux valgus occurs at the interphalangeal joint of the great toe in some adolescents and adults. Frequently, the great toe crosses under the second toe (Fig. 7.44). In these cases I have done an osteotomy-arthrodesis with a medially based wedge of bone removed at the interphalangeal joint and fixation with a threaded pin.

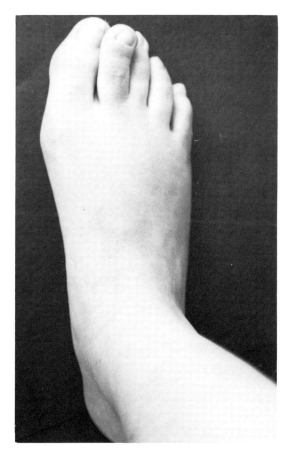

Fig. 7.44. The great toe is adducted due to a spastic adductor hallucis and crosses under the second toe. The additional deformity is adduction of the distal phalanx. This needs correction by a closed wedge osteotomy arthodesis at the distal interphalangeal joint.

The operative technique I would recommend for bunion and hallux valgus in *adolescents and adults* with cerebral palsy is: (1) tenotomy of the adductor hallucis insertion on the proximal phalanx of the great toe; (ii) a crescentric osteotomy of the proximal end of the first metatarsal (Mann 1986); a motorized crescentric-shaped saw is used, with the convexity of the crescent proximal. The metatarsal is then abducted and the osteotomy secured with a single transverse screw, obliquely directed from the proximal medial cortex laterally to cross the osteotomy: fixing the screw is easier if the drill hole and screw is placed in the shaft of the metatarsal distal to the intended osteotomy before the saw cut is made; (iii) for residual hallux valgus, a medially based closed-wedge osteotomy of the proximal phalanx. Before the bone is cut, two drill holes are placed proximally and distally just beyond the intended osteotomy. Then after the osteotomy is completed and the wedge removed, a strong suture (*e.g.* No. 0 Vicryl) is passed through these holes and tied on the medial cortex of the phalanx to secure the osteotomy.

In children I have not considered osteotomies of the bones to correct hallux valgus. Their hallux valgus is usually asymptomatic and secondary to the pes

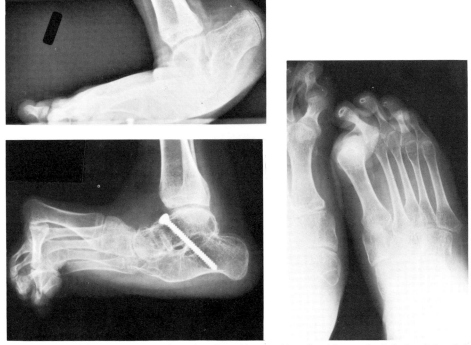

Fig. 7.45. *Top left:* severe pes equinovalgus in a 14-year-old male with spastic diplegia. *Below left:* lateral radiograph of foot after triple arthrodesis. The screw between the talus and calcaneus was used to maintain their proper alignments. Postoperative dorsiflexion of the first metatarsal caused a dorsal bunion. *Right:* anterior-posterior postoperative radiograph after triple arthrodesis; dorsal bunion and hallux valgus; great toe crosses under the second toe.

valgus, which should be corrected with a subtalar extra-articular arthrodesis when hallux valgus is observed. In these children's feet, a tenotomy of the insertion of the adductor hallucis muscle is probably sufficient. 10° of hallux valgus is not likely to cause significant symptoms.

Dorsal bunion

The *pathogenesis* of dorsal bunion in cerebral palsy is dorsiflexion of the first metatarsal due to spastic anterior tibial muscles, and acute flexion of the great toe due to spasticity of the flexor digitorum longus and flexor hallucis brevis muscles. I have seen it occur after a triple arthrodesis for severe pes equinovalgus in which the mid- and forefoot are dorsiflexed and the hind-foot plantar-flexed ('rocker bottom') (Fig. 7.45). In cerebral palsy it is not associated with a weak peroneus longus muscle, as it was in cases of poliomyelitis. The dorsal bunion is the prominent head of the first metatarsal on the dorsum of the foot. With shoes it is most uncomfortable.

The *management* of dorsal bunion is surgical. The only conservative management possible is to relieve the pressure on the prominence with extra large

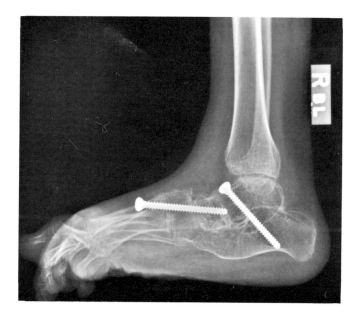

Fig. 7.46. Lateral radiograph of same foot after correction of dorsal bunion with closed wedge osteotomy-arthrodesis of the first metatarsal cuneiform and cuneiform navicular joints. The screw crossing both joints afforded firm fixation of the correction while healing occurred.

toe-caps in the shoes or the elimination of enclosing footwear (*e.g.* sandals or heavy stockings).

The operative technique is based upon the cause. The first metatarsal must be plantar-flexed, the spasm of the anterior tibial relieved and the toe-flexion deformity corrected. To accomplish this, Goldner (1981) transferred the anterior tibial tendon to the second metatarsal, did an osteotomy at the base of the first metatarsal and transferred the flexor hallucis longus to the extensor hallucis longus. In 26 feet of 16 patients it was not necessary to perform an arthrodesis of the metatarsal phalangeal joint.

The operations I have done in *skeletally mature* patients have followed Goldner's principles (1981): (i) z-lengthening of the anterior tibial tendon; (ii) arthrodesis of the metatarsal-cuneiform joint from which a dosrally based wedge of bone was removed and an arthrodesis of the cuneiform-navicular joint. A single screw directed from the shaft of the first metatarsal across both joints gave secure fixation; (iii) a z-lengthening of the flexor hallucis longus tendon and if required, a tenotomy of the insertions of the flexor hallucis brevis muscle. With this correction the dorsal bunion disappears. It is not necessary to remove any of the bone from the dorsum of the metatarsal head (Fig. 7.46). Plaster immobilization is presumed.

If the articular cartilage of the metatarsal-phalangeal joint has degenerative changes, an arthrodesis of the joint (or maybe a removal of the proximal half of the proximal phalanx) may prevent a painful joint after correction of the dorsal bunion. I have not done either procedure.

In children with cerebral palsy, dorsal bunion must be rare. McKay's (1983) procedure for dorsal bunion in children (24 patients) was applied to only two

274

patients with cerebral palsy at ages 14 and 15 years. Most of his patients had either poliomyelitis or club foot. McKay's successful procedure was to wrap the muscle-tendon units of the adductor hallucis, abductor hallucis and then flexor hallucis brevis around the neck of the first metatarsal. The mean age of the patients was 10.5 years.

Flexion deformity of the toes
Flexion deformities of the toes are more common in adolescents and adults than in children. When these cause discomfort, tenotomy of the flexor tendons of the toes at their proximal skin creases usually solves the problem. Menalaus (1984) successfully treated 'curly' and hammer toes in children (not necessarily those who had cerebral palsy) with toe-flexor tenotomy. He made the point to be sure that preoperatively the metatarsal-phalangeal joint could be flexed. If not, then it is a claw toe which I have not found in my patients with cerebral palsy. Claw-toe correction would need more than a simple flexor tenotomy.

Knee-flexion and hyperextension deformities
Knee-flexion deformities in hemiplegia are managed as described in the following chapter on spastic diplegia. The results of surgery are often better in hemiplegia than in diplegia because of normal function in the opposite limb.

Spastic knee hyperextension during gait is more often found in patients whose hemiplegia is due to a cerebral vascular accident or a head injury. Because the knee does not flex sufficiently in swing phase of gait, the lower limb circumducts in order for the foot to clear the ground. The spasticity in the quadriceps can be partly relieved with a rectus femoris tenotomy at its origin.

Orthotic management of knee hyperextension may be found in the plastic ankle-foot orthosis, in which the ankle is dorsiflexed above the neutral position (Rosenthal et al. 1975).

Hip-flexion and internal rotation deformity
As with the knee deformities, the management of the hip-flexion and internal rotation deformities are the same as in spastic diplegia (Chapter 8). The most common pitfall of femoral derotation osteotomy in this child with spastic hemiplegia is the failure to recognize concomitant excessive compensatory external tibial-fibular torsion ($>30°$). When only a femoral derotation osteotomy is done in this circumstance, the external rotation of the foot is greatly exaggerated. To prevent this undesirable change in the limb posture and gait, it is necessary to do an internal derotation tibial and fibular osteotomy at the time of the femoral osteotomy. Another less common pitfall of femoral derotation osteotomy is overcorrection so that no internal rotation of the hip is preserved. Then the pelvis cannot externally rotate during gait and remains in an anteriorly rotated position. I try to leave 30° to 45° of internal rotation of the hip in femoral derotation osteotomies.

Leg-length discrepancy
Stunting of linear growth in the hemiplegic limb is common; however, the

discrepancy rarely exceeds 1.5cm at the time of skeletal maturity. If serial measurements during growth show the discrepancy to be increasing, with a projected shortening of more than 2cm leg length, equalization by epiphyseal arrest or stapling of the distal femoral (and if need be, proximal tibial) physes is indicated.

Shoe lifts are not necessary. They prevent the child from participating fully in sports and games. Short legs do not cause scoliosis. Spinal curvatures in hemiplegia result from unknown causes (idiopathic scoliosis) or are due to congenital anomalies of the vertebrae and are independent of a leg-length discrepancy. The child with spastic hemiplegia is already burdened with an abnormal gait. Why add to the disability by prescribing shoe lifts? If anything, the shoe lift will prevent sometimes a desirable compensation for the inability of the ankle to dorsiflex and the toes to clear the ground during the swing phase of gait.

REFERENCES

Adler, N., Bleck, E. E., Rinsky, L. A. (1985) 'Decision making in surgical treatment of paralytic deformities of the foot with gait electromyograms.' *Orthopedic Transactions*, **9**, 90-91.
Aitken, J. (1952) 'Deformity of the elbow joint as a sequel to Erb's obstetrical paralysis.' *Journal of Bone and Joint Surgery*, **34B**, 352-365.
Baker, L. D. (1954) 'Triceps surae syndrome in cerebral palsy.' *Archives of Surgery*, **68**, 216-221.
—— (1956) 'A rational approach to the surgical needs of the cerebral palsy patient.' *Journal of Bone and Joint Surgery*, **38A**, 313-323.
—— Hill, L. M. (1964) 'Foot alignment in the cerebral palsy patient.' *Journal of Bone and Joint Surgery*, **46A**, 1-15.
Banks, H. H. (1975) 'The foot and ankle in cerebral palsy.' *In:* Samilson, R. L. (Ed.) *Orthopaedic Aspects of Cerebral Palsy. Clinics in Developmental Medicine, Nos. 52/53.* London: S.I.M.P. with Heinemann; Philadelphia: J. B. Lippincott.
—— (1977) 'The management of spastic deformities of the foot and ankle.' *Clinical Orthopaedics and Related Research*, **122**, 70-76.
—— (1983) 'Equinus and cerebral palsy.' *Foot and Ankle*, **4**, 149-159.
—— Green, W. T. (1958) 'The correction of equinus deformity in cerebral palsy.' *Journal of Bone and Joint Surgery*, **40A**, 1359-1379.
—— Panagakos, P. (1966) 'Orthopaedic evaluation in the lower extremity in cerebral palsy.' *Clinical Orthopaedics and Related Research*, **47**, 117-125.
Barenfeld, P. A., Weseley, M. D., Shea, J. M. (1971) 'The congenital cavus foot.' *Clinical Orthopaedics and Related Research*, **79**, 119-126.
Barnett, J. G., Holly, R. G., Ashmore, C. R. (1980) 'Stretch-induced growth in chicken wing muscles: biochemical and morphological characterization.' *American Journal of Physiology*, **239**, C39-C46.
Bassett, F. H. III, Baker, L. D. (1966) 'Equinus deformity in cerebral palsy.' *In:* Adams, J. P. (Ed.) *Current Practice in Orthopaedic Surgery, Vol 3.* St. Louis: C. V. Mosby. pp. 59-74.
Bennet, G., Rang, M., Jones, D. (1982) 'Varus and valgus deformities of the foot in cerebral palsy.' *Developmental Medicine and Child Neurology*, **24**, 499-503.
Berman, A., Gartland, J. J. (1971) 'Metatarsal osteotomy for the correction of adduction of the forepart of the foot in children.' *Journal of Bone and Joint Surgery*, **53A**, 498-506.
Bisla, R. S., Louis, H. H., Albano, P. S. (1976) 'Transfer of the tibialis posterior tendon in cerebral palsy.' *Journal of Bone and Joint Surgery*, **58A**, 497-500.
Bleck, E. E. (1967) 'Spastic abductor hallucis.' *Developmental Medicine and Child Neurology*, **9**, 602-608.
—— (1971) 'The shoeing of children: sham or science?' *Developmental Medicine and Child Neurology*, **13**, 188-195.
—— (1983) 'Metatarsus adductus: classification and relationship to outcomes of treatment.' *Journal of Pediatric Orthopedics*, **3**, 2-9.
—— (1984) 'Forefoot problems in cerebral palsy—diagnosis and management.' *Foot and Ankle*, **4**, 188-194.

—— Berzins, U. L. (1977) 'Conservative management of pes valgus with plantar flexed talus flexible.' *Clinical Orthopaedics and Related Research*, **122**, 85-94.

Braun, R. M., Vise, G. T., Roper, B. (1974) 'Preliminary experience with superficialis-to-profundus tendon transfer in the hemiplegic upper extremity.' *Journal of Bone and Joint Surgery*, **56A**, 466-472.

Carr, C. R., Boyd, B. M. (1968) 'Correctional osteotomy for metatarsus primus varus and hallux valgus.' *Journal of Bone and Joint Surgery*, **50A**, 1353-1367.

Chait, L. A., Kaplan, I., Stewart-Lord, B., Goodman, M. (1980) 'Early surgical correction in the cerebral palsied hand.' *Journal of Hand Surgery*, **5**, 122-126.

Coleman, S. S. (1983) *Complex Foot Deformities in Children.* Philadelphia: Lea & Febiger.

Colton, C. L., Ransford, A. D., Lloyd-Roberts, G. C. (1976) 'Transposition of the tendon of the pronator teres in cerebral palsy.' *Journal of Bone and Joint Surgery*, **58B**, 220-223.

Craig, J. J., Van Voren, J. (1976) 'The importance of gastrocnemius recession in the correction of equinus deformity in cerebral palsy.' *Journal of Bone and Joint Surgery*, **58B**, 84-87.

Crenshaw, A. H. (1963) *Campbell's Operative Orthopaedics, Vol. 2, 4th edn.* St. Louis: C. V. Mosby Co. p. 1052.

Dillin, W., Samilson, R. L. (1983) 'Calcaneus deformity in cerebral palsy.' *Foot and Ankle*, **4**, 167-170.

Edmonson, A. S., Crenshaw, A. H. (1980) *Campbell's Operative Orthopaedics, Vol.2, 6th edn.* St. Louis: C. V. Mosby Co. pp. 1426-1428.

Elliott, J. M., Connolly, K. J. (1984) 'A classification of manipulative hand movements.' *Developmental Medicine and Child Neurology*, **26**, 283-296.

Feldkamp, M., Güth, V. (1980) 'Operative Korrekturn an der Hand des Zerebralparetikers.' *Zeitschrift für Orthopedie*, **118**, 256-264.

Filler, B. C., Stark, N. H., Boyes, J. H. (1976) 'Capsulodesis of the metacarpophalangeal joint of the thumb in children with cerebral palsy.' *Journal of Bone and Joint Surgery*, **58A**, 667-670.

Funk, D. A., Cass, J. R., Johnson, K. A. (1986) 'Acquired adult flat foot secondary to posterior tibial-tendon pathology.' *Journal of Bone and Joint Surgery*, **68A**, 95-102.

Gaines, R. W., Ford, T. B. (1984) 'A systematic approach to the amount of achilles tendon lengthening in cerebal palsy.' *Journal of Pediatric Orthopedics*, **4**, 488-451.

Goldner, J. L. (1954) *Personal communication.*

—— (1955) 'Reconstructive surgery of the hand in cerebral palsy and spastic paralysis from injury to the spinal cord.' *Journal of Bone and Joint Surgery*, **37A**, 1141-1154.

—— (1975) 'The upper extremity in cerebral palsy.' *In:* Samilson, R. L. (Ed.) *Orthopaedic Aspects of Cerebral Palsy, Clinics in Developmental Medicine Nos. 52/53.* London: S.I.M.P. with Heinemann: Philadelphia: J. B. Lippincott. pp. 221-257.

—— (1981) 'Hallux valgus and hallux flexus associated with cerebral palsy: analysis and treatment.' *Clinical Orthopaedics and Related Research*, **157**, 98-104.

—— (1983) 'Surgical treatment for cerebral palsy.' *In:* Evarts, C. McC. (Ed.) *Surgery of the Musculoskeletal System, Vol.2.* Edinburgh: Livingstone. pp. 439-469.

—— Ferlic, D. C. (1966) 'Sensory status of the hand as related to reconstructive surgery of the upper extremity in cerebral palsy.' *Clinical Orthopaedics and Related Research* **46**, 87-92.

—— Keats, P. K., Bassett, F. H. III, Clippinger, F. W. (1974) 'Progressive talipes equinovalgus due to trauma or degeneration of the posterior tibial tendon and medial plantar ligaments.' *Orthopaedic Clinics of North America*, **5**, 39-50.

—— Goodman, W. B., Bookman, M. (1977) 'The long term results of soft tissue elbow releases for improved elbow and forearm function in children with cerebral palsy.' *Paper read at Annual meeting, American Academy for Cerebral Palsy and Developmental Medicine, Atlanta.*

Gräbe, R. P., Thompson, P. (1979) 'Lengthening of the Achilles tendon in cerebral paresis.' *South African Medical Journal*, **56**, 993-996.

Green, N. E., Griffin, P. P., Shiavi, R. (1983) 'Split posterior tibial tendon transfer in spastic cerebral palsy.' *Journal of Bone and Joint Surgery*, **65A**, 748-754.

Green, W. T., Banks, H. H. (1962) 'Flexor carpi ulnaris transplant and its use in cerebral palsy.' *Journal of Bone and Joint Surgery*, **44A**, 1343-1352.

Gritzka, T. L., Staheli, L. T., Duncan, W. R. (1972) 'Posterior tibial tendon transfer through interosseus membrane to correct equinovarus deformity in cerebral palsy.' *Clinical Orthopaedics and Related Research*, **89**, 201-206.

Hadad, R. J. (1977) 'Upper limb surgery in cerebral palsy.' *Regional Course, American Academy for Cerebral Palsy and Developmental Medicine, New Orleans.*

Heyman, C. H., Herndon, C. H., Strong, J. M. (1958) 'Mobilization of the tarso-metatarsal and intermetatarsal joints for the correction of resistant adduction of the forepart of the foot in congenital clubfoot or congenital metatarsus varus.' *Journal of Bone and Joint Surgery*, **40A**, 299-310.

Hirasawa, Y., Katsumi, Y., Tokioka, T. (1985) 'Evaluation of sensibility after sensory reconstruction of the thumb.' *Journal of Bone and Joint Surgery*, **67B**, 814-819.

Hoffer, M. M. (1976) 'Basic considerations and classification of cerebral palsy.' *American Academy of Orthopaedic Surgeons: Instructional Course Lectures*, **25**, 96-106:

—— (1985) 'Tendon transfer to the extensors of the wrists and fingers in cerebral palsy.' *Paper No. 35 presented at the Annual Meeting of the Pediatric Orthopaedic Society of North America, San Antonio, Texas.*

—— Reswig, J. A., Garrett, A. M., Perry, J. (1974) 'The split anterior tibial tendon transfer in treatment of spastic varus of the hindfoot in childhood.' *Orthopedic Clinics of North America*, **5**, 31-38.

—— Perry, J., Melkonian, G. J. (1979) 'Dynamic electromyography and decision-making for surgery in the upper extremity of patients with cerebral palsy.' *Journal of Hand Surgery*, **4**, 424-431.

—— —— Garcia, M., Bullock, D. (1983) 'Adduction contracture of the thumb in cerebral palsy.' *Journal of Bone and Joint Surgery*, **65A**, 755-759.

—— Barakat, G., Koffman, M. (1985) '10-year follow-up of split anterior tibial tendon transfer in cerebral palsied patients with spastic equinovarus deformity.' *Journal of Pediatric Orthopedics*, **5**, 432-434.

—— Holstein, A. (1980) 'Hallux valgus—an acquired deformity of the foot in cerebral palsy.' *Foot and Ankle*, **1**, 33-38.

Horstmann, H. H., Eilert, R. E. (1977) 'Triple arthrodesis in cerebral palsy.' *Paper presented at annual meeting of the American Academy of Orthopaedic Surgeons, Las Vegas.*

House, J. H. (1975) 'A dynamic approach to the "thumb-in-palm" deformity in cerebral palsy.' *Instruction Course Syllabus, American Academy for Cerebral Palsy.*

—— Gwathney, F. W., Fidler, M. O. (1981) 'A dynamic approach to the thumb-in-palm deformity in cerebral palsy.' *Journal of Bone and Joint Surgery*, **63A**, 216-225.

Huet de la Tour, E., Tardieu, C., Tabary, J. C., Tabary, C. (1979) 'Decrease of muscle extensibility and reduction of sacromere numbers in soleus muscle following local injection of tetanus toxin.' *Journal of the Neurological Sciences*, **40**, 123-131.

Inglis, A. E., Cooper, W. (1966) 'Release of flexor-pronator origin for flexion deformities of the hand and wrist in spastic paralysis: a study of eighteen cases.' *Journal of Bone and Joint Surgery*, **48A**, 847-857.

Inman, V. T. (1976) *The Joints of the Ankle.* Baltimore: Williams & Wilkins.

Ireland, M. L., Hoffer, M. M. (1985) 'Triple arthrodesis for children with spastic cerebral palsy.' *Developmental Medicine and Child Neurology*, **27**, 623-627.

Jahss, M. H. (1980) 'Tarsometatarsal truncated-wedge arthrodesis for pes cavus and equinovarus deformity of the forepart of the foot.' *Journal of Bone and Joint Surgery*, **62A**, 713-722.

Japas, L. M. (1968) 'Surgical treatment of pes cavus by tarsal V-osteotomy.' *Journal of Bone and Joint Surgery*, **50A**, 927-943.

Johnson, K. A. (1983) 'Tibialis posterior tendon rupture.' *Clinical Orthopaedics and Related Research*, **177**, 140-147.

Jones, M. (1976) 'Differential diagnosis and natural history of the cerebral palsied child.' *In*: Samilson, R. L. (Ed.) *Orthopaedic Aspects of Cerebral Palsy. Clinics in Developmental Medicine Nos. 52/53* London: S.I.M.P with Heinemann; Philadelphia: J. B. Lippincott.

Keats, S. (1965) 'Surgical treatment of the hand in cerebral palsy: correction of the thumb-in-palm and other deformities.' *Journal of Bone and Joint Surgery* **47A**, 274-284.

—— (1974) 'Congenital bilateral dislocation of the head of the radius in a seven year old child.' *Orthopaedic Review* **111**, 33-36.

Kettlekamp, D. B., Alexander, H. H. (1969) 'Spontaneous rupture of the posterior tibial tendon.' *Journal of Bone and Joint Surgery*, **514**, 759-764.

Kling, T. F., Kaufer, H., Hensinger, R. N. (1985) 'Split posterior tibial-tendon transfers in children with cerebral spastic paralysis and equinovarus deformity.' *Journal of Bone and Joint Surgery*, **67A**, 186-194.

Lake, D., Moreau, M., Rittenhous, B. (1985) 'Outpatient percutaneous heel cord lengthening for the treatment of equinus contractures in children.' *Paper read at the annual Meeting of American Academy for Cerebral Palsy and Developmental Medicine, Seattle.*

Lee, C. L., Bleck, E. E. (1980) 'Surgical correction of equinus deformity in cerebral palsy.' *Developmental Medicine and Child Neurology*, **22**, 287-292.

Lester, E. L., Johnson, W. L. (1985) 'Posterior tibial tendon transposition/rerouting (Baker's slide procedure).' *Paper read at the Annual Meeting of Shrine Surgeons,* 1985.

Lipp, E. B., Jones, D. A. (1984) 'Flexor carpi ulnaris transfer in cerebral palsy.' *Orthopaedic Transactions,* **8,** 101.

Mann, R. A. (1986) 'Surgery of hallux valgus and bunions.' *Orthopaedic Grand Rounds,* Stanford University School of Medicine.

—— Soecht, L. H. (1982) 'Posterior tibial tendon ruptures—analysis of eight cases.' *Foot and Ankle, (abstract)* **2,** 350.

Manske, P. R. (1984) 'Extensor pollicis longus re-routing for treatment of spastic thumb-in-palm deformity.' *Orthopaedic Transactions,* **8,** 95.

Matev, I. (1963) 'Surgical treatment of spastic "thumb-in-palm" deformity.' *Journal of Bone and Joint Surgery,* **45B,** 703-708.

Mayer, L. (1937) 'The physiological method of tendon transplantation in the treatment of paralytic drop-foot.' *Journal of Bone and Joint Surgery,* **19,** 389-394.

McBride, E. D. (1928) 'A conservative operation for bunions.' *Journal of Bone and Joint Surgery,* **10,** 735-739.

McKay, D. W. (1983) 'Dorsal bunions in children.' *Journal of Bone and Joint Surgery,* **65A,** 975-980.

McKeever, D. C. (1952) 'Arthrodesis of the first metatarsophalangeal joint for hallux valgus, hallux rigidus, and metatarsus primus varus.' *Journal of Bone and Joint Surgery,* **34A,** 129-134.

Menalaus, M. B. (1984) 'The management of curly and hammer toes by flexor tenotomy.' *Orthopaedic Transactions,* **8,** 447.

Meyer, R. D., Gould, J. S., Nicholson, B. (1981) 'Revision of the first web space: technics and results.' *Southern Medical Journal,* **74,** 1204-1208.

Miller, G. M., Hsu, J. D., Hoffer, M. M., Rentfro, R. (1982). 'Posterior tibial tendon transfer: a review of the literature and analysis of 74 procedures.' *Journal of Pediatric Orthopedics,* **2,** 363-370.

Mital, M. A. (1979) 'Lengthening of the elbow flexors in cerebral palsy.' *Journal of Bone and Joint Surgery,* **61A,** 515-522.

Mitchell, C. L., Fleming, J. L., Allen, R., Glenney, C., Sanford, G. A. (1958) 'Osteotomy-bunionectomy for hallux valgus.' *Journal of Bone and Joint Surgery,* **40A,** 41-60

Moberg, E. (1962) 'Criticism and study of methods for examining sensibility in the hand.' *Neurology,* **12,** 8-19.

—— (1976) 'Reconstructive hand surgery in tetraplegia, stroke, and cerebral palsy: some basic concepts in physiology and neurology.' *Journal of Hand Surgery,* **1,** 29-34.

—— (1984) *Splinting in Hand Therapy.* New York: Thieme-Stratton; Stuttgart-New York: Georg Thieme. pp. 17-21.

—— (1985) 'The surgery of the spastic, stroke and tetraplegic hand.' *(Unpublished paper.)*

Mowery, C. A., Gelberman, R. H., Rhoades, C. E. (1985) 'Upper extremity tendon transfers in cerebral palsy: electromyographic and functional analysis.' *Journal of Pediatric Orthopedics,* **5,** 69-72.

Nather, A., Balsubramaniam, P., Bose, K. (1984) 'Tendon lengthening—an experimental study in rabbits.' *Orthopaedic Transactions,* **8,** 109.

Patella, V., Martucci, G. (1980) 'Transposition of the pronator radio teres muscle to the radial extensors of the wrist, in infantile cerebral paralysis. An improved operative technique.' *Italian Journal of Orthopaedics and Traumatology,* **6,** 61-66.

Perlstein, M. A., Hood, P. M. (1956) 'Infantile spastic hemiplegia, intelligence, oral language and motor development.' *Courrier,* **6,** 567.

Perry, J. (1985) *Personal communication.*

—— Hoffer, M. M., Giovan, P., Antonelli, D., Greenberg, R. (1974) 'Gait analysis of the triceps surae in cerebral palsy. A preoperative clinical and electromyographic study.' *Journal of Bone and Joint Surgery,* **56A,** 511-520.

—— —— (1977) 'Preoperative and postoperative dynamic electromyography as an aid in planning tendon transfers in children with cerebral palsy.' *Journal of Bone and Joint Surgery,* **59A,** 531-537.

Pletcher, D. F.-J., Hoffer, M. M., Koffman, D. M. (1976) 'Non-traumatic dislocation of the radial head in cerebral palsy.' *Journal of Bone and Joint Surgery,* **58A,** 104-105.

Rang, M., Silver, R., de la Garza, J. (1986) 'Cerebral palsy.' *In:* Lovell, W. W., Winter, R. B. (Eds.) *Pediatric Orthopaedics Vol. 1.* 2nd edn. Philadelphia: J. B. Lippincott. p. 345.

Renshaw, T., Sirkin, R., Drennan, J. (1979) 'The management of hallux valgus in cerebral palsy.' *Developmental Medicine and Child Neurology,* **21,** 202-208.

Roberts, W. M. (1953) *Personal communication.*

Root, L., Kirz, P. (1982) 'The result of posterior tibial tendon surgery in 83 patients with cerebral palsy.' *Developmental Medicine and Child Neurology,* **24,** 241-242. (Abstract.)

Rosenthal, R. K., Deutsch, S. D., Miller, W., Schumann, W., Hall, J. E. (1975) 'A fixed ankle below-the-knee orthosis for the management of genu recurvatum in spastic cerebral palsy.' *Journal of Bone and Joint Surgery*, **57A**, 545-547.

Ruda, R., Frost, H. M. (1971) 'Cerebral palsy spastic varus and forefoot adductus, treated by intramuscular posterior tibial tendon lengthening.' *Clinical Orthopaedics and Related Research*, **79**, 61-70.

Sakellarides, H. T., Mital, M. A., Lenzi, M. D. (1981) 'Treatment of pronation contractures of the forearm in cerebral palsy by changing the insertion of the pronator radii teres.' *Journal of Bone and Joint Surgery*, **63A**, 645-652.

Samilson, R. L. (1966) *Personal Communication.*

—— (1976) 'Crescentric osteotomy of the os calcis for calcanealcavus feet.' *In:* Bateman, J. E. (Ed.) *Foot Science*, Philadelphia: W. B. Saunders. pp. 18-25.

——Morris, J. M. (1964) 'Surgical improvement of the cerebral palsied upper limb; electromyographic studies and results of 128 operations.' *Journal of Bone and Joint Surgery*, **46A**, 1203-1216.

Schneider, M., Balon, K. (1977) 'Deformity of the foot following anterior transfer of the posterior tibial tendon and lengthening of the Achilles tendon for spastic equinovarus.' *Clinical Orthopaedics and Related Research*, **125**, 112-117.

Schwartz, J. R., Carr, W., Bassett, F. H., Coonrad, R. W. (1977) 'Lessons learned in the treatment of equinus deformity in ambulatory spastic children.' *Orthopaedic Transactions*, **1**, 84.

Sequist, J. L. (1977) 'Surgical correction of hallux valgus in cerebral palsy'. *Paper submitted to program committee of the American Academy for Cerebral Palsy and Developmental Medicine (unpublished).*

Sharrard, W. J. W., Bernstein, S. (1972) 'Equinus deformity in cerebral palsy.' *Journal of Bone and Joint Surgery*, **54B**, 272-276.

Silfverskiold, N. (1923-24) 'Reduction of the uncrossed two-joint muscles of the leg to one-joint muscles in spastic conditions.' *Acta Chirurgica Scandinavica*, **56**, 315-330.

Silver, C. M. (1977) Instructional course on management of spastic hemiplegia, Las Vegas: American Academy of Orthopaedic Surgeons.

—— Simon, S. D. (1959) 'Gastrocnemius-muscle recession (Silfverskiold operation) for spastic equinus deformity in cerebral palsy.' *Journal of Bone and Joint Surgery*, **41A**, 1021-1028.

—— —— Spindell, E., Lichtman, H. M., Scala, M. (1967) 'Calcaneal osteotomy for valgus and varus deformities of the foot in cerebral palsy.' *Journal of Bone and Joint Surgery*, **49A**, 232-246.

—— —— Lichtman, H. M., Motamed, M. (1976) 'Surgical correction of spastic thumb-in-palm deformity.' *Developmental Medicine and Child Neurology*, **18**, 632-639.

Sirna, E., Sussman, M. D. (1985) 'Immediate mobilization of patients following tendo Achilles lengthening in short leg casts.' *Paper read at Annual Meeting of American Academy for Cerebral Palsy and Developmental Medicine, Seattle, Washington.*

Smith, R. J. (1982) 'Flexor pollicis longus abductor-plasty for spastic thumb-in-palm deformity.' *Journal of Hand Surgery*, **7**, 327-334.

Strayer, L. M. (1950) 'Recession of the gastrocnemius.' *Journal of Bone and Joint Surgery*, **32A**, 671-676.

—— (1958) 'Gastrocnemius recession. Five year report of cases.' *Journal of Bone and Joint Surgery*, **40A**, 1019-1030.

Sutherland, D. H., Cooper, L., Daniel, D. (1980) 'The role of the ankle plantar flexors in normal walking.' *Journal of Bone and Joint Surgery*, **62A**, 354-363.

Swanson, A. B. (1982) 'Surgery of the hand in cerebral palsy.' *In:* Flynn, J. E. (Ed.) *Hand Surgery, 3rd edn.* Baltimore: Williams & Wilkins. pp. 476-488.

—— Browne, H. S., Coleman, J. D. (1960) 'Surgery of the hand in cerebral palsy and the swan-neck deformity.' *Journal of Bone and Joint Surgery*, **42A**, 951-964.

—— —— —— (1966) 'The cavus foot-concepts of production and treatment by metatarsal osteotomy.' *Journal of Bone and Joint Surgery*, **48A**, 1019. *(Abstract.)*

Tachdjian, M. O. (1972) *Pediatric Orthopaedics.* Philadelphia: W. B. Saunders.

Tardieu, C., Tabary, J. S., Huet de la Tour, E., Tabary, C., Tardieu, G. (1977) 'The relationship between sarcomere length in the soleus and tibialis anterior and the articular angle of the tibia-calcaneum in cats during growth.' *Journal of Anatomy*, **124**, 581-588.

Throop, F. B., DeRosa, G. P., Reeck, C., Waterman, S. (1975) 'Correction of equinus in cerebral palsy by the Murphy procedure of tendo calcaneus advancement. A prelimary communication.' *Developmental Medicine and Child Neurology*, **17**, 182-185.

Truscelli, D., Lespargot, A., Tardieu, G. (1979) 'Variation in the long-term results of elongation of the tendo achilles in children with cerebral palsy.' *Journal of Bone and Joint Surgery*, **61B**, 466-469.

280

Turner, J. W., Cooper, R. R. (1972) 'Anterior transfer of the tibialis posterior through the interosseus membrane.' *Clinical Orthopaedics and Related Research,* **83,** 241-244.

Vulpius, O., Stoffel, A. (1913) *Orthopädische Operationslehre, 1st edn.* Stuttgart: Ferdinand Enke. (2nd edn. 1920), Stuttgart: Ferdinand Enke.

Watkins, M. B., Jones, J. B., Ryder, G. T., Brown, T. H. (1954). 'Transplantation of the posterior tibial tendon.' *Journal of Bone and Joint Surgery,* **36A,** 1181-1189.

White, J. W. (1943) 'Torsion of the Achilles tendon.' *Archives of Surgery,* **46,** 784-787.

White, W. F. (1972) 'Flexor muscle slide in the spastic hand. The Max Page operation.' *Journal of Bone and Joint Surgery,* **54B,** 453-459.

Wilcox, P. G., Weiner, D. S. (1985) 'The Akron midtarsal dome osteotomy in the treatment of rigid pes cavus: a preliminary review.' *Journal of Pediatric Orthopedics,* **5,** 333-338.

Williams, P. F. (1976) 'Restoration of muscle balance of the foot by transfer of the tibialis posterior.' *Journal of Bone and Joint Surgery,* **58B,** 217-219.

Wu, K. K. (1986) *Surgery of the Foot.* Philadelphia; Lea & Febiger.

Zancolli, E. A. (1979) *Structural and Dynamic Bases of Hand Surgery, 2nd edn.* Philadelphia; J. B. Lippincott.

—— Goldner, J. L., Swanson, A. B. (1983) 'Surgery of the spastic hand in cerebral palsy; report of the committee on spastic hand evaluation.' *Journal of Hand Surgery,* **8,** 766-772.

—— Zancolli, E. R. (1981) 'Surgical management of the hemiplegic spastic hand in cerebral palsy.' *Surgical Clinics of North America,* **61,** 395-406.

Ziv, I., Blackburn, N., Rang, M., Koreska, J. (1984) 'Muscle growth in normal and spastic mice.' *Developmental Medicine and Child Neurology,* **26,** 94-99.

8
SPASTIC DIPLEGIA

General characteristics

Spastic diplegia associated with prematurity now appears to be the most common type of cerebral palsy in the United States. In 1965, in an unpublished survey of the types of cerebral palsy in our patient population, we found that 47.5 per cent of all patients with cerebral palsy had spastic diplegia associated with premature birth. In a 1981 study of 423 patients with cerebral palsy, 66 per cent had spastic diplegia. Table 8.I lists the etiologies of spastic diplegia in our study of 119 children with spastic diplegia (Miranda 1979). Diplegia is defined as grossly spastic muscles in the lower limbs, with minor motor deficits in the upper limbs. In contrast, paraplegia involves just the lower limbs, with no deficits in the upper limb. If encountered, high spinal-cord lesions should be considered especially if the patient has urinary bladder problems. Hereditary spastic paraplegia must also be included in the differential diagnosis.

The general characteristics in the child with spastic diplegia are as follows:

1. Upper-limb gross motor function is good, with only minor inco-ordination of the fingers on fine motor-skill testing (*e.g.* approximating each fingertip to the thumb in sequence).

2. The lower-limb muscles are definitely spastic; the typical pattern is shown in Figure 8.1:
(a) Hip-flexion spasm and contracture
(b) Hip internal rotation with excessive femoral anteversion
(c) Hip-adduction spasm and contracture

TABLE 8.I
Etiology of 119 spastic diplegic children (Miranda 1979)

Associated with:		No.	Per cent
1. Prematurity		78	65.54
2. Unknown		22	18.48
3. Prematurity and hydrocephalus		2	1.68
4. Prematurity and Rh incompatability		3	2.52
5. Low birthweight (small for dates)		3	2.52
6. Hypoxia		2	1.68
7. Rubella		3	2.52
8. Head trauma		1	0.84
9. Encephalitis		1	0.84
10. Hydrocephalus and spina bifida		1	0.84
11. LSD during pregnancy		1	0.84
12. Neonatal respiratory distress syndrome		1	0.84
13. Cerebral embolism with heart surgery		1	0.84
	Total	119	99.98

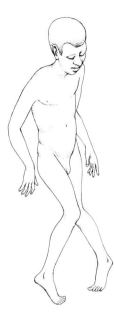

Fig. 8.1. Typical posture lower limbs: spastic diplegia.

(d) Knee flexor or extensor spasticity predominate or are equal in the degree of spasticity

(e) Equinus of the ankle

(f) Pes valgus with a plantar flexed talus and hind-foot equinus.

3. Speech and intellect are usually normal or only slightly impaired.

4. Esotropia and perceptual and visual-motor deficits are common.

5. The neurological examination shows hyperactive lower-limb reflexes, positive Babinski signs, no infantile automatisms, and deficient posterior equilibrium reactions.

6. Most children can walk independently. Those who have deficient anterior equilibrium reactions need crutches, and a few who are deficient in these reactions in all planes require walkers. The functional ambulatory status of 119 patients with spastic diplegia is delineated in Table 8.II. The mean age at follow-up was 14 years; 53 per cent were older than 14, with a mean age of 23 years and a range up to 39 years.

TABLE 8.II

Functional ambulatory status of 119 spastic diplegia children > six years

Status	N	%
Independent — community walker	94	78.9
With crutches — community walker	15	12.6
With walker — household walking	8	6.7
Not walking	2	1.7
Total	119	99.9

Natural history

Most of these children walk by 48 months. The deficient posterior equilibrium reactions seem to persist throughout life, but independent walking continues. I have observed that some children can discard crutches and get about the household when puberty begins. Why this occurs is a matter of speculation, but it may be related to the increased sex-hormone levels and their influence on the neuro-muscular system at this time.

Almost all can be 'integrated' into regular school by the age of seven or eight years. These days, Californian children with spastic diplegia rarely begin in a special school. The usual track is from preschool programs into regular school.

Almost all should be able to lead independent and useful lives provided they have not been conditioned or segregated into the 'handicapped' population through well-intentioned 'treatment' of their neurological defect. We can give parents of this group an optimistic prognosis on long-term function, but we must avoid talking about the disease which cannot be cured. Among the adult patients in our study, many diverse occupations were represented: computer programmer, mother and housewife, soap salesman, pizza cook, banker, secretary, teacher of physically handicapped children, insurance agent, recreation playground director, librarian and amusement-park worker. Of 44 who were 18 years or older (37 per cent of the group) only one was unemployed or not in school; only one was in a sheltered workshop.

The one predominant disability in adolescents and adults that blocks development of adult independence has been anxiety neurosis (in the 18+ age-group, two required intensive psychiatric care when breakdown occurred). It may be that parental and professional overtreatment, and excessive striving to remedy deficits rather than compensate for them, is the cause of the mental distress. Examples of such remedial efforts include: (i) 'practising to walk better'; (ii) attempting to learn philosophy when the grasp of abstractions is not possible, and (iii) trying to improve handwriting when typewriting or word-processing on a computer is more efficient.

Non-surgical management

The services that physical and occupational therapists and orthotists can give have been discussed in Chapter 6. In this group, as in spastic hemiplegia, physical and occupational therapy services need not be prolonged and should be functionally oriented. These children need preparation for fun and games in regular school so that they can be properly integrated with their peer groups. Physical therapy is certainly useful to restore gait function after orthopaedic surgery, by means of therapeutic exercise and joint mobilization, but usually should not last more than six months.

Time of orthopaedic surgery

Surgery for improvement of gait cannot be performed until the child has actually developed a gait pattern that can be observed and, if facilities are available, measured in a laboratory. Although the mature gait pattern develops at about the

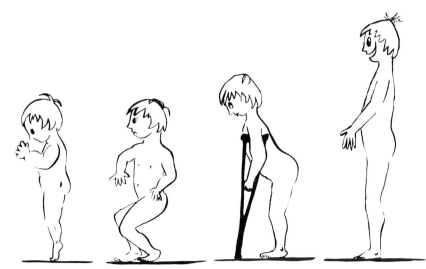

Fig. 8.2. Usual staging of orthopaedic surgery in spastic diplegia to be avoided. *From left to right:* talipes equinus; crouch after Achilles tendon lengthening; crouch corrected by hamstring lengthening; final erect posture after hip-flexion contracture corrected. (Drawing reproduced courtesy of the artist, Mercer Rang MD, Toronto.)

age of seven years (Sutherland *et al.* 1980), it is reasonably close to the mature pattern before this age. The consensus is that most of the surgical treatment can be accomplished between the ages of four and eight years (Rang *et al.* 1986). In spastic diplegia I strive to finish the more formal and intensive treatment program by this age.

Surgery should only be done earlier if there are structural changes such as subluxation of the hip, contracture of the knee joint due to spastic hamstrings and, in rare cases, a contracture of the gastrocnemius-soleus muscles.

Surgery should not be regarded as the last resort or as 'something that can be done when all other methods have failed'. The increased incidence of postoperative psychological problems in adolescents (Williams 1977), and the sudden disruption of the body-image which appears to reach its peak during adolescence, are probably related to the more frequent emotional upheavals and slow recovery from surgery in this age-group. Nor should surgery be unduly staged so that the phenomenon of marking birthdays with surgery and hospitalization becomes the predominant feature of life for the child with cerebral palsy (Figs. 6.23, 8.2).

In spastic diplegia surgery is confined to the lower limb. In order to describe the complex functional and structural deformities and their surgical management, it is necessary to discuss each as a separate entity even though they almost always coexist. The surgeon must carefully examine and re-examine the patient's gait, joints and muscles so that the appropriate surgical procedures can be combined and excessive staging avoided (Fig. 8.2). Examination techniques have been described in Chapter 2 and measurement methods (gait analysis) in Chapter 3.

Hip-adduction deformity

Anatomy, physiology and biomechanics

The adductor muscles of the hip originate from the pubis anteriorly and insert on the femur medially. Strange (1965) has proposed that anatomically the hip adductors function as external rotators. They are innervated by the obturator nerve, except for one half of the adductor magnus which is supplied by the tibial division of the sciatic nerve. The anterior branch of the obturator nerve supplies the adductor longus and gracilis and usually the adductor brevis; the posterior branch distributes branches to the adductor magnus and brevis when the brevis does not receive a branch from the anterior division (Gray 1942, Gardner *et al.* 1969).

Electromyograms of the adductors during level gait in normal persons have demonstrated that they contract at the end of stance phase (Fig. 8.9). Murray and Sepic (1968) showed that the maximum output of the gluteus medius and minimus muscles (hip adductors) occurs when the hip is in 5° of adduction. Matsuo *et al.* (1984, 1986), in a clinical study of the results of adductor myotomy with and without obturator neurectomy, concluded that the adductor brevis is an important antigravity muscle in quadripedal and bipedal locomotion, and essential for a stable erect posture.

The function of the hip abductors during gait has been well established (Inman 1947, Saunders *et al.* 1953); these muscles are essential for energy conservation because they prevent excessive lateral shift of the trunk during the single-limb phase of stance when their action pulls the pelvis down on the weight-bearing limb. Approximately 2cm of lateral trunk shift occurs quickly from limb to limb during level walking. Without good functioning of abductor muscles, a lurching gait occurs which expends high levels of energy.

The base of the gait in normal subjects measures 5 to 10cm from heel to heel, though in some individuals it may be as narrow as 1cm (mean in children 7.6cm, according to Scrutton 1969). These measurements are correlated with the need to keep the femora in slight adduction for efficient gait. Consequently, in children with spastic diplegia and adductor spasticity, the goal of treatment should be to keep the base of the gait within normal limits.

Are the hip adductors the main cause of the hip internal rotation gait pattern so common in children with spastic diplegia? Most surgeons reject the theory that the hip adductor muscles are the culprit responsible for the in-toed gait pattern in these patients. The former controversy probably arose because of differences in the perception of what constitutes hip internal rotation during gait—one surgeon's hip adduction may be another's internal rotation (Fig. 8.3). Furthermore, adduction spasticity usually can be found simultaneously with hip-flexion spasticity and internal rotation during gait. I have observed the gait of spastic hemiplegic children who internally rotated only the involved limb while walking. In these children no hip adduction spasticity or contracture or the adductors could be found. As will be discussed in the section on hip internal rotation, the major deforming force appears to be excessive femoral anteversion and, at times, a spastic gluteus medius which is the major internal rotator of the hip described by Duchenne a century ago (Duchenne 1867, 1959).

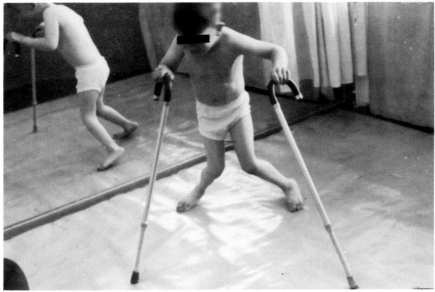

Fig. 8.3. Spastic diplegia, age six years. Does he have hip internal rotation or adduction? Ranges of motion each hip: abduction 30°, extension –35°, internal rotation 90°, external rotation 10°.

Banks and Green (1960), in their report of 89 patients who had adductor myotomy and anterior branch obturator neurectomy, found that 15 had persistent hip internal rotation gait patterns postoperatively. I have observed the same results even after intrapelvic obturator neurectomy.

While it is true that direct stimulation of the obturator nerve in surgery appears to cause hip internal rotation, a more careful observation shows that these patients have the knees flexed, so that as the heel rests on the table it acts merely as a pivot point which allows gravity to rotate the limb internally when adduction occurs. This phenomenon can be observed in normal unanesthetized children who have femoral torsion and whose knees are splinted in flexion. When asked to bring the knees together voluntarily, they internally rotate the limb.

Clinical examination
When the child walks, adduction spasticity is obvious and characterized by close approximation of the knees and thighs and a short stride-length. More severe adduction spasticity causes 'scissoring', with one limb crossing over the other.

The measurement of hip-adduction contracture is made with the child supine and the pelvis level. More accurate is the range of abduction of each hip, made with the hips in extension. When abducting one limb, the other needs to be held securely to prevent the pelvis from moving. The degree of abduction is determined with one limb of the goniometer placed along the line between the anterior superior iliac spines, and the other along the femur. With the hips flexed 90° the pelvis must be kept level by holding the other limb secure, otherwise the pelvis will rotate to the

287

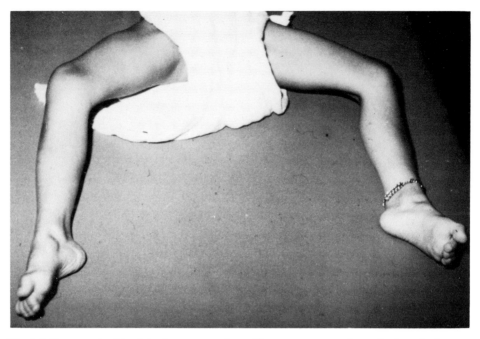

Fig. 8.4. Postoperative hip abduction posture after adductor myotomy and anterior branch obturator neurectomy, bilateral. Five-year-old patient with tension athetosis and dystonia.

side of the abducted limb to cause a false measurement of hip abduction. Athetosis and dystonic posturing must be differentiated from spasticity. With slow passive movements combined with relaxation of the patient, the lack of contracture of the muscle will be evident. In athetosis, particularly dystonic posturing, surgery to relieve the apparent adduction deformity may result in an abduction deformity (Fig. 8.4).

As might be expected, the electromyographic examination will show almost continuous activity of the adductor muscles during both phases of the gait (Fig. 8.5).

Indications for surgery
In the ambulatory patient, surgery to relieve adduction spasticity is indicated when each hip is limited in abduction to 20° or less with the hip extended, or when there is scissoring (Sharrard 1975). Hoffer (1986) states that the limit of passive abduction of the hip should be 30° or less. Given the errors in accurate measurement, I will compromise and state that the limits are between 20° and 30°.

When in doubt about the need for surgery and what its effects might be, myoneural blocks of the adductor longus with 45 per cent alcohol may help (see Chapter 3). In children this can be done under brief general anesthesia by injecting the belly of the adductor longus in three or four locations with 10cc of the 45 per cent alcohol; an injection deep to the belly of the adductor longus in its proximal

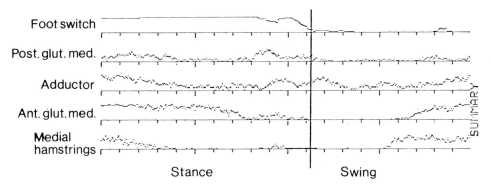

Fig. 8.5. Gait EMG of eight-year-old spastic diplegic: shows continuous firing of adductor muscles (surface electrodes); gluteus medius appropriate stance-phase activity (fine wire electrodes). Medial hamstring activity normal.

portion may block the anterior branch of the obturator nerve. The resulting paralysis of the adductor muscles will last between two and six weeks, which gives the physician, therapist, parents and patient sufficient time to observe the gait and make a decision for or against surgery. Lidocaine (1 per cent) can also be used in older children and adults. However, the drug seems to cause light-headedness often enough for a detailed and valid observation of the gait to be compromised.

Types of adductor 'release'
'Release' has become a general term to describe surgery in cerebral palsy. But the term is meaningless when the results of surgery demand specificity.

1. Adductor longus and gracilis myotomy with anterior branch obturator neurectomy used to be the recommended approach (Keats 1957, Banks and Green 1960, Silver *et al.* 1966, Samilson *et al.* 1967). However, in spastic diplegia a more critical appraisal of results has led to abandonment of the obturator neurectomy, which causes paralysis not only of the adductor longus but also of the adductor brevis (in the majority of cases where the anterior branch of the nerve supplies the adductor brevis). The results were judged quite adequate, but the effects of widening the base of the gait beyond normal and the need for adduction of the femur for the maximum pelvic stabilization of the hip during the stance phase of gait were not appreciated. I have abandonded this procedure for most patients, except those who definitely scissor in addition to having a contracture. Those who scissor rarely are independent ambulators who need no external support.

We have not performed posterior branch obturator neurectomy for the past 30 years. The posterior and anterior branch obturator neurectomies produce too much weakening of the adductors. The broad-based hip-abducted gait pattern might appear to be 'stable' (like an A-frame), but it is definitely not functional. If a patient continues to scissor after anterior branch obturator neurectomy, an intrapelvic obturator neurectomy is easier to perform and obviates operating through scarred tissue resulting from previous surgery.

289

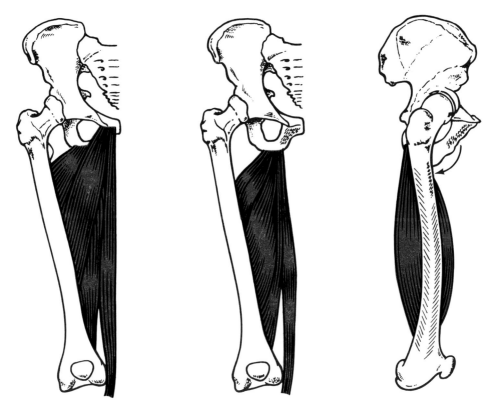

Fig. 8.6. Adductor origin transfer.

2. Adductor origin transfer to the ilium (Fig. 8.6). The credit for suggesting this operation in cerebral palsy has been given to Jacqueline Perry, who used it in patients who had poliomyelitis and required reinforcement of weakened hip extensor muscles (Garrett 1976). Westin (1965) also performed adductor transfers in patients who had paralysis of the hip extensors due to poliomyelitis.

After Stephenson and Donovan (1971) reported their results of transfer of the origins of the adductor longus, brevis and gracilis to the ischium in cerebral palsy, other surgeons also reported their results (Baumann 1972, Couch *et al.* 1977, Griffin *et al.* 1977, Baumann *et al.* 1978). Whereas Couch *et al.* (1977) transferred the origins of the adductor longus and brevis and the gracilis plus release of the origins of the adductor magnus, Evans (1977) transferred *only* the adductor longus and gracilis. Hoffer (1977) transferred the adductor longus, brevis and gracilis to the fascia overlying the adductor magnus, but limited the transfer to the longus and gracilis in less severe cases.

In the end-result studies of this operation, one criterion of success appeared to be improvement of the hip internal rotation gait. Krom (1969) found that in 50 per cent of his patients, the hip-rotation posture was converted to neutral or external rotation postoperatively (14 of his 20 patients also had iliopsoas tenotomy). Of the

35 patients analyzed by Couch *et al.* (1977), failure to correct internal rotation occurred in only five.

Another criterion for success was the measurement of the base of the gait. In the study by Couch *et al.* (1977), the mean preoperative measurement was 13.5cm and the postoperative mean was 24cm (range: 12 to 37cm). If the normal range is 5 to 10cm, is the broad-based gait a satisfactory goal for optimum function?

Other more recent studies on the results of adductor transfer have focused on the improvement of hip radiographs which assessed the degree of subluxation and/or acetabular dysplasia, utilizing the center edge (CE) angle method or the migration index of the femoral head (Reimers and Poulsen 1984, Schultz *et al.* 1984). Radiographs were also used to assess the results of adductor tenotomy and anterior branch obturator neurectomy by Wheeler and Weinstein (1984). None of these studies segregated potentially ambulatory patients from those who were ambulatory with or without support or were non-ambulatory. The importance of these functional differences in analyzing the results of surgery in prevention of subluxation and dislocation of the hip will be discussed in Chapter 9. The independently walking child with spastic diplegia rarely dislocates, if ever, and only those who have partial weightbearing with crutches or walkers subluxate.

Root and Spero (1981) did the only study which attempted to compare the results of adductor origin transfer with adductor tenotomies (with or without obturator neurectomy). In their study, 50 patients had adductor origin transfer to the ischium and 52 had 102 adductor myotomies with or without the obturator neurectomy. Their assessment was based upon changes in function, range of passive motion of the hip and radiographic stability. The need to transfer the origins of the adductor longus, brevis and gracilis to the ischium was challenged by Goldner (1981), who reported equally satisfactory results by merely recessing the detached muscles distally and anchoring them with a suture to the epimyesium overlying the adductor brevis.

Matsuo *et al.* (1984, 1986) made the point that the adductor brevis is the main hip stabilizer, and the loss of its strength results in overabduction of the hip. In an analysis of their 42 cases, they recommended cutting only the adductor longus to improve gait efficiency and preserve the function of the adductor muscles which keep the femur slightly adducted during the stance phase of gait. Based upon the physiology of the gluteus medius muscle and the need to maintain its tension for maximum strength during gait, this recommendation makes sense. Thus it does not seem logical to cut the anterior branch of the obturator nerve in patients who are ambulatory; to do so risks paralysis of the adductor brevis in the majority of patients.

3. Adductor longus tenotomy, allowing its proximal end to slide distally with a suture to anchor it to the underlying brevis, is my choice for most patients with spastic diplegia. According to long-standing recommendations and traditions of most orthopaedic surgeons, we also do a myotomy of the proximal portion of the gracilis in patients who are walking independently. For those who have scissoring, anterior branch obturator neurectomy seems indicated: and if under anesthesia the hip cannot be abducted 30° to 40° after the adductor longus tenotomy and gracilis

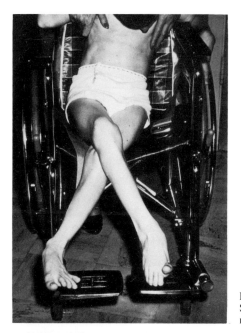

Fig. 8.7. Total body involved (spastic diplegia). Severe adductor spasticity; intrapelvic obturator neurectomy usually indicated.

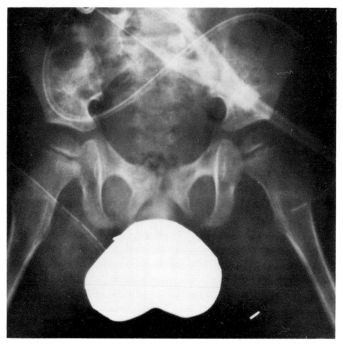

Fig. 8.8. Anterior-posterior radiographs of pelvis and hips made 18 hours postoperative bilateral adductor longus and gracilis transfer to ischium. Michele metallic clips placed at site of transfer; the clip on the left has retracted far distally from the ischium, while the right has remained in place. Results: identical on both sides.

myotomy, then an adductor brevis myotomy will be necessary to relieve the contracture. I have found this to be necessary only rarely in spastic diplegia.

4. Intrapelvic obturator neurectomy is indicated in those patients in whom an anterior branch obturator neurectomy has failed to relieve a sufficient amount of adductor spasticity, and its only indication will be in the total body involved non-ambulatory patient (Fig. 8.7). It must be combined with adductor tenotomy and myotomy to correct the adduction contracture of the hips (Samilson *et al.* 1967). I have never done the operation in spastic diplegia.

So, what to choose for adduction deformity of the hip in the child with spastic diplegia? For functional improvement of gait in these children, adductor longus tenotomy and gracilis myotomy seems quite sufficient for the majority. The temptation to do the quick and easy subcutaneous adductor longus tenotomy should be resisted. Not only can one inadvertently cut the saphenous vein or one of its branches, one can also incur a recurrence of the adduction contracture in 75 per cent (Feyen *et al.* 1984).

Adductor transfer appears to have no advantages, and in the few in which I have tagged the transferred origin with a metal clip, it was interesting (and dismaying) to see that the clip had moved distally from the ischial tuberosity in a radiograph made 24 hours postoperatively (Fig. 8.8). In effect the spasticity had performed Goldner's adductor origin recession postoperatively.

Anterior branch obturator neurectomy in the ambulatory child does not appear to offer any advantages, judging from a study of 163 such procedures by Kling (1984). Kling also noted that neither the adductor tenotomy nor its combination with obturator neurectomy improved the hip internal rotation gait of the children.

Operative technique for adductor tenotomy and gracilis myotomy (and anterior branch obturator neurectomy when indicated)
The linear incision begins about 2cm distal to the origin of the adductor longus and continues along the longus for 5cm. The deep fascia is incised, and with blunt dissection the posterior portion of the muscle is clearly defined and separated from the adductor brevis. The longus is lifted away from the brevis with a curved hemostat. This maneuver is crucial to avoid cutting the anterior branches of the obturator nerve when the adductor longus is sectioned at its musculotendinous junction with electrocoagulation. The gracilis muscle is also cut. The hip is abducted to about 40°, and the proximal cut ends of the distally retracted adductor longus and gracilis are sutured to the underlying adductor brevis. I do not cut the adductor brevis unless there is a severe contracture and passive hip abduction is less than 30° after the adductor longus and gracilis are cut. Adductor brevis myotomy seems rarely necessary in spastic diplegia.

To avoid the postoperative wound hematoma, all bleeding points are electrocoagulated and large veins ligated. Closed suction irrigation is routinely used. Wound closure is with absorbable subcutaneous and subcuticular sutures, reinforced with sterile adhesive tapes. In young children, who may urinate uncontrollably after surgery, sealing of the wounds with a collodian dressing prevents infection, maceration and delayed wound healing.

If anterior branch obturator neurectomy is thought necessary, the nerve and its branches can be seen within the veil of connective tissue on the surface of the adductor brevis. The branches are stimulated by pinching with the hemostat or by an electric stimulus to make sure these are indeed the nerves. Then with a hemostat the nerves are isolated, picked up and cut distal to the hemostat and dissected proximally for about 2cm to the point where the main anterior branch is cut.

Postoperative care

In children, postoperative immobilization with long leg plasters connected with a stick to keep each hip in 30° to 40° of abduction for three weeks is sufficient. Forced overabduction can lead to compression of the articular surfaces of the hip joints and may result in postoperative stiffness. After the plasters have been removed, the patients can be mobilized in parallel bars with graduation to crutches or a walker, and if they have adequate equilibrium reactions can resume independent walking.

Some people advocate the use of abduction splints at night to maintain the correction. Houkom *et al.* (1986) studied the incidence of hip subluxation with and without nap- and night-bracing after surgery for an average of 10.5 months. They concluded that bracing lowered the incidence of recurrent subluxation of the hip. However, 10 of 21 braced patients developed abduction contractures; two of 36 unbraced children had abduction contractures. Their recommendation was to use a Lorenz-type brace with a thoracic extension for nap- and night-time use for at least one year. This brace holds the thighs in 90° flexion and 60° abduction. Perhaps this degree of desired abduction obtained at surgery and the postoperative regimen might apply to non-ambulatory total body involved children with hip subluxation. In their series of 57 patients, only nine were classified as 'assisted ambulators'. Consequently, in spastic diplegic children, postoperative night-splinting (especially with the hips flexed 90°) might not be applicable or necessary. I do not recommend it. Early mobilization, active hip-abduction exercise (preferably in a swimming pool) and early ambulation seem more physiological in spastic diplegia.

Furthermore, we are not absolutely certain that the braces are really used as specified. Compliance in the Houkom *et al.* study (1986) was assessed by interview with the parents. Only a long-term in-patient study could really prove the point; but given the costs of hospitalization and the large numbers of children in various functional categories that would be needed to do an adequate study, it will probably never be done.

Early mobilization and ambulation without any postoperative immobilization has been used and found very satisfactory by Sussman (1984). He used Buck's skin traction on the lower limbs for a few days after surgery (to overcome the flexor spasms as the result of the first few days of postoperative pain), and then began an intensive physical therapy program which used passive positioning devices between therapy sessions.

In young adults who needed only a relief of their adductor spasticity and contracture by adductor tenotomy and anterior branch obturator neurectomy, I have not used plaster immobilization postoperatively. I found that the foam or sheepskin padded triangular wedge, used for postoperative total hip-joint replacement surgery, was easily tolerated and satisfactory for the first six weeks when combined with early resumption of ambulation and active and passive exercise.

Problems with adductor tenotomy with or without anterior branch obturator neurectomy

1. Failure to prevent continued subluxation and dislocation of the hip with adductor weakening alone. This problem will be discussed fully in Chapter 9.

2. Recurrence of the adduction contracture. Samilson *et al.* (1967) noted reattachment of the adductor tendons in only 23 of 178 adductor tenotomies. Recurrence is probably more related to increasing adductor strength as the result of increased function in walking and sports. In the 119 spastic diplegic children we studied (Miranda 1979), there was no need for additional adductor surgery in 25 who had adductor longus tenotomy, gracilis myotomy and anterior branch obturator neurectomy, nor in three who had adductor longus and gracilis transfer to the ischium with a mean follow-up of six years. However, these were all performed in conjunction with other surgery—either iliopsoas recession and/or hamstring lengthening.

Since 1980 I have not done obturator neurectomies, but only the adductor longus and gracilis myotomies as described in the operative technique. I have not seen the need to perform additional adductor weakening in this highly selected group of ambulatory spastic diplegic children.

3. Failure to correct the hip internal rotation gait. This 'failure' is actually due to excessive expectations of surgeon, parents, patient and therapist. It must be appreciated that internal rotation during gait is a complex activity, and depends upon the degree of femoral torsion and/or gluteus medius dysfunction.

4. A broad-based gait with marked trunk lurch may result from too much adductor weakening. In most cases the adductor brevis and the anterior branch of the obturator nerve can be left intact. Certainly there can be few indications for posterior branch obturator neurectomy in spastic diplegia. The worst lurching gaits have been seen in referred patients who had intrapelvic obturator neurectomy which resulted in a distance of 12 to 18 inches from heel to heel.

5. A permanent postoperative 'frog leg' or abduction deformity. This might be avoided by immobilization no longer than three to six weeks, and by not immobilizing the hips in exaggerated and forced abduction. Forced abduction can cause pressure necrosis of the articular cartilage of the hip joint (Salter and Field 1960). Samilson *et al.* (1967) had 13 patients whose hips were stiff in the 'frog-leg' position; 10 of these patients had been immobilized in double hip spica plasters for 2.4 months.

Abduction deformities have been seen in patients who had athetosis and/or dystonic posturing, and adductor 'releases' with obturator neurectomies. Although preoperatively they probably had dynamic excessive adduction of the hips, the contracture was minimal. Before adductor-weakening surgery is performed on this type of patient, it is prudent to use myoneural blocks of the adductor longus and/or the anterior branch of the obturator nerve.

6. Wound infection. Samilson *et al.* (1967) had an increased infection rate with a transverse incision (of the 14 patients who had wound infection in a series of 189 operations, 12 had a transverse incision in the groin). The longitudinal incision is preferred. Also, careful hemostasis by the use of electrocautery and closed suction drainage of the wound for 24 to 48 hours should help reduce the infection rate.

Adductor tenotomy, anterior branch obturator neurectomy and other adductor-muscle weakening procedures are probably the most overused operations in cerebral palsy. Now, with a better understanding of the physiology of normal gait and the mechanisms of the various hip deformities, more critical assessments are being done. The result seems to be fewer but more selective operations, and a decrease in unexpected and unwanted postoperative results.

Hip-flexion deformity
Anatomy, physiology and biomechanics
The sartorius, tensor fascia femoris, rectus femoris, adductors and the iliopsoas are all considered to be flexors of the hip (Duchenne 1867, 1959; Brunnstrom 1962). Although these muscles act synergistically and vary with joint position, a consideration of their probable isolated function helps to determine the specific muscle or muscles that might produce flexion deformities in spastic paralysis.

The sartorius and rectus femoris flex the hip up to 90°, but are weak flexors. The rectus femoris is more effective if the knee flexes simultaneously. Our studies have shown that spasticity of the rectus femoris is not an isolated one, and that the vastus medialis and lateralis (and probably the vastus intermedius) share in the spasticity of the entire quadriceps (Csongradi *et al.* 1979).

The pectineus adducts the hip and also flexes it, though not beyond 90°. The adductor longus, brevis and magnus act as hip flexors from the hyperextended position, but not beyond 50° to 70°. After these ranges the adductors become extensors. In the erect position, the lower portion of the adductor magnus is an extensor and this function increases as the joint is flexed. In the extended position, the adductor longus is a weak internal rotator. The gracilis acts as a flexor up to 20° to 40° of flexion, and then it becomes an extensor.

I have observed pure adductor spasticity in spastic diplegia in only 10 patients. In these patients the amount of hip-flexion deformity was no greater than 10°. Furthermore, in three patients wtih a preoperative hip-flexion deformity of greater than 15°, I noted no decrease in the hip-flexion contracture after adductor myotomy and anterior branch of obturator neurectomy. Severe hip-flexion deformities in two patients who had bilateral intrapelvic obturator neurectomies were unchanged postoperatively.

The iliopsoas is the main and powerful flexor of the hip. It is composed of the iliacus muscle, arising from the medial wall of the ilium, and the psoas portion, which originates from the transverse processes and sides of the bodies of all the lumbar vertebrae and the intervertebral disc annular ligaments from the 12th thoracic to the fifth lumbar interspaces. This psoas major muscle ends below the pelvic brim as a broad tendon which inserts into the lesser trochanter of the femur.

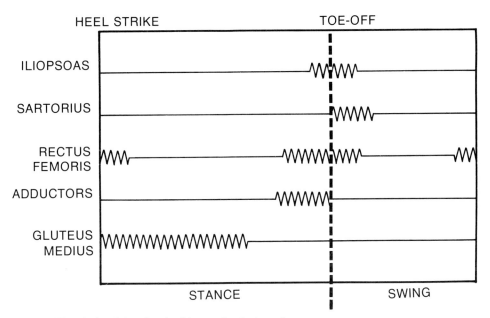

Fig. 8.9. Electrical activity of major hip muscles during gait.

The fibers of the iliacus muscle join this tendon at its lateral edge. The psoas tendon is the most medial structure crossing the hip-joint capsule, and is obscured from view laterally by overlapping bulky fibers of the iliacus.

The psoas minor muscle is slender, anterior to the psoas major, and arises from the sides of the bodies of the 12th thoracic and first lumbar vertebra and the intervening intervertebral disc. It inserts into the arcuate (or terminal) line of the iliac fossa and the iliopectineal eminence of the pelvis and sometimes it extends its lateral border into the iliac fascia. Because of its anatomy, this little muscle would seem unimportant in hip-flexion deformities. I mention it only because a reviewer of my paper on iliopsoas recession mentioned it in his critique (I do not know why), and because its tendon could be mistaken for the psoas tendon in surgery (Bleck 1971a).

Because the psoas major originates from the lateral aspect of the lumbar spine, its function in level gait may be to bring the trunk over the head of the femur at the beginning of the swing phase of gait (Strange 1965). Based upon observations of paralysis of the iliopsoas, walking on a level surface is possible without the muscle; the gait of a patient with a bilateral iliopsoas paralysis resulting from poliomyelitis was characterized by an anterior tilt of the pelvis and lumbar lordosis, and lacked speed and smoothness (Brunnstrom 1962). Without an iliopsoas to flex the hip, the person cannot lift the foot more than a few inches from the ground, cannot climb stairs and cannot run or jog. Basmajian (1962) recorded continous slight electrical activity of the iliacus while subjects were standing, and large action potentials in all degrees of hip flexion. A recognition of its function and the inability of the other hip flexors to substitute completely should make the surgeon cautious in

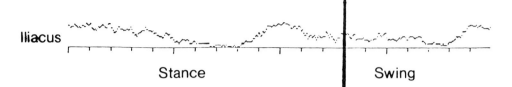

Stance | Swing

Fig. 8.10. Gait EMG, iliacus, fine wire electrodes; 10-year-old spastic diplegic with 10° hip-flexion contracture. Computer plot is summary of seven gait cycles.

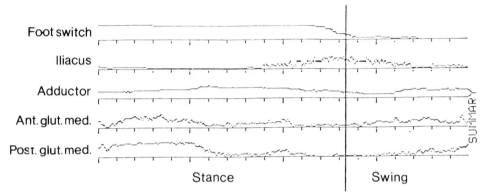

Foot switch

Iliacus

Adductor

Ant. glut. med.

Post. glut. med.

Stance | Swing

Fig. 8.11. Gait EMG of 20-year-old spastic diplegic. No previous surgery; 50° hip-flexion contracture and hip internal rotation gait. Iliacus activity normal; adductors continuous activity; anterior and posterior gluteus medius contract in both stance and swing phases.

performing iliopsoas tenotomy in patients who can walk or who have the potential to do so based upon the prognostic signs for walking as described in Chapters 1 and 5.

Electromyographic analyses of the psoas major while walking have shown that it contracts during heel rise and the first 40 per cent of the swing phase (Keagy *et al.* 1966, Morinaga 1973). The iliacus has a similar pattern (Hagy *et al.* 1973). We have found this true as well in our laboratory at Children's Hospital at Stanford (Fig. 8.9).

In patients who had spastic diplegia and hip-flexion deformities, Perry *et al.* (1976) used gait electromyograms to document abnormal and prolonged electrical activity of the iliacus. In 11 separate gait electromyograms of the iliacus muscle in spastic diplegic patients, we found normal electrical activity in five; in six the activity was prolonged and out of phase (Fig. 8.10). In two patients who had iliopsoas recession the contractions were normal (Bleck 1980) (Fig. 8.11).

Biomechanical adaptation to the hip-flexion deformity occurs as compensation in two ways, depending upon the position of the knee, the degree of spasticity of the quadriceps and hamstrings, and the strength of the gastrocnemius-soleus:

1. Posterior inclination of the pelvis. When the knees are flexed due to predominant hamstring spasticity and contracture, the pelvis inclines posteriorly and the lumbar spine flattens (Fig. 8.12). The patient assumes a sitting posture

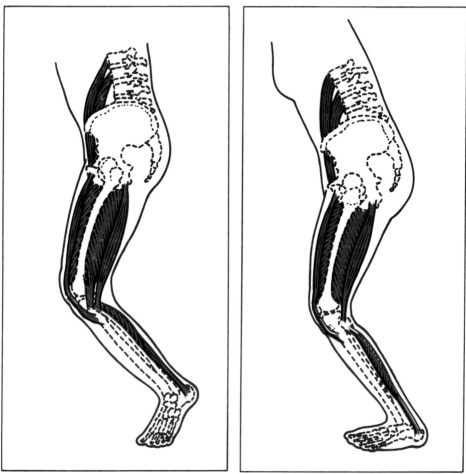

Fig. 8.12. Compensation for hip-flexion deformity by posterior pelvic inclination, flattening of lumbar spine and flexed knees.

Fig. 8.13. If a patient with the posture in Figure 8.12 has overlengthening of Achilles tendons, crouch becomes worse.

while trying to stand erect.

If the patient also suffered excessive weakening of the gastrocnemius-soleus muscle as a result of overlengthening of the Achilles tendon or a neurectomy of the muscle, the crouch is more exaggerated (Fig. 8.13).

If this same patient had lengthening or transfer of the hamstrings to the femur and retained the same hip-flexion deformity, the compensating effect of knee flexion is lost. The pelvis then inclines anteriorly and lumbar lordosis increases. Because there are limits to extension of the lumbar spine, the patient may have to lean his trunk forward to bring the trunk's center of gravity anterior to the ankle joint between the base of support (Fig. 8.14).

2. Anterior inclination of the pelvis. When the knees cannot be flexed due to quadriceps spasticity, the pelvis increases its anterior inclination and the lumbar

299

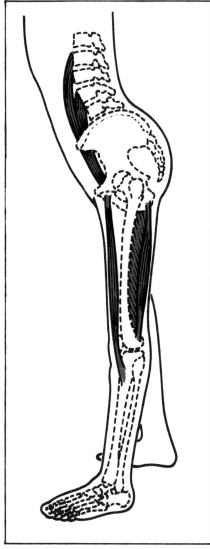

Fig. 8.14. If patient with the posture in Figures 8.12 or 8.13 has hamstring lengthening, hip-flexion contracture is compensated by increased anterior pelvic inclination, lumbar lordosis and forward lean of trunk.

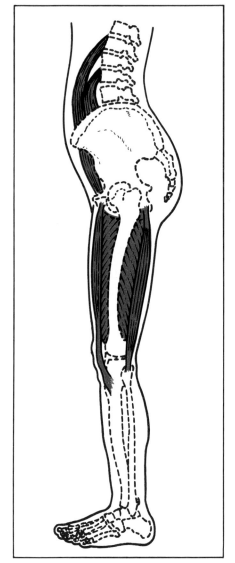

Fig. 8.15. Effect of spastic quadriceps and extended knees with hip-flexion contracture; increased anterior inclination of pelvis and lumbar lordosis.

spine becomes more lordotic (Fig. 8.15).

The correction of these undesirable postural adaptations of the pelvis and lumbar spine is relief of the hip-flexion deformity (Fig. 8.16).

Radiographic analyses of the pelvic and spinal compensatory mechanisms have been done using lateral radiographs of the lumbar spine, pelvis and proximal femur

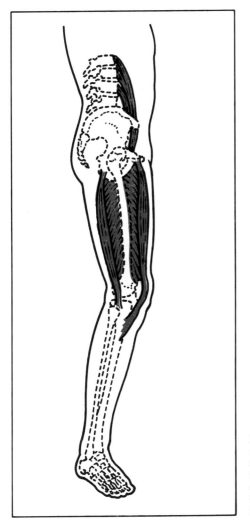

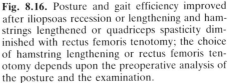

Fig. 8.16. Posture and gait efficiency improved after iliopsoas recession or lengthening and hamstrings lengthened or quadriceps spasticity diminished with rectus femoris tenotomy; the choice of hamstring lengthening or rectus femoris tenotomy depends upon the preoperative analysis of the posture and the examination.

with the patient standing as erect as possible (Bleck 1971*a*, *b*). On the radiograph a line is drawn along the top of the sacrum to locate the pelvic inclination (for all practical purposes the sacrum moves with the pelvis; its independent motion is no more than 4°). A second line is drawn along the shaft of the femur. The angle formed by the intersection of these two lines is called the *sacrofemoral angle*. In normal children and adolescents this angle measures between 50° and 65° (Fig. 8.17).

In the patient with a hip-flexion deformity and flexed knees, the femora were horizontally parallel with the sacrum and the sacrofemoral angle was less than 50° (Fig. 8.18).

In the patient with a hip-flexion deformity and spastic quadriceps muscles and

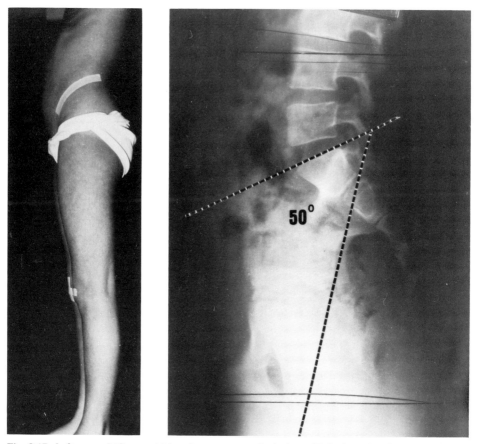

Fig. 8.17. *Left:* normal 13-year-old female; posture, sagittal plane. *Right:* lateral radiograph of lumbar spine, pelvis and proximal femora; same subject standing. Sacrofemoral angle is within normal limits (45° to 60°).

extended knees with a hip-flexion deformity, the femora were vertically parallel with the sacrum and the sacrofemoral angle was less than 50° (Fig. 8.19).

With acceptable compensation of the hip-flexion deformity, the sacrofemoral angle, although less than normal, was 35° to 45° (Fig. 8.20).

Almost all *lordosis* of the lumbar spine was confined to the lumbosacral joint. When the degree of lordosis between the first and fifth lumbar vertebrae was measured by the Cobb method, the resultant angles were between 45° and 65° and within the limits of normal for children (Propst-Proctor and Bleck 1983). These spinal measurements did not vary either with the degree of the hip-flexion deformity or with the sacrofemoral angle (Bleck 1975) (Fig. 8.21).

Excessive *anterior bowing of the femoral shaft* does not seem to occur in response to the hip-flexion deformity. In 27 patients who had spastic hip-flexion deformities and sacrofemoral angles that ranged from 15° to 48°, the anterior bow of the femur as measured on the lateral radiographs had a mean of 8° (range 1° to

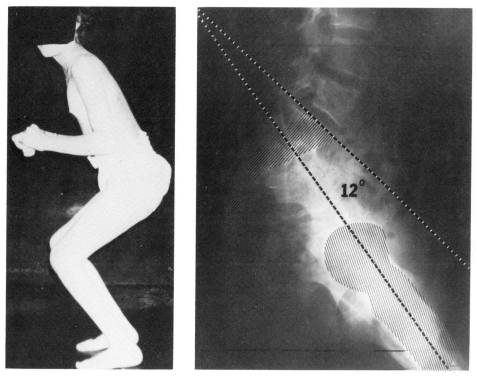

Fig. 8.18. *Left:* posture, sagittal plane, 13-year-old spastic diplegic, postoperative Young-Ober fasciotomy. Hip-flexion contracture 50°. *Right:* lateral radiograph of lumbar spine, pelvis and proximal femora; patient standing. Sacrofemoral angle 12°; with flexed knees the femora become more horizontally parallel with the top of the sacrum.

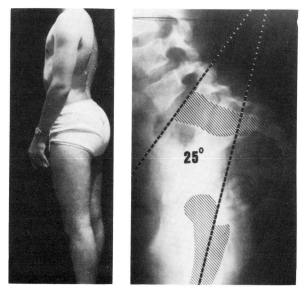

Fig. 8.19. *Left:* posture, sagittal plane, of 16-year-old spastic diplegic. Spastic quadriceps, lumbar lordosis. *Right:* lateral radiograph of lumbar spine, pelvis and proximal femora, same patient standing. Sacrofemoral angle 25°; with knees extended the femora become more vertically parallel with the top of the sacrum.

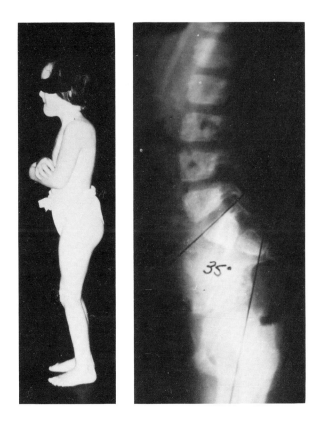

Fig. 8.20. *Left:* acceptable posture, sagittal plane, seven-year-old spastic diplegic: 15° hip-flexion contracture and slightly flexed knees (15°). *Right:* lateral radiograph of lumbar spine, pelvis and proximal femur with same patient standing. Sacrofemoral angle 35°.

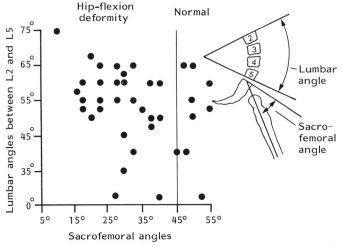

Fig. 8.21. Correlation between lumbar lordosis measured by Cobb method between second and fifth lumbar vertebrae, sacrofemoral angles and hip-flexion contracture in spastic diplegia and normal children without hip-flexion deformity. No correlation between hip-flexion deformity and lordosis from L2 to L5 vertebrae. There is a correlation of the hip-flexion deformity and the sacrofemoral angle. Conclusion: most, if not all, of the lumbar lordosis occurs at the lumbosacral joint.

304

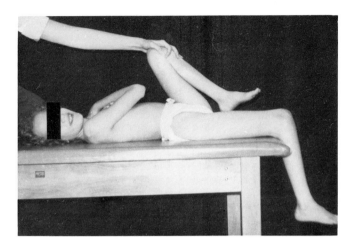

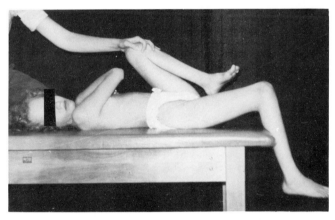

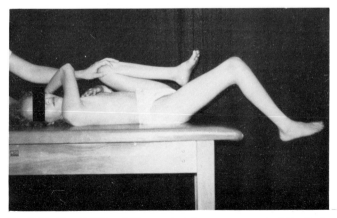

Fig. 8.22. Unreliability of Thomas test for measurement of hip-flexion contracture in cerebral palsy. One can obtain a range of 0° to 45° in the same patient. This is apt to occur when the hamstrings are contracted. Also note movement of right leg!

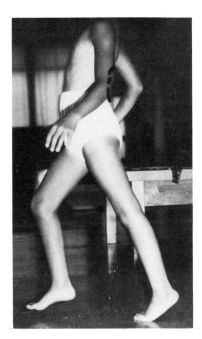

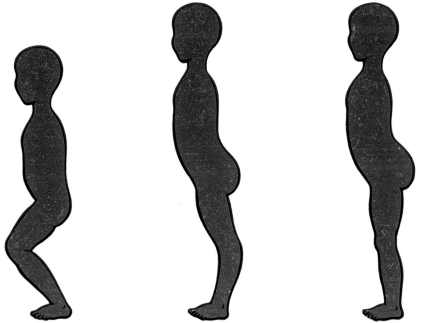

Fig. 8.23. Sagittal view of gait in spastic diplegia, age eight years. Hip extension very important; stance is 60 per cent of the gait cycle. With a hip-flexion contracture, part of the limited hip extension can be compensated by increased pelvic motion and mobility of the lumbosacral joint.

Fig. 8.24. Three gait patterns in spastic diplegia. *From left to right:* flexed hips and flexed knees; flexed hips and hyperextended knees; flexed hips and balanced hamstring and quadriceps function (often cospasticity exists). Almost all have hip internal rotation during stance and swing phases. Some have increased pelvic rotation which depends upon the amount and extent of spasticity in the hip musculature.

306

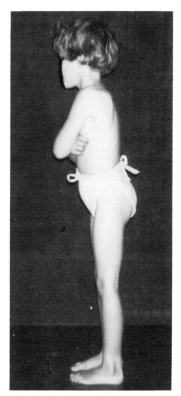

Fig. 8.25. Patient CR. Posture, sagittal plane, of seven-year-old spastic diplegic. Very acceptable compensation for the hip-flexion deformity; knee position functional. No need for surgical correction.

20°). The normal mean femoral shaft anterior bow is considered to be 7°.

The *clinical measurement* of the hip-flexion deformity has been described in Chapter 2. The Staheli prone extension method is most accurate. The Thomas test can be an inaccurate measurement of the hip-flexion contracture in spastic paralysis of the lower limbs (Fig. 8.22).

Pelvic-femoral fixation is another factor that can account for the gait abnormality. It can be demonstrated by asking the child to stand on one limb and hold onto a table with one hand while swinging the other limb back and forth. The femur moves with the pelvis as a unit. This partial pelvic-femoral fixation is due to spasticity and contracture of the hip musculature. The flexion deformity limits hip extension that is so essential to gait (stance is 60 per cent of the gait cycle) (Fig. 8.23). The lumbar spine absorbs this limited hip extension mainly at the lumbosacral articulation. These patients walk with an anterior and posterior pelvic motion as well as an increase in transverse pelvic rotation. Their gait is similar to that of patients who have had an arthrodesis of the hips.

Three spastic gait patterns can be described in children with spastic diplegia (Bleck 1971*a, b*) (Fig. 8.24):

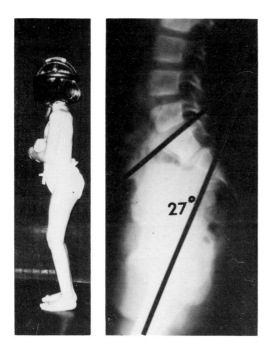

Fig. 8.26. *Left:* patient ES. Posture, sagittal plane, six-year-old spastic diplegic. Unacceptable posture due to hip-flexion contractures, spastic hamstrings with knees flexed 30°. Surgery indicated. *Right:* lateral radiograph of lumbar spine, pelvis and proximal femur of patient ES. Sacrofemoral angle conforms an increased anterior pelvic inclination and lumbar lordosis at the lumbosacral articulation. Persistent low back pain is likely after age 18 years and independent walking.

1. Flexed internally rotated hips and flexed knees—spastic hamstrings.

2. Flexed internally rotated hips and hyperextended knees—spastic quadriceps.

3. Flexed internally rotated hips and balanced knee function—neither hamstring nor quadriceps spasticity predominates. These children walk with an in-toed gait almost identical to that of normal children who have excessive femoral anteversion (Crane 1959).

Indications for surgery in hip-flexion deformity
When measurements of the hip-flexion deformity were made in children with spastic paralysis (particularly using the prone extension test recommended), we never observed a decrease in the hip-flexion deformity by passive stretching, prone lying, any physical therapeutic methods or by orthotics. Instead compensation with increased pelvic anterior or posterior inclination has been observed. If this compensation appears to be satisfactory, there is no need to apply direct surgical treatment (Fig. 8.25). In general, if the hip-flexion deformity is more than 15° to 20°, surgical correction is indicated (Fig. 8.26).

Orthopaedic surgeons in the past applied the same procedures used in poliomyelitis to spastic paralysis with disappointing results. For hip-flexion deformity in spastic paralysis, the Ober-Yount fasciotomy of the tensor fascia femoris and of the adjacent muscles and the distal iliotibial band is no longer used because it consistently failed to correct the deformity. The Soutter or Campbell muscle-slide operation, which detaches the origins of the sartorius, rectus femoris and tensor fascia femoris muscles and displaces them distally, has also failed to provide significant correction. Lamb and Pollock (1962) reported a 66 per cent recurrence rate with this operation.

Proximal rectus femoris tenotomy has not corrected the hip-flexion deformity. This operation detaches the rectus femoris from its origin on the anterior inferior iliac spine and allows this tendon to retract distally. It should not be done just because the surgeon feels it is 'tight'. Normal rectus femoris tendons are tight. The release of this muscle proximally weakens the quadriceps; if hamstring spasticity is present then it will overpower the quadriceps so that a flexed knee posture can result within six months to one year postoperatively.

Myotomy of the anterior fibers of the gluteus medius as an addition to the release of the sartorius and tensor fascia femoris origins for correction of spastic hip-flexion deformities was reported by Roosth (1971). It is probable that when the hip-flexion contracture is great enough, the anterior fibers of the gluteus medius appear to be one of the deforming forces. Certainly, as Roosth reported, the procedure diminished the hip internal rotation during gait because the major internal rotator of the hip is the gluteus medius. Although Perry and Hoffer (1977), in their gait electromyograms of the gluteus medius in patients with cerebral palsy and adult stroke, noted no abnormal contractions of the muscle (its major electrical activity is in the beginning of stance) (see Fig. 8.9), our electromyographic studies did show that the anterior fibers had more activity when normal children internally rotated the hip, and in nine of 11 children with cerebral palsy the muscle had prolonged abnormal contractions (Csongradi *et al.* 1980).

Hip internal rotation in gait is not necessarily unphysiological. A more important function for energy conservation during gait is the pelvic stabilization by the gluteus medius when weight-shifting from limb to limb during the stance phase of gait. It does not seem worthwhile to use surgery to comprise this function of the hip abductor muscles, which would incur excessive lateral displacement of the body for the sake of appearance.

Iliopsoas tenotomy, lengthening, or recession? Some type of surgical lengthening of the iliopsoas has been accepted because this muscle is the major flexor of the hip, and in spastic paralysis with contracture is the major contributor to the flexion deformity. The iliopsoas also has a function in walking, and for this reason it appears desirable not only to decrease the contracture but also to preserve its strength and function. *Tenotomy* of the iliopsoas tendon does not seem advisable in the ambulatory patient. In the non-ambulatory patient, or in one whose prognosis for walking is poor, iliopsoas tenotomy is satisfactory. Tenotomy is a far simpler operation than either recession or lengthening.

Bleck and Holstein (1963) performed iliopsoas tenotomy in 17 patients with cerebral palsy and spastic paralysis. All had a permanent loss of hip-flexion power that did not return in 13 years of follow-up. Fortunately, the patients who were ambulatory and selected for the procedure were dependent on crutches which always can compensate to some degree for deficiencies in hip muscle function. Hoffer (1969) and I tagged the end of the iliopsoas tendons with a metallic clip at the time of tenotomy. Postoperative radiographs revealed cephalad retraction of

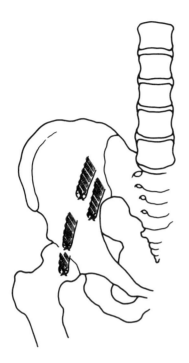

Fig. 8.27. Graphic representation from radiographs of pelvis and hips after iliopsoas tenotomy in cerebral palsy. Metallic clips put on iliopsoas tendon proximal to the cut. Note variation in levels of retraction of the tendon.

the tendon to unpredictable and varying levels. Some tendons retracted to the level of the femoral head, and others to the mid-ilium (Fig. 8.27).

In normal non-spastic children in whom tenotomy of the iliopsoas has been routinely performed, as part of the procedure for open reduction of a congenital dislocation of the hip, no functional loss of hip flexion has been noted. However, in cerebral-palsied children the muscle is spastic and can retract too far superiorly, depending upon the degree of spasticity; in effect the muscle is overlengthened by tenotomy.

Aponeurotic lengthening of the iliopsoas has recently been proposed by Tylkowski and Price (1986), who reported their results in 10 patients with spastic hip-flexion deformities. They described 'aponeurotic lengthening' as an incision made in the fascia of the psoas just after it crossed over the brim of the pelvis (similar to the psoas incision done with an innominate osteotomy for congenital dislocation of the hip—see Salter 1961). Presumably this 'aponeurosis' is the broad beginning of the psoas tendon which at this level, by its fusion with the fibers of the iliacus muscle, prevents inordinate retraction of the tendinous portion. Tylkowski's careful gait analyses and measurements showed improvement of the flexion contracture (mean 12°) and no loss of function. Rinsky (1985) reported that he does the same procedure, and finds it easier to do and just as effective as z-lengthening or recession.

Even with these early results of incision of the tendon within the fibers of the iliacus, there may be an occasional patient in whom excessive retraction of the proximal tendon occurs. In one 25-year-old patient in whom I recommended

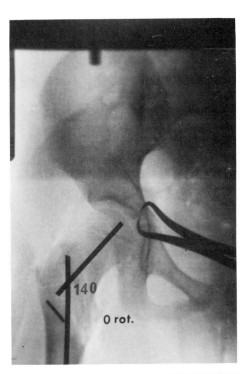

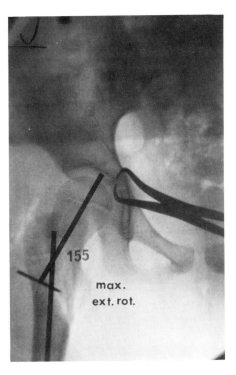

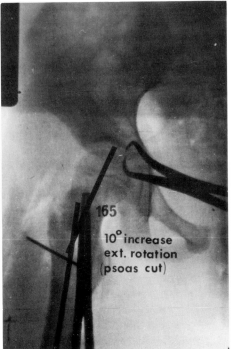

Fig. 8.28. Anterior-posterior radiographs of the hip made in the operating room at the time of iliopsoas recession. Metal pin in greater trochanter to mark rotation obtained: hip in neutral rotation (*above left*); maximum external rotation with hip extended (*above right*); and increased external rotation with hip extended after iliopsoas tendon cut (*left*).

bilateral iliopsoas tendon z-lengthenings for a 45° flexion contracture in order to relieve constant disabling low back pain, the tendon was inadvertently cut completely through on one side at the level of the femoral head. The proximal portion retracted about 10cm into the pelvis. Hip flexion on this side was extremely weak for approximately a year, after which normal strength returned; on the z-lengthened side there was no weakness. After five years the flexion contractures on both hips were 0° and strength was normal. The low back pain was relieved immediately postoperatively and never returned during the five-year follow-up.

Lengthening by the z-method still seems preferable if recession does not appear indicated. z-lengthening may be preferable to recession in adults and children who do not have subluxation of the hip and whose flexion contractures of the hips are unacceptable. These patients will almost always be independent fully weight-bearing community walkers who need neither crutches nor walkers. Lengthening was reported by Anthosen (1966) and Baumann (1970) with apparent good results. Anthosen's postoperative regimen entailed a prolonged hospital stay where the patient was kept prone and the hips maintained in extension.

I have learned that z-lengthening is quite satisfactory in ambulatory patients, and it may not risk as much hip-flexion weakness as does iliopsoas recession. I have followed for a mean of four years 10 patients who had bilateral lengthenings. Nine were aged between six and 14 years (mean nine years), and one was an adult age 25 years. The mean preoperative flexion contracture was 26° (range 15° to 45°) and the mean postoperative contracture was 10° (range 0° to 30°). The 30° preoperative flexion contracture of one girl at age six years was the same postoperatively at age eight years. None had any evidence preoperatively or postoperatively of subluxation, lateral migration of the femoral head or an abnormal CE angle of the hip.

Lengthening of the iliopsoas tendon appeared theoretically disadvantageous because:

1. When I performed an iliopsoas tenotomy, we could passively externally rotate the extended hip about 10° more (Fig. 8.28). This observation seemed to confirm Ferguson's concept of the iliopsoas tendon compressing the hip-joint capsule medially, and thereby acting as an obstruction to reduction of subluxations and dislocations of the hip—a concept that is now accepted in the treatment of congenital dislocation of the hip (Ferguson 1973, 1975). For this reason, in spastic paralytic subluxation of the hip I prefer to remove the tendon from its medial capsular position and preserve the strength of the muscle rather than increase the risk of additional postoperative compression of the medial-joint capsule that would be anticipated in the subsequent healing and scar formation when the tendon is z-lengthened. This was and remains the rationale for iliopsoas recession.

This rationale appears confirmed by Griffith *et al.* (1982) in a review of their original 131 patients who had 255 adductor transfers. After an average of three years follow-up, they found a need for secondary surgery for subluxation in 13 per cent, while 11 per cent required secondary acetabuloplasties. These results caused them to add iliopsoas recession to the adductor transfer surgery in 30 patients (60 hips), with the result that secondary surgery for subluxation dropped to 7 per cent and there was no need for secondary acetabuloplasties.

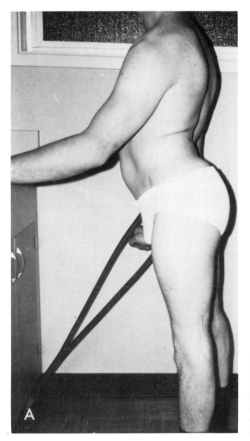

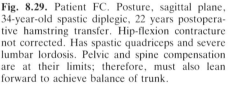

Fig. 8.29. Patient FC. Posture, sagittal plane, 34-year-old spastic diplegic, 22 years postoperative hamstring transfer. Hip-flexion contracture not corrected. Has spastic quadriceps and severe lumbar lordosis. Pelvic and spine compensation are at their limits; therefore, must also lean forward to achieve balance of trunk.

2. After z-lengthening of the tendon, healing must be by scar formation. As with all cicatrix formation, contracture of the fibrous tissue occurs. Hence early recurrence of the flexion contracture is a risk with lengthening. The patients must be carefully supervised postoperatively to ensure that they do not sit upright for long periods during the day. In one of my first patients in whom we did a lengthening on one side and a recession on the other, contracture recurred on the side of lengthening within three weeks postoperatively. Fortunately aggressive hip extension, passive and active exercise, together with strict prone positioning in bed, overcame this complication in six weeks.

Iliopsoas recession. The indications for iliopsoas recession are the same as with lengthening, except that I would recommend the recession in particular for those who have a subluxation of the hip. It is especially important to reduce the hip-flexion deformity if the flexed knee gait is to be corrected by lengthening of the hamstring muscles. If the hamstrings alone are weakened in such patients, increased pelvic inclination and lumbar lordosis can be anticipated as a compensatory mechanism (Fig. 8.29). This postural adaptation does not resolve with time, and low back pain occurs as the patient ages. Preoperative lateral radiographs of

313

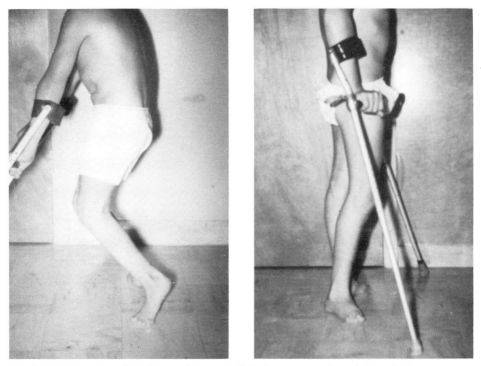

Fig. 8.30. *Left:* patient CR. 12-year-old spastic diplegic, postoperative sciatic and obturator nerve 'crushes'. Has typical posture of flexed hips and knees with increased posterior pelvic inclination and a flat lumbar spine. *Right:* patient CR, now aged 18, six years postoperative bilateral iliopsoas recession, hamstring lengthening, Achilles tendon lengthening and subtalar extra-articular arthrodeses for pes valgus. At 15 years postoperatively had severe constant retropatellar pain in right knee, patella alta and spastic quadriceps. Extensive chondromalacia of the patella. Patellectomy relieved pain; function remained the same.

the spine in such patients might disclose a silent spondylolisthesis which can be exaggerated if the hip-flexion deformity is not corrected at the time of hamstring lengthening. The incidence of spondylolisthesis in Caucasian males is 5 to 6 per cent, and in females 2 to 3 per cent; in black people it is less than 3 per cent, but as much as 50 per cent in Eskimos (Moe *et al.* 1978).

The best results of iliopsoas recession have been achieved in children between the ages of five and seven years. Ilipsoas recession can be combined with other surgical procedures on the lower limbs at the same time as the need dictates—*e.g.* adductor longus tenotomy, hamstring lengthening or rectus femoris tenotomy, Achilles tendon lengthening and tendon transfers or stabilization of the feet. One-stage surgeries demand very detailed and repetitive examinations preoperatively. The preoperative examinations (including gait analysis when available) should take at least as much time as the operation itself. Even orthopaedic surgeons need to use 'cognitive skills', which are currently claimed to be the exclusive province of internal medicine.

TABLE 8.III
Results of iliopsoas recession in spastic diplegia (61 patients, 116 hips)

Mean age of surgery (years)	Follow-up (years)	Flexion contracture preop.	Flexion contracture postop.	Hip internal rotation preop. postop.	
7.4	6.8	30°	10°	76°	59°
Range 3-18	3-14	15°-60°	0°-30°	65°-90°	30°-90°

TABLE 8.IV
Correction of sacrofemoral angles by iliopsoas recession

Patient	Sacrofemoral angles (degrees)		% improvement
Number	Preoperative	Postoperative	
1	17	10	−58
2	35	20	−57
3	20	45	56
4	25	50	50
5	38	30	7
6	30	45	34
7	20	30	34
8	25	45	45
9	30	40	25
10	25	22	−1
11	32	50	36
12	24	35	32
13	50	57	13
14	20	45	56
15	27	45	40
16	27	42	36
17	56	55	−1
18	40	50	20
19	45	55	19
20	30	50	40
21	15	30	50

From Bleck 1971*a*; first 25 patients who had iliopsoas recession, four of whom did not have preoperative radiographs to measure the sacrofemoral angle.

Results of iliopsoas recession (Table 8.III). The results are based upon 61 patients (116 hips) who could be followed longer than three years. Of the 61 patients, 55 had bilateral iliopsoas recessions and six were unilateral for a total of 116 hips. The mean age of surgery was 7.4 years in a range of three to 18 years (median 6 years). All patients over age four years were ambulatory except five (age two to three years) who had a good or fair prognosis but had a subluxation of one or both hips. Of the 56 who were walking, 51 did so without support; none of these had hip subluxation. The five who had a hip subluxation walked with crutches or walkers.

The follow-up was for a mean of 6.8 years, ranging from three to 14 years. The preoperative flexion contracture was a mean of 30° in a range of 15° to 60°. The postoperative flexion contracture was reduced to a mean of 10° in a range of 0° to

30°; the average correction was 48 per cent. Additional surgery consisted of adductor myotomy and anterior branch obturator neurectomy in 11 patients; hamstring lengthening was performed in 27 (Fig. 8.30).

In the 10 who had a subluxation of the hip, the mean age of surgery was 4.3 years (range two to nine years) and the follow-up was for a mean of 7.3 years (range two to 15 years). In six the subluxation was reduced at follow-up; in four it persisted and secondary procedures were performed.

Postoperative standing lateral radiographs of the lumbar spine, pelvis and proximal femur were compared with preoperative radiographs. The sacrofemoral angles decreased an average of 32 per cent in 21 who had these examinations (Table 8.IV).

Hip-flexion power was lost in all patients, but within the limits of manual muscle testing in spastic paralysis the grade in all except three was good to fair in a range of active hip flexion 115°. The flexion power was poor in two patients, and zero in another. This postoperative weakness might have been due to the sutures pulling out from the site of reattachment of the psoas tendon on anterior-lateral capsule of the hip; however, in one patient with severe spasticity no voluntary control of any muscle in the lower limb could be elicited.

In those patients in whom hamstring lengthening was performed for a flexed knee gait, the iliopsoas recession prevented the excessive lumbar lordosis postoperatively. With the exception of the three patients (and within the past two years a fourth who had marked weakness of the hip-flexor muscles) all patients were able to climb stairs, ride bicycles and engage in sports that were consistent with the amount of spasticity remaining and the adequacy of their equilibrium reactions. In the relatively recent patient who had marked postoperative weakness of hip flexion, the preoperative gait electromyograph showed very low voltage of the action potential received from the iliacus muscle. Electromyograms are not regarded as quantitative, but I believe that the weak signals received when fine wire electrodes are used in the muscle might have some validity.

Temporary postoperative quadriceps paralysis was reported to me by a surgeon. This can be avoided by gentle and minimal retraction of the femoral nerve during the procedure.

Correction of the hip-flexion deformity failed in some patients over the age of 11 years. Anterior incision of the joint capsule, while theoretically logical, has not in practice resulted in additional correction. In the few patients in whom I used this procedure, I noted a limited passive flexion of the hip to 90°—possibly due to the increased anterior cicatrix formation of the joint capsular incision.

Operative technique of iliopsoas recession (Fig. 8.31). The patient is supine. An incision is made, beginning about 1.5cm distal and lateral to the anterior superior iliac spine and continuing distally, medially and obliquely parallel with the groin crease. The incision terminates approximately at the junction of the medial one-third and lateral two-thirds of the anterior surface of the thigh.

The medial border of the sartorius muscle is identified and retracted laterally with the lateral femoral cutaneous nerve. The tendinous origin of the rectus femoris is noted (the 'silver fish'). Medial to this, and blending with the fascia surrounding

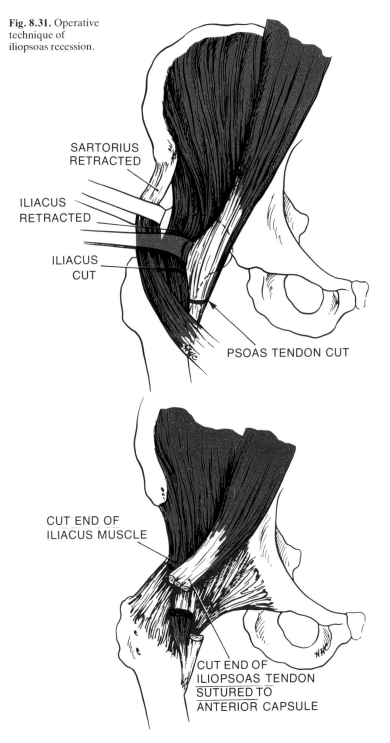

Fig. 8.31. Operative technique of iliopsoas recession.

SARTORIUS
RETRACTED

ILIACUS
RETRACTED

ILIACUS
CUT

PSOAS TENDON CUT

CUT END OF
ILIACUS MUSCLE

CUT END OF
ILIOPSOAS TENDON
SUTURED TO
ANTERIOR CAPSULE

317

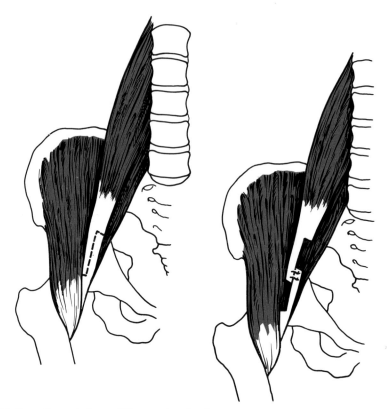

Fig. 8.32. Operative technique of iliopsoas lengthening.

the rectus tendon, is the iliacus muscle which is dissected free from this fascial
envelope and then from the anterior capsule of the hip. A blunt instrument (muscle
dissector or elevator) is placed between the iliacus muscle and the joint capsule,
and pushed medially so that it underlies the psoas tendon. The femoral nerve on
the anterior surface of the iliacus is found and freed-up so that it can be gently
retracted medially. The bulky iliacus fibers are retracted laterally to expose the
broad psoas tendon over the anterior capsule of the hip. The hip is then externally
rotated and flexed. The psoas tendon is cleansed of fatty connective tissue so that it
can be clearly visualized almost to the lesser trochanter.

The distal iliacus muscle fibers are then cut from lateral to medial in an oblique
line as far as the psoas tendon, which is then cut off close to the lesser trochanter.
The tendon is brought up into the wound. After exposure of the anterior capsule of
the hip with a blunt dissector, the tendon is sutured near the base of the femoral
neck on the anterolateral surface of the joint capsule. Two heavy absorbable
synthetic sutures are used. The iliacus fibers are then tacked down over the psoas
tendon with a suture or two.

If the patient walks with an hyperextended knee-gait pattern, the rectus
tendon origin is sectioned and the tendon allowed to retract distally. Otherwise the
tendon is not disturbed.

Because this is a deep wound, closed suction irrigation is always used. We close all wounds with absorbable synthetic sutures in the subcutaneous layer, and a subcuticular suture to close the skin which is reinforced with sterile adhesive tapes.

Postoperative care. No spica plasters are necessary. Additional plaster immobilization with long-leg plasters is used only if other procedures have been done at the same time: adductor myotomy, hamstring lengthening, Achilles tendon lengthening and/or reconstructive foot surgery.

The patient is kept in bed; sitting is not permitted for three weeks except in a position of 30° to 40° of trunk elevation during meals. During this period of bed rest, bed exercises are instituted: hip extension, abduction and external rotation three times a day. I recommend regular exercise of the upper limbs with the resistance of weights consistent with the age and strength of the child. At the end of three weeks, gait training should start: first in parallel bars, then graduating to crutches as balance improves, and finally leading to independent walking, if this was feasible preoperatively. Usually this process is complete in six weeks. Supervised exercise and balance training are continued for an average of six months after surgery.

Operative technique for iliopsoas lengthening (Baumann 1970). The same incision and approach as described for iliopsoas recession is used, except that it is not necessary to dissect the muscle from the anterior capsule of the hip. It is necessary to retract the femoral nerve medially and to identify the psoas tendon. Kocher clamps placed distally and proximally, with one on the medial half of the tendon and the other on the lateral half, prevent the unwanted retraction of the tendon into the pelvis when it is z-lengthened (Fig. 8.32). The lengthened ends are sutured together.

The postoperative care is the same as described for iliopsoas recession.

Hip internal rotation deformity
Anatomy, physiology and mechanisms
The internal rotator muscles of the hip are considered to be the gluteus medius and minimus, semitendinosus, adductors and the tensor fascia femoris (Duchenne 1867, 1959; Brunnstrom 1962).

Anatomists and physiologists have established that the anterior portion of the gluteus medius is the main internal rotator of the hip (Duchenne 1867, 1959; Hollinshead 1951; Grant 1952; Brunnstrom 1962). Clinical experience confirms these observations; if the tendon is cut or transferred (Steel 1980), the femur no longer internally rotates. Direct measurements of transverse rotations of the segments of the lower limb during level gait show that the pelvis, femur and tibia all internally rotate during swing phase and continue to do so until mid-stance, when abrupt shift to external rotation occurs and continues until toe-off as swing phase begins (Fig. 3.15). The gluteus medius contracts at the beginning of stance and continues to contract until mid-stance (Fig. 8.9). This early stance-phase activity correlates with internal rotation of the entire limb.

In a gait electromyographic telemetry study using fine wire electrodes in the anterior and posterior portions of the gluteus medius, Csongradi *et al.* (1980) were

TABLE 8.V

EMG gluteus medius during gait cycles (Csongradi *et al.* 1980)

	Anterior gluteus medius		Posterior gluteus medius	
	% activity	SD	% activity	SD
Normal-normal gait	64	11.3	62	16.2
Normal-internal rotation gait	87	11.6 p<0.001	70	17.4 NS
Spastic cerebral palsy	73	20.6 p<0.05	66	22.4 NS
Increased antetorsion	50	10.9 p<0.01	55	15.0 NS

able to demonstrate biphasic activity of both the anterior and posterior portions, with one phase lasting from late swing to mid-stance and a shorter phase at toe-off in 15 normal subjects aged five and over (Table 8.V). In the normal subjects who simulated the hip internal rotation gait, the activity of the anterior gluteus medius lasted significantly longer than normal (p<0.001); the posterior part was also of longer duration, but not significantly. In nine children with cerebral palsy and hip internal rotation gaits, the anterior fibers had a longer period of firing than the posterior, and the duration of firing was longer than normal (p<0.05). Surprisingly, in normal children who had femoral antetorsion, the duration of both anterior and posterior gluteus medius activity was less than the normals and the children with cerebral palsy (p<0.01). The results of the study by Csongradi *et al.* (1980) seem to indicate that overactivity or spasticity of the gluteus medius is not the etiology of excessive femoral anteversion (femoral antetorsion). These data also suggest that the anterior fibers of the gluteus medius in both normal and spastic children account for the hip internal rotation gait patterns.

The *semitendinosus* internally rotates the thigh medially when the knee is extended, but this rotation diminishes as the knee flexes (Duchenne 1867, 1959). The strength of the semitendinosus is much less than the biceps femoris, which is a powerful lateral rotator of the leg. The semimembranosus has no rotator function, but it is the strongest of the hamstring muscles in flexing the knee. Sutherland *et al.* (1969) studied gait electromyograms and transverse rotation of the lower limbs in seven patients with spastic paralysis and hip internal rotation; all patients consistently had prolonged contraction of the semitendinosus in the stance phase. Chong *et al.* (1978) recorded electromyographic activity in 12 cerebral-palsied children who had lower-limb internal rotation gaits. Spasticity of the medial hamstrings was deemed the most important causative factor. Our own studies of spastic gait patterns (not exclusively in-toed walking) in 32 children demonstrated dysphasic and prologed activity of the medial hamstrings (Csongradi *et al.* 1979).

These data do not contradict the suggestion that the semitendinosus may contribute to the in-toed gait, but they do indicate that other factors may account for hip internal rotation gait. Recorded overactivity of a muscle does not necessarily correlate with the abnormal motion observed. Only by removing the muscle function by surgery or isolated paralysis, and by observing the effects, can one be certain it is the prime cause of the gait abnormality. In other words, clinical observations still have an important rôle.

320

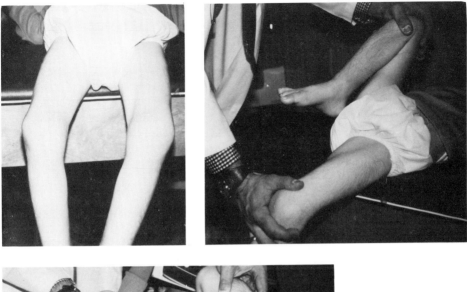

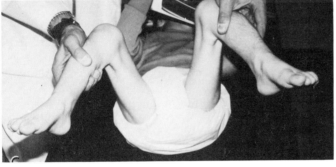

Fig. 8.33. *Above left:* patient AM, six-year-old spastic quadriplegic, with hip abductor spasticity. *Above right:* Thomas test: mild hip-flexion contracture, 5°. *Left:* hip internal rotation within internal limits.

The *adductors* were described as lateral rotators by Duchenne (1867, 1959). The lower portion of the adductor magnus is thought to be an internal rotator. Electromyographic studies of the adductors show contraction in late stance (Mann and Hagy 1973); an additional burst of activity in early stance occurs according to Brunnstrom (1962). Most electrical activity occurred after heel contact. These investigators considered the adductors to be weak internal rotators.

In cerebral-palsied patients who had no flexion contracture of the hip (measured with the prone hip extension method) and only adducted lower limbs during gait, no internal rotation was noted. Conversely, one can find children who have hip internal rotation gaits and no significant limitation of abduction (>40° each hip); these children invariably have clinical evidence of excessive femoral anteversion (range of hip internal rotation >60° and external rotation <30°) and a hip-flexion contracture.

The *tensor fascia femoris* was noted to be a weak internal rotator by Duchenne (1867, 1959). The fact is confirmed by the disappointing results of transfer of its origin posteriorly with the intent of correcting the in-toed gait in spastic paralysis in children (Majestro and Frost 1971).

321

I have observed four children who had spastic hip abduction contractures; they had large bulging tensor fascia femoris muscles. These children did not have an internally rotated hip posture, and the passive range of internal rotation and external rotation of their hips was within normal limits (Fig. 8.33).

The rotary function of the *iliopsoas* can be discounted, according to electromyographic evidence in several studies (Basmajian 1962, Close 1964, Guillot *et al.* 1977). In one study of the psoas major during gait (Keagy *et al.* 1966) the contraction of the muscle at the time of heel rise, and continuing through the first 40 per cent of the swing phase, correlated well with Strange's concept (1965) that the psoas major contracts to counteract the lateral rotation of the pelvis. When weight is placed on the hip as the body is propelled forward, the force generated leaves the pelvis behind. The iliopsoas muscle probably prevents excessive lateral pelvic rotation, and even rotates a little medially.

Increased transverse rotation of the pelvis has frequently been seen and photographed in cerebral-palsied patients who have pelvic-femoral fixation due to the marked spasticity of the muscles of the hip and thigh (Bleck 1975).

Tylkowski *et al.* (1982), in a massive and detailed motion-analysis study of hip internal rotation gait patterns in cerebral palsy, depicted the complexity of the problem and delineated three groups of patients who had some distinct gait analysis characteristics to account for the problem. Group I children had the least involvement; internal rotation gait was primarily the result of abnormal muscle activity (gluteus medius, adductors, hamstrings) and pelvic and femoral rotation. In this group, muscle surgery and and correction of the coexisting femoral rotation appeared logical to correct the in-toed walking. Group II children were more severely involved, had abnormal muscle activity and dissociated pelvic-femoral motion, and depended on assistive devices; in this group, hip internal rotation was not consistently found and femoral rotation was not an indicator of the hip rotation. In this pattern, soft-tissue surgery would have a limited effect. I gather that in this group the main problem was pelvic rotation. Group III children had no measurable rotation movements of the femur and pelvis, and the hip appeared fixed in internal rotation position. This group comprised the most severely neurologically involved. Their walking pattern was one of falling and catching oneself—a description of poor equilibrium reactions. In this group there may be no surgical procedure that would significantly improve their gait.

In view of the lack of convincing evidence of spastic muscles as the only cause of excessive hip internal rotation gait, some other mechanism must be responsible. This mechanism, which has been studied and verified by several investigators, is excessive femoral anteversion for the age of the child.

Excessive femoral anteversion

A more correct term is antetorsion ('version' is the normal; 'torsion' is abnormal rotation 2SD above or below the mean value). However, common usage is 'anteversion' and I use it here so that the subject will not be even more confusing to the reader.

Clinical and anatomical analyses support the concept that the one consistent

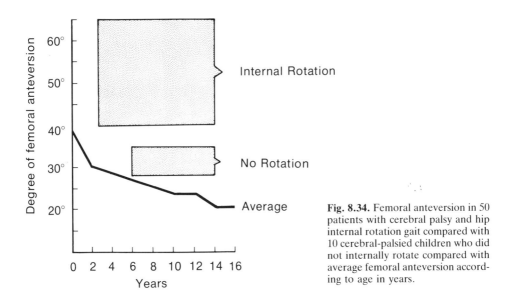

Fig. 8.34. Femoral anteversion in 50 patients with cerebral palsy and hip internal rotation gait compared with 10 cerebral-palsied children who did not internally rotate compared with average femoral anteversion according to age in years.

deformity associated with femoral internal rotation in the gait of cerebral-palsied patients is excessive femoral anteversion. The anatomical feature is a twist forward of the head, neck and trochanteric region of the femur with respect to the transcondylar axis of the knee beyond the range expected for normal humans at a given age.

Radiographic measurements using the Magilligan (1956) or the Ryder-Crane technique (1953, 1972) for determining femoral anteversion in ambulatory children who had hip internal rotation gaits demonstrated femoral anteversion beyond the range of normal for their age. I also studied 10 cerebral-palsied children who did not have hip internal rotation gait, and found that they did not have excessive femoral anteversion (Fig. 8.34). Lewis *et al.* (1964), Staheli *et al.* (1968), Beals (1969) and Fabry *et al.* (1973) have documented excessive femoral anteversion in cerebral palsy patients. It is also found in non-ambulatory patients.

Coxa valga (a femoral neck-shaft angle >145°) is a radiographic finding that is mistaken for femoral anteversion. This perceptual error is not surprising, inasmuch as radiographs are mere shadows of the bones projected in two dimensions. I measured the true angles of inclination of the femoral necks in 60 hips of cerebral-palsied children who had excessive femoral anteversion, and found only three femoral neck-shaft angles above the normal range for age as reported by Shands and Steele (1958). In the study of femoral anteversion in cerebral palsy by Lewis *et al.* (1964), the average anteversion was 54.8° and femoral neck-shaft angle average was 147°; if 145° is accepted as the upper limit of normal, this is not significant coxa valga.

Natural history of femoral anteversion
At birth, infants have angles of femoral anteversion from 10° to 60°; the mean is

323

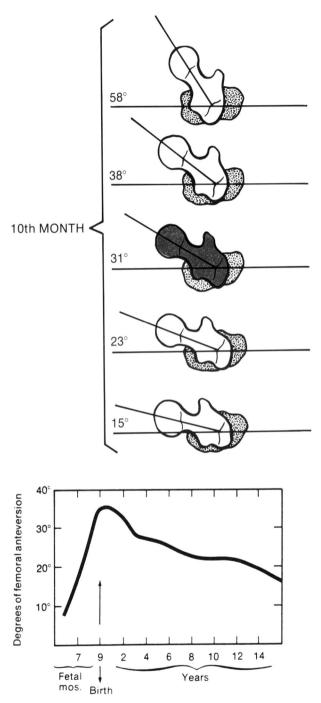

10th MONTH

58°

38°

31°

23°

15°

Fig. 8.35. Mean values of ranges of femoral anteversion at birth (redrawn from Michele 1962).

Degrees of femoral anteversion

40°

30°

20°

10°

7   9   2   4   6   8   10   12   14

Fetal mos.   Years

Birth

Fig. 8.36. Normal mean values of femoral anteversion from sixth month of fetal life to age 16 years. Note gradual decrease with advancing skeletal maturity.

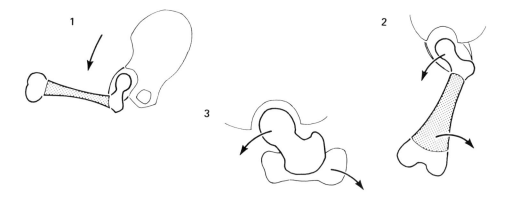

Fig. 8.37. Hypothetical explanation of decreasing femoral anteversion with hip extension and external rotation. With extension and external rotation of the hip in fresh stillborn specimens we found external rotation of the proximal cartilagenous portion of the femur; the joint capsule was intact.

variously given as 31° (Michele 1962) and 38° (Shands and Steele 1958) (Fig. 8.35). During skeletal maturation, this angle decreases to the adult value of 19° (Shands and Steele 1958, Crane 1959, Fabry *et al.* 1973) (Fig. 8.36). This spontaneous decrease in most normal children probably has a biomechanical basis.

Experimental data on femoral anteversion
At birth the proximal end of the femur (head, neck and greater trochanteric region) is entirely cartilaginous and pliable; this proximal segment is fixed to a rigid osseous diaphysis that terminates at the subtrochanteric level. When we manipulated fresh stillborn specimens of the femur, the proximal cartilaginous end could be made to rotate on the rigid osseous diaphysis. Mechanically and mathematically, the point of femoral torsion has been located in the subtrochanteric region of the femur (Michele 1962). With progressive ossification of the femoral head, neck and greater trochanteric region, the more elastic cartilage is replaced by bone and no further derotation can occur. Fabry *et al.* (1973) documented no further reduction of normal femoral anteversion after the age of eight years. In Fabry's (1977) study of 180 hips in 91 children with spastic diplegia and hemiplegia, the femoral anteversion did not decrease after the age of three years.

Lee (1977*a*) studied the possible mechanisms of derotation of the proximal femur in the hips of fresh stillborn specimens. The muscles were dissected from the hips leaving only the capsule intact; the newborn hip-flexion contracture was entirely in the capsule and not in the muscles. He found that a 2° to 4° external torque strain was needed to derotate the proximal end of the femur at the cartilaginous-osseous subtrochanteric junction. This derotation occurred as the hips were extended and externally rotated. The torque strains in external rotation were absent when the hips were flexed 90° (Fig. 8.37).

Wilkinson (1962) used skeletally immature rabbits whose hips were immobilized internally rotated for several weeks in plaster to create femoral anteversion; in the same experimental method, retroversion resulted when the hips were held in external rotation. These data strongly suggest that in humans the mechanisms necessary for the natural reduction of newborn femoral anteversion are: (i) external rotation of the hip, and (ii) hip extension to produce optimal derotation.

The experiments of Arkin and Katz (1956) on the pressure effects of epiphyseal growth demonstrated that this growth responded to stress on the physis. Torque caused torsional growth. All changes in bone shape were due to new bone laid down by the cartilage cells aligned in the stressed pattern.

Measurements of newborn hip passive extension and internal rotation confirm that all newborn children have a flexion contracture of the hip of 28° (Haas *et al.* 1973). At six weeks the flexion contracture decreases to a mean value of 19°, and at three to six months it decreases to 7° (Coon *et al.* 1975). Phelps *et al.* (1985) used the prone hip extension test rather than the Thomas test to measure hip extension at ages nine and 24 months in normal infants: a 10° flexion contracture was present at nine months and at 24 months it decreased to 3°. Internal rotation of the hip decreased from the age of six weeks to three months as this hip extended ($p=0.005$, Coon *et al.* 1975). In the study by Phelps *et al.* (1985), at age nine to 24 months hip internal rotation increased from 41° (sd=7.8) to 52° (sd=10.1), and external rotation decreased from 56° (sd=6.6) to 47° (sd=8.5). These serial measurements of the passive range of hip rotation were thought to confirm Pitkow's description (1975) of the spontaneous reduction of the hip external rotation contracture of the newborn.

A hypothesis to explain excessive femoral anteversion in cerebral palsy with spastic paralysis of the lower limbs can be constructed with the experimental and clinical data available. These children are born with spastic paralysis that results in spasticity of the iliopsoas muscle so that the newborn hip-flexion contracture persists. The persistent pull of spastic hip flexor muscle does not permit the stretching of the anterior capsule of the hip joint as in normal infants when the hip extends. The lack of hip extension decreases the torque strains on the proximal end of the femur, and derotation cannot occur. We might then deduce that persistent flexion contracture of the hip from birth causes persistence of the infantile femoral anteversion which generally exceeds that of the skeletally mature human.

In-toed gait and femoral anteversion

Why does excessive femoral anteversion cause the in-toed gait seen in some normal and cerebral-palsied children? The best explanation was offered by Merchant (1965), who constructed a mechanical model to study the function of the gluteus medius. This muscle is a major stabilizer of the pelvis, and by its contraction during the stance phase of gait allows the shift of the trunk and its center of gravity over the head of the femur. With Merchant's model the hip abductors exerted optimum force when the insertion of the abductor muscles on the greater trochanter were in a neutral relationship to their origins on the ilium. In femoral antetorsion the greater trochanter is in a posterior position with the femur in neutral rotation; thus, in order to gain optimum strength of the hip abductor during the stance phase of gait, the greater trochanter must shift from its posterior position by internal rotation of the femur. This internal rotation of the femur is necessary to shift the trunk laterally during the stance phase for optimum efficiency and energy conservation during forward progression. Clinical observations seem to confirm this explanation. Normal children who in-toe due to excessive femoral anteversion often do so more toward the end of the day when they are fatigued.

Radiographic measurements of the degree of femoral anteversion can be made with a variety of techniques. In the Magilligan technique (1956), an anterior-posterior radiograph of the hips is made with the hips and pelvis in neutral rotation; the femoral neck-shaft angle is measured on the film. Next, a true lateral radiograph is made with the hip in neutral rotation and with the film cassette held on the lateral aspect of the pelvis and femur, and parallel to the neck angle as measured on the first film. The projected angle of anteversion on this second film is obtained by drawing one line along the shaft and another along the center of the neck. Based upon a trigonometric calculation, the angle of rotation of the neck can be worked out. Magilligan constructed a chart so that the true angles of femoral anteversion could be determined without calculations, using the angles of femoral inclination derived from the two films.

In the Ryder-Crane technique (1953), an anterior-posterior radiograph with the hips and pelvis in neutral rotation is made to measure the neck-shaft angle on the film. The second radiograph is an anterior-posterior projection with the hips abducted exactly 30° and flexed 90°; the limb is held on a special frame (MacEwen 1972). The projected angle of femoral neck anteversion is measured by a line through the neck and a second line along the horizontal reference marker of the frame. Trigonometry calculates the true angle of anteversion. Ryder (1972) produced computer-generated tables so that the true angles of anteversion and femoral neck-shaft could be easily determined from the two measurements obtained. This method is reasonably accurate, with a reported error of ±10°.

The disadvantage of the Magilligan technique is the demand for a true lateral radiograph of the hip. The disadvantage of the Ryder-Crane technique is the requirement for the hip to be abducted 30°; in cerebral palsy this might not be possible if the child has spastic and contracted hip adductor muscles.

Other techniques are fluoroscopic (LaGasse and Staheli 1972), axial tomographic (Hubbard and Staheli 1972), computerized axial tomographic (Peterson *et al.* 1981) and ultrasonographic (Graf 1983, Phillips *et al.* 1985). All methods have been compared for accuracy. Ruby *et al.* (1979) studied the fluoroscopic and biplane methods and concluded that both were comparable in accuracy, but he favoured the Ryder-Crane technique. Computerized axial tomography has the advantage of a more direct visualization, and the radiation can be justified in special problem cases, but its routine use is questionable.*

*At the Stanford University Medical Center the mean skin dose from CT scan is 2.4rads to the adult pelvic area, 0.6rads to the male gonads and 2.6rads to the bladder. Compared with plain radiographs using earth-filtered screens, the active bone-marrow dose from a radiograph of the pelvis of a

Now that we know excessive femoral anteversion exists and can explain the in-toed gaits of children with spastic diplegia, is radiographic confirmation necessary in every case? It seems unlikely that more studies are needed to prove the point. A more prudent policy would be to rely on the published data and the clinical examination; the radiographic examinations could be reserved for special structural problems in the hip as part of the preoperative planning. Horstmann and Mahboubi (1986) have recommended CT scans of the hip in planning reconstructive surgery. The passive range of rotation of the hips, with the hips extended, will show internal rotation greater than 60° and external rotation less than 30°. A range of internal rotation of the femur in the 70° to 90° range, and external rotation of less than 20°, is good evidence of excessive anteversion. Computerized axial tomography, as well as magnetic resonance imaging, can be of enormous value in defining the location and integrity of the femoral head in relationship to the acetabulum in the analysis of structural changes in the hip joint.

Surgical procedures to correct hip internal rotation

Posterior transposition of the origin of the tensor fascia femoris was originally described by Durham (Edmonson 1963). I have never performed the procedure, but saw negative results from it many years ago. Majestro and Frost (1971) documented that this operation failed to correct the deformity.

Adductor myotomy with anterior branch obturator neurectomy or *transfer* of the adductor origins to the ischium has not been uniformly successful in overcoming hip internal rotation (Majestro and Frost 1971, Baumann 1972).

Neurectomy of the superior gluteal nerve was tried by Majestro and Frost (1971); this also failed.

Gluteus medius and minimus tendon transfer was the innovation of Steel (1980), who described the method and his results in 26 patients (42 hips) with a follow-up period from three to 11 years. Only six hips were failures, because they had a severe Trendelenburg gait and sign; none had this gait and sign preoperatively. Four of these five patients had a postoperative avulsion of the transferred greater trochanteric fragment and tendon; three of these were re-explored, and the avulsed fragment of bone with the tendon was reattached with a good final result. One patient had a severe Trendelenburg gait after a bilateral transfer without evidence of avulsion of the tendon. Steel also followed the course of femoral antetorsion in 10 patients (13 hips) who had the procedure between the ages of five and eight years. The femoral anteversion decreased from a range of 43° and 64° to between 18° and 36° at skeletal maturity. Although Steel had no postoperative subluxations or dislocations, one of three patients on whom I performed the procedure for severe hip internal rotation, and who had an excellent result, developed a painful subluxation three years postoperatively. Was this due to the anteverted head and neck of the femur (and possibly hyperelasticity of the

---

one-year-old child is 3 millirads (millirad=$\frac{1}{1000}$ of a rad) for an anterior-posterior view, and 2 millirads for a lateral view. At age five years an anterior-posterior view of the pelvis delivers 5 millirads (Bleck 1984). The ultrasonographic technique was studied by Phillips *et al.* (1985), who concluded it was too inaccurate to be useful.

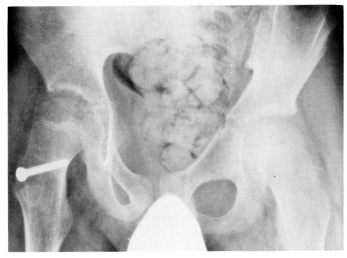

Fig. 8.38. Gluteus medius and minimus tendon insertion transfer to the anterior-lateral aspect of the proximal femur. Screw used to secure fixation. Note: three years postoperative this patient developed a painful subluxation of the hip. He was partially weight-bearing in a walker.

joints as well) gradually rotating out of the acetabulum, due to the change from internal to external rotation? This patient walked with an assistive device and thus was consistent with all other patients who develop subluxation of the hip. Independent walkers with hip-flexion contractures and femoral antetorsion do not subluxate; they internally rotate, and thus keep the hip located.

The operation consists of removing the tendinous insertion of the gluteus medius and minimus with a thin sliver of bone from the greater trochanter. The tendon and muscle is freed on all surfaces and then anchored to the bone of the femoral shaft just distal to the intertrochanteric line exposed by distal stripping of the vastus intermedius origin. The fixation can be done with two crossed pins, staple or screw. I prefer the latter (Fig. 8.38). A plaster spica holds the hip in external rotation and in 10° less than the maximum range of abduction for six weeks.

Although this ingenious approach to in-toed gait in cerebral palsy produced dramatic and excellent results, as shown in his motion pictures, I have not found very many patients who fit his criteria in patient selection. I am also fearful of the postoperative Trendelenburg gait. My criteria for selection of the patient are:

1. Severe in-toeing due to femoral internal rotation throughout the stance phase and bad enough to impair function: *e.g.* tripping and/or recurrent varus strain of the ankle.

2. A hip-flexion contracture less than 10°, no adduction contracture, hamstrings lax enough to permit 30cm stride length and a plantigrade foot (Steel 1980). This combination is difficult to find in most of my patients with spastic diplegia. A hip-flexion contracture could conceivably be made worse because the transferred muscles and tendons pass anterior to the hip.

329

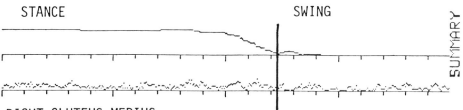

STANCE   SWING

RIGHT GLUTEUS MEDIUS

Fig. 8.39. Gait EMG. Summary computer plot of seven gait cycles in patient with spastic diplegia and hip internal rotation gait. Gluteus medius continuous activity in stance and swing.

3. A positive increased stretch reflex in the gluteus medius and minimus elicited with the patient prone and the knee flexed 90°. The involved limb is pushed sharply into external rotation from which a rebound into internal rotation connotes a positive test (Steel 1980). I have found interpretation of this test rather equivocal.

4. At least 20° of external rotation passively with the hip extended, and prolonged electrical activity of the gluteus muscle throughout the stance phase at least in the gait electromyogram and with a fine wire electrode in the muscle (Fig. 8.39). Most of my in-toeing patients have limited external rotation to 20° or less due to the excessive femoral anteversion.

5. I would *not* recommend the procedure if compensatory increased tibial-fibular torsion has developed. In these patients the knees turn in but the feet turn out or are straight ahead, so that the subjective disability is minimized (if trousers or slacks are worn to hide the gait abnormality); the objective disability is not usually significant.

6. The in-toeing must be due to femoral internal rotation and not the pelvis, as pointed out by Tylkowski *et al.* (1982).

7. Those patients who have more severe defects in their equilibrium reactions (usually good side-to-side but borderline anteriorly and completely deficient posteriorly as described in Chapter 2) may be poor candidates. They might fit into Tylkowski *et al.*'s (1982) group III patients delineated in the preceding paragraphs.

Their inability to stand on one leg is accompanied by the whole body falling to the unsupported side plus a Trendelenburg drop of the pelvis which is due to lack of proprioceptive 'awareness' and selective motor control. The true positive Trendelenburg sign is due to abductor muscle weakness and the pelvis drops on the unsupported side; the trunk may lean but the whole body does not. There is awareness of the instability, and the child tries to adjust and prevent a fall. Neither case seems to be appropriate for the operation, which may risk a postoperative Trendelenburg gait.

To correct the crouch gait, Steel uses the prone-lying rectus femoris test in which the knee is sharply flexed and a rise of the buttocks connotes a positive test. If so, Steel does a tenotomy of both heads of the rectus femoris (1980). In conjunction with the operation, Steel also performed Achilles tendon lengthening, adductor myotomies and hamstring lengthenings. It is probably too much to expect a single operation to correct all the defects.

330

TABLE 8.VI

Passive ranges of hip internal and external rotation preoperatively and postoperatively iliopsoas recession at follow-up of six years (range three-14 years)

Age at surgery (years)	Preoperative IR ER (degrees)		Postoperative IR ER (degrees)	
11	80	40	50	30*
9	80	5	80	20
5	80	30	80	10
13	70	15	65	15
5	75	20	45	40*
6	80	45	80	10
12	70	20	45	15*
10	90	20	70	20*
9	80	0	70	20*

IR = internal rotation; ER = external rotation
*Significant decrease in internal rotation >10°

Semitendinosus transfer to the anterior-lateral femur (Baker and Hill 1964, Sutherland *et al.* 1969) has had unpredictable results in my experience. If the patient has underlying quadriceps spasm, the removal of one hamstring may be sufficient to unbalance the spasticity between the hamstrings and quadriceps so that a postoperative spastic quadriceps gait with little or no knee flexion results. This gait will be more disabling and more energy-consuming than walking with hip internal rotation. I have deleted this procedure from my roster of operations in cerebral palsy.

Iliopsoas recession. In the follow-up of my patients who had this procedure, I noticed that some gradually decreased their passive range of hip internal rotation in a period of three to five years, and the objectionable in-toed gait diminished; further surgery to reduce this in-toeing was unnecessary (Bleck 1971*a*). In the original series of 25 patients who had iliopsoas recession, 21 were followed up for between seven and 10 years. In this group, seven had subsequent derotaton subtrochanteric femoral osteotomies; three were bilateral and four were unilateral. In those who did not have sufficient in-toeing during gait to recommend an osteotomy, the mean age at the time of the iliopsoas recession was seven years. The 61 patients (116 hips) had a mean preoperative hip internal rotation of 76° (range 65° to 90°) and a postoperative mean of 59° (range 30° to 90°). A sample of nine patients whose age at surgery was a mean of 8.9 years (range five to 13 years), and who were followed for a mean of six years (range three to 14 years), indicates in more detail what might be expected regarding hip internal rotation postoperatively. Table 8.VI lists the preoperative and postoperative passive ranges of hip internal and external rotation in this group. Five decreased the range of hip internal rotation more than 10°, and four had no change. This piece of data reconfirmed my original findings (Bleck 1971*a*) that after iliopsoas recession in spastic diplegic children who walked unassisted, there was about a 50 per cent chance of hip internal rotation during gait decreasing to an acceptable degree in three to four years. Only one patient had a bilateral derotation femoral osteotomy six years postoperatively because, although his gait was functional, the appearance was disturbing to him. I have preferred to wait and ask the patient, who is usually over age 10 years, to make the decision for femoral rotation osteotomy. This decision is obviously a value judgement.

Preoperative radiographic measurements of femoral anteversion were made with the Ryder-Crane technique in only six patients; these ranged from 55° to 73°. I have not performed postoperative radiographic measurements because of the common fear of excessive radiation. In my original series reported (Bleck 1971a) two patients had preoperative and postoperative radiographic measurements of femoral anteversion with the Magilligan technique. At follow-up ($4\frac{1}{4}$ years and $2\frac{2}{3}$ years) the anteversion decreased 8° (right hip) and 10° (left hip) in one and 24° (right hip) and 13° (left hip) in the other. No definitive statement can be made regarding the reduction of the angle of femoral anteversion, except that the passive range of internal rotation beyond 60° and the limitation of external rotation to less thn 30° does correlate with the anatomical change in rotation of the proximal end of the femur and with the observed internal rotation of the femur throughout the stance phase of gait.

After the correction of a hip-flexion deformity before the age of seven to eight years, my policy of waiting for spontaneous decrease of femoral anteversion is based upon the data that femoral torsion does not change in normal children after the age of eight years (Fabry *et al.* 1973, Fabry 1977). Our own study on the possible mechanism of derotation of the proximal end of the femur on extension and external rotation of the hip indicates that the earlier hip extension is obtained, the more likely correction of the torsion will occur. Certainly the data show exceptions to the decrease in hip internal rotation after correction of the hip-flexion contracture. In Table 8.V are six patients (aged nine to 13) who had significant decreases in their range of hip internal rotation on follow-up. This could be due to greater ligamentous laxity, which does vary in degree within the population; we did not test for this in these patients (Wynne-Davies 1970, Bleck *et al.* 1981). Increased laxity of the capsular ligaments might allow some children's hips to gain a greater degree of rotation in extension after the flexion contracture has been partly corrected. Also chronological age does not always correlate with skeletal age; children who have cerebral palsy, in particular, may have growth retardation (Horstmann 1986).

Derotation femoral osteotomy has produced definite and permanent results (Majestro and Frost 1971, Bost and Bleck 1975, Tylkowski *et al.* 1980, Hoffer *et al.* 1981). My policy has been to perform this operation in children in whom a marked in-toed gait persists after the age of eight, whose major deformity is femoral rotation and not pelvic rotation, and whose passive range of hip internal rotation is 70° to 90°, and whose external rotation is limited to less than 30° with the hip extended.

The site of the osteotomy is either subtrochanteric or supracondylar. Hoffer *et al.* (1981) prefer the supracondylar level because the femur can be sectioned here through a very small incision, blood loss is minimal and a long-leg plaster rather

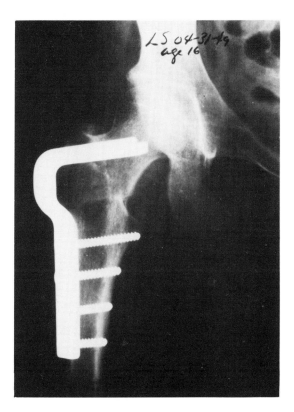

Fig. 8.40. Hip compression nail-plate (ASIF) for subtrochanteric derotation osteotomy.

than a hip spica, which would be necessary for osteotomies at the subtrochanteric level, secured with pin fixation. Threaded pins were inserted through the lateral to the medial cortices of the femur above and below the osteotomy site, with the distal pin at an angle to the proximal for the intended correction, so that the foot during gait would not exceed 15° of external rotation from the line of progression. The pins were removed after four to eight weeks and the long-leg plaster replaced. Early weight-bearing was encouraged; the usual time of immobilization was eight weeks.

Supracondylar osteotomy does have some complications. In Hoffer *et al.*'s 1981 report of 11 patients, three had pin-tract infections which subsequently healed; two had a 10° limitation of knee extension which resolved in six months; one required wedging of the plaster before healing was secure to correct anterior-posterior angulation of the distal fragment.

Thompson *et al.* (1986) made an even smaller incision to derotate the femur at the supracondylar region. Their operation also used two threaded Steinman pins above and below the osteotomy site. The method was percutaneous in that they drilled the cortices of the supracondylar region of the femur, performed a manual osteoclasis, derotated to the desired degree and immobilized in a long-leg or spica plaster five to nine weeks. Of their 19 patients, 11 had a 'gait abnormality'; 14 patients had cerebral palsy. They reported good results with only two complica-

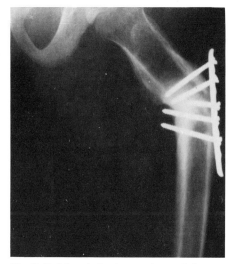

Fig. 8.41 *(above)*. Inadequate internal fixation for femoral derotation osteotomy.

Fig. 8.42 *(right)*. Persistent anterior rotation of pelvis after overcorrection on femoral internal rotation with derotation osteotomy. 0° of hip internal rotation = 0° of pelvic external rotation.

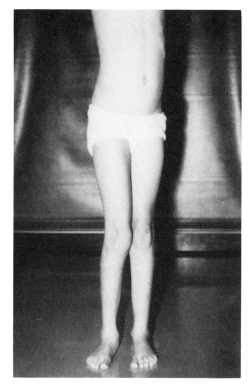

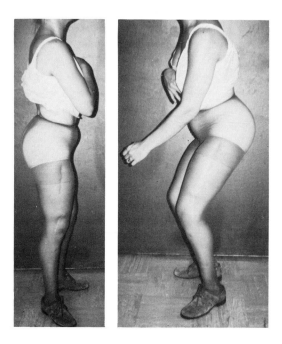

Fig. 8.43. Spastic diplegia, age 16 years, postoperative bilateral subtrochanteric derotation osteotomy. *Left:* hip-flexion contracture increased; spastic quadriceps; lumbar lordosis. *Right:* compensation for hip-flexion contracture only with knee flexion.

334

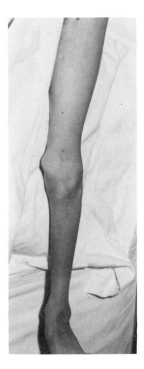

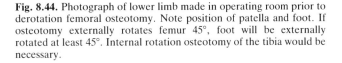

Fig. 8.44. Photograph of lower limb made in operating room prior to derotation femoral osteotomy. Note position of patella and foot. If osteotomy externally rotates femur 45°, foot will be externally rotated at least 45°. Internal rotation osteotomy of the tibia would be necessary.

tions: 5° of varus angulation and one pin breakage. An additional patient required knee manipulation under anesthesia.

There can be little argument with these good results of supracondylar osteotomy. I have preferred the subtrochanteric osteotomy with secure internal fixation: originally with the Jewett nail but in the last 20 years the right-angled hip compression nail (ASIF) (Fig. 8.40). My fears concerning supracondylar osteotomy were: (i) immobilization of the knee and subsequent stiffness when we know the knee is more determinant of gait; (ii) posterior angulation of the distal fragment causing genu recurvatum, and (iii) pin-tract infection. Staheli *et al.* (1980) reported a 15 per cent complication rate with derotation subtrochanteric femoral osteotomy in children who had femoral torsion, which does occur with indequate internal fixation (Fig. 8.41): but we had no infections or failures of fixation using the hip-compression nail in 24 spastic diplegic patients (31 hips) (Bost and Bleck 1975). Complications noted early in my experience (not always in patients on whom I had performed the procedure) were: (i) overcorrection of the internal rotation so that the toe-out was excessive and disabling: (ii) overcorrection of the internal rotation which prevented external rotation of the pelvis on the hip and resultant persistent anterior rotation of the pelvis evident in unilateral osteotomies (Fig. 8. 42); (iii) an increase in the hip-flexion contracture postoperatively (Fig. 8.43), and (iv) failure to recognize concomitant compensatory external tibial torsion (+30°), resulting in markedly excessive lateral rotation of the foot from the line of progression (Fig. 8.44).

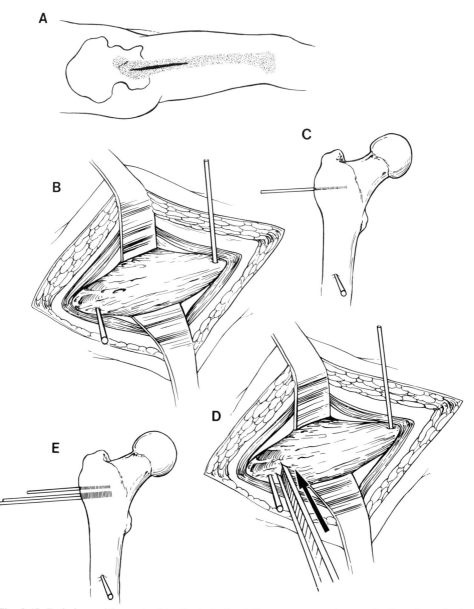

Fig. 8.45. Technique of femoral subtrochanteric derotation osteotomy. *A:* posterior-lateral proximal femur from trochanter and extended distally. *B:* fascia lata split and vastus lateralis separated in its posterior portion to expose femoral shaft subperiosteally. *C:* two Steinman pins inserted at appropriate angle of derotation desired. *D, E:* blade guide inserted distal to the guide pin. Localization and blade length determined with fluoroscopy image intensifier.

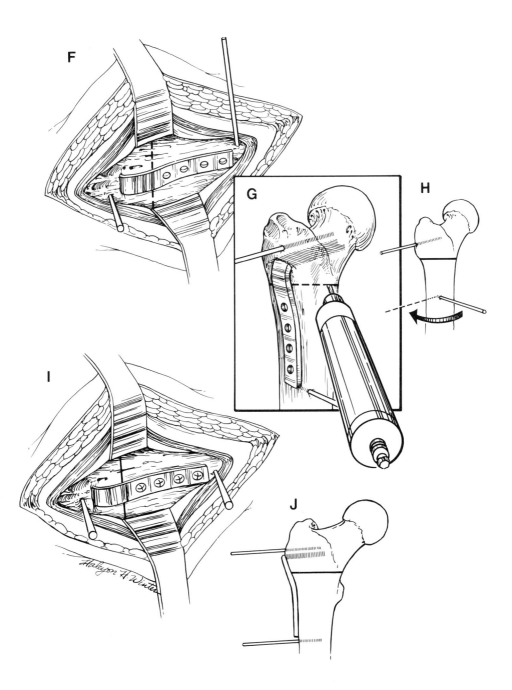

Fig. 8.45, *contd. F:* blade and plate portion inserted. *G:* osteotomy through subtrochanteric region is made parallel with the blade. *H:* proximal fragment held in internal rotation and distal portion of femur externally rotated the desired degree. *I:* pins now parallel and plate fixed to femoral shaft with screws. *J:* schematic representation of completed osteotomy. Pins, if used, are removed. Note that blade portion of device is parallel to osteotomy to assure compression forces, secure fixation and rapid union.

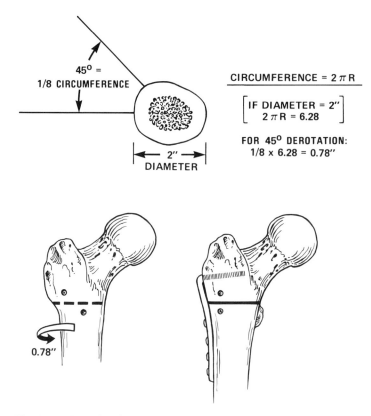

$$\text{CIRCUMFERENCE} = 2\pi R$$

$$\left[\begin{array}{l} \text{IF DIAMETER} = 2'' \\ 2\pi R = 6.28 \end{array}\right]$$

FOR 45° DEROTATION:
1/8 × 6.28 = 0.78''

45° =
1/8 CIRCUMFERENCE

2''
DIAMETER

0.78''

Fig. 8.46. Rinsky (1980) method of determining degree of rotation for derotation osteotomy: measure diameter of femoral shaft; calculate circumference = 2πR; then divide circumference by amount of rotation desired; *e.g.* if 45° = ⅛ circumference (360°). Then mark proximal portion of femur with drill hole; measure calculated distance and drill second hole distal to intended site of osteotomy. After the osteotomy, rotate so that the two drill holes are in alignment.

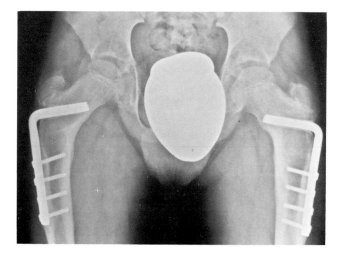

Fig. 8.47. Modified 90° hip-compression nail (Ted Nichols MD, Palo Alto, California). This avoids the lateral bump of the ASIF nail, which can cause a trochanteric bursitis and tent the skin of thin patients. Radiograph is of a healed bilateral subtrochanteric osteotomy of a 12-year-old boy with spastic diplegia.

338

Operative technique of derotation subtrochanteric femoral osteotomy

Because a hip-flexion contracture is inevitably found in spastic diplegic patients who have excessive femoral internal rotation during gait, I perform an iliopsoas recession or lengthening at the time of the osteotomy unless the flexion contracture has been previously corrected (Fig. 8.45).

The subtrochanteric osteotomy is done through the usual lateral approach to the proximal femoral shaft; the incision extends proximally to the tip of the greater trochanter. The origin of the vastus lateralis is detached, and through the posterior portion of this muscle the femur is stripped subperiosteally to expose the entire shaft all around. It is necessary to detach the posterior intramuscular septum from the linea aspera.

I no longer use Steinman pins in the proximal and distal fragments to determine the angle of derotation desired. With the hip in internal rotation, a guide pin is introduced into the basal region of the femoral neck at a 90° angle to the shaft; this pin is placed slightly more superior to the intended line where the blade of the hip-compression nail is to be inserted. Radiographic control with the image intensifier is used throughout the procedure. The special chisel for the nail is then inserted to create the channel for the blade portion and, if in the correct position on both anterior-posterior and lateral radiographic fluoroscopic projects, the blade of the nail is driven into the bone. The holding device which is used to drive in the blade is kept on it so that the hip can be maintained internally rotated.

To determine the degree of external rotation of the femur distal to the osteotomy, the preoperative passive ranges of motion need to be remembered. We strive to maintain 30° to 40° of hip external rotation after the osteotomy has been secured. The degree of external rotation can be reasonably estimated by marking the femoral shaft anteriorly with a visible line crossing the proximal and distal portions; an osteotome works best for this. Then, if the femoral shaft is almost a 360° circle, one quarter will represent 90° and one eighth will be 45°. So if the range of hip internal rotation is 80°, derotation of 50° will be about right. Rinsky (1980) has a more elegant and accurate method of determining the exact degree of derotation—a testimony to a superior mathematical mind (Fig. 8.46).

A transverse osteotomy at the subtrochanteric level about 1cm from the blade of the nail in the femoral neck is completed with a reciprocating saw. Bone-holding forceps (the c-type seem to work best) grasp the side-plate and femoral shaft, which is then rotated externally the desired degree while an assistant holds the proximal end with the nail-plate driver. The bone-holding forceps are clamped as securely as possible to secure the fixation. At this point the hip can be abducted so that the knee can be flexed over the edge of the table, with the range of internal rotation remaining checked. If satisfactory, the self-compressing plate is fixed to the shaft with the screws using the appropriate and particular technique. After two screws have been placed (out of a usual four to five) the range of hip internal rotation can be checked again. Closed suction drainage is used and wound closure is usual.

We have modified the original AO hip-compression nail by eliminating the lateral offset of the nail to a simple 90° 'L' hip-compression nail (Fig. 8.47). These are manufactured in infant, child, adolescent and adult sizes. The reason for eliminating the lateral protruded part of the original nail was to avoid discomfort over the greater trochanter in patients and tenting of the skin in especially thin children. In this way we are not forced to remove the nail before full recovery has occurred and at a time when schooling would be disrupted. In those patients who are near or beyond skeletal maturity, I see no need to remove the internal fixation unless it is causing discomfort.

The postoperative care is non-weightbearing for eight weeks. If iliopsoas recession or lengthening has been done, then bed rest with sitting up only for meals is instituted for three weeks, during which time bed exercises (quadriceps, hip external rotation, abduction and extension, foot dorsiflexion) are performed three times a day. The same exercises should be performed even if no iliopsoas surgery has been necessary. In most patients, even those who have unilateral osteotomies, a bed-wheelchair regime has been required; in bilateral cases this need is obvious; in unilateral osteotomies in spastic diplegia, crutch-walking and non-weightbearing on the operated limb risks falling down in some children because of the commonly associated deficient equilibrium reactions, particularly the posterior ones, which are lacking in almost all.

At the end of eight weeks, union is secure enough to permit resumption of full weight-bearing: beginning in parallel bars, graduating to crutches or walkers within two to five days, and without external support (for those who have never needed it) in one month (12 weeks postoperatively). No plaster immobilization has been used except for three weeks in those who had hamstring lengthenings at the same time, or short- or long-leg plasters when foot surgery was also done.

The advantage of this approach to subtrochanteric osteotomy has been the obvious ability to maintain muscle strength and joint range of motion while healing occurs. The disadvantages, in contrast to supracondylar osteotomy, are a longer and more precise operation, more blood loss (usually 350 to 500ml), a long lateral scar (10 to 15cm) on the proximal thigh, and the need for children to have a second operation a year or two later to remove the internal fixation.

An important preoperative observation is the degree of external tibial-fibular torsion. If it is a compensatory torsion of 35° to 45°, the derotation of the femur will make the out-toeing excessive, and can cause foot discomfort due to a compensatory pes varus. In these cases, therefore, an internal rotation osteotomy of the tibia and fibula should be planned at the same time as the femoral osteotomy or at a later date (Fig. 8.82). It may be that with the prospect of four osteotomies in the lower limbs, the patient and family will elect to do nothing.

The other preoperative assessment should include the measurement of the hip-flexion contracture which seems to increase after rotation osteotomy of the femur at any level. I believe this is due to increasing the tension on iliopsoas when the lesser trochanter is rotated in either direction (Fig. 8.48). If I discern a definite hip-flexion contracture of even 15° to 20°, and a femoral derotation osteotomy is contemplated, then a separate incision to lengthen the iliopsoas tendon is necessary. In the past several years, I have favoured lengthening rather than recession in these instances.

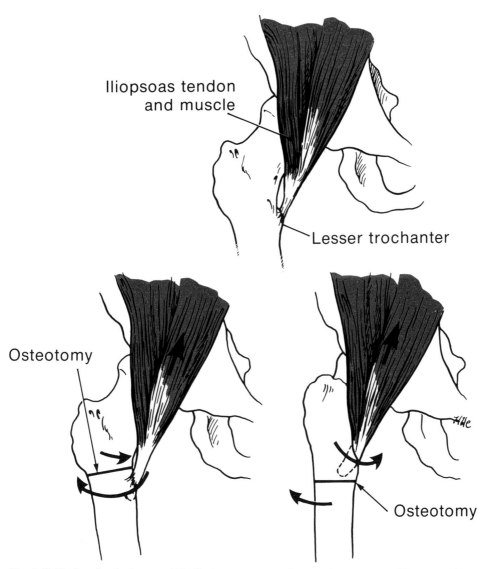

Fig. 8.48. Explanation for increased hip-flexion contracture after rotation osteotomy. No matter where the osteotomy is located, increased tension on the iliopsoas seems to occur.

Hip subluxation and acetabular dysplasia

Subluxation of the hip occurs in spastic diplegia when the child is only partly weight-bearing with the use of crutches or walkers. Dislocation rarely occurs in this kind of patient who at least has independent mobility with assistive devices to compensate for the deficient anterior and posterior equilibrium reactions. I have seen one patient who did have an acetabular dysplasia and dislocation of the hip at age three years. Because acetabular dysplasia in cerebral palsy is secondary to the dislocation, the etiology of the dislocation is probably congenital with superim-

341

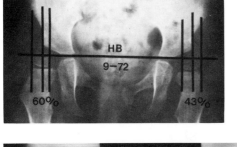

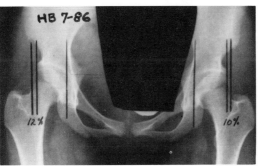

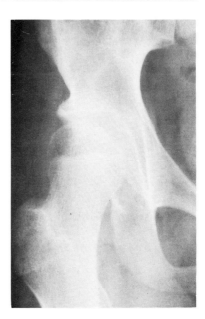

Fig. 8.49. Anterior-posterior radiographs of pelvis and hips. Patient HB, spastic diplegia. *Top left:* age three years, non-ambulatory; subluxation of both hips. Hip-flexion contracture 30°; abduction each hip 35°; internal rotation 90°. *Top right:* age 11 years. Eight years postoperative bilateral iliopsoas recession only. Patient now ambulatory. *Bottom left:* age 17 years, 14 years postoperative. *Bottom right:* age 17 years. Detailed radiograph of right hip. Ilium seems to hypertrophy laterally to cover femoral head. No apparent need for acetabular reconstruction.

posed spastic paralysis. This combination is rare, because the incidence of congenital dislocation of the hip is reported to be between eight and 10 per 10,000 births (Coleman 1978).

In spastic diplegia, full weight-bearing without support and the frequent hip internal rotation gait pattern prevents subluxation. The possible mechanisms for the development of subluxation and dislocation of the hip are delineated in Chapter 9.

From our data and experience on the prevention of spastic paralytic subluxation and dislocation of the hip, it seems apparent that reducing the spasticity and contracture of the major deforming muscles before the age of five years results in success in the majority of patients (Kalen and Bleck 1985). We found that adductor myotomy with anterior branch obturator neurectomy even before the age of five years did not necessarily prevent later subluxation or dislocation. We do have patients who did not have serious limitation of hip abduction but did have flexion contractures and subluxation of the hip before the age of five years; iliopsoas recession resulted in long-lasting reduction of the

342

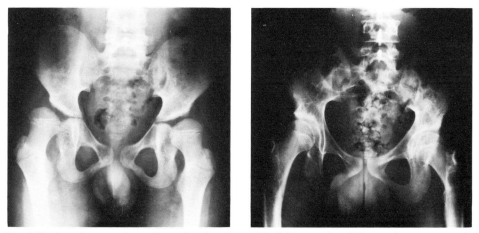

Fig. 8.50. Anterior-posterior radiographs of pelvis and both hips, patient PC, age nine years, crutch walker with spastic diplegia. *Left:* preoperative, and *right:* postoperative bilateral iliopsoas recession and derotation subtrochanteric osteotomy, eight years follow-up. Acetabular reconstruction not required.

subluxation and well-located hips without acetabular dysplasia on follow-up examination (Fig. 8.49).

Reimers (1980, 1985) disputed that the iliopsoas had any effect, on the basis of his results of iliopsoas lengthening in 11 patients to effect reduction of the subluxation and prevent dislocation of the hip. However, as pointed out in my letter to the editor on the subject (Bleck 1985), no study other than the one by Kalen and Bleck (1985) took into account the ambulatory status of the patient. None of our 99 patients walked independently; 48 walked with crutches, canes or walkers; 51 were non-walkers. In those who had adductor myotomy and iliopsoas recession the success rate in preventing further subluxation and additional surgery was 72 per cent, but for those who had adductor myotomy (with or without anterior branch obturator neurectomy) the success rate was only 36 per cent. In addition we found a 100 per cent success rate after iliopsoas recession and adductor myotomy in those who were ambulatory with assistive devices. The success of the soft-tissue surgery alone was in children younger than age five years. The median age in Reimers' 11 patients was 9.9 years. We never did answer the question posed by Reimers of whether the declining birth-rate in Denmark correlated with the decline in the stork population (Reimers 1985).

In summary, I would recommend iliopsoas recession or lengthening alone in spastic diplegic children under age five who have a subluxation of the hip, a flexion contracture of the hip and a range of abduction of each hip more than 30°, and either are ambulatory or have a good prognosis to walk. If this type of child has a range of abduction of the hip less than 30°, adductor myotomy should be added. If there is no flexion contracture and only an asymmetrical adduction contracture, the hip on the adducted side will *appear* uncovered. In these cases, release of the adduction contracture to correct the resultant pelvic obliquity will reduce this apparent 'subluxation'.

343

Varus and mainly derotation subtrochanteric osteotomy should be considered for children who have hip subluxation discovered after the age of five years (recognising the differences in skeletal age) and acetabular reconstruction for dysplasia, after age eight or nine years; femoral osteotomy by itself is not likely to result in acetabular remodeling toward normal coverage after this age (Tylkowski *et al.* 1980) (Fig. 8.50).

Knee
Knee-flexion deformity
The mechanism of the knee-flexion deformity may be due to spastic and contracted hamstring muscles, or secondary due to weakened triceps surae muscles. It is often accompanied by a hip-flexion deformity. As the result of the persistent knee-flexed posture, secondary contractures of the posterior capsule of the joint and shortening of the sciatic nerve occur.

The literature is replete with reports on the management of knee-flexion deformities in cerebral palsy (Keats and Kambin 1962, Hein 1969, Porter 1970, Hyashi 1970, Frost 1971, Banks 1972, Reimers 1974, Feldkamp and Katthagen 1975, Fixen 1979, Ray and Ehrlich 1979, Baumann *et al.* 1980, Sullivan *et al.* 1984, Simon *et al.* 1986). Because the knee flexion and extension are more important major determinants of an energy-efficient gait, and because a long 'reach' and stride-length are necessary for this efficiency, it is no wonder that the spastic hamstrings have received so much attention.

Knee-flexion contracture increases the energy requirements of gait. When the knee-flexion posture is 40°, calculations show an increase in energy requirements from the normal in men of 0.101kcal/m to 0.265kcal/m in cerebral palsy (Sutherland and Cooper 1978, Sutherland 1980).

ASSESSMENT

The clinical examination of the gait, hamstring spasticity and contracture have been described in Chapter 2. Of all the tests for hamstring contracture, the measurement of the popliteal angle with the hip flexed 90° is the best (normal <20°). Contracture of the posterior joint capsule is likely if the knee cannot be completely extended when the thigh is extended to rest on the examining table-top.

Gait electromyography of the hamstring muscles will demonstrate prolonged and out-of-phase action potentials, often throughout most of the stance phase. Our electromyographic studies have shown concomitant quadriceps prolonged and dysphasic contractions with the hamstring abnormal activity. This has been the case in most of our ambulatory patients with spastic diplegia. It seems that the two antagonistic muscle groups frequently balance one another, so that neither excessive knee flexion nor extension dominate (see Figs. 3.10, 3.12).

The clinical tests for quadriceps spasticity are: (i) to sharply flex the knee when the patient is prone—the increased resistance to knee flexion will be readily appreciated; (ii) with the patient seated and the knees flexed over the table edge—those with marked quadriceps spasticity will not be able to allow the knees to flex to 90°; passive knee flexion quickly done reveals the resistance of the

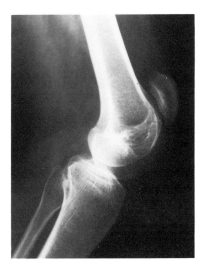

Fig. 8.51. Lateral radiograph of knee of 25-year-old female with spastic diplegia; severe knee pain, retropatellar. Patella alta due to spastic quadriceps. Both hamstring lengthening and proximal rectus femoris tenotomy relieved symptoms, and walking resumed without discomfort.

quadriceps due to spasticity. Voluntary knee extension from the flexed position indicates that the patient may have a good result from appropriate correction of the knee-flexed posture. In such patients a manual muscle test may possibly indicate the residual strength of the quadriceps. However, a more important concept is that surgery to weaken the hamstrings is essentially a 'balancing act', in which just enough quadriceps spasm will predominate to keep the knee extended at initial stance and to mid-stance and still allow the knee to flex in initial swing (normal 35°) to complete swing (normal 70°). In most patients this ideal result does not occur; but usually there is sufficient quadriceps spasticity to maintain correction so that postoperative orthoses are not required. Knee-ankle-foot orthoses with locked knee joints have only been necessary in older patients who have not only contracted hamstrings but also a joint capsule contracture which required a posterior capsulotomy of the knee joint.

Patients who have had weakening of the gastrocnemius-soleus muscle, following lengthenings or neurectomies, will have a 'crouch' position of knee flexion and ankle dorsiflexion. The function of the gastrocnemius-soleus is to prevent forward acceleration of the tibia in the stance phase of gait. When these muscles are too weak, ankle dorsiflexion increases and the strength and/or spasticity of the quadriceps is insufficient to maintain knee extension. To assess the effect of this weakness on knee flexion, the wearing of short-leg walking plasters with the ankle in neutral dorsiflexion can be helpful.

A lateral radiograph of the knee will often show the patella superiorly displaced and riding above its femoral articulation, often with elongation or fragmentation of its inferior pole. Special measurements of 'patella alta' in otherwise normal persons do not seem necessary in cerebral palsy. The structural change will be obvious. Patella alta in cerebral palsy seems to occur primarily because of a spastic quadriceps (vastus intermedius and rectus femoris) and secondarily to the flexed posture of the knee (Fig. 8.51).

Surgical weakening of the hamstring muscles is indicated if the knee-flexion deformity is greater than 15° during the stance phase of gait. This recommendation is based not only on clinical observations but on experimental studies as well. Patients who can tolerate the 15° of knee flexion are those who have good hip extension that locks the knee and brings the trunk forward anterior to the knee. In addition, the ankle plantar flexors serve to overcome the flexed knee at midstance and beyond (Perry *et al.* 1975).

Perry and associates (1975) in their study of knee-flexion posture during gait, measured the quadriceps force needed to stabilize the knee: in 15° of flexion, 75 per cent of the load on the femoral head was taken up by the knee; at 30° of flexion, 210 per cent; at 60°, 400 per cent. The quadriceps muscle force exerted at 15° of flexion was equivalent to 20 per cent of the maximal quadriceps strength; at 30° of flexion, this equivalent force was 30 per cent of the quadriceps strength. The quadriceps force needed when the knee is flexed beyond 15° is greatly increased because the weight-bearing surfaces of the femoral condyles are relatively flat in the first 15° of flexion; beyond this point the condyles are rounder and thus more muscle strength is required to maintain extension.

Biomechanical calculations have shown that a 70kg person who stands with the knee flexed 50° increases the quadriceps force to 752.4kg and the joint pressure to 1038.4kg (Kottke 1966). When patients who walk with flexion contractures of the knee are seen in the adult years, pain in the knee joint and inability to tolerate walking occurs due to degenerative arthritis of the knee joint. Adult patients whom I have seen with this disability had unremitting knee-joint pain; the initial stage of the degenerative arthritis began with patellar chondromalacia.

SURGICAL PROCEDURES

Because flexed knees are so obvious, the surgeon might be tempted to treat this deformity without considering the associated hip-flexion and equinus deformities. If there are structural deformities at the hip and ankle, these should be corrected at the same time as the knee-flexion deformity. If the hamstrings are weakened and a hip-flexion deformity of any degree exists, increased lumbar lordosis due to increased anterior inclination of the pelvis can be anticipated. If the hip-flexion contracture is over 15°, unacceptable pelvic and spinal compensation may be expected (Fig. 8.14). Studies of the sacrofemoral angle measured on the standing radiographs after hamstring lengthening have consistently shown a decrease in this angle which indicated the pelvic and lumbar spine adaptations to the hip-flexion deformity when the knee flexion was corrected (Bleck 1966).

HAMSTRING TENOTOMY, TRANSFER OR LENGTHENING?

Tenotomy of the hamstrings in spastic diplegia is almost certain to risk overcorrection in knee extension and a loss of knee flexion. The disability will be worse than with knee flexion.

Transfer of the hamstring tendon insertion to the femoral condyle has not fulfilled the promise that these muscles would then act as hip extensors (Eggers

1952). The procedure was progressively modified from transferring all the hamstrings to just transferring two and finally one medial hamstring. The total transfer often resulted in a straight knee which could not flex. The partial transfers of two hamstrings (usually the medial only) preserved more function, but knee flexion during gait was limited due to the unopposed action of the spastic quadriceps. The transfer of the semitendinosus only improved the results when the semimembranosus was lengthened. The only advantage that I could find with this latter procedure was perhaps that the semitendinosus could not retract promixally into the middle third of the femur, as occurred with tenotomy or if the z-lengthened tendon suture was too weak (Evans 1975). Because of the risk of knee hyperextension due to too much hamstring weakness, I have abandoned all hamstring transfers and the z-lengthening of the semimembranosus. The loss of the semimembranosus tendon strength probably accounts for the loss of its 'check rein' function and the resultant recurvatum of the joint.

FRACTIONAL LENGTHENING OF THE HAMSTRINGS

This is the technique that most surgeons now employ (Green and McDermott 1942). This method allows some control over the degree of lengthening, and although the muscles are weakened, some flexion power is preserved to begin initial swing during gait. Gage *et al.* (1987) quoted Perry's studies (1985) that initial swing is provided by the gracilis, short head of the biceps and sartorius. The usual hamstring lengthening does not include the short head of the biceps or sartorius, but very often the gracilis is tenotomized. Perhaps we should leave the gracilis intact in less severe cases.

Generally the results of fractional hamstring lengthening have been satisfactory. Rab (1985), in a three-dimensional study of hip musculature, determined the length of 27 hip muscles. The passive range of motion was correlated with known muscle excursion. Straight leg raising to 40° precluded normal gait. In his gait studies of children with a crouch gait, hamstring lengthening improved the gait; hamstring excursion did not change and in others it did increase as expected. In those in whom there was no change in hamstring excursion, dynamic overpull rather than 'tethering' was surmised.

Simon *et al.* (1986) analyzed the results of medial hamstring lengthening in 30 patients with a crouch gait. The preoperative gait analysis, compared with the postoperative studies, demonstrated that the greatest improvement averaged 20° in knee extension at heel contact. However, there was no change in the total knee motion from maximum flexion to extension.

Sullivan *et al.* (1984) also had success with medial hamstring lengthening in 39 children: 28 per cent were excellent, 68 per cent good and 4 per cent were unchanged. On follow-up from one to five years they noted a disturbing degree of out-toeing during gait which ranged from 15° to greater than 30° and noted the development of hind-foot valgus. I believe these results may be due to the unopposed action of the biceps femoris, which is known to be a strong lateral rotator of the tibia (Duchenne 1867, 1959). I have noted this in my patients in whom I did only medial hamstring lengthening prior to 1977. Bassett *et al.* (1976), in a long follow-up study on patients who had a medial hamstring transfer, found external tibial torsion in 79 per cent. Because of development of external tibial-fibular torsion beyond the normal, I have consistently lengthened the biceps femoris as well as the medial hamstrings using the technique of fractional lengthening (see below).

Others have reported success with hamstring lengthening. Feldkamp and Katthagen (1975) stated that 33 of 48 children under age nine years were improved; Ray and Ehrlich (1979) had 91 per cent improved walking after 23 patients had transfer of the semitendinosus to the lateral intramuscular septum; Hsu (1986) did z-lengthenings of the semitendinosus and gracilis and aponeurotic lengthenings of the semimembranosus and biceps femoris in 49 patients, 40 of whom improved their crouch position, while nine recurred and one developed recurvatum.

Hsu's method of hamstring lengthening is practically the same as mine has been for the past nine years. In my series of 33 patients who had a mean age of seven years (range three to 13 years), and were followed an average of 4½ years (range three to 11 years), had good results in correcting the flexed knee posture during stance phase; three had a recurrence of the knee flexion; two had slight hyperextension of the knee. One patient not in this series, who had only a semitendinosus lengthening, developed a severe hyperextended knee pattern almost immediately postoperatively (after the three-week plaster immobilization was removed). I had ignored the preoperative gait electromyograph which showed continuous activity of the quadriceps all through the stance phase of gait (some experts have interpreted this constant firing of the quadriceps as a response to the knee-flexed posture and not to the spasticity—see Mann 1983). Most of the patients in whom I have lengthened hamstrings for a flexed knee gait gained extension on stance phase but usually had only the minimum knee flexion on initial swing phase (20° to 30°). Can we improve these results and come closer to the normal function?

CO-SPASTICITY OF THE QUADRICEPS AND HAMSTRINGS

The 'stiff-legged' gait after hamstring lengthening has been recognized by Gage *et al.* (1987). These surgeons found that in gait analysis there is spasticity of both the quadriceps and hamstrings. To solve the problem of insufficient knee flexion on the swing phase, they performed the corrective surgery based on Perry's observations that inadequate initial knee flexion in gait might be due to inadequate function of the sartorius, gracilis and short head of the biceps. The surgical principle was derived from the experience of Waters *et al.* (1979) in their management of the 'stiff-legged' gait of adult hemiplegic patients. Gage *et al.* (1987) transferred *the distal insertion of the rectus femoris tendon* to the sartorius; the results have been quite satisfactory in most, although the transfer to the sartorius did not change the foot-progression angle to external rotation. In some patients more success in correcting the externally rotated limb was obtained by transfer of this distal rectus tendon to the iliotibial band. In the videotape of one patient who had a flexed knee gait, the postoperative improvement in both knee extension and initial flexion in swing phase was dramatic and approached normal.

Gage *et al.* (1987) did state that transfer of the rectus tendon to the sartorius was difficult because this soft and pliable muscle precluded a secure anchoring suture. They commented that perhaps the procedure was no more than a *distal rectus femoris release*. I would tend to agree. Recently (1986), I did a bilateral hamstring lengthening and a distal rectus femoris tendon recession in a 28-year-old spastic diplegic who was disabled with patellar pain, progressive 'sagging' of the knees into flexion, a short stride-length and only 10° to 15° of knee flexion on swing phase. EMG and clinical studies demonstrated both hamstring and quadriceps spasticity (vastus medialis and lateralis and rectus femoris; vastus intermedius not done) and contracture. The early postoperative result has been a dramatic improvement approaching a more normal gait.

Long ago we demonstrated co-spasticity of the quadriceps and hamstring muscles in spastic diplegia (Csongradi *et al.* 1979). Distal rectus femoris tendon recession might be considered in patients who have flexed knee gait patterns, definite findings of hamstring contracture, definite increased stretch reflexes of the quadriceps as well as resistance to complete knee flexion and confirmation with gait electromyography of prolonged and abnormal contraction of both groups of muscles. A crouch posture due to over-weakened calf muscles must be recognized before doing the above procedures. In addition, a contracture of the posterior capsule of the knee joint will limit extension despite hamstring lenthening and must also be dealt with. The more cautious surgeon may want to recommend the distal rectus femoris recession (or transfer to the sartorius) only for those patients who had limited knee flexion after hamstring lengthening and confirmation of quadriceps spasticity with gait electromyography.

The technique of distal rectus femoris recession is to expose the distal quadriceps tendon above the superior pole of the patella through a 4 to 5cm transverse incision. The insertion of the tendon on the patella is cut and the tendon cut away proximally from the adjoining fibers of the vastus medialis and lateralis so that when the knee is flexed 90° the rectus tendon slides proximally for an estimated 2 to 3cm. A few sutures can anchor it in this position. I favour commercially available knee immobilizers (foam-padded canvas aluminum-stave reinforced circular splints), which are somewhat similar to long leg cylinder plasters, but lighter and easier to apply, and which support the knee in extension. Walking and weight-bearing can begin in two or three days postoperatively. At the end of three weeks this support can be removed. As a precaution against falling, I recommend that the patient uses crutches for another three weeks while strength and knee mobility are regained (if the patient used crutches preoperatively, the operation will not eliminate their need postoperatively).

I must state that I do not have many cases like the above to report, and no long-term follow-up. However, based upon Gage *et al.*'s (1987) experience with the rectus femoris distal tendon transfer to the sartorius or iliotibial band, and their good results carefully analyzed with gait analysis techniques, either operation (recession or transfer of the distal rectus tendon, or to be precise, quadriceps tendon) seems logical in the selected patient with the criteria delineated in the preceding paragraphs. I have lengthened the quadriceps tendon in patients who had severe extension contractures of the knee after almost total hamstring

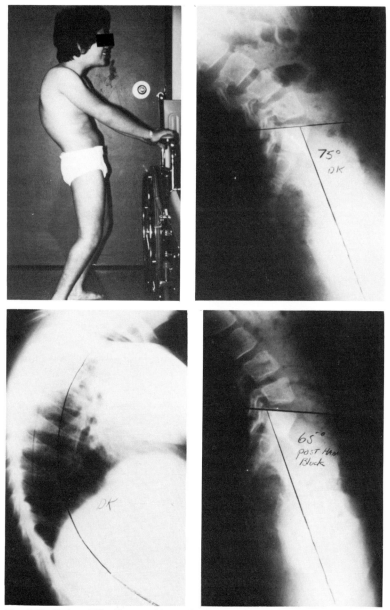

Fig. 8.52. Patient PK, 12-year-old spastic diplegic. *Top left:* photograph of posture, sagittal plane; thoracolumbar kyphosis. *Top right:* lateral radiograph of spine, pelvis and proximal femur with measurement of sacrofemoral angle indicating considerable posterior inclination of pelvis. *Bottom left:* lateral radiograph of spine, kyphosis. *Bottom right:* lateral radiograph demonstrating reduction in sacrofemoral angle after infiltration of hamstring muscles with 0.5 per cent lidocaine. Posture improved and sacrofemoral angle decreased 10°. Proximal hamstring myotomy would appear beneficial. Postoperative result: good correction of kyphotic posture. 10 years postoperative, had intractable patellar pain due to a spastic quadriceps. Symptoms relieved with distal rectus femoris tendon recession. Lesson: one change anticipates another.

350

obliteration, either by transfers to the femoral condyles or tenotomies. Quadriceps tendon lengthening did improve their ability to flex the knee, thus helping not only gait but also sitting.

PROXIMAL HAMSTRING MYOTOMY

Proximal myotomy of the hamstring origins was proposed by Seymour and Sharrard (1968). Their indications were a strong quadriceps, 'tightness' of the hamstrings which limited flexion of the hip, a short stride-length, straight leg raising limited to 30° or less and inability to sit upright with the knees extended. In nine children the results were satisfactory. These surgeons saw no advantage to this procedure over distal elongation of the hamstrings if there was a knee-flexion deformity. Drummond *et al.* (1974) thought the procedure quite satisfactory in 14 patients who had a 'tight hamstring gait' manifested by a short stride-length and who accomplished 'swing-through' by pelvic motion. Fixen (1979) thought the procedure was very effective. Reimers (1974) also seemed to prefer proximal myotomies, even though he had success with the distal lengthenings of the hamstrings. Hoffer (1972) had two patients whose knee-flexion contracture was not corrected after proximal hamstring release.

I would recommend this procedure mainly in the total body involved patient when adductor myotomy and iliopsoas tenotomy is done; the proximal origins can be sectioned through the same medial incision over the proximal femur (Rang *et al.* 1986).

There may be a rare patient who would benefit from proximal myotomy of the hamstrings. This is the patient who does not have a hip-flexion deformity but does have both spastic hamstrings and a strong quadriceps that does not allow knee flexion, so that the hamstrings extend the pelvis posteriorly with a secondary kyphosis of the thoracolumbar spine. A myoneural block of the hamstring muscles with 0.5 per cent lidocaine may help in evaluating the potential effects of the proximal myotomy. If the pelvis inclines anterior after the temporary paralysis of the hamstring muscles, a proximal myotomy may help to restore pelvic balance and decrease the compensatory and flexible kyphosis (Fig. 8.52).

POSTERIOR CAPSULOTOMY OF THE KNEE JOINT

In a knee-flexion deformity due to spastic and contracted hamstrings, the knee will completely extend when the limb is brought into extension and rests on the table-top. If the knee joint will not go into complete extension in this position, a contracture of the posterior capsule is likely. In these circumstances I am always prepared to do a posterior capsulotomy of the knee joint in addition to the hamstring lengthenings. In this case the hamstring lengthenings and posterior capsulotomy can be done through medial and lateral incisions over the distal femur and knee joint. I have found that relying on wedging casts to correct a residual knee-flexion contracture after hamstring lengthening risks posterior subluxation of the tibia, continued knee-flexed posture and recurrence of the flexion posture. When the knee is absolutely in complete extension, no quadriceps force is required to stand erect.

351

I have done this procedure for the past 10 years. Westin (1973) introduced the incision and the supine position to me and I have used it since. We always lengthen the biceps femoris as well as the medial hamstrings (this seems to have avoided the late development of excessive lateral rotation of the tibia). I do not use the incision described below if the patient has evidence of a contracture of the posterior capsule of the knee joint.

With the patient supine, an assistant flexes the hip 90° and extends the knee to its limit but not beyond and without force. A straight incision is made in the midline to the distal one third of the thigh, ending at the popliteal crease. We try to z-lengthen the semitendinosus. In little children with small tendons this is often not possible and a tenotomy results (by design or inadvertently). On follow-up evaluations it is not possible to ascertain the difference between those who had tenotomies or lengthenings of the semitendinosus. Others have made the same observation (Diamond 1978). The lateral aspect of the semimembranosus distally is freed of fat and connective tissue to expose the whole of its aponeurosis, which is incised in a v or delta manner. As the knee is extended, the ends of the aponeurosis pull apart and the muscle fibers also glide apart; some may tear but continuity is maintained. The aponeurosis on the lateral aspect of the biceps femoris is exposed and similarly incised as the knee is extended. Extreme force should not be exerted, to avoid stretching the sciatic nerve; a 20° popliteal angle is within the limits of normal. In severe contractures the gracilis tendon is also cut. However Perry (1985) recommends it should be saved, because of the rôle it plays in initiating the swing phase of gait (together with the sartorius and short head of the biceps).

If the knee cannot be completely extended and 5° to 10° of knee-flexion contracture remains, it is safer to apply a plaster to be wedged and gradually to extend the knee to the neutral position. Sudden forced extension risks a sciatic neuropathy.

A proximal rectus femoris tenotomy has been performed at the same time if the patient has evidence of a spastic quadriceps and chronic pain at the lower pole of the patella. The indications for distal rectus femoris tendon transfer or recession have been discussed in the preceding sections.

The *postoperative* immobilization is a cylinder plaster or fiberglass cast. A long leg plaster incorporating the foot is necessary if foot or ankle surgery has been done. If a slight flexion contracture of 5° to 10° remains (confirmed by lateral radiographs of the knee to measure the femoral-tibial angle), a long-leg plaster (not the plastic fiberglass type) will be necessary to permit gradual and repeated wedging of the knee to obtain complete extension. The patient is permitted to stand and walk beginning on the first postoperative day. The immobilization is removed in three weeks; walking is resumed as the best therapy.

Postoperative knee-ankle-foot orthoses with a drop lock at the knee are rarely necessary in children under age 12 after hamstring lengthening. Orthoses to prevent knee flexion while quadriceps strength is restored seem essential in older children and adolescents who have long-standing hamstring and posterior capsular contractures corrected by surgery.

If a flexion contracture of the posterior capsule of the knee joint is suspected preoperatively (as determined by the examination described previously in this section) then the midline posterior distal thigh incision to lengthen the hamstrings cannot be used. Instead the hamstrings are fractionally lengthened through medial and lateral longitudinal incisions over the distal thigh and knee joint. The approach to the capsule is from the lateral incision (Wilson 1929, cited by Crenshaw 1963); the iliotibial band can be divided and the biceps aponeurosis incised as previously described. Through the medial incision, the semitendinosus tendon is z-lengthened and the semimembranosus aponeurosis is incised in a v fashion. The hip is then flexed 90° and the knee gradually extended but not forced (this is no place for a 'macho' surgeon demonstration). The residual knee-flexion contracture will be apparent.

The hamstring tendons are reflected posteriorly together with the neurovascular bundle. The heads of the gastrocnemius muscle origins are detached from the femur and stripped distally to expose the joint capsule which is completely incised to obtain additional knee extension. Again do not use undue force. The sciatic nerve is contracted as well.

We also cut the insertion of the anterior cruciate ligament (Rinsky 1977). This helps prevent posterior subluxation of the tibia as the knee is extended (Somerville 1960). He maintained that in long-standing flexion contractures of the knee, such as occur in rheumatoid arthritis, the anterior cruciate ligament shortens and prevents the last few degrees of extension. We had not observed any instability of the knees postoperatively as a result of sectioning the anterior cruciate ligament in the intercondylar notch posteriorly.

The *postoperative care* entails a long leg plaster with ample soft padding over the anterior and posterior aspects of the knee and dorsum of the foot in order to bring the knee gradually into complete extension by progressive wedging of the plaster. This is accomplished by making a linear anterior hinge 7.5cm long in the plaster over the knee and the supracondylar region of the femur, where a circular cut is made in the plaster from medial to lateral. Usually on the third day postoperatively the plaster is cut for wedging, the patient placed prone and the knee extended to the point of pain tolerance and absence of paresthesias in the foot. A block of plastic or wood holds the wedge open; a single roll of cast padding around the area followed by plaster secures the position. It is simple then to remove this plaster, extend the knee again and hold the wedge open in the same manner. A lateral radiograph, using a large film with the knee joint in the center, permits more accurate measurement of the degree of extension of the tibia on the femur.

In all cases of posterior capsulotomy with hamstring lengthening, I plan to use a knee-ankle-foot orthosis (KAFO) with a drop-lock at the knee joint in six weeks postoperatively when the plaster is removed. It is important for the orthosis to be ready as soon as the plaster is removed. To delay application of the orthosis risks recurrence. In three to four weeks postoperatively, when the knee is straight, we remove the plaster and ask the orthotist to make the negative plaster mold of the limb. From this mold a positive plaster is made, from which the orthosis can be

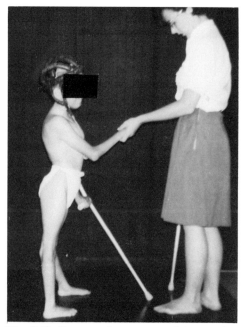

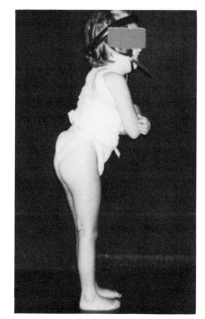

Fig. 8.53. Postoperative posture of knees after bilateral hamstring transfer. Preoperatively had a 40° knee-flexion posture. Genu recurvatum evident. Knee flexion limited to 30° due to quadriceps spasticity. A recurrence of knee-flexion contracture is preferable to this result.

Fig. 8.54. Posture of eight-year-old girl with spastic diplegia, postoperative bilateral semitendinosus transfer (I no longer do this procedure), semimembranosus lenthening and gracilis tenotomy. Untreated hip-flexion contracture causes lordosis and forward trunk lean to bring center of gravity of trunk anterior to ankle joint for stability.

constructed. The long-leg plaster is reapplied while the orthosis is being made in the two additional weeks of immobilization. As long as the knee is in extension, weight-bearing in the plaster can be encouraged.

After the orthosis is applied, active and active assisted knee-flexion and extension exercises can be done by unlocking the knee joint of the orthosis at least three times a day. The patient walks with the knee joints locked until the knee maintains extension at heel contact and throughout mid-stance of gait. Once this occurs, there will be no further need for the orthosis.

If the knee-flexion posture has been aggravated by weakening of the gastrocnemius-soleus muscles and excessive dorsiflexion of the ankle, the knee-ankle-foot orthosis can be converted to an ankle-foot orthosis (AFO) which will block the dorsiflexion of the ankle.

RESULTS AND PROBLEMS

Recurrence of the knee-flexion contracture has been the dominant concern of surgeons. Lottman (1976) examined 152 patients three years postoperative hamstring surgery, and found a 32 per cent recurrence rate: but this high a relapse rate is not the usual experience. We had a 9 per cent recurrence in a 4.5 year follow-up. Hsu (1986) reported 18 per cent recurred. In our first nine patients (18 knees) with cerebral palsy who had the additional posterior capsulotomies and anterior cruciate ligament insertion incisions for a flexion deformity of the knee, none recurred and there were no posterior subluxations of the tibia or anterior instability of the knee in a mean follow-up of two years (Page 1982). Problems other than recurrence have been more prominent and disabling:

1. Increased postoperative lumbar lordosis (Bleck 1975); to avoid this result the hip-flexion deformity should be corrected either before or during hamstring lengthening. Perhaps a hip-flexion contracture of less than 15° to 20° might be tolerated, but not 45° (Fig. 8.53).

2. Hyperextended knee gait. When the hamstrings are weakened the quadriceps spasticity becomes evident and can help maintain correction of the flexion contracture of the knees. However, too much quadriceps spasticity and overweakening of the hamstrings will lead to postoperative limited knee flexion on swing phase and genu recurvatum (Fig. 8.54). This straight knee gait will be more disabling than a knee-flexion contracture of 15°.

3. Failure to correct the knee-flexion deformity. This discouraging result is more common when the deformity has been allowed to persist in children older than 10 years. Possible reasons for this failure are: (i) inability to achieve complete extension of the knee due to secondary contracture of the posterior capsule— capsulotomy is required; and (ii) quadriceps weakness with lack of terminal extension and insufficient quadriceps spasticity to take up the slack in the stretched-out muscle. This is a rare result and confined mostly to older children who have walked with knees flexed more than 30°. Perhaps there is a case here for quadriceps augmentation by patellar tendon advancement.

4. Crouch position due to weakness and increased length of the triceps surae. It is better to underlengthen an Achilles tendon and have a bit of residual equinus or recurrence.

5. Sciatic neuropathy. A postoperative sciatic stretch paralysis may occur in patients with severe and long-standing knee-flexion contractures if too much force is exerted in extending the knee at the time of surgery. It may not be entirely avoidable, because how far to stretch the hamstrings is a matter of judgement. It could also occur by zealous passive straight leg-raising exercises postoperatively. If in doubt as to how much to extend the knee after hamstring lengthening, with or without posterior capsulotomy, it is probably better to plan on wedging casts postoperatively to extend the knee gradually. Health-care management types will have to realize that hospitalization will be longer than the statistical graphs and charts indicate to be the norm.

The symptoms of sciatic neuropathy include pain in the plantar aspect of the foot, paresthesias and hyperesthesia of the toes. A stretch paralysis usually recovers, but may take six months to a year.

PATELLAR TENDON ADVANCEMENT
This technique (Chandler 1933, Roberts and Adams 1953, Baker 1956, Keats and Kamblin 1962) no longer seems popular. The decline in interest possibly stems

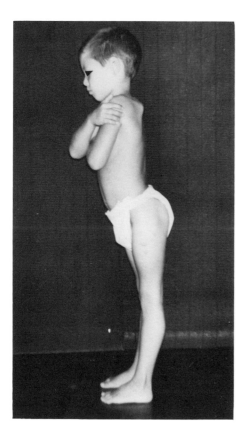

Fig. 8.55. Posture of seven-year-old with spastic diplegia. Hip-flexion contractures, spastic quadriceps with hyperextended knee gait pattern.

from the lack of need to restore the tension in the quadriceps muscle when hamstring lengthening is done early enough to avoid years and years of a persistent flexed knee gait. Furthermore, the operation of transfer of the patellar tendon distally, in children with open epiphyses, risks premature closure of the proximal anterior portion of the tibial physis when the patellar tendon is detached from its insertion. It has occurred even with the Baker modification (1956), in which the tendon was skived off its insertion rather than removed with block of bone.

Another possible problem with patellar advancement is the aggravation of chondromalacia patellae and accompanying knee pain. When the patella has been chronically displaced proximally and is out of contact with its opposite femoral area, degeneration of its articular cartilage occurs. Radiographs may reveal spur formation at the poles of the patella, fragmentation of its lower pole and elongation of the distal end (Kaye and Freiberger 1971, Rosenthal and Levine 1977). In children with spastic diplegia who have both flexed knees and a spastic quadriceps, patellar pain can be constant. In these cases lateral radiographs of the knee often show fragmentation of the distal pole of the patella (the mechanism appears to be the same as in 'jumper's knee').

I no longer do patellar advancements. I tried augmentation of the quadriceps with a transfer of the semitendinosus to the patella in spastic diplegia in a few patients, but dropped this operation too because the results were never better than neutral.

SUPRACONDYLAR CLOSED WEDGE OSTEOTOMY OF THE FEMUR

An osteotomy of the femur in the supracondylar region is an effective and safe correction for a flexion deformity of the knees in adults with spastic diplegia. The hamstrings are lengthened as usual. A wedge of bone with its base anterior is removed from the supracondylar region of the femur. The amount of bone to be removed is calculated preoperatively. The wedge is closed, and secure internal fixation can be obtained with a contoured lateral plate and screws (the two cancellous bone screws are best in the condylar area distal to the osteotomy) or an external fixator can be applied with appropriate fixation pins (lacking an external fixator, threaded Steinman pins joined with methylmerthacrylate cement can be used, but the pins should be incorporated in a long leg plaster).

A closed wedge extension supracondylar osteotomy will result in a loss of knee flexion equal to the amount of correction. The advantage of the osteotomy is that it shortens the thigh and relaxes the neurovascular structures. Sciatic stretch paralysis and vascular insufficiency are minimized.

Spastic hyperextension deformity of the knee

MECHANISMS

Two explanations for the hyperextended knee gait have been offered: (i) a spastic quadriceps (Csongradi *et al.* 1979), and (ii) poor regulation of ankle plantar-flexion power (Simon *et al.* 1978) (Fig. 8.55).

Although the spastic rectus femoris muscle was once thought to be an isolated entity (Duncan 1955, Sutherland *et al.* 1975) it is now clear that all segments of the quadriceps muscle can be spastic (Gage *et al.* 1987). In normal subjects, all four portions of the quadriceps contribute to knee extension; the vastus intermedius is a strong extensor (Perry and Lieb 1967).

The sophisticated study of genu recurvatum in spastic paralysis by Simon *et al.* (1978) pointed to a number of factors responsible. The most important factor was poor ankle plantar flexion; this caused an abrupt halt in tibial motion in early stance if the calf muscles were weak, and in late stance if they were strong. From this study Simon *et al.* recommended a rigid plastic ankle-foot orthosis to overcome the genu recurvatum.

INDICATIONS FOR SURGERY

If the patient has hyperextension of the knee during the stance phase of gait, and the knee does not flex sufficiently in swing phase to allow the foot to clear the floor, the gait is functionally disabling. Confirmation of the spasticity of the quadriceps is obtained by the clinical tests described in Chapter 2 and in this chapter. Electromyography will demonstrate the continuous and out-of-phase activity of the various parts of the quadriceps during level walking.

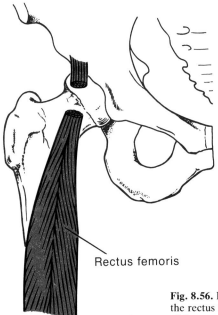

Rectus femoris

Fig. 8.56. Proximal rectus femoris tenotomy. The straight head of the rectus tendon is cut; the distal portion retracts to lessen some of the quadriceps spasm.

OPERATIVE PROCEDURES

Operative procedures to correct the hyperextended knee gait are the rectus femoris origin tenotomy (Duncan 1955) and, for more severe cases, the distal rectus femoris tendon resection or recession or transfer (Waters *et al*. 1979, Gage *et al*. 1987).

The operative technique for rectus femoris origin tenotomy is simple. The tendon can be approached through an oblique incision in the groin region about 1.5cm between the anterior superior iliac spine. The sartorius is retracted laterally, and after removing the investing iliacus fascia from the medial border of the tendon and clearing the tendon of the overlying fatty connective tissue, the direct head of the tendon can be picked up and cut near its origin and allowed to retract distally (Fig. 8.56).

The *results of rectus femoris tenotomy*, although not extraordinary, have improved gait by allowing a bit more knee flexion on initial swing (Sutherland *et al*. 1975). In more severe cases of quadriceps spasticity, the distal rectus femoris tendon transfer to the sartorius (or iliotibial band) or a recession may give much better results (see pp. 248–249).

Quadriceps tendon lengthening has been performed in patients (N=4) who had no knee flexion during gait due to severe quadriceps spasticity after total hamstring release; when seated they could barely bend their knees.

The operation was quite direct. Through a transverse incision the quadriceps tendon was z-lengthened and sutured with the knee flexed 45°. Plaster immobilization was for six weeks with the knees in 30° of flexion.

358

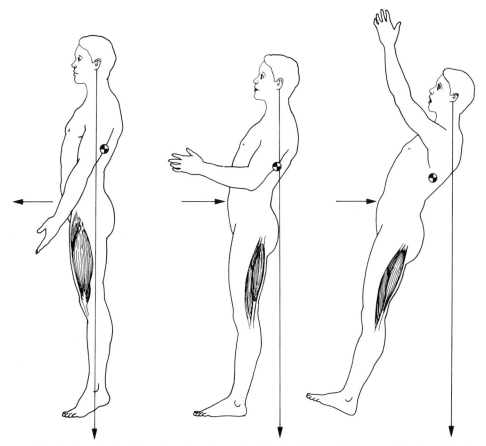

Fig. 8.57. Explanation for dynamic equinus in spastic diplegic children. *Left:* center of gravity of trunk anterior to the 10th thoracic vertebra. Line of weight-bearing falls anterior to ankle joint and between feet for stability. The equinus is necessary to bring line of weight-bearing anterior to center of gravity. *Center:* spastic hamstrings pull body posteriorly when feet are dorsiflexed and flat on floor. *Right:* patient falls backwards. Equinus necessary for stable posture.

The results have been satisfactory in permitting the knee to flex 75° to 90° when the patient was seated; their gaits, while not normal, were improved. A flexed knee posture did not result.

Foot and ankle

Equinus deformity

In spastic diplegia equinus is usually bilateral and almost always dynamic when the child begins to walk. Surgical lengthening at this age when no contracture of the triceps surae can be demonstrated is to be resisted. The risk is of weakening the calf muscle and a crouch posture for the physiological and mechanical reasons already given in the preceding section and in Chapter 7.

Dynamic equinus in some children with spastic diplegia appears related to

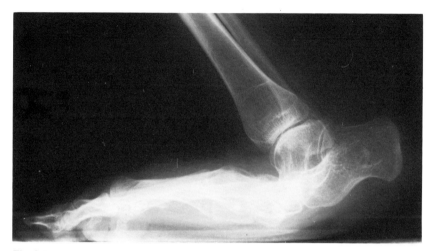

Fig. 8.58. Lateral radiograph on weight-bearing, spastic diplegia. Severe pes valgus; plantar-flexed talus and calcaneal equinus.

hamstring spasticity and contracture; the equinus is secondary. These children need the equinus to bring the center of gravity of their trunks anterior to the ankles and through the base of support between the feet. Their equilibrium reactions are deficient, especially posteriorly. The hamstrings pull the child backward and the center of gravity is then posterior to the base of support; this instability causes a backward fall and can only be corrected by assuming equinus to bring the center of gravity anteriorly (Fig. 8.57). In this type of equinus the child can place his feet firmly on the floor with at least neutral dorsiflexion of the ankles by flexing the knees so that he is in a sitting posture while trying to maintain the erect posture (see Chapter 2, Fig. 2.12).

It may be that in these cases of equinus the 'inhibitive casts' and their

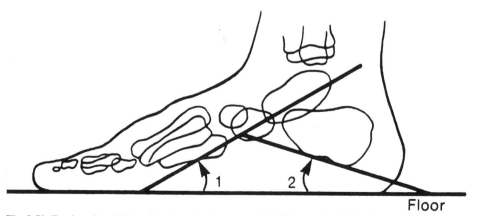

Fig. 8.59. Tracing of weight-bearing lateral radiograph of child's foot. Angle 1 is plantar-flexion angle of talus (normal mean 26.5°, SD 5.3); angle 2 is the dorsiflexion angle of the calcaneus (normal mean 16.8°, SD 5.6).

companion plastic ankle-foot orthoses can buy time until the equilibrium reactions are more developed, and thus overcome the equinus contracture. When the equinus persists and no contracture of the triceps surae can be found, the hamstrings are usually at fault. Fractional lengthening of the hamstrings does resolve the dynamic equinus more often than not. If in doubt about the mechanisms, one should use short-leg walking plasters to inhibit the equinus and then observe the knee posture and balance. Additionally, doubts on the efficacy of proposed gastrocnemius lengthening can be resolved by myoneural blocks of the muscle using 45 per cent alcohol injecting 3 to 4ml into four quadrants of the gastrocnemius (see Chapter 3, Fig. 3.19).

Pes valgus
Pes valgus is more common in spastic diplegia than pes varus. In one study of 230 patients, 94 per cent of hemiplegic children had pes varus; 64 per cent of the spastic diplegics and quadriplegics had pes valgus (Bennet *et al.* 1982). Of course, children with spastic diplegia have varus deformities of the foot; the management of these is discussed in Chapter 7.

Anatomy
The spastic pes valgus foot has an eversion and equinus inclination of the calcaneus and abduction of the midfoot which results in a prominence of the head of the talus medially. It is a flexible deformity until adolescence. Until that time of fixed changes, the foot can be passively manipulated into the corrected position by plantar flexion of the ankle and inversion of the foot.

Lateral radiographs of the foot when the patient is standing show greater than normal plantar flexion of the talus and varying degrees of loss of dorsiflexion of the calcaneus (Fig. 8.58). According to our studies, the normal plantar flexion of the talus is 26.5° (SD 5.3°). In children younger than five years, the normal plantar flexion of the talus can be as much as 35° so that a line through the center of the talar neck and body falls just inferior to the first metatarsal shaft. The normal calcaneal dorsiflexion angle is 16.8° (SD 5.6°) (Bleck and Berzins 1977) (Fig. 8.59).

On the anterior-posterior radiograph of the foot with the patient weight-bearing, the normal angle formed by a line bisecting the talar neck and another line parallel to the lateral border of the calcaneus is a mean of 18° (SD 5°). If this angle is greater than 25°, valgus is present; if less than 15°, the heel is in varus (Fig. 8.60).

Mechanisms
The *axis of rotation of the subtalar joint* has been compared to a mitered hinge; its axis is more horizontal than oblique, accounting for the greater degree of eversion than inversion of this joint. The mean angle of inclination of this joint projected on the sagittal plane when measured on anatomical specimens was 42°, with a great variation ranging from 20.5° to 68.5° (Inman 1976).

Spastic peroneal muscles abduct the mid- and forefoot excessively and continuously; this abnormal movement pulls the navicular laterally and with it the supporting plantar ligaments for the talar head. The result is plantar flexion of the

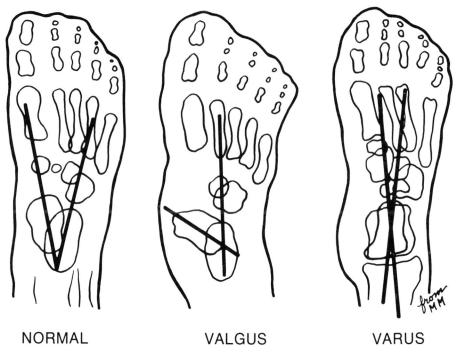

| NORMAL | VALGUS | VARUS |

Fig. 8.60. Tracings of anterior-posterior weight-bearing radiographs of children's feet. Talar-calcaneal divergence angles: normal mean 15; heel neutral; varus: less than 15°; valgus: more than 25°.

talus. Skinner and Lester (1985) analyzed the dynamic electromyograms in 13 CP children to observe their hind-foot valgus deformities. They described three different patterns of muscle activity to account for the valgus: (i) hyperactive peroneal muscles with a strong posterior tibial muscle; (ii) hyperactive peroneals with a weak posterior tibial; (iii) hyperactive extensor digitorum longus muscles (Fig. 8.61).

Orthopaedic surgeons have recognized the spastic peroneals as the major deforming force, and have lengthened the peroneus brevis in an attempt to prevent further deformity in young children (Nather *et al.* 1984). An electromyographic study of the posterior tibial muscle in spastic pes valgus came to the opposite conclusion: in five of six spastic diplegic children, the posterior tibial muscle was electrically silent. This led to the conclusion that without the counterbalancing effect of the posterior tibial muscle, valgus occurred (Bennet *et al.* 1982). Accordingly, transfer of the peroneus brevis to the posterior tibial tendon was proposed.

STANCE   SWING

Gastroc
Tibialis posterior
Peroneals

Fig. 8.61. Gait EMG. Computer plot of leg muscles in spastic pes valgus. Peroneals active in stance and swing phase. Posterior tibial also firing in both phases. Gastrocnemius normal activity.

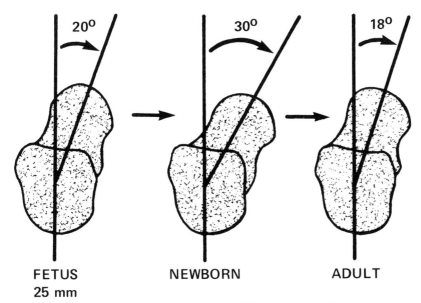

Fig. 8.62. Talar neck angles increasing from fetal life to newborn and normally decreasing at maturity.

Calcaneal plantar flexion due to gastrocnemius-soleus contracture contributes to the deformity but unfortunately cannot be the sole cause. If it were, Achilles tendon lengthening would not only prevent but also correct the flexible pes valgus. This we know does not occur. Equinus deformity is seen without valgus and also with varus deformities.

Variations in *ligamentous laxity* among children may account for the early development of severe pes valgus in some and not in others. This variation in laxity of connective tissues among individuals has been ascribed to defects in the cross-linking of collagen (Eyre 1984).

Persistent fetal medial deviation of the talar neck is an anatomical departure from the norm and may account for the internal axial rotation of the foot that is sometimes observed after arthrodesis of the talonavicular joint when the navicular is placed in its anatomical alignment on the talar head. The newborn talus has a greater degree of medial deviation of its neck at birth than in the adult form (Lisowski 1974) (Fig. 8.62). I believe that persistence of the newborn talar neck angle is one cause of in-toeing in children (Bleck and Minaire 1983). Some normal children who at first merely have in-toeing may develop pes valgus with a prominent head of the talus on the medial aspect of the foot.

Assessment

In addition to the examination of the deformity, the surgeon must confirm the flexibility and correctibility of the foot by passive manipulation. The foot will have to be brought into varying degrees of equinus before it can be placed in the corrected position. If in doubt about the mobility of the talus, a lateral radiograph

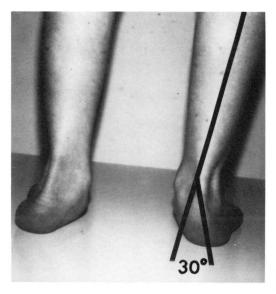

Fig. 8.63. Clinical measurement of hind-foot valgus to judge severity.

of the foot held in equinus and inversion resolves the question and differentiates a fixed from a flexible deformity.

It is essential to obtain anterior-posterior and lateral radiographs of the foot with the patient weight-bearing and, most importantly, an anterior-posterior radiograph of the ankle when weight-bearing. The ankle radiographs are necessary to determine any valgus tilt of the talus in the ankle mortice. If so, reconstructive surgery of the foot only will be insufficient to correct all of the valgus deformity.

Indications and timing of surgery
An obvious and severe pes valgus in spastic diplegia can be corrected only with surgery. One possible classification of severity is the degree of valgus of the heel in relation to the longitudinal alignment of the tibia: less than 10° is mild; 10° to 15° is moderate, and greater than 15° is severe (Fig. 8.63).

The measurement of the degree of plantar flexion of the talus on the lateral radiograph, made when weight-bearing, may be an additional way to assess severity: 35° to 40° is mild; 40° to 50° is moderate, and greater than 50° is severe. The lateral radiograph of the foot may also show a decrease in the calcaneal dorsiflexion angle of less than 10° and is an indicator of additional severity.

Pes valgus thought to be 'severe' in children under age four years may not be as severe at age six to seven years. This decrease in severity seems to occur as the foot equilibrium reactions reverse from the primitive infantile eversion reaction to the more mature inversion foot reaction (Gunsolus *et al.* 1975). Another natural phenomenon to account for a decrease in pes valgus is decreasing ligamentous laxity with age, presumably due to more cross-linking of the collagen.

Because of these observations, I am reluctant to advise early surgical treatment of pes valgus (generally younger than age five years). We know that the

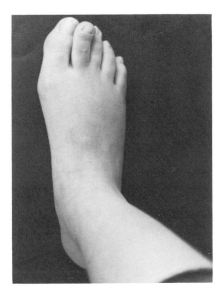

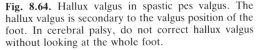

Fig. 8.64. Hallux valgus in spastic pes valgus. The hallux valgus is secondary to the valgus position of the foot. In cerebral palsy, do not correct hallux valgus without looking at the whole foot.

mature gait parameters emerge at about the age of seven years (Sutherland *et al.* 1980). I prefer to delay surgery until about seven years. Occasionally I have operated for a severe deformity of a more skeletally mature foot in children between the ages of 5.5 and 6.5 years. Early surgery seems to bring a risk of late pes varus. Lee (1977*b*) found failures in 11 of 13 of my patients who had extra-articular subtalar arthrodesis under the age of seven years. This type of arthrodesis is difficult to achieve in young children, owing to the smallness and cartilagenous bulk of their tarsal bones.

Though premature surgery seems to create problems, delaying surgery until adolescence is not wise either. The moderate and severe pes valgus seen in cerebral palsy eventually becomes rigid and impossible to correct with passive manipulation. At this time a triple arthrodesis is the procedure of choice. At this later age, however, correction is not so satisfactory: and because bone and articular cartilage must be removed from the subtalar joint, the height of the foot is decreased. This results in uncomfortable impingement of the malleoli on the top edge of the lower quarter shoe (Banks 1976).

Special shoes, sole and/or heel wedges, arch supports and orthotics have not been successful in prevention of pes valgus or in treatment. It might be a sort of psychological placebo for the physician, therapist and parents. The only orthosis with which I have had occasional success in patients under age six years was the single medial tubular steel upright type described in Chapter 6 (Fig. 6.15, p. 180).

Correction by extra-articular subtalar arthrodesis is indicated by incipient development of hallux valgus, which indicates excessive pressure on the medial aspect of the foot on weight-bearing. Hallux valgus will often get worse and become painful due to callosities on the medial border of the great toe and the first metatarsal head (Fig. 8.64).

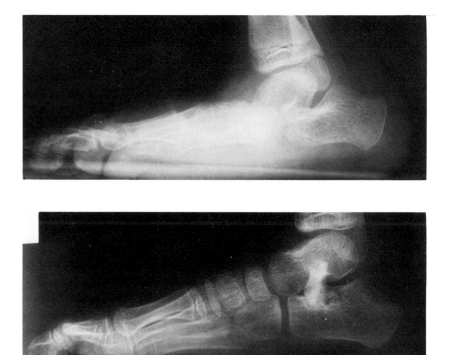

Fig. 8.65. Lateral radiographs, weight-bearing, spastic pes valgus. *Top:* preoperative. *Bottom:* postoperative subtalar extra-articular arthrodesis with a tibial bone graft almost in parallel alignment with tibia—the classic Grice procedure (1952).

Surgical procedures

There are several choices for correction of pes valgus in cerebral palsy. I use only two of these: one for correction before adolescence and the other in adolescents or adults. But first a full review of these choices and a critique seems appropriate.

1. *Peroneal tendon transfer* seems logical. Unfortunately, pes varus has been the frequent result (Keats 1974).

Bennet *et al.* (1982) found no electromyographic activity in five or six posterior tibial muscles in spastic pes valgus. This evidence encouraged them to try transfer of the peroneus brevis to the posterior tibial tendon, with good preliminary results. Time will tell. The electromyograph is not so much quantitative as qualitative. Low-voltage output may be the result of fewer motor units in the area of muscle sampled, and electrical silence can be due to technical adjustments in an attempt to eliminate background noise so that only the strongest signals are recorded. In my own experience, lengthening of the peroneus brevis at the time of extra-articular subtalar arthrodesis caused a reversal to varus deformities in five of seven feet (Lee 1977*b*).

2. *Peroneus brevis intramuscular tenotomy* was reported in 30 cases of spastic pes valgus by Nather *et al.* (1984). The mean age of 20 patients was six years (range two to 14 years). Severity was graded by the eversion angle of the heel: mild, less

than 10° (N=14); moderate, 10° (N=12); severe, greater than 10° (N=4). Using these criteria, the postoperative results on hind-foot valgus were: 14 decreased, 12 were unchanged and 4 increased. Mild cases showed the most improvement. Experimental lengthenings of leg tendons in rabbits and the effects of immobilization did demonstrate that intramuscular tenotomy did not require immobilization to maintain the separation of tendons ends while healing occurred (Nather *et al.* 1986).

Perhaps intramuscular tenotomy of the peroneus brevis could be considered in children under age seven years with mild spastic pes valgus. I wonder if mild pes valgus is any more disabling in a child with cerebral palsy than it is in normal children who seem to tolerate and often 'outgrow' mild hind-foot valgus; and, with moderate deformities, will reversal to varus occur in time when the peroneus brevis spasticity has been reduced with lengthening? In more severe cases this simple operation is not likely to work. These statements are not a criticism—only a shared perspective.

3. *Extra-articular subtalar arthrodesis* has been the standard operation to correct spastic pes valgus in children. Grice (1952) originated this operation for valgus foot deformities in the residuals of poliomyelitis. The objective was to prevent eversion of the hind-foot by permanently eliminating subtalar joint motion with an arthrodesis exterior to the articular surfaces (Fig. 8.65). Thus children under age 13 years would have preservation of the tarsal bone growth; growth arrest of the tarsal bones would occur with intra-articular arthrodesis; each articular surface is comparable to a growth plate in a long bone.

After Grice published his technique and results (1952), some surgeons saw the operation as a solution to correct pes valgus in CP children and avoid the very severe valgus feet seen in adults (Baker and Dodelin 1958, Baker and Hill 1964). Since that time there have been many reports on the efficacy of the procedure, not only in poliomyelitis but also in cerebral palsy and meningomyelocele (Pollack and Carrell 1968; Banks 1977; Moreland and Westin 1977, 1986; Ross and Lyne 1980; Aronson *et al.* 1983; Mohaghegh and Stryker 1983; McCall *et al.* 1985).

Banks (1977) had the best results: 86 per cent successful and 63 per cent excellent. Other surgeons have not had as much success in cerebral palsy: Pollack and Carrell reported a 31 per cent failure rate (15 per cent had graft failure); Ross and Lyne reported 64 per cent failure and 28 per cent complications. Moreland and Westin (1977) had satisfactory results in 73 per cent, but in 1986 they had unpredictable results with pes valgus except in cases due to poliomyelitis. 21 per cent were fused in an unacceptable position; in cerebral palsy the non-union rate was 31 per cent. McCall *et al.* had unsatisfactory results in 46 per cent; 25 of 75 feet in cerebral palsy had bone-graft failure.

My own results were studied by Lee (1977*b*). Of 44 Grice procedures in cerebral palsy, only 50 per cent had good corrections. Eventually, with secondary procedures, the poor results were converted to satisfactory results in 85 per cent. The procedures used for postoperative varus were posterior tibial tendon transfer or lengthening or anterior tibial tendon transfer in dynamic varus deformities; if the varus was fixed, a closed wedge lateral calcaneal osteotomy sufficed. For dynamic

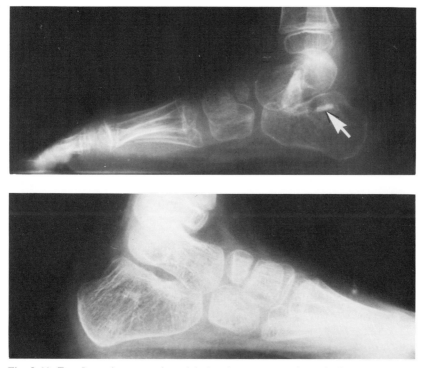

Fig. 8.66. *Top:* Lateral radiograph, weight-bearing, postoperative subtalar extra-articular arthrodesis with tibial bone graft and calcaneal osteotomy (Baker). The arrow points to the white horizontal density beneath the posterior calcaneal facet. This is the horizontal osteotomy, open wedge and its bone graft. *Bottom:* lateral radiograph, weight-bearing, same foot as *top*, one year postoperative. Despite dissolution of the tibial bone graft in the sinus tarsi, correction has been maintained, probably the result of the added horizontal calcaneal osteotomy.

Fig. 8.67. Correct alignment of cortical tibial bone graft in the Grice procedure. It should cross the oblique axis of rotation of the subtalar joint and not be parallel with it. The mean axis of this joint is 42°, with wide variations (Inman 1976).

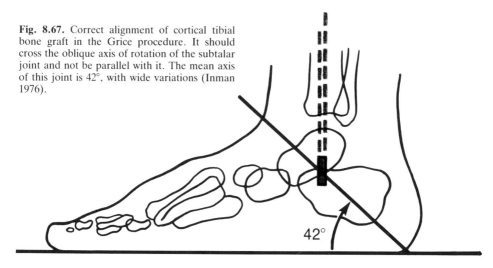

368

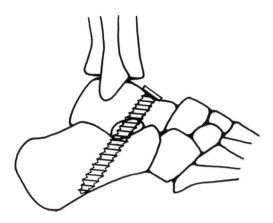

Fig. 8.68. A single screw can hold the corrected position of the talus and calcaneus; however, referring to Figure 8.67, one can easily see that the screw is in the same axis of rotation of subtalar joint and, similar to a bone graft used in the same manner, is liable to break or come loose. The screw can be used temporarily while extra-articular fusion occurs.

forefoot valgus, peroneus brevis tendon lengthening alleviated this problem which occurred in only two feet.

4. *Modifications of extra-articular subtalar arthrodesis.* Baker (1986) used rib homografts and not the original tibial cortical bone grafts. Baker and Hill (1964) did laterally based open wedge osteotomies of the posterior calcaneal facet, holding the wedge open with a cortical bone graft, to block eversion of the subtalar joint. I used Baker's modification in conjunction with the Grice procedure as originally described, and my results improved dramatically. With the tibial cortical grafts alone in the sinus tarsi the failure was 83 per cent, but with the Grice and Baker combined procedures only 25 per cent failed. The rationale for combining the two was that if the tibial bone graft in the sinus tarsi failed to unite or was resorbed, the calcaneal facet osteotomy would hold the correction (Fig. 8.66).

Brown (1968) and Seymour and Evans (1968) used a fibular bone graft in a method Brown learned from Mr J. S. Batchelor at Guy's Hospital in London (unpublished). The fibular shaft bone graft was driven through a hole in the neck of the talus and into the calcaneus to maintain the correction of the pes valgus. Graft failure and breakage occurs with this method because the graft is inserted almost exactly parallel with the axis of rotation of the subtalar joint. Ideally, all grafts should be placed perpendicular to this axis (Fig. 8.67); they will then be under compression and rotation will be minimal.

Hsu *et al.* (1986) used the fibular graft method devised by Batchelor, but added another fibular graft parallel to the tibial shaft as originally recommended by Grice. The risk of fibular shaft removal for a bone graft is failure of reformation of the fibula, which results in valgus of the ankle joint (Wiltse *et al.* 1972, Hsu *et al.* 1974).

Mohaghegh and Stryker (1983), applying the principle of stopping eversion by extra-articular arthrodesis, used a dowel graft from the calcaneus in the sinus tarsi.

To simplify the technique of extra-articular arthrodesis, Cahuzac (1977) and the orthopaedic surgeons of Montpellier, France, used the technique of Cavalier and Judet (cited by Trouillas 1978). After the valgus foot was manipulated into the correct position, a single screw was inserted from the superior surface of the talar neck obliquely into the calcaneus (Fig. 8.68). Only 10 per cent bad results were

369

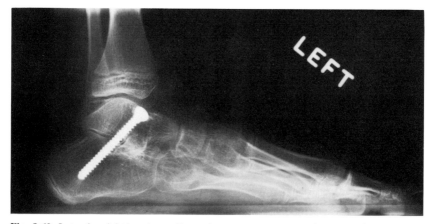

Fig. 8.69. Lateral weight-bearing radiograph, one year postoperative correction of spastic pes valgus with screw fixation and iliac bone graft in the sinus tarsis (Dennyson and Fulford 1976).

reported in 50 feet. The presumption apparently is that the corrections will be sustained, either because of arthrofibrosis of the subtalar joint secondary to immobilization, or because of a possible redirection of the tarsal bone growth. Since this screw is in the axis of rotation of the subtalar joint, the risk of failure in time seems likely. During gait the subtalar joint does rotate in order to absorb the torques generated between the foot and the floor. It seems more logical to add a bone graft to assure solid extra-articular fusion while the screw holds the correction.

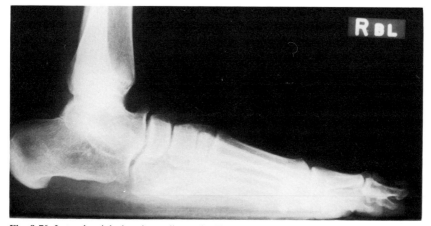

Fig. 8.70. Lateral weight-bearing radiograph, 15 years postoperative subtalar extra-articular arthrodesis, 22-year-old male. Foot discomfort. Degenerative arthritis has occurred in the talonavicular and calcaneal-cuboid joints. Could this be a frequent long-term result? No one knows. This is one reason why I continue to be very selective in recommending subtalar arthrodesis in children with spastic diplegia and pes valgus. 'Mild' valgus needs no correction and 'moderate' may need correction if hallux valgus and medial callouses on the head of the first metatarsal and great toe are developing.

Dennyson and Fulford (1976) used the same screw fixation but added an iliac bone graft to the sinus tarsi. They had good results, with a 93.7 per cent fusion rate. An additional advantage of the procedure is that it allows a shorter period of plaster immobilization and earlier weight-bearing than the classic Grice procedure. I was first introduced to this method by Cary (1978) at the Newington Children's Hospital, Newington, Connecticut, and have used it since. Barrasso and surgeons (1984) of this hospital have reported results that parallel my own: in 40 feet (26 patients), 95 per cent were rated good or excellent with no poor results. Union of the iliac bone graft with the talus and calcaneus was reported to occur within a mean time of 10 weeks. In 25 feet I have had one failure of correction, and have had to remove only one screw (Fig. 8.69).

Other ways to 'skin the cat' were described by Rang *et al.* (1986) and Rinsky (1985). Rang also uses internal fixation and a dowel graft from the calcaneus, rather than an iliac graft. He drives the screw upward from the lateral aspect of the calcaneus into the talus. Rinsky (1985) uses a Steinman pin from the lateral aspect of the calcaneus to the talus; the pin holds the correction until fusion with the iliac bone graft occurs; then the pin is extracted.

Extra-articular subtalar stabilization without arthrodesis has been introduced by Crawford and associates (1986). In this operation the spastic valgus foot is placed into the corrected position which is secured by a laterally placed staple across the subtalar joint in the body of the talus and the calcaneus. The mean age of their patients was three years. In 18 patients (28 feet), followed for an average of 3.5 years, the results were good in 20, fair in six and poor in two. At the time of this follow-up report, many of the children were over age six years with satisfactory results and no evidence of staple extrusion. Crawford's original intent was to use the staple as a temporary correction until the child was old enough to have an extra-articular arthrodesis with a bone graft. Crawford now believes that this secondary procedure will be unnecessary.

I have not performed this procedure because the subtalar joint movement would loosen the staple. In the follow-up radiographs I saw the bone around the staple prongs was resorbed; nevertheless correction was maintained. Was this due to arthrofibrosis of the joint and/or cartilage degeneration due to the immobilization? I am still reluctant to recommend surgical correction of pes valgus under the age of six to seven years (the mean age in Crawford's series was three years) because mild and moderate pes valgus (less than 15° of heel eversion) may not be any more significant in spastic diplegia than it is in non-paralytic static pes valgus. If surgery is reserved only for severe cases, will the stapling alone be sufficient for sustained correction?

5. *Open wedge calcaneal osteotomy* (Silver *et al.* 1967, 1974, 1977) was proposed to preserve the mobility of the subtalar joint and correct the valgus by shifting the weight-bearing area of the calcaneus from an everted to an inverted position (Fig. 8.70). A sterile slice of cadaver cortical bone kept the laterally based osteotomy open while healing occurred (Fig. 8.71). Silver had success with this procedure. From a study of the radiographs in Silver's publications, it appeared to me that this osteotomy will realign the valgus foot if the talus has moderate plantar

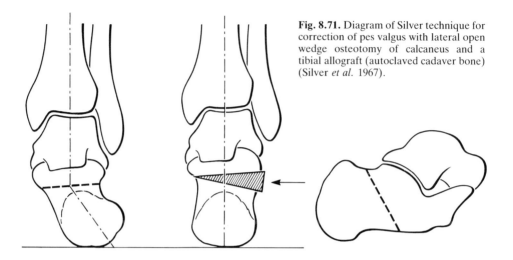

Fig. 8.71. Diagram of Silver technique for correction of pes valgus with lateral open wedge osteotomy of calcaneus and a tibial allograft (autoclaved cadaver bone) (Silver *et al.* 1967).

flexion of 45° to 55°. If plantar flexion of the talus is greater than this (60° to 80°), calcaneal osteotomy may not suffice for an adequate correction (Samilson 1972, Sage 1977) (Fig. 8.72).

A medial displacement osteotomy of the calcaneus was mentioned by Coleman (1983) as yet another way to overcome pes valgus. This oblique osteotomy in the coronal plane of the calcaneus made through a lateral approach can shift the heel directly medially. It brings the heel into direct alignment with the tibia. Correction of the valgus of the hind-foot can occur. I do not think it will correct the mid- and forefoot pathological anatomy characteristic of pes valgus in spastic diplegic children.

6. *Triple arthrodesis* is the standard operation for severe pes valgus in adolescents and adults. If performed before adolescence when skeletal maturity begins (age 13 years and older), foot growth will not be significantly stunted by removal of the articular surfaces of the talus, calcaneus, navicular and cuboid bones. Although triple arthrodesis offers good correction of the varus deformities, the results have not been as pleasing for valgus deformities (Horstmann and Eilert 1977, Duckworth 1977). All too often the postoperative foot still has the appearance of pes valgus. The talus usually returned to its plantar-flexed position and the calcaneus remained in relative equinus (less than 10° of dorsiflexion). To improve these results, I have added Grice's principle to the procedure; the talus is brought out of its plantar-flexed position and secured while healing with solid arthrodesis occurs (Fig. 8.73).

Operative techniques

I prefer two operations which have been reliable in a reasonable restoration of the normal anatomy and configuration of the foot. Given the obvious discrepancies between chronological and skeletal age, a general policy is to recommend the extra-articular arthrodesis before age 13 years and the intra-articular arthrodesis after that age.

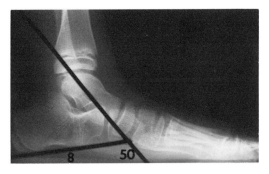
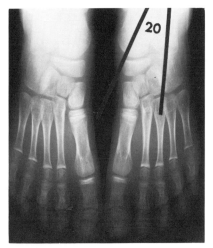

Fig. 8.72. *Left:* lateral weight-bearing radiograph, spastic diplegia, moderate pes valgus. Talar plantar-flexion angle 50°. Upper limits of normal 30°–35°. *Right:* anterior-posterior weight-bearing radiograph, same foot as *left.* Talar-calcaneal divergence angle only 20°. Hind-foot valgus is not severe.

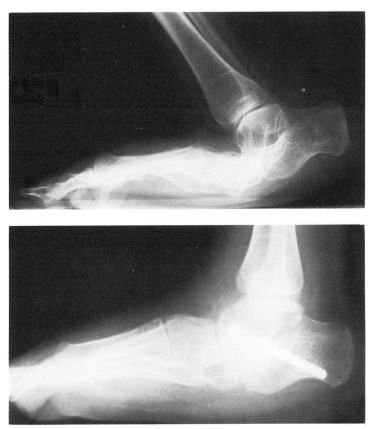

Fig. 8.73. *Top:* lateral weight-bearing radiograph, 16-year-old spastic diplegic with severe pes valgus. *Bottom:* lateral weight-bearing radiograph postoperative triple arthrodesis with screw fixation to maintain a reasonable correction of the plantar-flexed talus, one year postoperative.

Extra-articular subtalar arthrodesis with internal fixation (Dennyson and Fulford 1976, Barrasso *et al.* 1984). With the patient anesthetized, the foot is inverted and dorsiflexed. If the heel remains in equinus, a sliding Achilles tendon lengthening (Hoke or White) is first performed. The foot is dorsiflexed with the foot held in varus just to the neutral position where the plantar surface of the heel is in 90° relationship to the tibia. Zealous dorsiflexion beyond this point should be avoided.

The superior surface of the talar neck and sinus tarsi are exposed through an oblique posteriorly directed incision beginning at the talar head to bisect the heel and ending at the peroneal tendon sheaths. The inferior aspect of the talar neck, sinus tarsi and superior surface of the calcaneus are denuded of all fat and fibrous tissue. It is desirable to preserve a thick posterior flap of skin and subcutaneous tissue. The bone surfaces are cleanly exposed and gently roughened with a curette and small osteotome.

The foot is then manipulated into the corrected anatomical position, which is confirmed by a lateral fluoroscopic view with the image intensifier. The foot is held securely and steadily in this position.

The spot for screw insertion on the superior aspect of the talar neck is found by blunt dissection of the soft tissue between the extensor digitorum longus tendons and the neurovascular bundle. A small dissecting elevator can be placed on either side of the talar neck. The space created should be just large enough to accommodate the cortical bone screw (threaded throughout). The screw length and direction can be estimated by overlaying a depth gauge on the lateral aspect of the foot, checking the position with the image intensifier fluoroscope, and marking the skin for the direction. Others (Barrasso *et al.* 1984) introduce a Kirschner wire as a guide pin driven posterior to the intended site of the screw. With the proper size drill to match the screw, and through a drill sleeve to protect the adjacent tissues, a hole is drilled from the center of the talar neck and through to the body of the calcaneus. The screw is then inserted to maintain the new position of the talus securely. The screw can end near the plantar surface of the calcaneus but not through it. A cortical cancellous bone graft and chips are removed from the outer wall of the ilium and packed into the sinus tarsi.

I use suction drainage of the wound in all cases. A long leg plaster, with the foot well padded and the knee slightly flexed, immobilizes the limb. At four weeks postoperative this plaster is removed and replaced with a short-leg plaster and walking boot. Weight-bearing to tolerance is permitted for the next four weeks. After plaster removal, supportive elastic bandages or elastic stockingette with temporary felt arch supports usually give more comfort to the patient for the next week or two while walking in ordinary low quarter-leather or sports shoes. Although some surgeons (Barrasso *et al.* 1984) have prescribed plastic ankle-foot orthoses as additional protection postoperatively, I use these custom-molded orthotics only in large and heavy children.

Foot-skin and soft-tissue tenderness persists for several weeks in children who have had overprotection of their feet preoperatively. The only way the skin and fat on the plantar aspect of the foot can hypertrophy enough to get rid of this

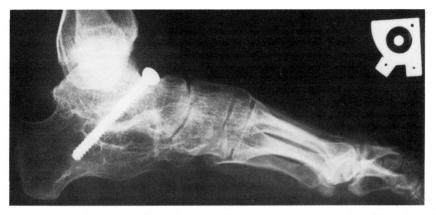

Fig. 8.74. Lateral weight-bearing radiograph of foot three years postoperative triple arthrodesis for pes valgus in a patient with spastic diplegia, age 18 years. Talar plantar-flexion correction well maintained.

hypersensitivity is through consistent and persistent weight-bearing. Walking barefoot on grass, sand or carpets seems to help.

Triple arthrodesis. If the hind-foot is in equinus when the foot is inverted and dorsiflexed, a sliding Achilles tendon lengthening to allow dorsiflexion just to the neutral position is necessary. The incision for the arthrodesis of the three joints is the same as described in the preceding section for extra-articular arthrodesis. The fibrous tissue and fat should be removed from the sinus tarsi in almost one piece and remain attached as a flap of the posterior skin of the incision to facilitate wound closure after the foot has been corrected.

The three joints (calcanealcuboid, talonavicular and subtalar) are denuded of articular cartilage to expose the subchondral bone (the details of the technique have been described for varus feet in Chapter 7). Medially based wedges of bone are cautiously removed as necessary to obtain good contact of the raw and roughened joint surfaces when the foot is manipulated into the corrected position in which the talus is brought out of its plantar flexion. Removal of large wedges of bone from the joint is not necessary. The foot is firmly held in its corrected position while another surgeon introduces the fixation screw from the talar neck into the calcaneus, as described for extra-articular arthrodesis (Fig. 8.74).

I use a Steinman pin from the plantar surface of the heel inserted anterior to its weight-bearing area into the calcaneus and talus. A second pin can be driven from the first metatarsal shaft to cross the talonavicular joint. With this combination of internal and external fixation, a bulky padding comprised of dorsal and plantar ABD pads secured with several layers of rolled padding prevents constriction by the plaster. A plaster should extend from the toes to the midthigh with the knee flexed 30° (unless the Achilles tendon has been lengthened, in which case only slight knee flexion is appropriate). Suction drainage of the wound for 24 to 48 hours is routine.

The pins and plaster are removed in four weeks and replaced with a short-leg walking plaster; weight-bearing to tolerance is permitted for the next four to six weeks. When the plaster is removed, elastic bandages or elastic support-hose

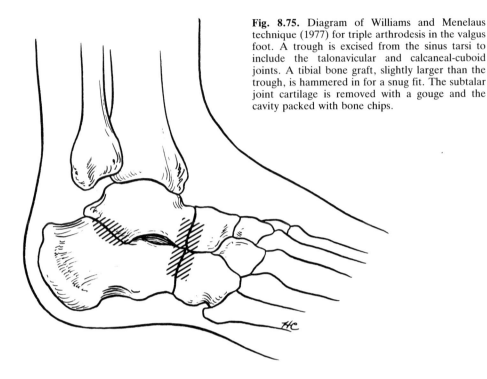

Fig. 8.75. Diagram of Williams and Menelaus technique (1977) for triple arthrodesis in the valgus foot. A trough is excised from the sinus tarsi to include the talonavicular and calcaneal-cuboid joints. A tibial bone graft, slightly larger than the trough, is hammered in for a snug fit. The subtalar joint cartilage is removed with a gouge and the cavity packed with bone chips.

control postoperative edema which can last for a month or more. Ordinary low quarter shoes or sturdy sports shoes are adequate.

Because fusion of the joints will not be evident radiographically from six months to one year postoperatively, both patient and surgeon can be relieved of anxiety if solid union is not seen at the time of final plaster removal.

Williams and Menelaus (1977) described an inlay bone graft for correction and arthrodesis of pes valgus. A vertical trough was created in the sinus tarsi to include

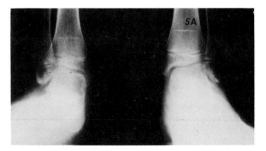

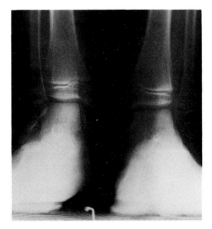

Fig. 8.76. *Left:* anterior-posterior radiographs of ankle joints in patient with spastic pes valgus. Ankle joints have a valgus deformity in addition to that of the feet. *Right:* anterior-posterior radiographs of ankle joints, weight-bearing. Normally tibial plafond and tibial articular surface of talus is parallel to floor.

376

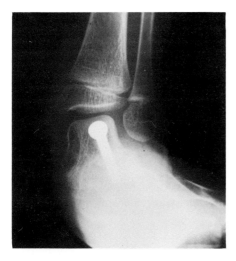
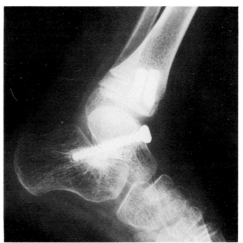
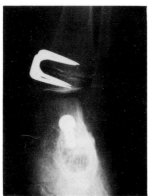

Fig. 8.77. *Top left:* anterior-posterior radiograph of ankle joint postoperative subtalar extra-articular arthrodesis (Dennyson-Fulford method) for pes valgus. Coexistent valgus of the ankle joint. *Top right:* stapling of the medial distal tibial physis for correction of ankle valgus. *Left:* result of stapling, one year postoperative; correction has occurred.

the talonavicular and calcanealcuboid joints. A slightly oversized tibial bone graft was then hammered into this trough. Subtalar joint cartilage was removed with a gouge, and the cavity packed with bone chips (Fig. 8.75). Though I have not tried this procedure, it has merit because the bone graft would act as a prop for the repositioned talus.

Problems with subtalar extra-articular or triple arthrodesis in pes valgus
The main problems are as follows:

1. Failure to recognize concomitant valgus of the ankle joint. If subtalar correction is done and valgus of the ankle is present, the foot will still be in valgus. A preoperative weight-bearing anterior-posterior radiograph of the ankle joints forewarns and allows additional operative planning (Fig. 8.76).

In young children who have valgus of the ankle, I have performed stapling of the distal medial tibial physis; restoration of a horizontal ankle joint has occurred without resort to a supramalleolar osteotomy (Burkus *et al.* 1983) (Fig. 8.77). In

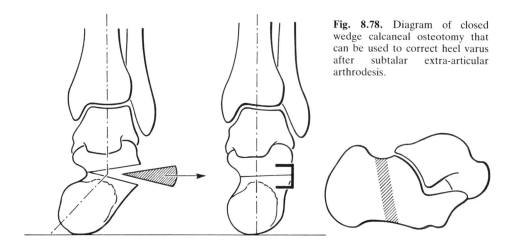

Fig. 8.78. Diagram of closed wedge calcaneal osteotomy that can be used to correct heel varus after subtalar extra-articular arthrodesis.

adolescents there may be insufficient growth potential for staples to be effective. Supramalleolar closed wedge tibial and fibular osteotomies will be required.

2. Overcorrection into varus with the extra-articular arthrodesis occurs most often in young children. This can be partly avoided by observing the position of the heel at the time of surgery when the foot is manipulated into the correct position before fixation. After fixation, the heel position can be checked in an anterior-posterior radiograph of the foot made in the operating room. The measured angle between the talus and calcaneus indicates heel position. A neutrally aligned heel will have an angle of approximately 15°. If this happens, and the joints are fused, the problem can be corrected by a laterally based closed wedge osteotomy of the calcaneus (Figs. 8.78, 8.79).

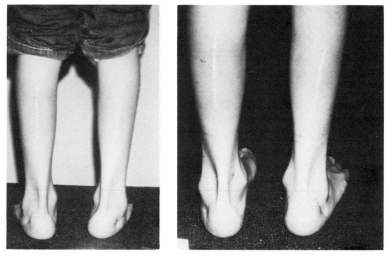

Fig. 8.79. *Left:* patient PL, spastic diplegia, postoperative varus after bilateral Grice procedure. Unacceptable varus of the left heel. *Right:* patient PL, postoperative correction of left heel varus with closed wedge calcaneal osteotomy.

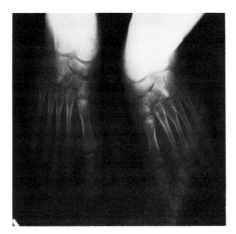

Fig. 8.80. Anterior-posterior radiograph of pes valgus in spastic diplegia. Typical lateral displacement of the navicular bone on the talar head. When the navicular is aligned anatomically with the talar head and the subtalar joint is stabilized by arthrodesis, the foot may be internally rotated.

3. Undercorrection and valgus of the hind-foot can be due in a triple arthrodesis to recurrence of plantar flexion of the talus. This return of the talus to its plantar-flexed position can be minimized with the internal fixation of the talus and calcaneus as described. Even with this extra fixation, I have not seen any normal-looking balanced feet after triple arthrodesis for severe spastic pes valgus.

What seems evident in these flat-looking feet after surgery is a calcaneal equinus which is not corrected by Achilles tendon lengthening. Posterior capsulotomy of the ankle might allow dorsiflexion of the calcaneus; however, in severe pes valgus of adolescents and adults, the tibial articular surface of the talus becomes limited in area anteriorly due to the deformity of the talus. Perhaps a crescentric osteotomy of the posterior portion of the calcaneus to simulate its dorsiflexed position might improve the result (Wu 1986). This osteotomy is the reverse of that described by Samilson (1976) for pes calcaneal cavus. Because I have not performed this additional procedure, it is only a suggestion and not based on results.

4. Varus of the mid-foot is a problem due to lengthening of one or both peroneal tendons. In this instance, lengthening or a split transfer of the posterior tibial tendon should resolve the problem. In some cases, a split anterior tibial tendon transfer may be the solution. The decisions should be based on the clinical examination and confirmed with dynamic electromyography if available.

5. Valgus deformity of the ankle postoperatively may result from removal of a segment of the fibular shaft to be used as a bone graft and reossification does not occur (Wiltse 1972, Hsu *et al.* 1974).

6. Postoperative in-toe gait can be confused with a dynamic varus. The gait problem is due to internal axial rotation of the entire foot. Preoperatively, either internal tibial-fibular torsion or persistent excessive medial deviation of the talar neck is not recognized as associated with the spastic pes valgus. The in-toeing becomes evident after surgical correction when the navicular bone is aligned in its normal position on the head of the talus. In spastic valgus feet the navicular bone is displaced laterally on the talar head (Fig. 8.80).

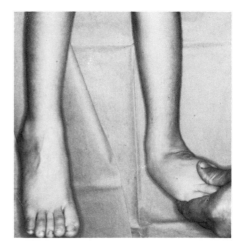

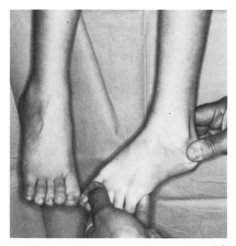

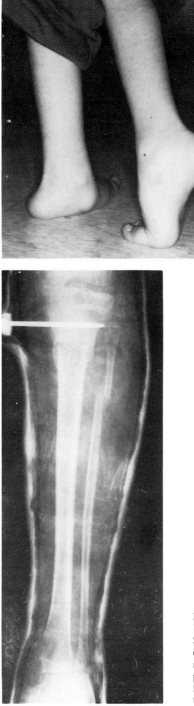

Fig. 8.81. *Top left:* severe spastic pes valgus left foot, age seven years. *Top right:* with patient seated and left foot dorsiflexed and in valgus. *Above:* when foot is manipulated into the corrected position, internal rotation of the entire foot is evident. This will be the position after subtalar extra-articular arthrodesis. Derotation osteotomy of the tibia and fibula also indicated.

Fig. 8.82 *(left).* Anterior-posterior radiograph of tibia. Proximal tibial and fibular rotation osteotomy. Proximal Steinman pin is inserted from medial side and engages both cortices but does not penetrate the lateral muscular compartment or skin. Note pin holder to be incorporated in the plaster; movement of the pin is prevented. Secure proximal fixation allows changing the osteotomy position by wedging the plaster at the osteotomy site.

380

This result might be avoided by careful preoperative evaluation. When the foot is passively manipulated into the desired corrected position, the internal rotation of the foot will be appreciated (Fig. 8.81). When this is observed, a derotation osteotomy of the tibia and fibula at the time of subtalar arthrodesis can be planned and accomplished at the same operation or at a second stage (Fig. 8.82).

Tibial-fibular torsion, internal or external
Excessive external tibial-fibular torsion is more common than internal in cerebral palsy as a compensation for femoral torsion or as the result of medial hamstring tendon lengthening (Bassett *et al.* 1976).

Internal tibial-fibular torsion is probably the congenital type superimposed on spastic diplegia. Spontaneous correction is dubious. It can be masked by spastic pes valgus. We have no evidence that orthotics correct the torsion in either direction.

Surgical correction of excessive external tibial torsion (greater than 30°) is indicated (i) if it causes symptoms in the foot or ankle as the result of excessive stress on the medial side of these joints, (ii) if the foot assumes a varus position in the attempt to rectify the abnormal position, or (iii) if a knee-ankle-foot orthosis cannot accommodate the degree of torsion either at the knee or ankle joints.

The indications for correction of internal tibial torsion in spastic diplegia are present when the patient walks in-toed so badly as to create a subjective disability. Usually the request for surgery comes from an emerging adolescent who has a fairly good gait pattern and is independent. The other indication has been mentioned in the previous section on in-toeing after extra-articular subtalar arthrodesis for spastic pes valgus.

Operative technique for derotation osteotomy of the tibia and fibula. The choice is either a proximal or distal osteotomy. I prefer the transverse osteotomy of the proximal tibia just below the tibial tubercle and a fibular osteotomy 1 to 2cm distal to the tibial site. The fibular osteotomy is done through a small lateral incision with an osteotome. The exact desired area of the tibia is located with the fluoroscope; the skin is marked and a straight 3cm incision is made on the center of the medial cortex of the tibia. The incision can be slightly oblique if one wants it to be straight after the rotation (oblique from lateral to medial for an external rotation osteotomy, and the opposite for the internal). To control the proximal tibial fragment and to enable wedging of the plaster to correct malalignment postoperatively, a Steinman pin is inserted medially to engage both cortices of the proximal tibia and parallel to the knee joint (Fig. 8.82). It is not necessary to penetrate the lateral muscular compartment or the skin. The tibia is exposed subperiosteally distal to the pin, and retractors are inserted around the entire bone to protect the posterior neurovascular structures. A power oscillating saw is used.

With the hip in neutral position (patella facing forward) and the knee extended, the correct degree of rotation can be determined by 10° of external axial rotation of the foot when the ankle is dorsiflexed to the neutral position.

The fascia of the anterior compartment is easily reached and routinely slit proximally and distally. Continuous suction drainage of the wound for 24 to 48 hours obviates a hematoma. After wound closure and dressing, the osteotomy site is dressed anteriorly and posteriorly with ABD pads secured with rolled cotton as usual. The first section of the plaster incorporates the thigh, knee, pin and the leg to its distal third. The knee is kept in almost complete extension, taking care not to overextend the leg and cause a posterior angulation at the osteotomy site. The pin is prevented from sliding with a slotted metal dial and screw-holding device, which is also incorporated in the plaster. When this section of the plaster has 'set', then rotation is manually checked and the foot and ankle are joined with plaster to the proximal portion. We then check the position of the osteotomy in the operating room with fluoroscopy. If unacceptable angulation is noted, the plaster can be cut at the osteotomy site, manipulated appropriately and replastered. Obviously a major portion of the operation depends upon who holds the limb while plaster is applied. The surgeon holds and the assistant wraps.

On the second or third day postoperatively, anterior-posterior and lateral radiographs are made of the limb with the knee centered on a large film (35 × 45cm). The alignment of the bones can be measured and the plaster cut if realignment is required.

The patient is non-weightbearing for four to five weeks, after which the pin and plaster are removed and replaced with a long-leg walking plaster. Standing and walking to tolerance are encouraged in plaster for an additional four to five weeks. At eight to 10 weeks postoperatively, radiographs usually show sufficient union to allow weight-bearing without plaster. Knee-flexion and extension exercises are necessary to restore function.

Osteotomy of the distal tibia and fibula has been heralded as a more satisfactory and cosmetic procedure (Bennett *et al.* 1985). A 1cm horizontal incision was made anteriorly over the distal tibia. With the aid of fluoroscopy and 'tactile sensation' of the surgeon's hands, multiple drill holes were made through a single hole in the anterior cortex. The osteotomy was completed with a small osteotome. The fibular osteotomy is similarly made through a 1cm incision 2cm proximal to the tibial site. With the knee flexed 90° the foot was rotated to the desired position with reference to the knee axis. A long-leg plaster was applied with the knee flexed 60° to 90°.

Postoperatively additional correction was obtained by circumferentially cutting the plaster at the osteotomy sites. After four to six weeks, a short-leg walking cast was applied until there was radiographic evidence of union (usually in four to six weeks).

Bennett *et al.* (1985) stated that the major reason to perform the distal osteotomies was to avoid the cosmetically objectionable scar of the proximal sites. Inasmuch as abnormal foot rotation is a subjective disability, they have a point. Their other reasons included a high complication rate reported with proximal tibial osteotomies (Steel *et al.* 1971, Jackson and Waugh 1974). Steel *et al.* reported that of 46 osteotomies in children for genu varum or valgum, nine had a serious complication which they attributed to compression or stretching of the anterior tibial artery; in studying this paper it now appears that these were all instances of anterior compartment syndromes due to a rise in compartment pressures—an entity that has been defined and become common knowledge in the past 10 years.

The report of Jackson and Waugh was exclusively about complications of proximal tibial osteotomy for osteo-arthritis in adults whose mean age was 59.9 years.

The complications reported with the distal osteotomies in 19 patients (32 rotation osteotomies) were remanipulation (9 per cent), posterior bowing in six (19 per cent), transient 'numbness' in three patients, delayed healing, tendonitis and a cast sore in one patient. Their mean healing-time necessitating plaster immobilization was 14.5 weeks (range 10 to 24 weeks). Most of their postoperative plasters required splitting to accommodate apparent swelling (70 per cent). These surgeons also believe that derotation of the tibia could be best accomplished with the knee flexed 90° rather than with the knee extended.

I have heard from other orthopaedic surgeons that they much prefer the distal method. I have used it in one case, an eight-year-old boy with spastic diplegia; healing was delayed beyond the usual eight weeks (for proximal osteotomy) to 16 weeks. I still favour the proximal osteotomy of the tibia because: (i) the operative scar is only 3cm long, and does not seem objectionable when closed with subcuticular synthetic absorbable sutures; (ii) healing is rapid with a range of eight to 10 weeks; (iii) rotation of the tibia with the knee extended is the position of the knee at heel contact and to mid-stance when the excessive rotation of the foot is noted; (iv) keeping the knee immobilized 60° to 90° from four to six weeks in spastic diplegia could aggravate hamstring contracture. Apparently this was not the case in Bennett *et al.*'s series (1985), even though seven of their patients had spastic diplegia; (v) genu valgum or varum of the tibia cannot be corrected with a distal osteotomy when these coexist with the rotational deformity; (vi) while posterior bowing of the tibia in six of the distal osteotomies reported did not adversely affect the result, it does not seem mechanically desirable unless it corrects ankle equinus. Proximal osteotomies can bow posterior and affect the result (genu recurvatum); (vii) anterior compartment syndromes are a complication with proximal tibial osteotomies of any kind. Since we have been routinely performing a lateral and anterior compartment fasciotomy for the past 13 years, I have not seen this problem; (viii) delayed union of the distal tibial osteotomy in older children near adolescence, in adolescents whose epiphyses have closed and in adults, can be expected as it is in fractures of the distal third of the tibia due to the lack of enveloping muscles and more tenous blood supply to the bone; (ix) with the heavy padding used under the plaster as described for proximal tibial osteotomies, and which is feasible because of the external pin fixation, we have almost never had to split a cast—I like to sleep nights and so do our residents.

In conclusion, if the proximal scar on the leg is the major objection and the surgeon has excellent 'tactile sensation' to avoid penetrating the cortex and winding up the posterior or anterior tibial nerve or artery, the distal 'peep-hole' osteotomies of the tibia and fibula are quite satisfactory. Several very good surgeons like the procedure (Morrissy 1985)—*nolo contende*.

REFERENCES

Anthosen, W. (1966) 'Treatment of hip flexion contracture in cerebral palsy patients.' *Acta Orthopaedica Scandinavica*, **37**, 387–393.

Arkin, A. M., Katz, J. F. (1956) 'The effects of pressure on epiphyseal growth.' *Journal of Bone and Joint Surgery*, **38A**, 1056–1076.

Aronson, J., Nunley, J., Frankovitch, K. (1983) 'Lateral talocalcaneal angle in assessment of subtalar valgus: follow-up of seventy Grice-Green arthrodeses.' *Foot and Ankle*, **4**, 56–63.

Baker, L. D. (1956) 'A rational approach to the surgical needs of the cerebral palsy patient.' *Journal of Bone and Joint Surgery*, **38A**, 313–323.

—— (1986) *Personal communication.*

—— Dodelin, R. A. (1958) 'Extra-articular arthrodesis of the subtalar joint (Grice procedure).' *Journal of the American Medical Association*, **168**, 1005–1008.

—— Hill, L. M. (1964) 'Foot alignment in the cerebral palsy patient.' *Journal of Bone and Joint Surgery*, **46A**, 1–15.

Banks, H. H. (1972) 'The knee and cerebral palsy.' *Orthopaedic Clinics of North America*, **3**, 113–129.

—— (1977) 'Management of spastic deformities of the foot and ankle.' *Clinical Orthopaedics and Related Research*, **122**, 70–76.

—— Green, W. T. (1960) 'Adductor myotomy and obturator neurectomy for correction of adduction contracture of the hip in cerebral palsy.' *Journal of Bone and Joint Surgery*, **42A**, 111–126.

Barrasso, J. A., Wile, P. B., Gage, J. R. (1984) 'Extra-articular subtalar arthrodesis with internal fixation.' *Journal of Pediatric Orthopedics*, **4**, 455–459.

Basmajian, J. V. (1962) *Muscles Alive*. Baltimore: Williams & Wilkins.

Bassett, F. H., Poehling, G. G., Moorefield, W. G., Riley, K., Minnich, J. (1976) 'Hamstring procedures in cerebral palsy. A: sequelae after long follow-up. B: recommendations for current practice.' *Journal of Bone and Joint Surgery*, **58A**, 725. (*Abstract*.)

Baumann, J. V. (1970) *Operative Behandlung der Infantilen Zerebralparesen*. Stuttgart: Georg Thieme.

—— (1972) 'Hip operations in children with cerebral palsy'. *Reconstructive Surgery and Traumatology*, **13**, 68–82.

—— Meyer, E., Schurmann, K. (1978) 'Hip adductor transfer to the ischial tuberosity in spastic and paralytic hip disorders.' (*German*.) *Archives of Orthopaedic and Traumatic Surgery*, **92**, 107–112.

—— Ruetsch, H., Schurmann, K. (1980) 'Distal hamstring lengthening in cerebral palsy. An evaluation by gait analysis.' *International Orthopaedics*, **3**, 305–309.

Beals, R. K. (1969) 'Developmental changes in the femur and acetabulum in spastic paraplegia and diplegia.' *Developmental Medicine and Child Neurology*, **11**, 303–313.

Bennet, G., Rang, M., Jones, D. (1982) 'Valgus and varus deformities of the foot in cerebral palsy.' *Developmental Medicine and Child Neurology*, **24**, 499–503.

Bennett, J. T., Bunnell, W. P., MacEwen, G. D. (1985) 'Rotational osteotomy of the distal tibia and fibula.' *Journal of Pediatric Orthopedics*, **5**, 294–298.

Bleck, E. E. (1966) 'Management of hip deformities in cerebral palsy.' *In:* Adams, J. P. (Ed.) *Current Practice in Orthopaedic Surgery*. St. Louis: C. V. Mosby.

—— (1971*a*) 'Postural and gait abnormalities caused by hip flexion deformity in spastic cerebral palsy.' *Journal of Bone and Joint Surgery*, **53A**, 1468–1488.

—— (1971*b*) 'The hip in cerebral palsy.' *In: Instructional Course Lectures, American Academy of Orthopaedic Surgeons*. St. Louis: C. V. Mosby.

—— (1975) 'Spinal and pelvic deformities in cerebral palsy.' *In:* Samilson, R. L. (Ed.) *Orthopaedic Aspects of Cerebral Palsy. Clinics in Developmental Medicine, Nos. 52/53*. London: S.I.M.P. with Heinemann. Philadelphia: J. B. Lippincott.

—— (1980) 'The hip in cerebral palsy.' *Orthopedic Clinics of North America*, **11**, 79–104.

—— (1984) 'Computerized axial tomography for developmental problems of the hip.' *Developmental Medicine and Child Neurology*, **26**, 231–235. (*Annotation*.)

—— (1985) 'Spastic paralytic disclocation of the hip.' *Developmental Medicine and Child Neurology*, **27**, 401–403. (*Letter*.)

—— Holstein, A. (1963) 'Iliopsoas tenotomy for spastic hip flexion deformities in cerebral palsy.' *Paper presented at the Annual Meeting American Academy of Orthopaedic Surgeons, Chicago*.

—— Berzins, U. J. (1977) 'Conservative management of pes valgus with plantar flexed talus flexible.' *Clinical Orthopaedics and Related Research*, **122**, 85–94.

—— Terver, S., Wheeler, R., Csongradi, J., Rinsky, L. A. (1981) 'Joint laxity in children: statistical correlations with scoliosis, congenital dislocations of the hip and talipes equinovarus'. *Orthopaedic Transactions*, **5**, 5–6.

384

—— Minaire, P. (1983) 'Persistent medial deviation of the neck of the talus: a common cause of in-toeing in children.' *Journal of Pediatric Orthopaedics*, **3**, 149–159.

Bost, F. W., Bleck, E. E. (1975) 'Rotation osteotomies for spastic paralytic internal rotation deformities of the femur.' *Paper read at the Annual Meeting American Academy for Cerebral Palsy, New Orleans.*

Brown, A. (1968) 'A simple method of fusion of the subtalar joint in children.' *Journal of Bone and Joint Surgery*, **50B**, 369–371.

Brunnstrom, S. (1962) *Clinical Kinesiology.* Philadelphia: F. A. Davies.

Burkus, J. K., Moore, D. W., Raycroft, J. F. (1983) 'Valgus deformity of the ankle in myelodysplastic patients. Correction by stapling of the medial part of the distal tibial physis.' *Journal of Bone and Joint Surgery*, **65A**, 1157–1162.

Cahuzac, M. (1977) *L'Enfant Infirme Moteur d'Origine Cérébrale.* Paris: Masson.

Cary, J. (1978) *Personal communication.*

Chandler, F. A. (1933) 'Re-establishment of normal leverage of patella in knee flexion deformity in spastic paralysis.' *Surgery, Gynecology and Obstetrics*, **57**, 523–527.

Chong, K. C., Vojnic, C. D., Quanbury, A. O., Eng, P., Letts, R. M. (1978) 'The assessment of the internal rotation gait in cerebral palsy: an electromyographic gait analysis.' *Clinical Orthopaedics and Research*, **132**, 145–150.

Close, J. R. (1964) *Motor Function in the Lower Extremity.* Springfield, Ill.: C. C. Thomas.

Coleman, S. S. (1978) *Congenital Dysplasia and Dislocation of the Hip.* St. Louis: C. V. Mosby.

—— (1983) *Complex Foot Deformities in Children.* Philadelphia: Lea & Febiger.

Coon, V., Donato, G., Houser, C., Bleck, E. E. (1975) 'Normal ranges of motion of the hip in infants six weeks, three months and six months of age.' *Clinical Orthopaedics and Related Research*, **110**, 256–260.

Couch, W. H., Jr., De Rosa, G. P., Throop, F. B. (1977) 'Thigh adductor transfer for spastic cerebral palsy.' *Developmental Medicine and Child Neurology*, **19**, 343–349.

Crane, A. (1959) 'Femoral torsion and its relation to toeing-in and toeing-out.' *Journal of Bone and Joint Surgery*, **41A**, 421–428.

Crawford, A. H., Bilbo, J. T., Schniegenberg, G. (1986) 'Subtalar stabilization by staple arthrodesis in the young child.' *Orthopaedic Transactions*, **10**, 152.

Crenshaw, A. H. (1963) *Campbell's Operative Orthopaedics, 4th Edn. Vol. 2.* St Louis: C. V. Mosby. pp. 1061–1062.

Csongradi, J., Bleck, E. E., Ford, W. F. (1979) 'Gait electromyography in normal and spastic children with special reference to the quadriceps femoris and hamstring muscles.' *Developmental Medicine and Child Neurology*, **21**, 738–748.

—— Terver, S., Mederios, J., Bleck, E. E. (1980) 'Electromyographic study of the gluteus medius during the gait of normal children and cerebral palsy children.' *Orthopaedic Transactions*, **4**, 72.

Dennyson, W. G., Fulford, R. (1976) 'Subtalar arthrodesis by cancellous grafts and metallic fixation.' *Journal of Bone and Joint Surgery*, **58B**, 507–510.

Diamond, L. (1978) *Personal communication.*

Drummond, D. S., Rogala, E., Templeton, J., Cruess, R. (1974) 'Proximal hamstring release for knee flexion and crouched posture in cerebral palsy.' *Journal of Bone and Joint Surgery*, **56A**, 1598–1602.

Duchenne, G. B. (1867) *Physiologie des Mouvements.* Paris: J.-B. Baillière et Fils. pp. 328–341.

—— (1959) *Physiology of Motion.* Kaplan, E. B. (translator). Philadelphia: W. B. Saunders, pp. 245–255.

Duckworth, T. (1977) 'The surgical management of cerebral palsy.' *Prosthetics and orthotics International*, **1**, 96–104.

Duncan, W. R. (1955) 'Release of rectus femoris in spastic children.' *Journal of Bone and Joint Surgery*, **37A**, 634.

Edmonson, A. S. (1963) *Campbell's Operative Orthopaedics.* St. Louis: C. V. Mosby.

Eggers, G. W. N. (1952) 'Transplantation of hamstring tendons to femoral condyles in order to improve hip extension and to decrease knee flexion in cerebral spastic paralysis.' *Journal of Bone and Joint Surgery*, **34A**, 827–830.

Evans, E. B. (1975) 'The knee in cerebral palsy.' *In:* Samilson, R. L. (Ed.) *Orthopaedic Aspects of Cerebral Palsy. Clinics in Developmental Medicine, Nos. 52/53.* London: S.I.M.P. with Heinemann; Philadelphia: J. B. Lippincott.

—— (1977) *Personal communication.*

Eyre, D. R. (1984) 'Collagen cross-linking in normal and diseased skeletal connective tissues.' *In:* Jacobs, R. R. (Ed.) *Pathogenesis of Idiopathic Scoliosis.* Chicago: Scoliosis Research Society. pp. 107–118.

Fabry, G. (1977) 'Torsion of the femur.' *Acta Orthopaedica Belgica*, **43**, 454–459.
—— MacEwen, G. D., Shands, A. R. (1973) 'Torsion of the femur. A study in normal and abnormal conditions.' *Journal of Bone and Joint Surgery*, **55A**, 1726–1738.
Feldkamp, M., Katthagen, E. W. (1975) 'Results of surgical correction of flexion contractures of the knee joint in cerebral palsy children.' *Zeitschrift fur Orthopädie und ihre Grenzgebiete*, **113**, 181–188.
Ferguson, A. B. (1973) 'Primary open reduction of congenital dislocation of the hip using a median adductor approach.' *Journal of Bone and Joint Surgery*, **55A**, 671–689.
—— (1975) *Orthopaedic Surgery in Infancy and Childhood.* Baltimore: Williams & Wilkins.
Feyen, J., Libricht, P., Fabry, G. (1984) 'Adductor myotomy, hamstring lengthening and Achilles tendon lengthening in cerebral palsy.' *Acta Orthopaedica Belgica*, **50**, 180–189.
Fixen, J. A. (1979) 'Surgical treatment of the lower limbs in cerebral palsy: a review.' *Journal of the Royal Society of Medicine*, **72**, 761–765.
Frost, H. M. (1971) 'Cerebral palsy, the spastic crouch.' *Clinical Orthopaedics and Related Research*, **80**, 2–8.
Gage, J. R., Perry, J., Hicks, R. R., Koop, S., Wrentz, J. R. (1987) 'Rectus femoris transfer as a means of improving knee function in cerebral palsy.' *Developmental Medicine and Child Neurology.* (*In press.*)
Gardner, E., Gray, D. J., O'Rahilly, R. (1969) *Anatomy-A Regional Study of Human Structure.* Philadelphia: W. B. Saunders.
Garrett, A. L. (1976) 'Discussion of papers by Couch *et al.* and Griffin *et al.* on adductor transfer.' *Paper presented at the Annual Meeting of the American Academy for Cerebral Palsy, Los Angeles.*
Goldner, J. L. (1981) 'Hip adductor transfer compared with adductor tenotomy in cerebral palsy.' *Journal of Bone and Joint Surgery*, **63A**, 1498. (*Letter.*)
Graf, R. (1983) 'New possibilities for the diagnosis of congenital hip joint dislocation by ultrasonography.' *Journal of Pediatric Orthopedics*, **3**, 354–359.
Grant, J. C. B. (1952) *A Method of Anatomy, 5th edn.* Baltimore: Williams & Wilkins.
Gray, H. (1942) *Anatomy of the Human Body, 24th edn.* Lewis, W. H. (Ed.) Philadelphia: Lea & Febiger.
Green, W. T., McDermott, L. J. (1942) 'Operative treatment of cerebral palsy of the spastic type.' *Journal of the American Medical Association*, **118**, 434–440.
Grice, D. S. (1952) 'Extra-articular arthrodesis of the subastragalar joint for correction of paralytic flat feet in children.' *Journal of Bone and Joint Surgery*, **43A**, 927–940.
Griffin, P. P., Wheelhouse, W. W., Shiavi, R. (1977) 'Adductor transfer for adductor spasticity: clinical and electromyographic gait analysis.' *Developmental Medicine and Child Neurology*, **19**, 783–789.
Griffith, B., Donavan, M. M., Stephenson, C. T., Franklin, T. (1982) 'The adductor transfer and iliopsoas recession in the cerebral palsy hip.' *Orthopaedic Transactions*, **6**, 94–95.
Guillot, M., Terver, S., Betrand, A., Vanneuville, G. (1977) 'Radiographie, electromyographie et approche fonctionnelle due muscle psoas-iliaque.' *Acta Anatomica*, **99**, 274.
Gunsolus, P., Welsh, C., Houser, C. E. (1975) 'Equilibrium reactions in the feet of children with spastic cerebral palsy and of normal children.' *Developmental Medicine and Child Neurology*, **17**, 580–591.
Haas, S. S., Epps, C. H., Adams, J. P. (1973) 'Normal ranges of hip motion in the newborn.' *Clinical Orthopaedics and Related Research*, **91**, 114–118.
Hagy, J. L., Mann, R. A., Keller, C. (1973) *Normal Gait Electromyograms and Lower Limb Ranges of Motion.* San Francisco: Shriner's Hospital for Crippled Children.
Hein, W. (1969) 'Surgical therapy of the knee contracture in cerebral paresis.' (*German.*) *Zeitschrift fur Orthopädie und ihre Grenzgebiete*, **106**, 755–759.
Hoffer, M. M. (1969) *Personal communication.*
—— (1972) *Personal communication.*
—— (1977) *Personal communication.*
—— (1986) 'Management of the hip in cerebral palsy.' *Journal of Bone and Joint Surgery*, **68A**, 629–631.
—— Prietto, C., Koffman, M. (1981) 'Supracondylar derotational osteotomy of the femur for internal rotation of the thigh in the cerebral palsied child.' *Journal of Bone and Joint Surgery*, **63A**, 389–393.
Hollinshead, W. H. (1951) *Functional Anatomy of the Limbs and Back.* Philadelphia: W. B. Saunders.
Horstmann, H. (1986) 'Skeletal maturation in cerebral palsy.' *Orthopaedic Transactions*, **10**, 152.
—— Eilert, R. E. (1977) 'Triple arthrodesis in cerebral palsy.' *Paper presented at annual meeting of the American Academy of Orthopaedic Surgeons, Las Vegas.*
—— Mahboubi, S. (1986) 'Use of CT scan in cerebral palsy hip reconstruction.' *Paper No. 20, Annual meeting of the Pediatric Orthopaedic Society of North America, Boston.*
Houkom, J. A., Roach, J. W., Wenger, D. R., Speck, G., Herring, J. A., Norris, R. N. (1986)

'Treatment of acquired hip subluxation in cerebral palsy.' *Journal of Pediatric Orthopedics,* **6,** 285–290.

Hsu, L. (1986) 'Results of hamstring lengthening at the Duchess of Kent Hospital, Hong Kong.' *Paper presented at Second Symposium on Cerebral Palsy, Singapore.*

—— O'Brien, J. D., Yau, A. C. M. C., Hodgson, A. R. (1974) 'Valgus deformities of the ankle in children with fibular pseudoarthrosis.' *Journal of Bone and Joint Surgery,* **56A,** 503–510.

—— Jaffray, D., Leong, J. C. Y. (1986) 'The Batchelor-Grice extra-articular subtalar arthrodesis.' *Journal of Bone and Joint Surgery,* **68B,** 125–127.

Hubbard, D. D., Staheli, L. T. (1972) 'The direct radiographic measurement of femur torsion using axial tomography.' *Clinical Orthopaedics and Related Research,* **86,** 16–20.

Hyashi, Y. (1970) 'The surgery of hamstring tendons for knee flexion contracture in cerebral palsy.' *Journal of the Kumamoto Medical Society,* **44,** 144–149.

Inman, V. T. (1947) 'The functional aspects of the abductor muscles of the hip.' *Journal of Bone and Joint Surgery,* **29A,** 607–619.

—— (1976) *The Joints of the Ankle.* Baltimore: Williams & Wilkins.

Jackson, J. P., Waugh, W. (1974) 'The technique and complications of upper tibial osteotomy.' *Journal of Bone and Joint Surgery,* **56B,** 236–245.

Kalen, V., Bleck, E. E. (1985) 'Prevention of spastic paralytic dislocation of the hip.' *Developmental Medicine and Child Neurology,* **27,** 17–24.

Kaye, J. J., Freiberger, R. H. (1971) 'Fragmentation of the lower pole of the patella in spastic lower extremities.' *Radiology,* **101,** 97–100.

Keagy, R. D., Brumlik, J., Bergin, J. L. (1966) 'Direct electromyography of the psoas major muscle in man.' *Journal of Bone and Joint Surgery,* **48A,** 1377–1382.

Keats, S. (1957) 'Combined adductor-gracilis tenotomy and selected obturator nerve resection for the correction of adduction deformity of the hip in children with cerebral palsy.' *Journal of Bone and Joint Surgery,* **39A,** 1087–1090.

—— (1974) 'Congenital bilateral dislocation of the head of the radius in a seven year old child.' *Orthopaedic Review,* **111,** 33–36.

—— Kambin, P. (1962) 'An evaluation of surgery for the correction of knee-flexion contracture in children with cerebral spastic paralysis.' *Journal of Bone and Joint Surgery,* **44A,** 1146–1154.

Kling, T. F., Jr. (1984) 'Adductor release with and without obturator neurectomy.' *Orthopaedic Transactions,* **8,** 112.

Kottke, F. J. (1966) 'The effects of limitation of activity upon the human body.' *Journal of the American Medical Association,* **196,** 825–830.

Krom, W. (1969) 'An evaluation of the posterior transfer of the adductor muscles of the hip in the ambulatory patient with cerebral palsy.' *Resident conference paper, unpublished. Downey, California: Rancho Los Amigos Hospital.*

LaGasse, D. J., Staheli, L. T. (1972) 'The measurement of femoral anteversion. A comparison of the fluoroscopic and biplane roentgenographic methods of measurement.' *Clinical Orthopaedics and Related Research,* **86,** 13–15.

Lamb, D. W., Pollock, G. A. (1962) 'Hip deformities in cerebral palsy and their treatment.' *Developmental Medicine and Child Neurology,* **4,** 488–497.

Lee, C. (1977a) 'Forces acting to derotate exaggerated femoral anteversion of the newborn hip.' *Unpublished thesis as part of a fellowship from the United Cerebral Palsy Research and Education Foundation, New York and the Children's Hospital at Stanford.*

—— (1977b) 'The Grice subtalar extra-articular arthrodesis.' *Unpublished thesis of fellowship from the United Cerebral Palsy Research and Education Foundation. Palo Alto, California: Children's Hospital at Stanford, Pediatric Orthopaedic-Rehabilitation Service.*

Lewis, F. R., Samilson, R. L., Lucas, D. B. (1964) 'Femoral torsion and coxa valga in cerebral palsy—a preliminary report.' *Developmental Medicine and Child Neurology,* **6,** 591–597.

Lisowski, F. P. (1974) 'Angular growth changes and comparisons in the primate talus.' *Folia Primatol (Basel),* **7,** 81–97.

Lottman, D. B. (1976) 'Knee flexion deformity and patella alta in spastic cerebral palsy.' *Developmental Medicine and Child Neurology,* **18,** 315–319.

MacEwen, G. D. (1972) *Adjustable Frame for the Lower Limb for Radiographs by the Ryder-Crane Technique.* Washington, Delaware: A. I. Dupont Institute.

Magilligan, D. J. (1956) 'Calculation of the angle of anteversion by means of horizontal lateral roentgenography.' *Journal of Bone and Joint Surgery,* **38A,** 1231–1246.

Majestro, T. C., Frost, H. M. (1971) 'Cerebral palsy: spastic internal femoral torsion.' *Clinical Orthopaedics and Related Research,* **79,** 44–56.

Mann, R. (1983) 'Biomechanics in cerebral palsy.' *Foot and Ankle,* **4,** 114–118.
—— Hagy, J. (1973) *Normal Electromyographic Data.* San Francisco: Shriner's Hospital for Crippled Children.
Matsuo, T., Hajime, T., Tada, S., Fujii, T., Hara, H. (1984) 'The role of hip adductors for adduction contracture of the hip in cerebral palsy.' *Seikeigeka (Orthopedic Surgery),* **35,** 1265–1272 *(Japanese.)*
——Shunsaku, T., Hajime, T. (1986) 'Insufficiency of the hip-adductor after anterior obturator neurectomy in forty-two chidren with cerebral palsy.' *Journal of Pediatric Orthopedics,* **6** (6). *(In press.)*
McCall, R. E., Lillich, J. S., Harris, J. R., Johnston, F. A. (1985) 'The Grice extra-articular subtalar arthrodesis: a clinical review.' *Journal of Pediatric Orthopedics,* **5,** 442–445.
Merchant, A. C. (1965) 'Hip abductor muscle force.' *Journal of Bone and Joint Surgery,* **47A,** 462–475.
Michele, A. A. (1962) *Iliopsoas.* Springfield, Ill.: C. C. Thomas.
Miranda, S. (1979) 'Outcomes of spastic diplegia.' *Unpublished study at Children's Hospital at Stanford, Palo Alto, California.*
Moe, J. H., Winter, R. B., Bradford, D. S., Lonstein, J. E. (1978) *Scoliosis and Other Spinal Deformities.* Philadelphia: W. B. Saunders. p. 538.
Mohaghegh, H. A., Stryker, W. (1983) 'Grice procedure using dowel iliac graft.' *Orthopaedic Transactions,* **7,** 166.
Moreland, J. R., Westin, G. W. (1977) 'Further experience with Grice subtalar arthrodesis.' *Orthopaedic Transactions,* **1,** 109.
—— —— (1986) 'Further experience with Grice subtalar arthrodesis.' *Clinical Orthopaedics and Related Research,* **207,** 113–121.
Morinaga, H. (1973) 'An electromyographic study on the function of the psoas major muscle.' *Journal of Japanese Orthopaedic Association,* **47,** 47 *(English abstract.)*
Morrissy, R. T. (1985) *Personal communication.*
Murray, M. P., Sepic, S. B. (1968) 'Maximum isometric torque of hip abductor and adductor muscles.' *Physical Therapy,* **43,** 1327–1335.
Nather, A., Fulford, G. E., Stewart, K. (1984) 'Treatment of valgus hindfoot in cerebral palsy by peroneus brevis lengthening.' *Developmental Medicine and Child Neurology,* **26,** 335–340.
—— Balasubramaniam, P., Bose, K. (1986) 'A comparative study of different methods of tendon lengthening: an experimental study in rabbits.' *Journal of Pediatric Orthopedics,* **6,** 456–459.
Page, J. (1982) 'Results of posterior capsulotomy of the knee with section of the anterior cruciate ligament insertion.' *Thesis for orthopaedic graduate education program in orthopaedic surgery, Stanford, California: Stanford University School of Medicine.*
Perry, J. (1985) 'Normal and pathological gait.' *In: Atlas of Orthotics: Biomechanical Principles and Application.* St. Louis: C. V. Mosby.
—— Lieb, F. J. (1967) 'A study of the quadriceps extension mechanism at the knee.' *Final Project Report, Downey, California: Rancho Los Amigos Hospital.*
——Antonelli, D., Ford, W. (1975) 'Analysis of knee joint forces during flexed-knee stance.' *Journal of Bone and Joint Surgery,* **57A,** 961–967.
—— Hoffer, M. M., Antonelli, D., Plut, J., Lewis, G., Greenberg, R. (1976) 'Electromyography before and after surgery for hip deformity in children with cerebral palsy.' *Journal of Bone and Joint Surgery,* **58A,** 201–208.
—— —— (1977) *Personal communication on electromyographic gait studies of the gluteus medius in patients with cerebral palsy and stroke.*
Peterson, H., Klassen, R., McLeod, R., Hoffman, A. (1981) 'The use of computerized tomography in dislocation of the hip and femoral neck anteversion in children.' *Journal of Bone and Joint Surgery,* **63B,** 198–208.
Phelps, E., Smith, L. J., Hallum, A. (1985) 'Normal ranges of hip motion of infants between nine and 24 months of age.' *Developmental Medicine and Child Neurology,* **27,** 785–792.
Phillips, H. O., Greene, W., Guilford, W. B., Mittelstaedt, C. A., Gaisie, G., Vincent, L. M., Durell, C. (1985) 'Measurement of femoral torsion: comparison of standard roentogenographic techniques with ultrasound.' *Journal of Pediatric Orthopaedics,* **5,** 546–549.
Pitkow, R. B. (1975) 'External rotation contracture of the extended hip: a common phenomenon of infancy obscuring femoral neck anteversion and the most frequent cause of out-toeing gait in children.' *Clinical Orthopaedics and Related Research,* **110,** 139–145.
Pollock, J. H., Carrell, B. (1964) 'Subtalar extra-articular arthrodesis in the treatment of paralytic valgus deformities.' *Journal of Bone and Joint Surgery,* **46A,** 533–541.
Porter, R. E. (1970) 'Hamstring transfers in cerebral palsy.' *New York State Journal of Medicine,* **70,**

388

1866–1867.

Propst-Proctor, S. L., Bleck, E. E. (1983) 'Radiographic determination of lordosis and kyphosis in normal and scoliotic children.' *Journal of Pediatric Orthopedics,* **3,** 344–346.

Rab, G. T. (1985) 'Static and dynamic muscle length model use in cerebral palsy.' *Paper No. 34, Annual Meeting of Pediatric Orthopaedic Society of North America, San Antonio, Texas.*

Rang, M., Silver, R., de la Garza, J. (1986) 'Cerebral palsy.' *In:* Lovell, W. W., Winter, R. B. (Eds.) *Pediatric Orthopaedics, 2nd edn. Vol I.* Philadelphia: J. B. Lippincott.

Ray, R. L., Ehrlich, M. G. (1979) 'Lateral hamstring transfer and gait improvement in the cerebral palsy patient.' *Journal of Bone and Joint Surgery,* **61A,** 719–723.

Reimers, J. (1974) 'Contracture of the hamstrings in spastic cerebral palsy.' *Journal of Bone and Joint Surgery,* **65B,** 102–109.

—— (1980) 'The stability of the hip in children. A radiological study of the results of muscle surgery in cerebral palsy.' *Acta Orthopaedica Scandanavica* (Supplement), **184,** 1–97.

—— Poulsen, S. (1984) 'Adductor transfer versus tenotomy for stability of the hip in spastic cerebral palsy.' *Journal of Pediatric Orthopedics,* **4,** 52–54.

—— (1985) 'Spastic paralytic dislocation of the hip.' *Developmental Medicine and Child Neurology,* **27,** 401. (*Letter.*)

Rinsky, L. A. (1977) *Personal communication.*

—— (1980) *Personal communication.*

—— (1985) *Personal communication.*

Roberts, W. M., Adams, J. P. (1953) 'The patellar-advancement operation in cerebral palsy.' *Journal of Bone and Joint Surgery,* **35A,** 958–966.

Root, L., Spero, C. R. (1981) 'Hip adductor transfer compared with adductor tenotomy in cerebral palsy.' *Journal of Bone and Joint Surgery,* **63A,** 767–772.

Roosth, H. P. (1971) 'Flexion deformity of the hip and knee in spastic cerebral palsy: treatment by early release of spastic hip-flexor muscles.' *Journal of Bone and Joint Surgery,* **53A,** 1489–1510.

Rosenthal, R. K., Levine, D. B. (1977) 'Fragmentation of the distal pole of the patella in spastic cerebral palsy.' *Journal of Bone and Joint Surgery,* **59A,** 934–939.

Ross, P. M., Lyne, D. (1980) 'The Grice procedure: indicators and evaluation of long term results.' *Clinical Orthopaedics and Related Research,* **153,** 195–200.

Ruby, L., Mital, M., O'Conner, J., Patel, U. (1979) 'Anteversion of the femoral neck. A comparison of methods of measurements in patients.' *Journal of Bone and Joint Surgery,* **61,** 46–51.

Ryder, C. T. (1972) *Computerized calculations for femoral anteversion with the Ryder-Crane technique. Personal communication.*

—— Crane, L. (1953) 'Measuring femoral anteversion: the problem and the method.' *Journal of Bone and Joint Surgery,* **35A,** 321–328.

Sage, F. (1977) *Personal communication.*

Salter, R. B. (1961) 'Innominate osteotomy in the treatment of congenital dislocation and subluxation of the hip.' *Journal of Bone and Joint Surgery,* **43B,** 518–539.

—— Field, P. (1960) 'The effects of continuous compression in living articular cartilage: an experimental investigation.' *Journal of Bone and Joint Surgery,* **42A,** 31–49.

Samilson, R. L. (1972) *Personal communcation.*

—— (1976) 'Crescentric osteotomy of the os calcis for calcanealcavus feet.' *In:* Bateman, J. E. (Ed.) *Foot Science.* Philadelphia: W. B. Saunders. pp. 18–25.

—— Carson, J. J., James, P., Raney, F. L. (1967) 'Results and complications of adductor tenotomy and obturator neurectomy in cerebral palsy.' *Clinical Orthopaedics and Related Research,* **54,** 61–73.

Saunders, J. B., Inman, V. T., Eberhart, H. D. (1953) 'The major determinants in normal and pathological gait.' *Journal of Bone and Joint Surgery,* **35A,** 543–558.

Schultz, R. S., Chamberlain, S. E., Stevens, P. M. (1984) 'Radiographic comparison of adductor procedures in cerebral palsied hips.' *Journal of Pediatric Orthopedics,* **4,** 741–744.

Scrutton, D. R. (1969) 'Foot sequences of normal children under five years old.' *Developmental Medicine and Child Neurology,* **11,** 44–53.

Seymour, N., Evans, D. K. (1968) 'A modification of the Grice subtalar arthrodesis.' *Journal of Bone and Joint Surgery,* **50B,** 372–375.

——Sharrard, W. J. W. (1968) 'Bilateral proximal release of the hamstrings in cerebral palsy.' *Journal of Bone and Joint Surgery,* **58B,** 274–277.

Shands, A. R., Steele, M. K. (1958) 'Torsion of the femur.' *Journal of Bone and Joint Surgery,* **40A,** 803–816.

Sharps, C. H., Clancy, M., Steel, H. H. (1984) 'A long-term retrospective study of proximal hamstring release for hamstring contracture in cerebral palsy.' *Journal of Pediatric Orthopedics,* **4,** 443–447.

389

Sharrard, W. J. W. (1975) 'The hip in cerebral palsy.' *In:* Samilson, R. L. (Ed.) *Orthopaedic Aspects of Cerebral Palsy, Clinics in Developmental Medicine Nos. 52/53.* London: S.I.M.P. with Heinemann; Philadelphia: J. B. Lippincott.

Silver, C. M. (1977) 'Calcaneal osteotomy results in 100 operations and 64 feet followed longer than 5 years.' *In: Instructional Course Lectures, American Academy of Orthopaedic Surgeons.* St. Louis: C. V. Mosby.

—— Simon, S. D., Lichtman, H. M. (1966) 'The use and abuse of obturator neurectomy.' *Developmental Medicine and Child Neurology,* **8,** 203–205.

—— —— Spindell, E., Lichtman, H. M., Scala, M. (1967) 'Calcaneal osteotomy for valgus and varus deformities of the foot in cerebral palsy.' *Journal of Bone and Joint Surgery,* **49A,** 232–246.

—— —— Lichtman, H. M. (1974) 'Long term followup observations on calcaneal osteotomy'. *Clinical Orthopaedics and Related Research,* **99,** 181–187.

Simon, S. R., Deutsch, S. D., Nuzzo, R. M., Mansour, M. J., Jackson, J. L. F., Koskinen, M., Rosenthal, R. K. (1978) 'Genu recurvatum in spastic cerebral palsy.' *Journal of Bone and Joint Surgery,* **60A,** 882–894.

—— Thometz, J., Rosenthal, R. K., Griffin, P. (1986) 'The effect of medial hamstring lengthening on the gait of patients with cerebral palsy.' *Orthopaedic Transactions,* **10,** 152.

Skinner, S. R., Lester, D. K. (1985) 'Dynamic EMG findings in valgus hindfoot deformity in spastic cerebral palsy.' *Orthopaedic Transactions,* **9,** 91.

Somerville, E. W. (1960) 'Flexion contractures of the knee.' *Journal of Bone and Joint Surgery,* **42B,** 730–735.

Staheli, L. T., Duncan, W. R., Schaefer, E. (1968) 'Growth alterations in the hemiplegic child.' *Clinical Orthopaedics and Related Research,* **60,** 205–212.

—— Clawson, D. K., Hubbard, D. D. (1980) 'Medial femoral torsion: experience with operative treatment.' *Clinical Orthopaedics and Related Research,* **146,** 222–225.

Steel, H. H. (1980) 'Gluteus medius and minimus insertion advancement for correction of internal rotation gait in spastic cerebral palsy.' *Journal of Bone and Joint Surgery,* **62,** 919–927.

—— Sandrow, R. E., Sullivan, P. D. (1971) 'Complications of tibial osteotomy in children for genu varum or valgum.' *Journal of Bone and Joint Surgery,* **53A,** 1629–1635.

Stephenson, C. T., Donovan, M. M. (1971) 'Transfer of hip adductor origins to the ischium in spastic cerebral palsy.' *Developmental Medicine and Child Neurology,* **13,** 247. (*Abstract.*)

Strange, F. G. St. Clair (1965) *The Hip.* Baltimore: Williams & Wilkins.

Sullivan, R. C., Gehringer, K. M., Harris, G. F. (1984) 'A computer assisted survey of the results of medial hamstring surgery in children with cerebral palsy.' *Orthopaedic Transactions,* **8,** 109.

Sussman, M. (1984) 'Adductor and iliopsoas releases: results after early mobilization.' *Orthopaedic Transactions,* **8,** 112.

Sutherland, D. H. (1980) *Lecture, International Pediatric Orthopaedic Seminar, San Francisco.*

—— Schottstaedt, E. R., Larsen, L. I., Ashley, R. K., Callander, J. N., James, P. M. (1969) 'Clinical and electromyographic study of seven spastic children with internal rotation gait.' *Journal of Bone and Joint Surgery,* **51A,** 1070–1082.

—— Larsen, L. I., Mann, R. (1975) 'Rectus femoris release in selected patients with cerebral palsy: a preliminary report.' *Developmental Medicine and Child Neurology,* **17,** 26–34.

—— Cooper, L. (1978) 'The pathomechanics of progressive crouch gait in spastic diplegia.' *Orthopaedic Clinics of North America,* **9,** 142–154.

—— Olshen, R., Cooper, L., Woo, S. K. (1980) 'The development of mature gait.' *Journal of Bone and Joint Surgery,* **62A,** 336–353.

Thompson, G. H., Shaffer, J. W., Zdeblich, T. (1986) 'Percutaneous distal femoral derotation osteotomy.' *Paper No. 19, Annual Meeting, Pediatric Orthopaedic Society of North America,* Boston.

Trouillas, J. (1978) 'La chirurgie des membres inferieurs chez l'infirme moteur cérébrale spastique. *Thesis for the Faculty of Medicine, Montpellier, France.*

Tylkowski, C. M., Rosenthal, R. K., Simon, S. R. (1980) 'Proximal femoral osteotomy in cerebral palsy.' *Clinical Orthopaedics and Related Research,* **151,** 183–192.

—— Simon, S. R., Mansour, J. M. (1982) 'Internal rotation gait in spastic cerebral palsy.' *Hip,* 89–125.

—— Price, C. T. (1986) 'Aponeurotic lengthening of the iliopsoas muscle for spastic hip flexion deformities-assessment by gait analysis.' *Paper No. 25, Pediatric Orthopaedic Society of North America Annual Meeting, Boston.*

Waters, R. L., Garland, D. E., Perry, J., Habig, T., Slabaugh, P. (1979) 'Stiff-legged gait in hemiplegia: surgical correction.' *Journal of Bone and Joint Surgery,* **61A,** 927–933.

Westin, G. W. (1965) 'Tendon transfers about the foot, ankle, and hip in the paralyzed lower extremity.' *Journal of Bone and Joint Surgery*, **47A,** 1430–1443.

—— (1973) *Personal communication.*

Wheeler, M. E., Weinstein, S. L. (1984) 'Adductor tenotomy-obturator neurectomy.' *Journal of Pediatric Orthopedics*, **4,** 48–51.

Wilkinson, I. (1962) 'Femoral anteversion in the rabbit.' *Journal of Bone and Joint Surgery*, **44B,** 386–397.

Williams, I. (1977) 'The consequences of orthopaedic surgery to the adolescent cerebral palsied: medical, educational and parental attitudes.' *Paper presented at the Study Group on Integrating the Care of Multiply Handicapped Children, St. Mary's College, Durham, England.* London: The Spastics Society Medical Education and Information Unit.

Williams, P. F., Menelaus, M. B. (1977) 'Triple arthrodesis by inlay grafting-a method suitable for undeformed or valgus foot.' *Journal of Bone and Joint Surgery*, **59B,** 333–336.

Wilson, P. D. (1929) 'Posterior capsuloplasty in certain flexion contractures of the knee.' *Journal of Bone and Joint Surgery*, **11,** 40–58.

Wiltse, L. L. (1972) 'Valgus deformity of the ankle. A sequel to acquired or congenital abnormalities of the fibula.' *Journal of Bone and Joint Surgery*, **54A,** 595–606.

Wu, K. K. (1986) *Surgery of the Foot.* Philadelphia: Lea & Febiger.

Wynne-Davies, R. (1970) 'Acetabular dysplasia and familial joint laxity: two etiological factors in congenital dislocation of the hip.' *Journal of Bone and Joint Surgery*, **52B,** 704–716.

9
TOTAL BODY INVOLVEMENT

Stereotyping is inversely proportional to familiarity (Robert L. Samilson 1981).

Characteristics

'Total body involved' is the term now commonly used to describe cerebral palsy in persons who have quadriplegia, trunk, head and neck dysequilibrium, speech and hearing deficits and a variety of intellectual dysfunctions (*e.g.* retardation, perceptual and visual defects). The most serious defect in many is an inability to orally communicate needs, thoughts and feelings. The over-all incidence of communication disorders in this group was estimated as 40 per cent unable to write, 10 per cent non-verbal and 20 per cent non-vocal (Bureau of Education for the Handicapped 1976). Non-verbal means the inability to think and talk; non-vocal indicates an ability to think but not talk.

Deafness is common in those whose cerebral dysfunction was due to maternal rubella or erythroblastosis fetalis. Deafness with cerebral palsy is now rare due to prevention of both these etiologies. Blindness due to retrolental fibroplasia, associated with the neonatal respiratory distress syndrome, has fortunately disappeared due to the discovery of the effects of hyperoxygenation. Convulsive disorders are common and add to the turmoil of existence and care. However, drug therapy has been successful in controlling most recurrent convulsions.

Mental retardation is not inevitable, even though first impressions can lead to rash judgements. Non-verbal persons who were taught to communicate with alternative methods were found to have normal intelligence (McNaughton 1975). Root (1977) reported that 55 per cent of his total body involved patients had IQs over 80; normal intelligence was documented in 36 per cent of those who had spastic paralysis and in 68 per cent involved with athetosis.

Head and trunk control are often deficient. Standing equilibrium reactions are usually nil. Total extensor patterns of the trunk and limbs predominate in some, while others have a mixture of flexor (usually in the upper limbs) and extensor (in the lower limbs) involuntary or spastic muscle activity. The upper limbs may be more involved in athetosis, and there are patients who have better foot and toe control than in their hands and fingers. Often one upper limb is not as involved as the other, which will have better voluntary control of some sort. Then we have patients whose only voluntary control is with their head and neck and/or eyes.

The most common skeletal problems are subluxation and dislocation of the hip, scoliosis, knee-flexion contractures and ankle equinus. If the skeletal changes are not corrected, particularly in the hip, degenerative changes cause pain and added disability as the person ages (see Chapter 5). Those who have athetosis seem especially prone to pain in the spine and limb joints due to the effects of continuous contorted motion as they grow older (Bleck 1975, Hirose and Kadoya 1984). Recurrent dislocation of the shoulder in athetosis has been observed occasionally.

Prognosis

Prognosis for function in communication, activities of daily living, mobility and walking have been discussed in Chapter 3.

Walking is almost always impossible or not functional. The level of wheelchair mobility can be categorized according to ability to transfer in and out of the chair:

(1) independent transfers
(2) assistive transfers
(3) totally dependent.

Mobility in the wheelchair is subdivided according to those who are able to use a manual chair efficiently or a motorized wheelchair effectively. Some can do neither and are dependent on another person to push them about. Most total body involved children and adults need motorized wheelchairs and can use them effectively with appropriate interfaces and control mechanisms.

Because most of these patients lack trunk balance, supportive sitting has become recognized as most important. Rang *et al.* (1981) has classified sitting as follows: (i) by ability—hands free, hand dependent, or propped; (ii) by pattern of deformity—asymmetrical slouch or windswept hips and pelvis; (iii) by severity of deformity—none, amenable to surgery, or beyond surgery. Do we remake the child to fit the seat or do we design the seat to fit the child (Rang 1986)? Interest in seating has exploded; more and more publications on seating analysis and construction have appeared in the past nine years (Ring *et al.* 1978, Trefler *et al.* 1978, Paul *et al.* 1980, Rang *et al.* 1981, Fulford *et al.* 1982, Holte and Siekman 1983). Seating clinics have been established in many centers. The physical therapist's interest in seating seems to have displaced inhibitive casts (Rang 1986).

Assessment, management and goals

These patients require all the clinical orthopaedic and neurological assessments delineated in Chapter 2, with added special assessments according to need (Chapter 3). Assessments for the senses and intellect will be required, depending upon the individual's deficits in function and physiology.

Management is based upon the goal-oriented approach according to the priorities for optimum independent living as described in Chapter 6. Because these persons present an almost overwhelming number of problems, efforts toward rehabilitation are apt to be truncated, individuals relegated to the waste-basket category of medical care and their potential as persons neglected.

A philosophy of care is needed. Samilson referred to the evils of stereotyping. So-called 'health-care providers, managers and economists' can have difficulty in acknowledging the differences in people. As the late Dr Samilson noted, with reference to orthopaedic surgery as part of the treatment of the total body involved and retarded person: 'I have found that the physicians most adamant about strict nonoperative management of the retarded cerebral-palsied patients are precisely the same physicians who rarely, if ever, see such patients' (Samilson 1981, p.89).

Goals need to be established and changed if repeated evaluations require reorientation of recommended management. To rely on one's own values and culture to judge the 'quality of life' of disabled persons would be highly subjective and prejudicial. Because of increasing life-expectancy due to advances in medicine and sanitation, we have a constant outpouring of rhetoric in medical journals and the mass media concerning cost-benefit ratios. It seems to me that Samilson was correct: 'The interpretation of what is cost and what is benefit varies from person to person and is dependent on individual interests and biases' (Samilson 1981, p.89). The only rational approach in this group of severely disabled persons is to focus on them as individuals who will need the resources to achieve optimum independence in function consistent with the limitations imposed by the neurological and orthopaedic condition. A happy and comfortable life exclusive of gainful employment can also be a reasonable goal. Achievement of independence and demedicalization should be 'cost effective' in the long run.

Orthopaedic surgery

The major orthopaedic problems which require orthopaedic surgery for prevention and reconstruction in the total body involved patient are dislocation of the hip and scoliosis. Structural deformities of other joints in the upper and lower limbs can be surgically treated depending upon the feasibility for improving function. An occasional patient may have hand function improved with surgery, as outlined in Chapter 7. Correction of knee-flexion contractures and severe foot deformities can be justified in wheelchair users if assistive or independent transfers will be facilitated. Reconstructive surgery for the lower-limb deformities are the same as described for spastic hemiplegia and diplegia (Chapters 7 and 8).

The most common problem in limb surgery in the total body involved is the preoperative differentiation of spasticity from athetosis of the dystonic type. Tenotomies or lengthenings in the athetoid patient can result in the opposite and more disabling deformity.

Hospitalization for orthopaedic surgery in this group has been two to four times longer than the average length of stay for spastic diplegia and hemiplegia (Hoffer and Bullock 1981). However, surgery for hip and knee deformities did produce gains, primarily in hygiene and sitting tolerance. Surgery can be complicated by compromised pulmonary function, urinary-tract infections and bed care at home, especially in patients who require postoperative plasters. In-patient preoperative preparation, and pulmonary function assessment and treatment, decrease postoperative complications. Discharge planning, to facilitate home nursing care, must be more detailed than with other types of patients. Since not all patients will be from traditional nuclear families, with the space for bed care and energetic caregiving family members, some sort of continuous inpatient care facility will be required during the time for healing of skeletal structures.

In all patients who have hip and/or spine surgery, the skills of the rehabilitation engineering team will be needed for assessment and fabrication of seating and mobility equipment.

Fractures in the severely total body involved patient are another complication of management and seem to occur more commonly in those in long-term care institutions. McIvor and Samilson (1966) had 92 patients who had 134 fractures in a 10-year period. The mechanism of fracture in 70 was undetermined. In others it was from falling, catching a limb in the railing of a bed, turning in bed or in a radiology department, or during a bath. Closed treatment was preferred: the healing time with closed treatment was 3.5 months, and with surgery 5.3 months. Plaster and splint application was adapted to the patient's particular limb deformity. Of 69 fractured femora, 45 had malunion but function was not compromised.

Supracondylar fractures of the femur occurred often, and always with osteopenia. Over-zealous and vigorous passive exercise of the knee by the physical therapist can cause the supracondylar fracture; however, the complication is not entirely avoidable nor should it be overdrawn as a catastrophic event. Osteopenia always occurs in the absence of gravity and the forces of weightbearing. It is one of the physiological changes in space travel. Calcium and vitamin D intake alone will not prevent it. All these fractures heal with simple immobilization. If there is a flexion contracture of the knee, extension of the distal femoral fragment will correct the contracture; or if there is an internal rotation deformity of the femur, external rotation of the distal fragment will be corrective. Paradoxically, one can use an opportunity to turn what seems bad into some good.

Hip and pelvic deformities
Adduction contractures
Adduction contractures that interfere with perineal hygiene and sitting can be corrected with adductor myotomies and, in this group, anterior branch obturator neurectomy. The operative techniques are described in Chapter 8.

When one leg is crossed over the other (see Fig. 8.9), intrapelvic obturator neurectomy can be considered—especially if scissoring recurs after anterior branch obturator neurectomy.

Asymmetrical adduction contractures cause pelvic obliquity and uncovering of the most adducted hip with apparent subluxation. If there is no flexion contracture, adductor myotomy and anterior branch obturator neurectomy alone will correct the pelvic obliquity, unless it is due to a scoliosis when the pelvis is part of the curve as another vertebra.

The 'windblown' or 'windswept' posture of the lower limbs is due to a combination of an adduction contracture of one hip and displacement of the other hip in abduction. It can be accompanied by a pelvic obliquity secondary to scoliosis. Apparent subluxation of one hip is usual (Fig. 9.1). Unilateral dislocation is often present, usually after the age of six to seven years (Samilson *et al.* 1972). The abducted hip may have a contracture of the iliotibial band. To prevent this deformity, Letts *et al.* (1984) recommended bilateral adductor myotomy and anterior branch obturator neurectomy in infancy or early childhood as soon as radiographs show evidence of a break in Shenton's line; an iliopsoas recession was also included if a flexion contracture coexisted. All such surgery was followed with long-term abduction seating.

I have observed the 'windswept' pelvic and hip deformity in patients who had only a unilateral adductor myotomy and anterior branch obturator neurectomy on the side where early hip subluxation was seen, even though both hips had identical adduction contractures. The rôle of the adductor, iliopsoas and hamstring muscles

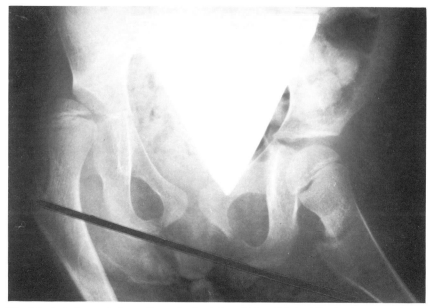

Fig. 9.1. Anterior-posterior radiograph of pelvis and hips. Pelvic obliquity due to persistent adduction contracture of right hip—'windswept pelvis'. Hip 'uncovered' on adducted side. Age nine years, female, total body involved.

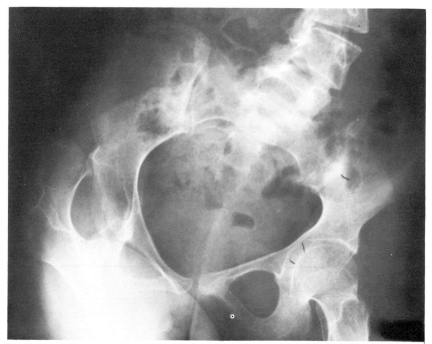

Fig. 9.2. Anterior-posterior radiograph of pelvis and hips. Pelvic obliquity due to scoliosis; pelvis is part of the curve. Hip dislocation independent of scoliosis.

in spastic dislocation of the hip will be discussed in the section on hip subluxation and dislocation.

Hip-flexion contractures

Hip-flexion contractures alone, without subluxation or dislocation in the total body involved patient, rarely need correction. After all, these patients are sitters. I can imagine surgical correction of hip-flexion contractures in wheelchair-bound patients if they stand for assistive transfers and have hamstring lengthenings to correct untenable knee-flexion contractures. Iliopsoas tenotomy to prevent severe and possible painful lumbar lordosis due to adaptive increased anterior inclination of the pelvis might be a necessary accompaniment to the correction of the knee-flexion posture.

Hip-extension and abduction contractures

Hip-extension and abduction contractures have been seen in total body involved patients most often after iliopsoas tenotomy and adductor myotomy with obturator neurectomy. The functional problem was the inability to sit in a wheelchair. Treatment was surgical, with release of the proximal hamstring muscle origins, gluteus maximus, hip external rotator muscles and, if necessary to gain flexion of the hip to 90° for sitting, the posterior capsule of the hip joint (Bowen *et al.* 1981, Szalay *et al.* 1986). Extension deformity of the hips with anterior dislocation has been reported (Copeliovitch *et al.* 1983).

This unusual contracture does not seem to occur as a primary deformity. As with the 'frog-leg' abduction deformity of the hips following adductor myotomy and anterior branch obturator neurectomy, iliopsoas tenotomy in a total body involved patient who has athetosis with dystonic posturing seems the likely cause. In these patients, alternating flexion and extension posturing without hip-flexion contracture can be found. The discernment of a true hip-flexion contracture is difficult. The Thomas test will be misleading. The repeated, careful and tedious examination with the prone hip-extension test may change the decision to perform an iliopsoas tenotomy. A calm and repetitive examination of the patient should assist in the diagnosis of athetosis.

If this type of patient has a flexion contracture and a hip subluxation, perhaps an iliopsoas lengthening or recession should be done to minimize the weakness of hip-flexion power and the risk of the postoperative hip-extension contracture.

Pelvic obliquity

Pelvic obliquity in the sagittal plane in the total body involved patient who sits is rarely as much of a problem as it is in spastic diplegia.

Pelvic obliquity in the coronal plane is frequent in the total body involved. In the coronal plane, pelvic obliquity can be due to contractures above and/or below the iliac crest. The most common cause is an adduction contracture of the hip (see above). The other frequent cause is scoliosis where the pelvis is part of the curve (Dubousset 1985) (Fig.9.2). Pelvic obliquity in the transverse plane also accompanies scoliosis when the curvature includes the pelvis (Dubousset 1985). Fixed

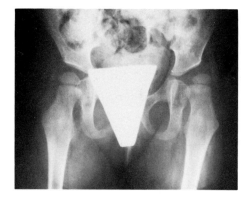

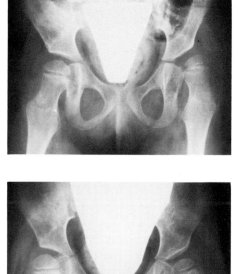

Fig. 9.3. Anterior-posterior radiographs of pelvis and hips. *Above left:* patient MS, age 18 months, total body involved. Subluxation of left hip and acetabular dysplasia, which is most unusual at this early age in cerebral-palsy acquired subluxation. *Above right:* MS, 18 months postoperative adductor myotomy and iliopsoas tenotomy. Subluxation the same. *Right:* MS, one year postoperative open reduction of hip, capsulorraphy and derotation subtrochanteric osteotomy with Wagner nail-plate fixation. Finally recognized this as a *congenital subluxation of the hip and cerebral palsy*.

rotation of the pelvis is usually first observed after scoliosis and pelvic obliquity correction by spinal instrumentation and arthrodesis.

The correction of pelvic obliquity with scoliosis will be discussed below (p.441).

Lonstein and Beck (1986) and Cristofaro *et al.* (1985) found no association between hip subluxation and dislocation and pelvic obliquity. Hip instability and scoliosis are separate entities, each with its own etiology in muscle imbalance. Prevention or correction of hip dislocation has no effect on scoliosis prevention, although the two often coexist.

Hip dislocation

INCIDENCE

Dislocation of the hip occurs almost exclusively in the total body involved non-ambulatory patient. Of 284 patients who had dislocated hip in Samilson's study (1972), 90 per cent had quadriplegia. Only 11 per cent had some limited ambulation. Baker *et al.* (1962) analyzed the incidence of subluxation and dislocation in 129 patients (258 hips), and found that 42 hips were subluxated and 31 were dislocated (28 per cent). Hoffer *et al.* (1972) reported dislocation of the hips in 75 per cent of 20 non-ambulatory total body involved patients.

Walking ability is directly related to the incidence of dislocation, and increasingly recognized by more recent observers (Le Foll 1980, Le Foll *et al.* 1981,

Vidal 1982). In an analysis of 85 patients with 'bilateral hemiplegia' (the term used by Howard *et al.* 1985 for quadriplegia or total body involved), 10.5 per cent were dislocated, 10.5 per cent had subluxation and 18 per cent had dysplastic acetabula. Of the 29 hemiplegics, only two had abnormal hip architecture; one had a bilateral dislocation. None of the hemiplegics had an abnormal hip joint. Of the 44 total body involved in this series, only nine walked unaided and nine used a rollator or frame walker; all the rest were non-walkers, 61 per cent of whom had abnormal hips. In our own study of 119 spastic diplegic children, none had hip dislocations at follow-up (Miranda 1979). In another review we did of 694 patients with cerebral palsy followed from 1957 to 1980, only the total body involved had dislocations.

It is possible to have a congenital dislocation of the hip and cerebral palsy. This combination is unlikely to occur in spastic hemiplegia or diplegia. In Western nations, the incidence of congenital dislocation is thought to be between 0.2 and 2.2 children per 1000 livebirths. Ethnic and racial differences are recognized. Con genital dislocation is rare in blacks, Koreans and Chinese, and more common in North American Indians, Lapps, and Hungarians (Coleman 1978).

The major radiological change, in distinguishing between a congenital and an acquired spastic paralytic dislocation, is the absence of any acetabular dysplasia in the infant and young child with cerebral palsy and a dislocated hip. In contrast, con genital dislocations of the hip will develop very early acetabular dysplasia, manifested in the radiograph by increased acetabular angles (Fig. 9.3).

NATURAL HISTORY
In the total body involved baby, the radiographs of the hips at first appear normal; then lateral subluxation without acetabular dysplasia occurs, and finally dislocation (see Fig. 9.19). The acetabular shallowing occurs as a response to the lack of contact of the femoral head in the acetabulum. The mean age of dislocation is thought to be about seven years (Samilson 1972).

The ability to walk by age four or five years profoundly influences the outcome. Those who are household and neighbourhood walkers, and use assistive devices for partial weight-bearing, retain the subluxation and acetabular dysplasia but do not dislocate. There is strong evidence that concentrically located femoral heads will have acetabular remodeling up to the age of four years (Harris *et al.* 1975). Subluxation of the hip discovered in spastic diplegic children under the age of five years, who have either adductor myotomies and/or iliopsoas lengthenings or recessions, will have excellent results as they become weight-bearing and functional walkers with aids to compensate for their lack of balance (Kalen and Bleck 1985) (Fig. 9.4).

MECHANISM
Two structural changes appear to be the major factors in spastic paralytic dislocation of the hip: persistence of the infantile hip-flexion contracture, and infantile excessive femoral anteversion. The existence of femoral torsion and its radiographic shadow called 'coxa valga' have been discussed in Chapter 8. The continuous spasticity of the iliopsoas muscle leads to its shortening and contracture,

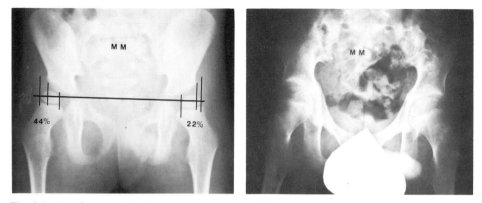

Fig. 9.4. Anterior-posterior radiographs of pelvis and hips. *Left:* MM, age two years, not walking, spastic subluxation of left hip (migration percentage = 44 per cent). Passive range of hip abduction = 40°, hip-flexion contractures = 30°. *Right:* MM, age 18 years. 16 years postoperative iliopsoas recession only. Community walker with crutches. Hips well located.

because it fails to have appositional growth as suggested by the experimental data reviewed by Rang *et al.* (1986) (see page 110 and page 248). The spastic adductor muscles have long been implicated as the major deforming force. Asymmetrical adduction contracture and pelvic obliquity does compound the problem, but the evidence does not point exclusively to these factors. The contracture of the medial hamstrings also contributes to the dislocation, as the femoral head drifts out of the acetabulum when the knee extends with hip adduction (Hiroshima and Ono 1979,

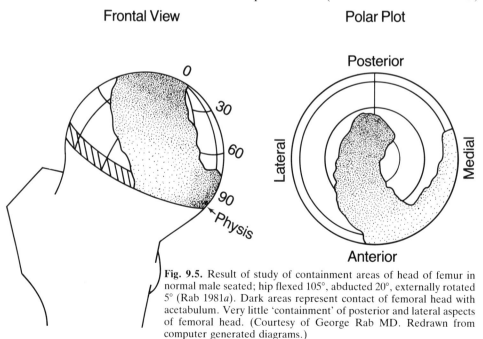

Fig. 9.5. Result of study of containment areas of head of femur in normal male seated; hip flexed 105°, abducted 20°, externally rotated 5° (Rab 1981*a*). Dark areas represent contact of femoral head with acetabulum. Very little 'containment' of posterior and lateral aspects of femoral head. (Courtesy of George Rab MD. Redrawn from computer generated diagrams.)

400

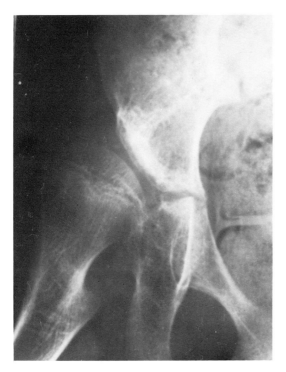
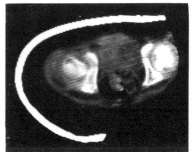

Fig. 9.6. *Left:* anterior-posterior radio-graph of hip; eight-year-old male, total body involved. Severe subluxation and acetabular dysplasia. *Above:* computer-ized axial tomography, transverse section through hips. Note lack of anterior and posterior acetabular development.

Vidal 1982).

The walking ability, as noted, has a major influence on hip dislocation. A synthesis of the combination of the flexion contracture of the hip due to iliopsoas spasticity and femoral torsion with walking ability can be expressed:

(1) Non-ambulatory, sitting patient = dislocation.

(2) Partial weight-bearing with canes, crutches or walkers, functional neighbour-hood walking = subluxation.

(3) Fully weight-bearing, functional neighbourhood walking = hip internal rotation gait and located hips.

It was presumed that sitting would 'contain' the hip. Using mathematical models of the hip and computerized simulations of the hip orientation and mobility, Rab (1981*b*) provided me with a model of femoral head containment with the subject seated. This study seems to refute the perception of increased femoral head contact with the acetabulum when sitting. The contact areas of the femoral head with the acetabulum are small, but seem less so on its posterior portions (Fig. 9.5). These findings correlate with transverse plane computerized axial tomograms of acetabula in spastic paralytic dislocations of the hip; the posterior acetabulum appears deficient (Fig. 9.6). Similar acetabular changes in paralytic dislocations have been described by Coleman (1983) and Lau *et al.* (1986).

The iliopsoas during gait acts at the very end of the stance phase and in the first 40 per cent of the swing phase (Fig. 9.7). It appears to act to bring the trunk over

TABLE 9.I

Electromyographic study of the psoas major; needle electrode inserted translumbar approach at level of third lumbar vertebra; six normal subjects (ages 19 to 32 years) non-weightbearing (from Guillot *et al.* 1977).

Motion of hip	Subjects					
	1	2	3	4	5	6
With hip flexed 90°						
Flexion against resistance	+++	+++	+++	+++	++	++
Abduction	0	0	0	+	±	±
Adduction	++	++	++	+++	++	++
Rotation internal	+	0	0	±	0	+
Rotation external	±	0	0	++	+	+
Flexion 90° to 110°		++	+	+	++	++
Flexion >110°	+++	+++	+++	+++	+++	+++
Hip extended						
Rotation internal	0	+	±	±	±	+
Rotation external	+	+	±	±	±	+
Flexion against resistance	++	++	+++	++	++	++
Extension against resistance	0	±	+	++	+	++
Abduction against resistance	+	±	±	+	±	±
Adduction against resistance	0	±	++	0	±	±
Subjects sitting						
Simple sitting	0	0	0	±	0	0
Sitting with holding a weight (*'en charge'*)	±	±	+	±	+	+
Sitting with flexion of the trunk	0	0	0	+	±	+

Symbols used for quality of EMG responses:
    0 = none
    ± = equivocal; not consistent
    + = mild
  ++ = moderate
+++ = strong

the advancing femoral head during level walking. In one study of normal subjects, the iliopsoas activity was recorded with wire electrodes in non-weightbearing and sitting postures (Guillot *et al.* 1977). With the hip flexed 90°, flexion against resistance at more than 110° created the greatest activity of the psoas major. The intensity was the same when the hip was extended and flexion resisted. Adduction of the hip when flexed 90° produced moderate contractions. When the subjects were tested standing, elevation of the pelvis on the same side resulted in moderate to strong action potentials in all but one subject. Electrical activity with hip-external rotation when the hip was flexed 90° was mild to moderate in five of the six subjects (Table 9.I). From these studies, Guillot *et al.* (1977) indicated that the iliopsoas was a stabilizer of the hip and not only a flexor but an adductor beyond 90° flexion. The muscle also contracted as the trunk was brought up into extension (*'redressement du tronc'*—straighten up) after hip flexion and extension was resisted.

Morigana (1973) also studied the function of the iliopsoas with needle electrodes inserted to a depth of 7cm from the back at the level of the third lumbar vertebra together with electrodes in the rectus abdominis and sacropinalis muscles. In

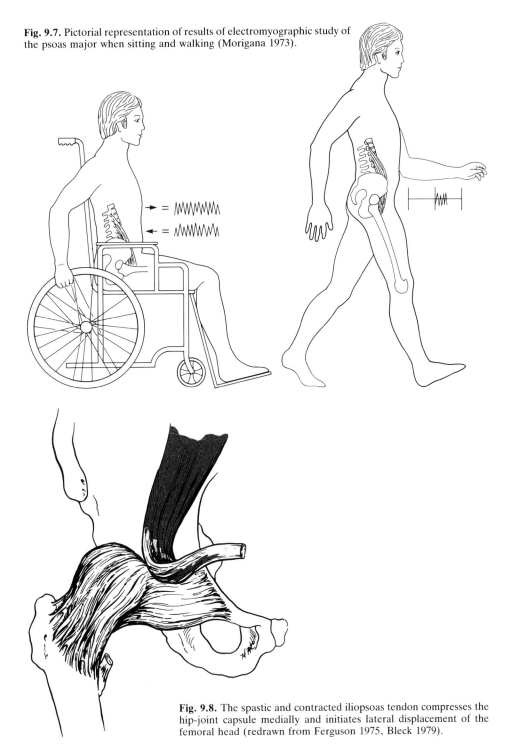

Fig. 9.7. Pictorial representation of results of electromyographic study of the psoas major when sitting and walking (Morigana 1973).

→ = \\/\/\/\/\/\/\/\/\
← = \\/\/\/\/\/\/\/\/\

Fig. 9.8. The spastic and contracted iliopsoas tendon compresses the hip-joint capsule medially and initiates lateral displacement of the femoral head (redrawn from Ferguson 1975, Bleck 1979).

403

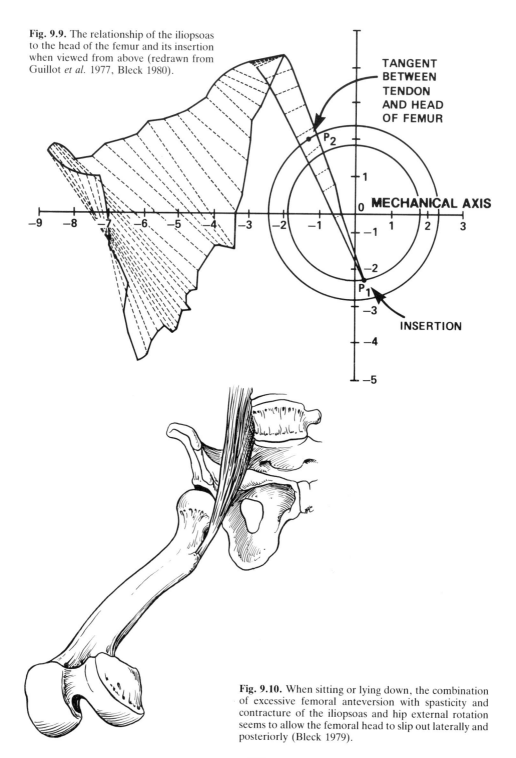

Fig. 9.9. The relationship of the iliopsoas to the head of the femur and its insertion when viewed from above (redrawn from Guillot *et al.* 1977, Bleck 1980).

TANGENT BETWEEN TENDON AND HEAD OF FEMUR

P_2

MECHANICAL AXIS

P_1

INSERTION

Fig. 9.10. When sitting or lying down, the combination of excessive femoral anteversion with spasticity and contracture of the iliopsoas and hip external rotation seems to allow the femoral head to slip out laterally and posteriorly (Bleck 1979).

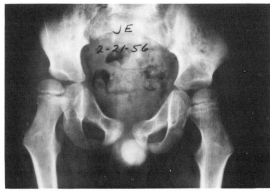
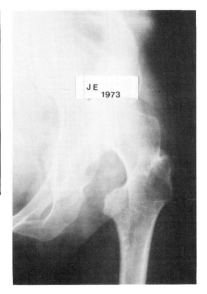

Fig. 9.11. Anterior-posterior radiographs of hips. *Above:* JE, age three years, total body involved. Preoperative bilateral adductor longus and gracilis myotomy and anterior branch obturator neurectomy. Note pelvis is level; subluxation of both hips. *Right:* JE, age 20 years. Postoperative 17 years. Dislocation of hip. Typical flattening of lateral aspect of femoral head from pressure of hip-abductor muscles.

easy standing and sitting upright, slight to moderate activity of the psoas was found in most of the 10 subjects. When leaning forward or backward, large amplitude action potentials were always evident from the iliopsoas. Flexion of the opposite hip also consistently recruited strong electrical activity from the iliopsoas. With other hip motions, the activity varied greatly among the subjects (Fig. 9.7).

The above electrical studies indicate that the iliopsoas probably contracts with trunk and opposite hip motions in the non-ambulatory total body involved patient when sitting or lying down as gravity is eliminated. As suggested by Ferguson (1973), in his studies of congenital dislocation of the hip, the iliopsoas tendon pushes the femoral head laterally when the muscle is contracted (Fig. 9.8). With femoral torsion and non-weightbearing in the total body involved patient, the hip obviously flexes and begins to rotate externally as the subluxation increases and the center of rotation shifts from the femoral head to the lesser trochanter (Somerville 1959, Sharrard *et al.* 1975) (Figs. 9.9, 9.10). Because of the lack of pressure by the femoral head, the acetabulum fails to deepen and dysplasia occurs (Smith *et al.* 1958, Salter 1966, Beals 1969). Finally, hip flexion and adduction pushes the head posteriorly to complete the dislocation. Eventually the femoral head comes to rest on the lateral superior and posterior aspect of the ilium. Usually, by the age of 13 years, the femoral head becomes flattened laterally due to the pressure of the overlying abductor muscles, and a deep groove appears on the center of the femoral head due to the pressure of the ligamentum teres (Samilson *et al.* 1972) (Fig. 9.11). In the end, cartilage of the femoral head degenerates completely.

PREVENTION

The controversy and confusion concerning prevention of the hip dislocation in

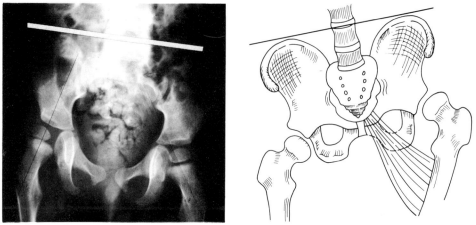

Fig. 9.12. *Left:* anterior-posterior radiograph pelvis and hips. Pelvic obliquity and subluxation of left hip. Spine straight. *Right:* drawing indicates pelvic obliquity due to adduction contracture of the hip. No flexion spasticity. This kind of case has a good result from adductor myotomies.

cerebral palsy can be resolved only if the data include precisely the functional ambulatory status of the patient and the age. Generalizing without these particulars can lead to misleading conclusions. I would summarize the types of subluxation at which stage preventative surgery is indicated as follows:

Type 1: with asymmetrical adduction contracture, without flexion contracture and a resultant pelvic obliquity (Fig. 9.12).

Type 2: symmetrical hip-adduction and hip-flexion contracture with a level pelvis (Fig. 9.13).

Type 3: a combination of an asymmetrical adduction, pelvic obliquity and a hip-flexion contracture (Fig. 9.14).

Type 4: with pelvic obliquity due to scoliosis and:

(a) only an asymmetrical adduction contracture;

(b) a hip-flexion contracture;

(c) both a hip-flexion and adduction contracture.

O'Brien and Sirkin (1977) described a patient with dislocated hips, and said that pain, perineal care and loss of functional status were not major problems, but the majority of experienced orthopaedic surgeons consider the problem to be of major importance in adolescents and adult patients (Hoffer *et al.* 1972, Samilson *et al.* 1972, Sharrard *et al.* 1975). In our study of 99 patients, 75 were seen for subluxation of the hip and 24 for dislocation; 8 per cent of those with subluxation and 24 per cent of those with dislocation had pain at a mean age of 18 years with a range from 9.8 to 24.8 years (Kalen and Bleck 1985). It takes long and consistent follow-up to make a judgement on pain incidence, and there is no way to predict which patients will have pain and when it will occur.

Orthotics and physical therapy methods have not been demonstrated to have any effect on prevention of subluxation or dislocation of the hip.

Surgery has been shown to be an effective preventative, with some

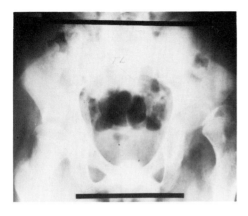

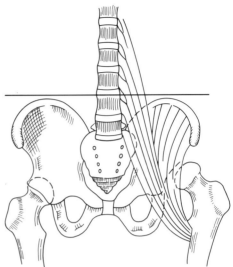

Fig. 9.13. *Above:* anterior-posterior radiograph of pelvis and hips. Pelvis level. Right hip dislocated. Spine straight. *Right:* drawing depicts that iliopsoas is the major deforming force. Spastic paralytic dislocation occurs without pelvic obliquity.

qualifications. Weakening of the adductor muscles was proposed in the studies of Tachdjian and Minear (1956), Phelps (1959), Sharrard *et al.* (1975), Reimers (1980), Reimers and Poulsen (1984), Schultz *et al.* (1984), Wheeler and Weinstein (1984), Parsch (1985), and James (1986). In these studies reported since 1980, the migration percentage and index devised by Reimers (1980) and/or the center edge angles of Wiberg (1939) were the radiographic criteria used to judge the efficacy of adductor myotomy with or without anterior branch obturator neurectomy or adductor origin transfer.

Success with adductor myotomy, with or without anterior branch obturator neurectomy or adductor origin transfer, seems limited if the ambulatory status of

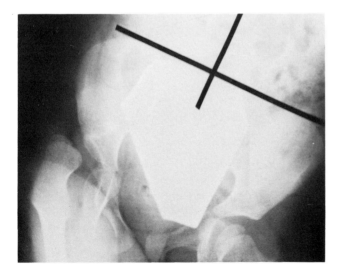

Fig. 9.14. Anterior-posterior radiograph of the pelvis and hips. Pelvic obliquity. Spine straight. Subluxation of left hip. A combination of hip adductor and iliopsoas spasticity.

407

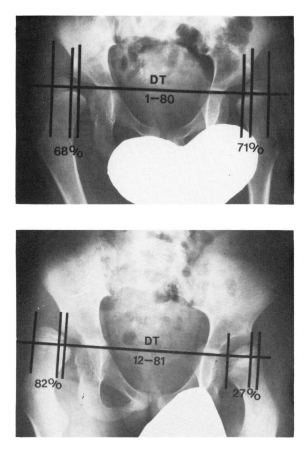

Fig. 9.15. Anterior-posterior radiographs of pelvis and hips. *Top:* DT, age three years, spastic paralysis, bilateral hip subluxation. Migration percentage measured according to Reimers (1980). *Bottom:* DT, one year postoperative bilateral adductor longus and gracilis myotomies and anterior branch obturator neurectomy; left hip worse, right hip improved from 71 per cent to 27 per cent lateral migration. (Reproduced with permission from Kalen and Bleck 1985.)

the patients is carefully defined. Sharrard *et al.* (1975) were able to achieve stability of the hips in 75 per cent of their cases with only one surgical procedure. These were adductor myotomy in 132 cases, additional anterior branch obturator neurectomy in 46 and iliopsoas tenotomy in only three. 48 per cent of their patients were independent walkers. Nevertheless, 25 per cent had unsuccessful surgery with the initial adductor weakening procedures.

Reimers (1980) maintained or improved hip stability in 57 per cent of 127 patients who had adductor surgery alone. The ambulatory status of his patients was not mentioned. Banks and Green (1960) had a 70 per cent success rate in preventing further subluxation with adductor myotomy and anterior branch obturator neurectomy; in 30 per cent subluxation increased or progressed to dislocation.

Samilson *et al.* (1972) had a failure rate of 25 per cent in preventing dislocation in 105 patients. Griffith *et al.* (1982) found a disappointingly high percentage of failures of their original adductor transfer operation (Stephenson and Donavan 1971) in prevention of subluxation of the hip. They improved their results 50 per cent with the addition of iliopsoas recession.

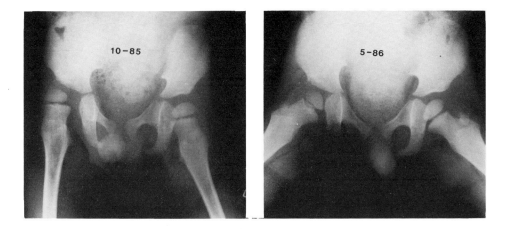

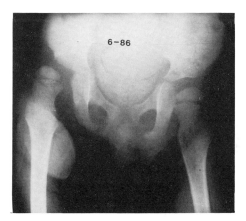

Fig. 9.16. Anterior-posterior radiographs of pelvis and hips. *Above left:* DN, total body involved, subluxation of left hip. October 1985, preoperative bilateral adductor myotomy and anterior branch obturator neurectomy. *Above right:* DN, May 1986, in abduction hips appear located. *Left:* DN June 1986, in adduction, left hip still subluxated. (Radiographs courtesy of Kamal Bose MD, Department of Orthopaedic Surgery, University of Singapore, School of Medicine.)

In the study by Kalen and Bleck (1985) adductor surgery alone had a 75 per cent failure rate for patients who walked with crutches or walkers and a 59 per cent for non-walkers (Figs. 9.15, 9.16).

The radiographic successes of adductor myotomy with or without anterior branch obturator neurectomy in improving or stopping progression of subluxation of the hip can be related to the ambulatory status of the child. There is 100 per cent success when the child is a fully independent walker. If partial or non-weightbearing is the functional status, the successes appear only if there is an asymmetrical adduction with pelvic obliquity and an 'uncovered' hip on the adducted side (Fig. 9.17).

Based upon our studies of the rôle of the iliopsoas in dislocation of the hip, we recommend an iliopsoas tenotomy for prevention of dislocation of the hip in total body involved children who are under the age of five years and have a poor prognosis for walking. In those who have a guarded prognosis for walking, an iliopsoas recession seems safer to preserve hip-flexion power which might be lost with tenotomy. In all young children who have early subluxation demonstrated by

409

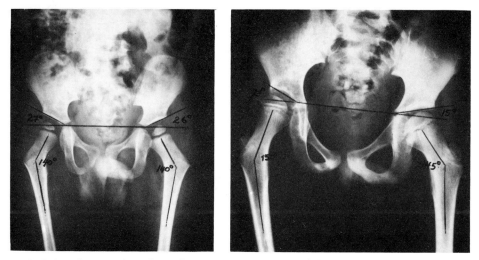

Fig. 9.17. Anterior-posterior radiographs of the pelvis and hips. *Left:* EN, age one year, normal hips and acetabular angles. Spastic paralysis, total body involved. *Right:* EN, age six years, slight subluxation left hip, pelvic obliquity due to adduction contracture. This is the kind of patient in whom adductor myotomy is likely to be successful in stopping the 'lateral migration' of the femoral head and in restoring the CE angle.

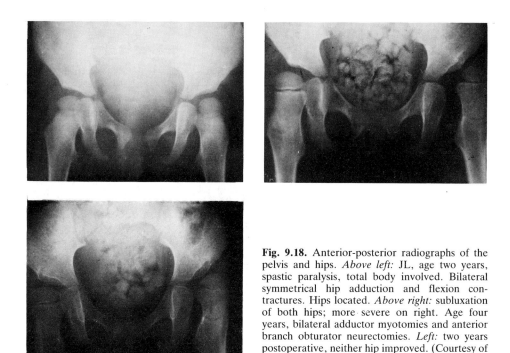

Fig. 9.18. Anterior-posterior radiographs of the pelvis and hips. *Above left:* JL, age two years, spastic paralysis, total body involved. Bilateral symmetrical hip adduction and flexion contractures. Hips located. *Above right:* subluxation of both hips; more severe on right. Age four years, bilateral adductor myotomies and anterior branch obturator neurectomies. *Left:* two years postoperative, neither hip improved. (Courtesy of Arthur Holstein MD, Berkeley, California.)

410

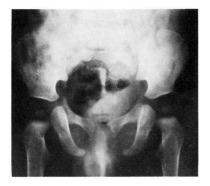

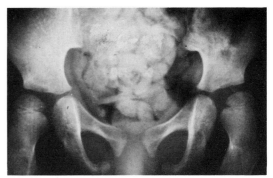

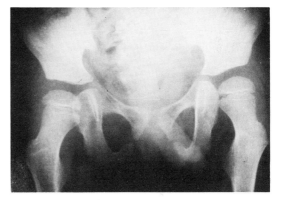

Fig. 9.19. Anterior-posterior radiographs of the pelvis and hips. *Above left:* HCK, age five months, spastic paralysis total body involved. Hips normal. *Above right:* HCK, age three years, subluxation of right hip. *Right:* HCK, age 6½ years, 3½ years postoperative bilateral adductor myotomies, anterior branch obturator neurectomies and iliopsoas tenotomies. Hips reasonably located. Patient non-ambulatory. (Courtesy of Arthur Holstein MD, Berkeley, California.)

radiographs of the hips and pelvis, a hip-flexion contracture found by the prone extension test on the clinical examination will be the indication for iliopsoas tenotomy or recession in addition to adductor myotomy (with anterior branch obturator neurectomy) to prevent dislocation in the total body involved child (Figs. 9.18, 9.19, 9.20).

Kalen and Bleck (1985), in their review of the effects of adductor surgery alone compared with adductor surgery and iliopsoas tenotomy or recession, reported a 100 per cent radiographic success rate in reduction of subluxation in the iliopsoas group of partial weight-bearing ambulators and a clinical success rate of 84 per cent (meaning that no further surgery was necessary). In contrast, the clinical failure rate in these ambulators with adductor surgery alone was 59 per cent. In the non-ambulators the clinical success rate in the iliopsoas group fell to 58 per cent and the radiographic result to 67 per cent; however, in those who had no pelvic obliquity, clinical success rose to 83 per cent and radiographic success to 95 per cent. The mean age of surgery with success in both groups was 4.4 to 4.9 years, and the failures had a mean age range of 5.3 to 6.0 years.

Radiographic success was determined by the migration percentage devised by Reimers (1980) (Fig. 9.15). If the last follow-up radiographs showed a ≥10 per cent increase in the migration percentage, progressive subluxation occurred and result

411

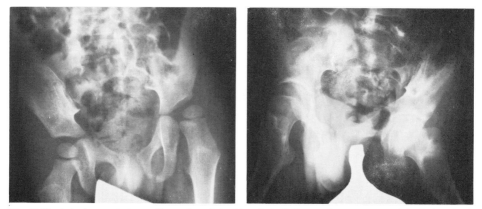

Fig. 9.20. Anterior-posterior radiographs of the hip. *Left:* DK, age four years, total body involved, non-ambulatory, pelvic obliquity, hip-flexion and adduction contractures and subluxation of right hip; at risk for dislocation. *Right:* DK, 12 years postoperative bilateral adductor myotomies, anterior branch obturator neurectomies and iliopsoas tenotomies.

was called a failure. The CE angles of Wiburg were not used because of their unreliability under the age of five years (Coleman 1978, Kalen 1985).

Sharrard *et al.* (1975) also had good results in prevention of dislocation of the hip in cerebral palsy in 101 of 134 hips which had iliopsoas elongation and adductor myotomy with anterior branch obturator neurectomy. Sharrard and Burke (1982) performed a transfer of the iliopsoas posterior laterally or anterior laterally with adductor release and open reduction of the hip when necessary in established dislocations or progressive subluxation of the hip in cerebral palsy. Of 23 patients' hips all become stable and pain-free. Fettweis (1979) also noted that adductor myotomy with obturator neurectomy did not always result in reduction of spastic subluxation of the hip and even cautioned against weakening the adductor muscles too much with intrapelvic obturator neurectomy. He found the iliopsoas to be an important deforming force in dislocation.

SUMMARY: SURGICAL PREVENTION OF PROGRESSIVE SUBLUXATION AND DISLOCATION
I recommend iliopsoas recession in potential ambulators and tenotomy in non-ambulators, plus adductor myotomy. Anterior branch obturator neurectomy improved the results from 56 to 69 per cent in our study (Kalen and Bleck 1985). These data suggest that it might be better in the total body involved child to do the neurectomy as well as the myotomy of the adductor longus and gracilis; myotomy brevis can be added if the range of each hip's abduction is limited to less than 40° to 45° after the longus and gracilis have been released, and the range of abduction of each hip determined while the child is still under anesthesia. The exception to performing the iliopsoas recession or tenotomy would be if no flexion contracture is demonstrated with the prone extension test (see Chapter 2).

Pelvic obliquity due to scoliosis was present in 66 per cent of our patients; the data indicate that this compromises the results of preventative surgery.

Muscle releases to prevent progressive subluxation have the best results under

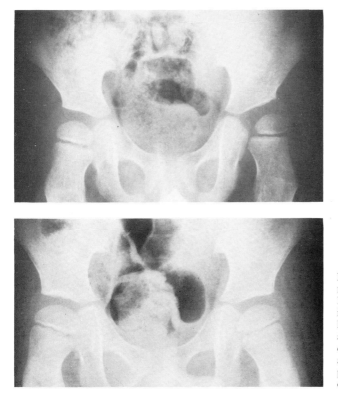

Fig. 9.21. Anterior-posterior radiographs of the hip. *Top:* FV, age three years, total body involved. Pelvis level, subluxation left hip. *Bottom:* FV, age five years, two years postoperative iliopsoas tenotomy; almost perfect hip joints. No postoperative night-splinting or orthosis used.

the age of five years. Generally, after this age, varus-derotation osteotomy and pelvic osteotomies are required.

Postoperative bracing with the Lorenz type of orthosis which held the hips in 90° flexion and 60° abduction, combined with a thoracic extension, was reported to have improved the results of reduction of hip subluxations in cerebral-palsied patients who had adductor myotomies with anterior branch neurectomies and iliopsoas 'releases'. Based upon the data of successful reduction of the subluxations, in children less than age six years, this postoperative bracing at nap and night time was recommended for a minimum of one year (Houkom *et al.* 1986). Their results in the 27 patients who were severe improved with bracing 69 per cent compared to 0 per cent without. The only complication of this regimen was a hip abduction contracture in 21 per cent.

I have been reluctant to impose additional burdens on the family by insisting on postoperative bracing for these total body involved children. It would mean application and removal of the device twice each during the 24 hours. Many of these children awaken frequently during the night even without bracing. I always doubt the compliance of night-bracing. Parents need sleep, to face the next day. Instead we have implemented functional goals of mobility, communication and activities of daily living. Our results without bracing had an 83 per cent success rate in those who did not have a pelvic obliquity and scoliosis, and with these additional

413

deformities a 60 per cent success—almost comparable to Houkom *et al.*'s (1986) good results with prolonged postoperative bracing (Fig. 9.21).

Iliopsoas tenotomy
Iliopsoas tenotomy for spastic hip-flexion contractures was first described in the American literature by Peterson (1950) in the surgical treatment of spastic paraplegia resulting from spinal-cord injury. Bleck and Holstein (1963) reported its use in cerebral palsy. The medial approach to the proximal femur was devised by Ludloff (Crenshaw 1963), and brought to my attention by Young (1954) as a way to expose the lesser trochanteric region of the femur. Keats and Morgese (1967) published a description of the operation.

The procedure should be performed bilaterally when both hips have spasticity and contracture, even though only one has a subluxation. In unilateral procedures, the opposite untreated hip is apt to dislocate postoperatively (Samilson 1970). Uematsu *et al.* (1977) performed, in effect, iliopsoas tenotomies when they did posterior iliopsoas transfers for hip instability in cerebral palsy. In the 30 hips in which this transfer was performed, they noted a marked tendency to convert unilateral to bilateral deformities.

In addition to iliospoas tenotomy, adductor longus and gracilis myotomy with anterior branch obturator neurectomy is usually necessary in most cases of early subluxation of the hip in the total body involved child. If the hamstrings are spastic and contracted (popliteal angle greater than 20°), lengthening of the hamstrings either by proximal origin myotomy or distal fractional lengthening may achieve a higher percentage of good results (Hiroshima and Ono 1979, Rang *et al.* 1986).

Operative technique—iliopsoas tenotomy
With the hip flexed, abducted and externally rotated an incision is begun 1 to 1.5cm distal to the origin of the adductor longus and extended directly over the adductor longus distally for 5cm (Fig. 9.22). If required, the adductor myotomy and anterior

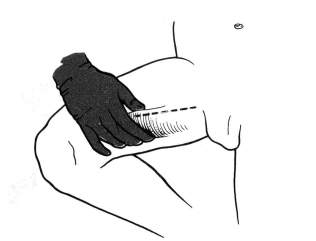

Fig. 9.22. Operative technique of iliopsoas tenotomy— medial proximal thigh approach. *Left:* incision over adductor longus. *Opposite, top:* adductor longus, brevis and pectineus muscles retracted to expose iliopsoas tendon insertion on lesser trochanter. *Opposite, bottom:* iliopsoas tendon cut and allowed to retract proximally.

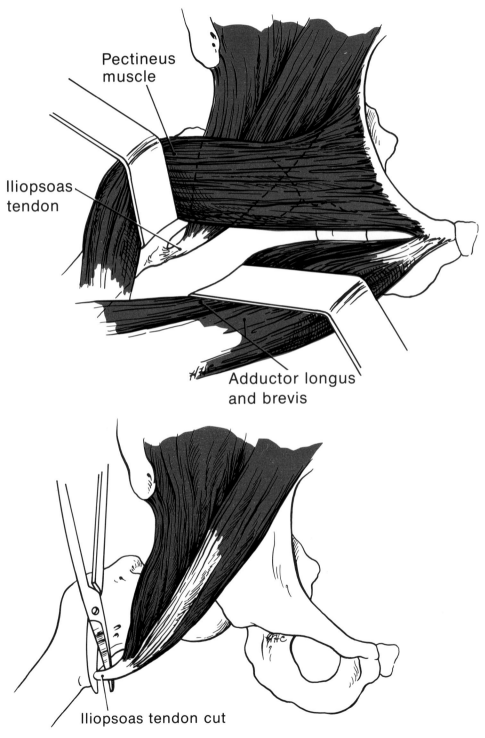

Pectineus
muscle

Iliopsoas
tendon

Adductor longus
and brevis

Iliopsoas tendon cut

415

branch obturator neurectomy are then performed. With finger dissection the interval between the pectineus and adductor brevis muscles is developed to palpate the lesser trochanter. A spade-type retractor (Chandler retractor) is placed medially around the lesser trochanter to retract the adductor magnus medially, and a similar retractor laterally retracts the pectineus. The veil of connective tissue and fat is swept off the psoas tendon under which is passed a 90°–angled forceps (Mixter type) and the tendon is cut as well as some of the fibers of the iliacus which accompany it a bit distal to the tendon. The tendon is freed by blunt dissection proximally; it then retracts.

The *proximal hamstring origin myotomy* can be done through the same incision (Gurd 1984, Rang *et al.* 1986). The gracilis origin is sectioned; then the blunt dissection is carried medially around the adductor magnus to the origins of the medial hamstring muscles on the ischium. The semitendinosus origin is partly tendinous and can cause concern because it is easily mistaken for the sciatic nerve or vice versa. When one is certain of the location of the sciatic nerve, then the semitendinosus is sectioned. The semimembranosus origin is cut. Use of the electrocautery lessens the bleeding and risk of a hematoma. Continuous suction of the wound is essential for 24 to 48 hours.

Postoperative care
I do not use hip spica plasters. Instead bilateral long-leg plasters connected with a stick, to abduct each hip 40° to 45°, has been sufficient for three weeks. After plaster removal, an abduction pillow splint or a triangular abduction wedge splint can be used for 10 to 12 weeks at night while the postoperative scar matures (although I have not routinely used night splinting). In small children (age 18 months to three years) who did not have hamstring spasticity or contracture, I have not always used the plaster immobilization, but rather the pillow hip-abduction splint. The number of cases who qualified for this sort of postoperative management is too small to give a data-based result.

Hip-abduction wedges in the wheelchair seat are routine. Early mobilization of the hip and knee joints with gentle and regular passive exercise allows an early return to comfortable sitting and resumption of functional goals. The hot-tub whirlpool at home (comparable to those used in many health clubs and modern hotels for the 'tired executive') has been the single most valuable relaxation and mobility device for these total body involved children.

Subluxation of the hip and acetabular dysplasia over age five years
The indications for a femoral osteotomy and acetabular reconstruction in addition to the myotomies or lengthening of the spastics, as delineated in the preceding paragraph, are age-related. Our data (Kalen and Bleck 1985) suggest that soft-tissue surgery to prevent dislocation is less successful after age five years. Remember, however, that skeletal and developmental ages may lag a year or two behind normal children (Horstmann 1986).

In all children under age six or seven years skeletal age, the surgeon can wait for a year after tenotomies and myotomies to determine whether or not additional

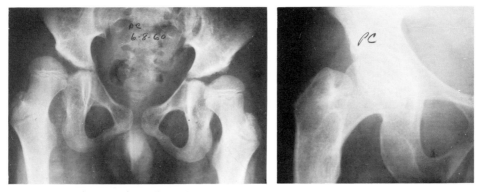

Fig. 9.23. Anterior-posterior radiographs of pelvis and hips. *Left:* PC, age nine years, spastic diplegia, crutch walker, bilateral hip subluxation, 45° flexion contracture of hips. *Right:* PC, age 19 years, 10 years postoperative adductor myotomies, anterior branch obturator neurectomies, iliopsoas recessions and varus-derotation subtrochanteric osteotomies. Community walker with crutches. Hips well located and formed. Iliac osteotomies not required. (NB even though age nine years at time of surgery, skeletal age apparently retarded one to two years.)

bone surgery will be required.

The femoral deformity to be corrected is excessive anteversion, although the common operation is referred to as a varus derotation subtrochanteric osteotomy. The procedure has had much approbation by many surgeons (Eilert and MacEwen 1977, Tylkowski *et al.* 1980, Steeger and Underlich 1982, Horstmann and Rosabal 1984, Vanderbrink *et al.* 1984, Bunnell 1985). Various internal fixation devices for the osteotomy have been recommended (Bleck 1979, Greene 1985, Alonso *et al.* 1986).

Although the varus component of the osteotomy seems superficially important, the coxa valga is more of a radiographic artifact due to the femoral torsion than actual valgus of the femoral neck. The major correction is derotation of the femur. The varus component should restore the femoral neck angle to about 135°. Too much varus in the femoral neck will create an adduction deformity of the hip. As with derotation osteotomy for hip-internal rotation gait, the derotation must not be overdone; a residual passive range of 20° to 30° of internal rotation is more functional even when sitting.

Acetabular dysplasia in children older than the skeletal age of four years is not likely to self-correct with growth in congenital dislocation of this hip after femoral osteotomy (Harris *et al.* 1975). In spastic paralytic dislocations one could wait a year or two when femoral osteotomies have been performed between the ages of five and seven years (Fig. 9.23). Tylkowski *et al.* (1980) found no acetabular remodeling after femoral osteotomies in children older than eight years.

Inasmuch as the posterior acetabulum is most often deficient in paralytic dislocations (Coleman 1983, Lau *et al.* 1986) (Fig. 9.24), I no longer perform innominate osteotomies that rotate the pelvis anteriorly and laterally. These are the single innominate osteotomy of Salter (1961), the double one of Sutherland and Greenfield (1977), and the triple type of Steel (1977). Molloy (1986) had good

417

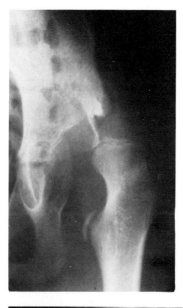

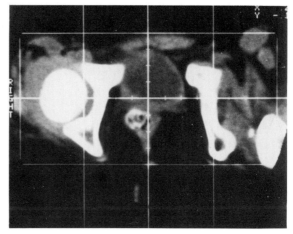

Fig. 9.24. *Left:* anterior-posterior radiograph of spastic paralytic dislocation of hip. *Above:* computerized axial tomography in transverse plane of same hip showing deficiency in the posterior acetabular wall.

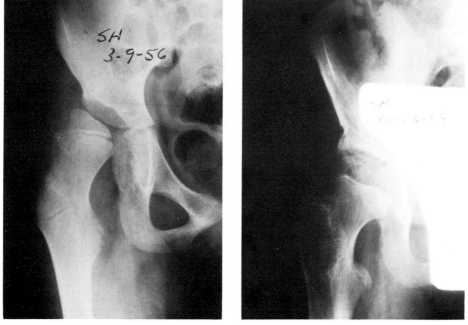

Fig. 9.25. *Left:* anterior-posterior radiographs of left hip, age eight years, female, spastic diplegia, crutch walker, 50 per cent subluxation of hip. *Right:* 3½ years postoperative adductor myotomy, anterior branch obturator neurectomy, iliopsoas recession, varus derotation osteotomy, and acetabuloplasty. Skeletal growth in long bones appears to be almost complete; thus result was probably permanent. (This patient was the author's first attempt at hip reconstruction and prevention of progressive subluxation in cerebral palsy.) The pelvic osteotomy was very similar to that described by Murbarak *et al.* (1986), who said it resembled a Pemberton osteotomy or the Dega technique.

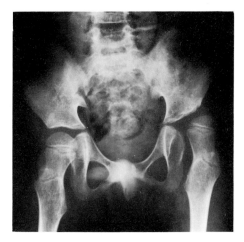

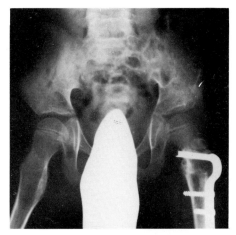

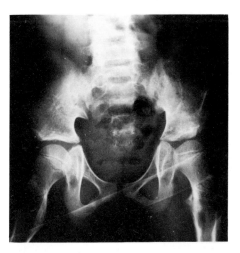

Fig. 9.26. Anterior-posterior radiographs of the pelvis and hips. *Above left:* GC, age 10 years, total body involved. Subluxation right hip with acetabular dysplasia. *Above right:* GC, six months postoperative, adductor myotomy, derotation subtrochanteric osteotomy (note very little varus component) and iliac osteotomy (Pemberton type). *Right:* GC, one year postoperative. Hip well located. Internal fixation removed. (Courtesy Henri Hornung, MD, Hôpital Heliol-Marin, Hyères les Palmiers, France.)

Fig. 9.27. Anterior-posterior radiographs of pelvis and hips. *Below left:* AA, age six years, total body involved. Subluxation of right hip. *Bottom right:* AA, one year postoperative, derotation subtrochanteric osteotomy and Pemberton iliac osteotomy.

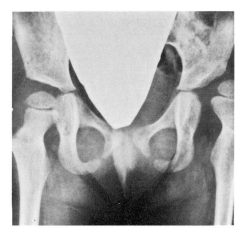

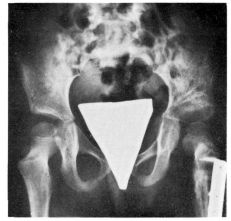

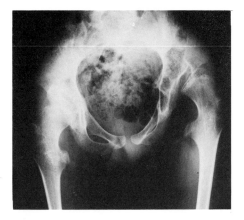

Fig. 9.28. Anterior-posterior radiographs of the hip, patient ST, total body involved, non-ambulatory. *Left:* age 13 years, subluxation of the hip. *Center left:* one month postoperative: bilateral adductor myotomy, iliopsoas tenotomy, hamstring lengthenings, tenotomies of rectus femoris and sartorius. Remarkable improvement. *Center right:* eight months postoperative. Began walking with a walker. *Bottom left:* hip stable in adduction. *Bottom right:* hip stable in abduction. (Courtesy of Akira Uehara MD, Chiba Rehabilitation Center, Department of Pediatric Orthopaedics, University of Chiba School of Medicine, Japan.)

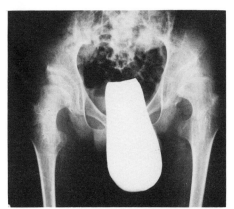

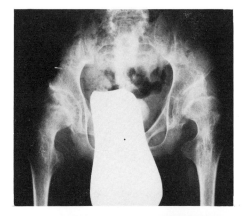

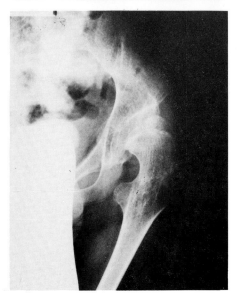

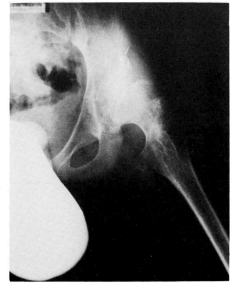

results in both flaccid and spastic paralytic subluxation or dislocation of the hip with the Salter innominate osteotomy combined with a femoral osteotomy and transiliac transfer of the iliopsoas posteriorly. Eight patients had cerebral palsy and 10 myelomeningocele. She found no differences in the results between these two groups.

However, the Salter innominate osteotomy has some biomechanical limits. It will not be sufficient if the head of the femur is not covered by the acetabulum, as shown by radiographic examination of the hip in 25° of flexion, neutral rotation, 10° abduction and the x-ray beam directed 25° posteriorly and caudally to the coronal plane (Rab 1978, 1981*b*).

Together with other surgeons I prefer the Pemberton iliac osteotomy in paralytic subluxation of the hip and acetabular dysplasia (Coleman 1983, Barry and Staheli 1986, Hoffer 1986). In a follow-up study of 30 subluxed hips in children, age 23 months to 12 years, with either cerebral palsy or myelomeningocele, Barry and Staheli (1986) had satisfactory results at the time of evaluation with an average of four years (range two to nine years) postoperatively.

Because the Pemberton iliac osteotomy depends upon the flexibility of the triradiate cartilage when prying down the roof of the acetabulum, the operation is most satisfactory in children at or under age seven years (Pemberton 1965, Eyre-Brook *et al.* 1978). However, age eight to nine is probably not too old. Again age is relative and depends upon the skeletal maturity of the child (Figs. 9.25, 9.26, 9.27).

In more skeletally mature children and certainly in adolescents, the Chiari iliac osteotomy seems the easiest and most effective operation (Chiari 1974, Bailey and Hall 1985).

The indications and techniques for varus derotation subtrochanteric and iliac osteotomies are the same for subluxation of the hip in children with spastic diplegia, triplegia or quadriplegia and who are dependent upon crutches or walkers for ambulation.

Are femoral and iliac osteotomies *always* necessary in the skeletally mature total body involved patient who has a 50 per cent or less subluxation of the hip? Based upon the preliminary results of Uehara (1986) and my own observations, the answer is a tentative 'no'. In this type of patient, iliopsoas and adductor tenotomy *plus proximal hamstring myotomy or distal hamstring lengthening,* seems to have resulted in pain relief and stability of the hip (Fig. 9.28). Uehara (1986), at the Chiba Rehabilitation Center in Japan, studied the results of adductor longus and gracilis myotomy (and, in severe cases, adductor brevis myotomy), iliopsoas tenotomy and hamstring lengthening in their cases of subluxation of the hip in non-ambulatory total body involved patients. His conclusions were: (i) if the femoral head coverage by the acetabulum was between one-half and two-thirds, the improvement in congruity was 72.5 per cent (N = 40 hips); (ii) if coverage was less than 50 per cent, good results were obtained in 55.8 per cent (N = 29 hips); and (iii) in lateral dislocation, the improvement after surgery dropped to 18.7 per cent (N = 16 hips). The objective to prevent further subluxation and dislocation without bone surgery seems to have been accomplished in a sufficient number of these patients to merit its use as a first-stage procedure. One undesirable effect of hamstring lengthening, either proximal or distal, would be to reinforce underlying quadriceps spasticity. In this event, knee flexion might be so restricted as to preclude sitting in a chair. Some consideration ought to be given in these cases to lengthening the quadriceps as well as the hamstrings. Time will tell.

Operative technique of varus derotation subtrochanteric osteotomy
Adductor myotomy and anterior branch obturator neurectomy, iliopsoas tenotomy and (when indicated) a proximal hamstring myotomy are first performed through the medial groin approach previously described.

The subtrochanteric osteotomy is performed through the straight lateral incision from the tip of the greater trochanter distally along the shaft of the femur for 10 to 12cm. Because the major femoral deformity is excessive anteversion, a derotation osteotomy is the major component.

I prefer the 90° osteotomy compression nail plates for fixation. The nail portion of the fixation device should be inserted into the femoral neck at an angle that will correspond with the degree of varus inclination desired. If a varus angle of 15° is wanted at the osteotomy, for example, the nail is inserted at a 15° angle to what would be the horizontal line of the osteotomy (this angle will be 90° + 15° = 105° to the femoral shaft). Radiographic control with guide pins is used throughout the operation.

The track for the nail is cut in the neck of the femur with the special chisel, and the nail is then inserted into the femoral neck just to the point where the plate portion abuts against the lateral aspect of the shaft. With a power saw, a transverse subtrochanteric osteotomy is performed at a 90° angle to the shaft. In the proximal fragment, an oblique cut is made parallel to the nail in the neck of the femur so that a wedge of bone with the base medial can be removed. The nail is then driven completely into the femoral neck. When the two surfaces are brought together, the distal shaft is rotated externally the appropriate amount. A linear mark crossing the osteotomy site is previously made with an osteotome so that the amount of rotation can be gauged. When the two surfaces are coapted, the nail in the neck of the femur should lie parallel to the osteotomy site so that compression of the bone surface is obtained (see Fig. 9.31).

Iliac osteomies can be done at the same time. If this is done, a separate oblique incision beginning 1–2cm medial and 1.5cm distal to the anterior superior iliac spine and continued laterally 1cm distal to the mid-portion of the iliac crest usually affords sufficient exposure for these osteotomies. (In complete dislocation of the hip, I use one single incision for both the femoral and iliac osteotomies described in the next section.)

Pericapsular iliac osteotomy operative technique
As with the Salter osteotomy, I prefer the transverse incision beginning medial to the anterior superior iliac spine and carried laterally over the anterior two-thirds of the ilium (Pemberton 1965, Coleman 1978). The usual anterior iliofemoral exposure of the lateral aspect of the ilium is then made after subcutaneous

reflection of the skin. The sartorius is sectioned at its origin and retracted distally. With a sharp elevator or an osteotome, the cartilaginous apophysis of the ilium is peeled off the crest and reflected medially. The iliacus muscle is easily dissected subperiosteally to expose the inner wall of the ilium. The gluteus medius is similarly stripped from the outer wall. Blunt retractors are placed on both sides of the ilium against the bone circumscribing the sciatic notch. The anterior aspect of the ilium is stripped to the origin of the rectus femoris muscle. The attachment of the capsule of the hip joint is exposed anteriorly and laterally.

The osteotomy of the outer wall of the ilium is curvilinear and parallels the capsule; it begins at the anterior inferior iliac spine just above the reflected head of the rectus femoris. The bone is cut posteriorly and inferiorly toward (but not into) the triradiate cartilage. The posterior cut is directed anterior to the sciatic notch and posterior to the hip-joint edge. The inner wall cut is made in the same line, and usually inferior to the outer wall cut, in order to provide more lateral coverage in the case of the paralytic dysplastic acetabulum.

The two cuts in the ilium are joined with a curved osteotome as far as the triradiate cartilage. The inferior portion of the cut ilium is then rotated laterally with a lamina spreader between the two osteotomized segments. With a small gouge, grooves are made in the opposing two slabs of the ilium. These help stabilize the bone graft, which is cut from the anterior-superior aspect of the ilium above the anterior-inferior iliac spine. The graft is wedged into place to hold the osteotomy open. No internal fixation is necessary. The image intensifier fluoroscope throughout the procedure with a radiopaque dye in the joint (30 per cent Renografin) can give the surgeon more assurance that the operation has accomplished the correction as intended.

Muscles are reapproximated as usual and the skin closed. Suction drainage should prevent hematoma formation. A 1½ spica plaster for six weeks is sufficient for bone healing so that early mobilization is possible.

PROBLEMS WITH PERICAPSULAR ILLAC OSTEOTOMY

As pointed out by Coleman (1978), one disadvantage of this osteotomy is that it is dependent upon the flexibility of the triradiate cartilage which is the hinge on which all the correction depends. Thus it works best in children with a skeletal age seven years or younger, and is progressively more difficult to do until it becomes impossible by 10 or 12 years.

It is a more technically difficult procedure than the Salter innominate osteotomy. The American Orthopaedic Association has produced a very helpful videotape on various iliac osteotomies.

A major pitfall of the Pemberton osteotomy would be growth arrest of the triradiate cartilage; this would result in a small acetabulum and a larger femoral head, which obviously would not be contained. This problem can be minimized by avoiding entrance into the triradiate cartilage during the procedure.

Too much anterior displacement of the distal segment will block hip flexion and uncover the posterior portion of the femoral head in paralytic subluxations. Therefore the major displacement of this distal segment should be lateral.

423

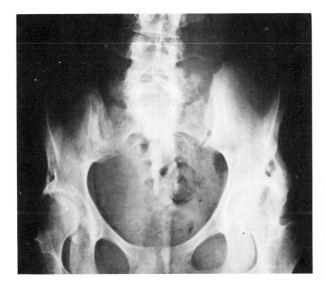

Fig. 9.29. Anterior-posterior radiograph of pelvis and hips. Adult total body involved, partial ambulation with crutches, 10 years postoperative bilateral acetabular augmentations (shelf procedures); joint space on left is narrow, and motion limited.

Another problem I have observed, in contrast to the Salter osteotomy, is postoperative stiffness that can persist for several weeks. Avoiding more correction than necessary, and restoring the acetabular roof to the right angle (20° to 25° acetabular angle) may prevent compression of the articular cartilage and resultant limited motion of the hip.

Acetabular augmentation ('shelf procedure') has been resurrected and greatly improved in technique by Staheli (1981) for congenital acetabular dysplasia. Zuckerman *et al.* (1984) reported good results from this procedure in subluxation of the hip in cerebral palsy in 17 patients (Fig. 9.29). These orthopaedic surgeons combined acetabular augmentation with additional procedures on 14 hips, including six varus derotation femoral osteotomies and, significantly, one Pemberton iliac osteotomy. Their institution also had good results with Pemberton iliac osteotomies in paralytic subluxations (Barry and Staheli 1985). Pous (1985) described an ingenious new method of acetabular augmentation by using a vascularized graft of the iliac crest which resulted in immediate stability of the hip in three children with cerebral palsy and subluxation. So there are choices. I have reserved acetabular augmentation for congenital acetabular dysplasias, where the round uncovered portion of the femoral head matches that equally round contour of the acetabulum. This is hardly ever the case in cerebral palsy.

Indications for relocation
Although it is true that not all dislocated hips in total body involved adolescents are painful (as discovered in an analysis of 3922 patients with cerebral palsy by Gandy and Meyer 1983), we cannot predict which ones will become painful. I agree that the painless dislocated hip in the skeletally mature patient can be left alone. There is no point in using surgery to produce a painful located hip. The mean age of dislocation of the hip is about seven years. Secondary changes occur as the

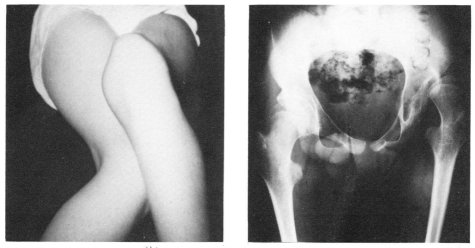

Fig. 9.30. *Left:* clinical appearance of patient with dislocation of left hip, flexed and adducted. *Right:* anterior-posterior radiograph of pelvis and hips; no scoliosis and no pelvic obliquity. Is this patient a candidate for the soft-tissue procedures alone as reported by Uehara 1986? (see Fig. 9.28).

dislocation persists, not only as acetabular development lags but also in the femoral head. The head becomes deformed and the cartilage degenerates as described in Chapter 5 (see Figs. 5.7, 5.9). It should be obvious that placing this deformed and degenerated femoral head in the acetabulum might be an unnecessary risk. If the dislocation is painless in these older mature patients, there is no need for salvage operations, unless performed to enhance sitting and perineal hygiene.

Given these perspectives and the inability to predict the painful adolescent or adult dislocated hip, then it seems logical to relocate these hips in children before skeletal maturity, preferably under age 12 years. There is no better substitute for a located and stable femoral head in a reconstructed acetabulum. Nor are 'simple' solutions, such as femoral head and neck resection, entirely satisfactory for pain relief (Cristofaro *et al.* 1977, Root 1977).

In older children with hip dislocation and deformation of the femoral head (flattening of its lateral surface) seen on the radiographic examination, I expose the femoral head first and inspect its articular cartilage and if it is intact I then proceed with the entire reconstructive operation (Fig. 9.30). If the cartilage has degenerated, then I proceed with a salvage procedure and make no attempt to do an elaborate reconstruction to relocate the femoral head.

The indications to relocate the dislocated hip in children and adolescents before skeletal maturity can be summarized as follows:
1. To prevent a painful hip in adult life; a painful hip can compromise their mobility and render their care more difficult.
2. To prevent and correct severe pelvic obliquity which interferes with sitting balance. However, if the pelvic obliquity is due to concomitant scoliosis, relocating the hip will not correct the pelvic obliquity.

3. To prevent painful bursal formation over the greater trochanter on the dislocated side and over the ischial tuberosity due to pelvic obliquity as the result of the dislocation only (*i.e.* no scoliosis).

4. To prevent and correct severe adduction of the femur that makes perineal hygiene difficult.

Dislocated hip and scoliosis

With this combination, the scoliosis should be corrected first, and then (if the femoral articular surface is intact) followed by surgical reconstruction to reduce the dislocation. If the hip is painful in the adolescent and the femoral head obviously deformed, I have performed a resection interposition capsular arthroplasty first and used the femoral head as part of the bone graft in the spinal fusion.

Operative plan of one-stage reconstruction

I have had satisfactory long-term results in spastic paralytic dislocations of the hip with the techniques performed at one stage as follows:

1. Adductor longus, gracilis and adductor brevis myotomy, anterior branch obturator neurectomy and iliopsoas tenotomy. If the hamstring muscles are contracted, I would add proximal hamstring myotomy. All this can be done through the medial thigh incision previously described.

2. Capsulotomy to inspect the femoral head before proceeding. As mentioned previously, if the articular cartilage is degenerated, proceed no further and perform a salvage operation.

3. Femoral shortening with a varus derotation subtrochanteric femoral osteotomy and internal fixation (90° hip osteotomy compression nail-plate).

4. Pemberton iliac osteotomy in patients under age 10 years. Chiari (1974) iliac osteotomy over age 10 years.

5. Capsulorraphy of the hip.

Femoral shortening has been used successfully for the reduction of congenital dislocation of the hip (Klisic and Janovic 1976). I have used the method in spastic paralytic dislocations since 1971, when Larsen introduced it to me (Bleck 1979, 1980). Of 20 dislocated hips in total body involved patients who had the one-stage procedure and a follow-up of five to 14 years, none have redislocated. Two had a recurrent subluxation, possibly due in one case to failure to perform a capsulorraphy, and in the other due to the unrelieved spastic and contracted hamstring muscles. The only complication was one patient who had a supracondylar fracture secondary to osteoporosis and immobilization in the postoperative plaster.

Using open reduction and femoral osteotomy, Sherk *et al.* (1983) successfully reduced 52 dislocations in 45 non-ambulatory patients with cerebral palsy. Soft-tissue surgery was always unsuccessful in 11 patients whose average age was 23 years. Abduction of the hip was prevented by the dislocated femoral head resting against the lateral wall of the ilium. These surgeons had the best results in relieving pain with extensive resection type arthroplasties.

Root and Broumann (1985) had success with the combined femoral shortenings and pelvic osteotomies for spastic dislocation of the hips in 23 patients. In the follow-up they also noted pain persisting in the hips of some patients for six to eight months. I too have had this experience. Gentle passive range-of-motion exercises, plus non-narcotic analgesics, have resolved this problem in all. Of the 29 hips Root and Broumann reduced with the one-stage operation, four had some residual subluxation and two had supracondylar fractures of the femur after plaster removal.

Gross *et al.* (1984) and Ibrahim *et al.* (1986) also had success with the one-stage procedure of femoral and Chiari osteotomies in 13 hips of 10 patients with cerebral palsy. Eight patients were relieved of hip pain; in two the pain was relieved after the iliac osteotomy fixation screws were removed.

Chiari iliac osteotomy

The Chiari iliac osteotomy (1974) alone has been used for painful subluxation and dislocation of the hip in cerebral palsy by Bailey and Hall (1985), but in only three of the five patients was pain relieved and secondary intertrochanteric osteotomies required. Grogan *et al.* (1986), in their study of 16 Chiari osteotomies in cerebral palsy, concluded it was a satisfactory procedure to obtain hip stability. In the majority of their patients, femoral osteotomies and the usual muscle weakening procedures were previously done or carried out at the time of the iliac osteotomy.

Since Chiari first described his innovative operation for congenital subluxation of the hip in 1955, a plethora of papers have reported successes, complications, modifications of the technique and biomechanical analyses (Colton 1972, Hoffman *et al.* 1974, Mitchell 1974, Salvati and Wilson 1974, Canale *et al.* 1975, Benson and Evans 1976, Drummond *et al.* 1979, Herold and Daniel 1979, Onimus and Vergnat 1980, Malefijt *et al.* 1982). In general the results have been good when assessed by the relief of pain. In ambulatory patients with congenital subluxation, a postoperative limp is usual. One issue has been the amount of medial displacement of the distal portion of the osteotomy. Colton (1972) recommended that it be no more than 55 per cent. Salvati and Wilson (1974) contended it should be enough to cover the femoral head completely with the proximal ilium, and Bailey and Hall (1985) would do even a 100 per cent displacement and used a cortical-cancellous bone graft between the two segments in order to achieve anterior femoral head coverage when necessary.

Onimus and Vergnat (1980) said that the iliac osteotomy did not hinge solely on the symphysis pubis, but that both sacroiliac joints moved to cause upward and lateral displacement of the iliac crest; the opposite acetabulum was displaced laterally, while that on the osteotomized side slid medially.

Benson and Evans (1976) used cadaver specimens and found that the sciatic nerve was stretched over the brim of the sciatic notch when displacement occurred. They surmised that when unwanted posterior drift of the distal segment of the osteotomy occurred, it prevented sciatic neuropathy. They also believed that splintering of the bone in the sciatic notch puts the nerve in jeopardy. Their radiographic study suggested that some poor results might be explained by a tendency for the iliac osteotomy to hinge posteriorly at the sciatic notch and open anteriorly like a book. Radiographs may give the illusion that the femoral head is covered.

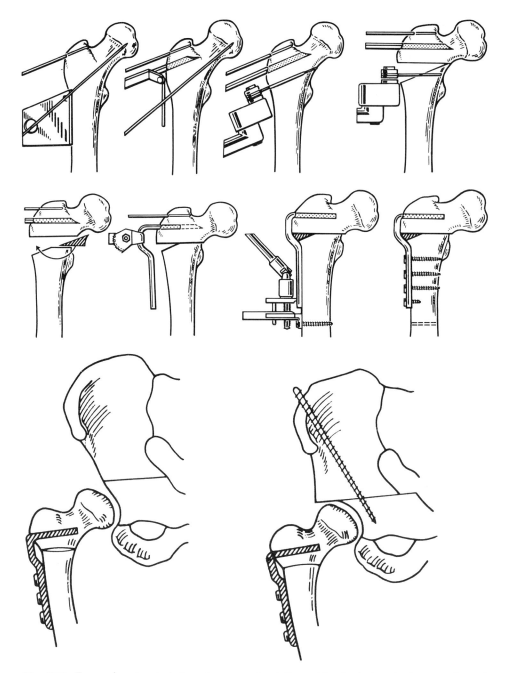

Fig. 9.31. *Top and center:* technique for varus derotation subtrochanteric osteotomy or femoral shortening for reduction of dislocation of the hip. Note: more recent ASIF nail-plate devices are self-compressing; however, at times in femoral shortening cases, the compression device is useful. (Redrawn from ASIF technique manual, Synthes Corporation.) *Bottom:* scheme for one-stage reconstruction: subtrochanteric osteotomy and Chiari iliac osteotomy (see text).

428

The important points of the technique of Chiari's osteotomy are: (i) the osteotomy must begin at the margin of the acetabulum—not too far above it or in it; (ii) the osteotomy must be ascending and directed 10° cephalad to end in the sciatic notch and not in the sacroiliac joint; (iii) if possible it should be curved slightly posteriorly in order to prevent posterior slippage of the distal segment. After observing my long follow-ups, it does not seem to make much difference in contouring of the acetabulum with growth if the osteotomy is almost straight and not curved. In postoperative computerized axial tomographs the proximal ilium overlies the femoral head 'like an umbrella' (Terver 1981), or perhaps more appropriately 'like a plank' (Hall 1981) under age 10 years.

Operative technique of one-stage reconstruction for spastic dislocation of the hip
1. The patient is supine. No towels or sandbags are used under the hip to rotate the pelvis. This position will distort the radiographic image. Fluoroscopy with image intensification and a video monitor help to achieve optimum accuracy in the techniques.

2. An anterior-medial groin incision and approach (as described above) is used for the myotomies of the adductors, anterior branch obturator neurectomy, iliopsoas tenotomy, and when indicated, proximal hamstring myotomy.

3. The anterior iliofemoral approach to the hip is made through an incision that begins at the mid-crest of the ilium and continues just below the crest to the anterior superior iliac spine, where it curves medially and then laterally toward the greater trochanter. There it turns distally over the lateral aspect of the proximal femoral shaft. The incision has the configuration of a question mark (?).

The proximal dissection is first done by detaching the origins of the sartorius and rectus femoris and the tensor fascia femoris and gluteus medius muscles. The latter is stripped off the outer wall of the ilium, and its fibers are separated from the joint capsule over the dislocated femoral head. The capsule is now opened and the articular cartilage inspected. If it is in reasonably normal condition, we proceed with the operation of relocation. If it is degenerated, a salvage procedure such as femoral head and neck dissection with capsular interposition is carried out.

4. The capsule is opened with a т incision, the ligamentum teres excised and the acetabulum visualized. In contrast to congenital dislocations, it is rarely necessary to remove fat and fibrous tissue from the acetabulum. The lateral aspect of the femur and subtrochanteric region is exposed by detaching the origin of the vastus lateralis and stripping the muscle subperiosteally from the femur, as well as stripping the periosteum circumferentially and including the insertion of the posterior-lateral intermuscular septum.

Next, using radiographic control, a guide pin is introduced from the greater trochanter into the head and neck of the femur and checked for position in both planes. It should be inserted superior to the site of intended nail insertion of the ASIF hip-compression nail-plate. The pin is inserted at a 70° to 75° angle to the femoral shaft in order to accomplish a 20° to 25° varus osteotomy (Fig. 9.31).

The special chisel, which matches the nail portion of the nail-plate, is introduced into the head and neck using the guidance of the pin. The length of the

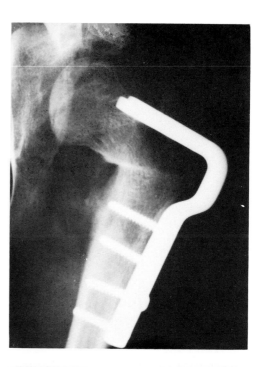

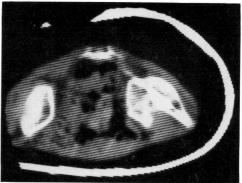

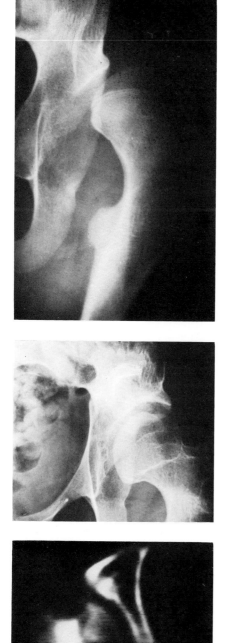

Fig. 9.32. Anterior-posterior radiographs of left hip, patient FC. *Top left:* age 16 years, total body involved, household walking with support, pain left hip. *Top right:* immediately postoperative, adductor longus myotomy, anterior branch obturator neurectomy, iliopsoas tenotomy, femoral shortening (1.5cm), varus derotation subtrochanteric osteotomy and Chiari iliac osteotomy. *Center left:* three years postoperative. Hip located. *Center right:* computerized axial tomography, transverse section through hip joint, postoperative Chiari illiac osteotomy. This osteotomy puts a 'plank' over the femoral head. *Left:* CAT of hip postoperative Chiari iliac osteotomy. Femoral head is concentrically reduced in acetabulum.

nail portion is determined and the chisel removed. The nail is driven into the chisel track until the distal portion of the plate abuts against the femoral shaft. With a power saw, an oblique osteotomy parallel to the nail is made in the subtrochanteric region, to end just inferior to the neck of the femur. The nail is then driven the whole way into the neck of the femur.

A second cut in the femur is made 1 to 1.5cm distal to the osteotomy and perpendicular to the femoral shaft. The bone fragment is removed. With the nail holder-driver in place the femoral head is easily placed in the acetabulum. The distal femoral fragment is then coapted to the proximal one and the femoral torsion corrected by externally rotating the distal femur, while keeping the proximal femur internally rotated with the holder driver attached to the nail-plate. Care must be taken to allow approximately 20° to 30° of hip internal rotation after the osteotomy is secured. Bone-holding forceps (I prefer the Richard's c-clamp type) secure the plate to the lateral femoral shaft. The modern ASIF hip-compression plates have offset holes to allow compression without the use of the special compression device. It can be used, however, if difficulty is encountered in closely approximating the osteotomy sites. The plate is fixed to the femoral shaft with the usual screw techniques.

5. To perform the iliac osteotomy, a guide pin is placed just at the edge of the acetabular margin below the anterior inferior iliac spine but above the site of intended osteotomy. To ensure that the osteotomy is neither too high nor too low, I visualize the articular cartilage of the joint through a tiny incision in the capsular attachment. The guide pin is inserted under radiographic control and directed 10° cephalad to end in the greater sciatic notch. Blunt retractors must be inserted on both sides of the ilium in the sciatic notch.

The osteotomy cut is made with a narrow osteotome in the lateral wall of the ilium, and must always ascend slightly toward the inner wall (Fig. 9.31). The cut can curve slightly posteriorly to follow the margins of the capsular attachment. 'Repeated checking of the osteotome position by x-ray is very helpful' (Chiari 1974, p. 58). When the osteotomy is completed, displacement can be attempted by holding the proximal ilium with a forceps while abducting and internally rotating the hip. Because of the previous femoral osteotomy and the relaxed abductor muscles, it is usually necessary and safer to push the femoral head medially by applying lateral pressure on the greater trochanter. At times the insertion of a dull spade elevator to act as a lever between the osteotomy surfaces is helpful to initiate the displacement.

If you need more displacement than is possible, iliac bone grafts can be added, similar to the technique used for acetabular augmentation described by Zuckerman *et al.* (1984) although I have not had occasion to do so. The main cause of inability to displace the distal segment medially is allowing the osteotomy to drift inferiorly during the procedure. Then the only remedial measure will be to recut the osteotomy sufaces so gliding can occur. This may produce a little gap in the site, but in growing children it will eventually fill in with new bone. The osteotomy is secured with oblique threaded Steinman pins or bone screws. The long cortical cancellous type are ideal, but only if the ilium is wide enough to accommodate. The screw direction needs checking with the fluoroscope to ensure that the fixation screw or pin in the proximal ilium enters the distal segment superiorly and medially to the acetabulum and not in it.

Suction drainage is used in all cases, and wound closure is in the routine manner.

6. A 1½ spica plaster with the hip in slight flexion, unstressed abduction and neutral rotation is applied and removed in six to eight weeks postoperatively. Because we use internal fixation, we extend the spica to below the rib margins so that the patient can be semi-reclining in a wheelchair with an adjustable back-rest rather than be forced to remain flat in bed for weeks. After plaster removal, passive range of motion of the joints and pool therapy, if available, speeds up the restoration of comfortable sitting. Wheelchair seating modifications may be required (Fig. 9.32).

The only significant complication has been sciatic neuropathy in two of the 20 patients. In one it gradually disappeared; in the other, I exposed the greater sciatic notch and found the nerve stretched tightly over it. Removing the underlying bone and wrapping the nerve in cellulose foam sponge relieved the symptoms of pain in the calf and foot. Chiari (1974) also reported a sciatic neuropathy, and presumed it was from stretching of the nerve; the femoral nerve was involved in one case, and six cases had peroneal neuropathies. Malefijt *et al.* (1982) had one case of postoperative sciatic neuropathy in 27 patients. Benson and Evans (1976), in an anatomical study using human cadavers, concluded that the sciatic nerve was angulated at the osteotomy site; bone splintering at the sciatic notch was also thought to be a contributing factor in the complication of postoperative neuropathies. They reasoned that the nerve was sometimes protected from over-stretching when the distal segment of the osteotomy slipped posteriorly.

Non-union of the osteotomy is a possibility. I have seen only one such case suspected in an adult who had the procedure for a congenital acetabular dysplasia. In one of my patients in whom the one-stage procedure was performed, we obtained a 100 per cent displacement of the osteotomy; but after four months of worry about union, healing occurred. I believe that 100 per cent is too much, although the addition of the interposed flat cortical iliac bone graft suggested by Bailey and Hall (1985) may be just right.

Salvage procedures for painful dislocated hips
When the head of the femur is deformed and the cartilage degenerated as usually occurs in the total body involved adolescent and adult who has a painful dislocated hip, four salvage procedures have been proposed: (i) subtrochanteric abduction osteotomy; (ii) femoral head and neck resection; (iii) hip arthrodesis; and (iv) total hip-replacement arthroplasty. Which to choose?

SUBTROCHANTERIC ABDUCTION OSTEOTOMY
I have had no experience with this procedure in which the femoral head is left dislocated and the femur abducted at the osteotomy distal to the lesser trochanter. It is an old operation for longstanding irreducible congenital dislocations of the hip

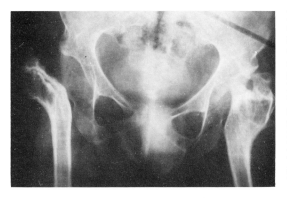

Fig. 9.33. Anterior-posterior radiograph of hips of 17-year-old total body involved male capable of wheelchair transfers. Originally had bilateral adductor myotomies and anterior branch obturator neurectomies for subluxation of the hips. Reduction did not occur. Then bilateral varus derotation subtrochanteric osteotomies performed (no ilopsoas tenotomies). Because of continued painful subluxation of the hips, bilateral femoral head and neck resections were combined with subtrochanteric abduction osteotomies. (Surgery performed in Milwaukee, Wisconsin, circa 1965.)

dating from Kirmisson (1894), modified by Lorenz (1918), Schanz (1922) and finally Hass (1943) (all cited by Crenshaw 1963, page 1738). Weinert and Ireland (1985) made a further modification, in that they used rigid fixation with the compression hip-screw system. They performed the operation in four total body involved patients who had severe contractures and hip dislocations, apparently with satisfactory results. Other surgeons seem to have tried this procedure in cerebral palsy, but have not published the results. One crutch-dependent ambulatory adolescent with spastic diplegia, whom I saw in consultation 15 years ago, had rather poor functional results; hip stability was nil (Fig. 9.33).

FEMORAL HEAD AND NECK RESECTION

Resection of the femoral head and neck has been the most commonly used

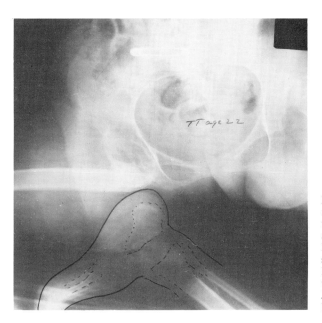

Fig. 9.34. Anterior-posterior radiograph of hip of 22-year-old total body involved non-ambulatory patient after femoral head and neck resection; hip was still painful and hyperabducted. Note that the resection was below the trochanters. (Courtesy of Jacob Sharp MD, Porterville State Hospital, California.)

433

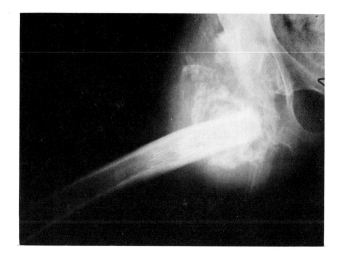

Fig. 9.35. Anterior-posterior radiograph of hip, postoperative femoral head and neck resection with commonly observed heterotopic ossification. (Courtesy of Jacob Sharp MD, Porterville State Hospital, California.)

operation to relieve the pain of a dislocated hip in a skeletally mature total body involved patient. The results seem to have been equivocal, and some surgeons have wondered if there is any good salvage procedure for this distressing condition (Koffman 1981). I too have wondered if the procedure is worthwhile. However, my colleagues (Kalen and Gamble 1984) re-examined the 18 hips in 15 patients in whom the operation was done at an average age of 17.5 years. They found pain was relieved in two-thirds; 89 per cent had heterotopic ossification and 28 per cent were ankylosed (Figs. 9.34, 9.35). Even though the radiographs were 'not pretty', the goals of pain relief, improved sitting ability and facilitation of nursing care were accomplished in the majority.

Castle and Schneider (1978) were specific in their directions; they resected not just the head and neck of the femur but the entire proximal end to below the lesser trochanter. This procedure was an interposition arthroplasty in which the hip-joint capsule was detached from the femur and then sutured across the acetabulum; the gluteus medius and minimus muscle insertion was sutured into the space between the proximal femur and the acetabulum; iliopsoas tenotomy was always performed. The quadriceps' origins were sutured over the end of the resected femoral shaft. Their 14 patients (14 hips) were placed in Russell's traction postoperatively for an unspecified duration. In three patients who had only the femoral head and neck resected, pain and deformity recurred. But in those who had the entire proximal end of the femur removed and the interposition arthroplasty, pain and deformity were relieved.

I think this is a satisfactory procedure. The results will be more sustained if the femur is kept in skeletal traction, using a Kirschner wire through the distal femur or proximal tibia, and balanced suspension with the limb resting on a posterior Thomas splint for two to three weeks. During this time, frequent passive range of motion of the hip would be indicated. This is the régime used by Murray *et al.* (1964) when they had very successful results of femoral head and neck resection as a salvage procedure for arthritis of the hip (Fig. 9.36).

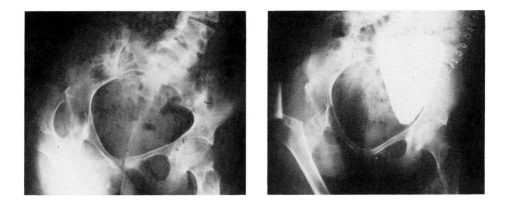

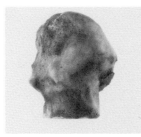

Fig. 9.36. Anterior-posterior radiographs of pelvis and hips. *Above left:* LS, age 19, total body involved, non-ambulatory. Left hip dislocated. Femoral head decreased density in lateral half. Pelvic obliquity with scoliosis. *Above right:* LS, postoperative excision of femoral head used an additional bone graft for spine fusion. Metallic clips on right side of trunk are wound closure for first stage anterior intervertebral disc excision and spinal fusion to correct scoliosis. *Left:* LS, photograph of femoral head removed. No articular cartilage on lateral aspect which has lost its spherical contour. Reconstructive surgery hopeless. Best chance for relief of pain was excision of the femoral head.

Raih *et al.* (1985) seemed to be satisfied with their results of proximal femoral resection in 30 patients; their resection varied from mid-neck to below the lesser trochanter. They used skeletal traction for three to four weeks postoperatively. Heterotopic ossification occurred in 18 per cent of the proximal resections and, curiously, in 85 per cent who had the more distal femoral resections. D'Astous and Baxter (1986) reported good results in four total body involved patients who had the procedure of Castle and Schneider (1978).

Hip arthrodesis or total joint arthroplasty?
Both arthrodesis of the hip and total hip replacement arthroplasty were the procedures of choice by Root (1977a, 1982).

Arthrodesis seems best performed both intra- and extra-articular. The Davis (1954) method of the muscle pedicle inlay graft from the iliac crest has assisted in obtaining better and more rapid fusion, plus some sort of internal fixation. The simple method of cancellous screws inserted from inside the pelvis into the femoral head seems to be a good method for intra-articular fixation (Mowery *et al.* 1986). The position of the hip can be set at the site of a subtrochanteric osteotomy performed at the same time. The osteotomy should be secured with a nail plate. The position of arthrodesis for these sitting patients is neutral rotation, 40° to 50° of flexion and 10° of abduction (Root *et al.* 1986).

I have had occasion to perform arthrodesis of the hip in only one patient with cerebral palsy. She was referred with a severe abduction deformity of the hip with

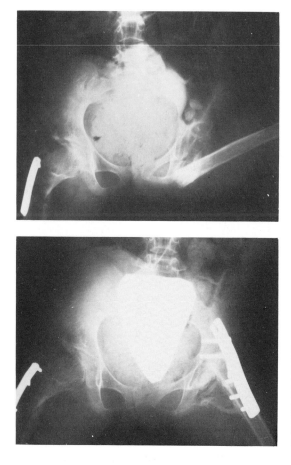

Fig. 9.37. Anterior-posterior radiographs of pelvis and hips. *Top:* AS, age 20, total body involved, postoperative femoral head and neck excision. Hip ankylosed in 120° of abduction. Impossible to sit and even to get through a door! *Bottom:* AS, postoperative. Solution was to perform a hip arthrodesis in 50° flexion, 30° abduction, neutral rotation. Comfortable sitting resumed.

pain after a proximal femoral resection for a dislocated hip. Her hip was so abducted that she could no longer sit in her wheelchair. Arthrodesis, although challenging, was accomplished with internal fixation; the hip was moved to a position of 45° flexion, 30° abduction and neutral rotation. Pain was relieved and her sitting became comfortable. Fortunately she had no scoliosis with a pelvic obliquity that would demand correction with spinal instrumentation, and fusion into the sacrum which would effectively remove the required mobility of the pelvis via the lumbosacral joint after hip arthrodesis (Fig. 9.37).

Total hip arthroplasty in 15 patients relieved the painful hip in 14 (Root *et al.* 1986). Preoperatively 12 of the patients had some ability to walk, most with external support. All were able to resume some functional walking after the arthroplasty. Four had spastic diplegia or paraplegia; three were listed as triplegic and the remaining eight were called quadriplegic. The postoperative complications were probably usual for total hip replacements, but in a greater incidence: bending of the femoral component; dislocation 12 days after surgery, then again at four months and 10 months; loosening of the femoral component after seven years but

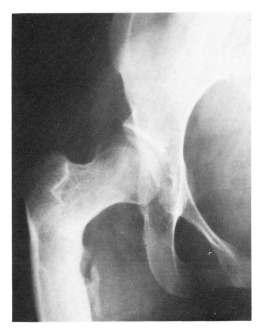

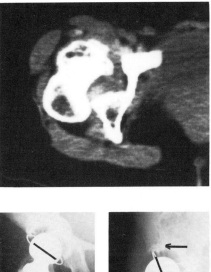

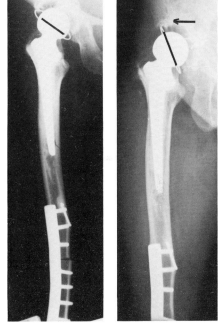

Fig. 9.38. *Top left:* anterior-posterior radiograph of left hip in TR, 19-year-old female with spastic diplegia, walked with crutches. Postoperative varus osteotomy for subluxation. Severe constant hip pain. *Top right:* CAT of left hip, transverse section. Note marked femoral torsion and extensive degenerative changes of the anterior aspect of the femoral head. *Bottom left:* TR, postoperative total hip arthroplasty. To correct the femoral torsion a derotation osteotomy in the distal femoral shaft was required and done at the same time as the arthroplasty. (The almost vertical and useless screw in the distal shaft medially is from a previous osteotomy performed 'elsewhere'.) *Bottom right:* two years postoperative. The acetabular component has shifted to a more vertical position due to the commonly observed acetabular loosening. Arrow indicates a radiolucent line along the lateral side of the cup at the cement-bone interface.

with mild symptoms; recurrent subluxation of the femoral component requiring its replacement six years postoperatively. 53 per cent had heterotopic ossification, but with no obvious clinical significance.

I have performed total hip replacement in only one patient with spastic diplegia who was a community walker with crutches. Because of severe unremitting hip pain due to extensive degeneration of the articular cartilage after varus and derotation osteotomies, she was wheelchair-bound and had pain even when sitting or lying down. Total hip arthroplasty and a distal femoral rotation osteotomy to correct 60° of femoral anteversion relieved her pain and restored her walking ability. Fortunately she uses crutches and restricts her walking to the household and neighbourhood. In a way, her functional walking is not much different from many adults who become, as they now say, 'couch potatoes'—*i.e.* never walking, jogging or running. For this sort of disabled person, swimming is the best exercise—has anyone thought of setting up a health club for the handicapped? (Fig. 9.38).

What is to be done, arthrodesis or arthroplasty?
In order to answer this, another question needs to be posed. Is this patient with cerebral palsy specifically total body involved? If so, sitting and standing equilibrium reactions will be deficient. If they are not absent, and the lateral equilbrium reactions are or have been fairly normal when standing, the patient is not total body involved and has the ability to be at least a household walker.

Given the above conditions, the total body involved person who might be a candidate for hip arthrodesis would be one who:
(1) is skeletally mature (and this will usually be the case if hip pain is disabling)
(2) has no evidence of subluxation or dislocation in the opposite hip
(3) has no pelvic obliquity due to scoliosis, or no evidence of a spinal curvature beyond 30° to 40° that may progress throughout life
(4) is able to perform minimally assistive or independent transfers from the wheelchair
(5) has a lower limb in an untenable position for sitting following resection arthroplasty of the proximal femur.

In the person with spastic diplegia or triplegia who was at least a household ambulator with crutches, and who has degenerative arthritis due to a subluxation of the hip, the first choice operation to be considered would be a varus (and medial displacement subtrochanteric osteotomy combined with a Chiari iliac osteotomy; an iliopsoas lengthening and adductor myotomies would be included). If the degenerative arthritis is far advanced in this type of patient, there is a case for total hip arthroplasty rather than arthrodesis.

One problem with arthrodesis is some compromise of sitting ability and more stress on the lumbosacral joint; this stress might be even greater in the spastic diplegic who has excessive lumbar lordosis due to long-standing hip-flexion contractures.

Even though very long follow-up studies of children who had hip arthrodeses revealed very satisfactory results, with sustained function for employment and almost all activities of living, I would not recommend arthrodesis of the hip in children who have cerebral palsy (Sponseller *et al.* 1984). The spasticity, and lack of normal patterns of control of knee-flexor and extensor muscles, would inevitably make walking less efficient. The knee is a more important determinant of gait than the hip. The reason why otherwise normal persons have good results with hip arthrodesis is preservation of knee function.

In conclusion, I can make the case for total hip replacement for painful subluxation of the hip in the adult with spastic diplegia or triplegia who has lost the ability for household walking with crutches. The spastic diplegic or triplegic who was more than a household walker and never used crutches and had a subluxation

438

of the hip would be rare indeed. If subluxation was found in this totally independent walking patient, coexistent congenital subluxation or dislocation of the hip would be the likely etiology.

If total hip replacement is performed, the patient should be told that revision and replacement of the arthroplasty may be necessary several years later. The patient should also know about postoperative complications such as dislocation and deep venous thrombosis, which may be more common in spastic paralysis than in normal persons.

I can imagine few indications for complete hip replacement in the total body involved person as defined in the preceding paragraphs. The magnitude of the current operation and its complications seem to outweigh the possible benefits of more comfortable sitting and sleeping. However, improvements in this surgery may occur and my statements should be seen only in the context of what we know in 1987 (*i.e.* I could be wrong).

We can hope that early surgery to prevent and correct subluxation and dislocation of the hip will continue to keep the numbers of cases in follow-up studies of salvage surgery very low.

Knee, foot and ankle deformities

Knee-flexion contractures in the total body involved patient need correction only if the flexed knee interferes with assistive transfers from the wheelchair, or if positioning in bed becomes uncomfortable. A knee-flexion contracture combined with the osteopenia due to non-weightbearing in these patients makes them prone to supracondylar fractures of the femur (Samilson *et al.* 1972). If the patient has transfer ability from the chair, a knee-flexion contracture beyond 15° to 20° is an indication for correction.

Fractional and prudent lengthening of the hamstring tendons, rather than tenotomy or transfer of all, should prevent the conversion of a flexed knee to a constantly extended posture. An underlying quadriceps spasticity is present in most of these patients. If the hamstring muscles are excessively weakened, the predominant extensor pattern which follows would make sitting in a chair more untenable than if the knees were left flexed. If knee flexion is severely limited after hamstring lengthening, quadriceps tendon recession or lengthening should restore knee flexion.

Very often these are long-standing contractures which involve the posterior capsule of the knee joint. If so, posterior capsulotomy and section of the anterior cruciate ligament insertion will be indicated. Sudden and forced extension of the knee under anesthesia may be inadvertent and cause a temporary sciatic neuropathy. In adolescents and young adults, soft-tissue surgery alone may not be feasible due to the shortening of the neurovascular structures. A closed wedged femoral condylar osteotomy with internal fixation and hamstring lengthening would be the preferred surgical treatment.

Foot and ankle deformities in this group of patients need correction only if they interfere with sitting posture or the mobility of the patient who is capable of transfers, either assistive or independent.

Given the stipulations for surgery with regard to functional potential, equinus, valgus and varus deformities of the foot and ankle can be corrected. Severe equinus, even if the person has no transfer abilities, can be disabling; shoeing is impossible and the foot cannot rest comfortably on the foot-rest of the wheelchair. Without the foot-rests, the equinus foot hangs down so that the toes drag on the floor or else the wheelchair seat has to be raised to a position beyond the usual table or desk height.

The surgical techniques for corrections of these deformities are identical to those described in Chapters 7 and 8.

Upper-limb deformities

Upper-limb deformities that are amenable to surgical correction for improved function are rare in the total body involved. As discussed in Chapter 7, hand or elbow surgery has been performed in very few patients with quadriplegia. Before surgery of the upper limb is considered in these patients, it is essential to obtain a detailed and repeated analysis of the potential for function, especially voluntary control. An occupational therapist can assess the patient's limited function decisions for surgery are made. As noted in Chapter 7, elbow-flexion contracture correction has been done to allow elbow extension and the use of crutches for at least household walking. The potential for walking can be determined largely based upon testing for infantile automatisms and the development of the normal parachute reactions. To use crutches or canes effectively, there must be good side-to-side equilbrium reactions. In our patient population of total body involved I have not found any who would benefit from correction of upper-limb deformities. Undoubtedly, other surgeons with different populations of cerebral palsy have found an occasional patient who can be improved with selective upper-limb surgery.

Spinal deformities

Spinal deformities are the other predominant skeletal problem in the total body involved patient. The two spinal problems are scoliosis and cervical spine degenerative changes which cause spinal-cord or nerve-root compression and superimpose a neurological condition on the motion disorder due to the brain malfunction.

Kyphosis and lordosis

Kyphosis of the thoracic spine is seen in many children with cerebral palsy when first sitting erect. This early kyphosis usually is not structural nor fixed. Bobath (1966) explained it as a compensatory mechanism in bringing the trunk over the pelvis in the child who has an extensor pattern of spasticity with resultant insufficient hip flexion.

Fixed kyphosis can be due to long-standing hamstring spasticity and contracture which is counterbalanced by quadriceps muscle spasticity, so that the pelvis is in constant posterior inclination when the child sits. Ambulatory patients with excessive lumbar lordosis may have a compensatory thoracic kyphosis.

TABLE 9.II
Summary of distribution of lordosis, kyphosis, and L5–S1 angle. (Patients: 104 normal, 114 scoliosis; two to >20 years)

| | Lordosis | | Kyphosis | | L5–S1 angle | |
	Normal	Scoliotic	Normal	Scoliotic	Normal	Scoliotic
Median	40	48.5	27	28	12	10.5
20 to 75%	31–49.5	40–55	21–33	16.5–36	9–16	6–14.5
10 to 90%	22.5–54	33.5–61.5	11.5–39.5	9–53	5–21	4–18

From Propst-Proctor and Bleck (1983)

Treatment of the thoracic kyphosis with the usual Milwaukee CTLSO (cervical-thoracic-lumbar-spinal-orthosis) brace has not been successful in the few patients for whom I have prescribed its use. The addition of a brace adds another handicap to the already seriously disabled person. Furthermore, I have seen no functional disability from kyphosis in the total body involved. The problem seems to alarm the physical therapist and family more than the patient. Lengthening of the hamstring muscles does not necessarily reduce the kyphosis in the wheelchair-bound patient, but instead is more likely to release the underlying extensor spasticity which prevents knee flexion and makes sitting comfortably more difficult.

In the sitting patient, lordosis is rarely a problem; in fact if it is eliminated by spinal fusion with straight rods, or anterior Dwyer instrumentation and fusion, sitting becomes a greater problem. The problem is that without lumbar lordosis, most of the pressure of the head, trunk and upper limbs when weight-bearing is concentrated on the small surface area of the coccyx and end of the sacrum. The surface area becomes much greater with lordosis, as weight is then on the posterior aspect of the thighs.

Measurement of the thoracic kyphosis and lumbar lordosis on lateral radiographs of the spine with the patient seated or standing is sometimes useful in the assessment of the presumed spinal problem. Measurements of what is considered to be normal have been published. The Cobb method of measurement has been used on the lateral radiographs; for the thoracic kyphosis we used the angle between the top of the fifth and 12th thoracic vertebrae and for lumbar lordosis between the first and fifth lumbar vertebrae (Table 9.II).

Although thoracic kyphosis of 40° is considered normal, 60° seems compatible with a long and useful life. At least one orthopaedic surgeon has recognized that 60° of thoracic kyphosis does not preclude Olympic championship (Nachemson 1980). Kyphosis of 80° and beyond does seem disabling but I have never encountered such a deformity in cerebral palsy. If I ever did, in an adolescent with a fixed structural deformity, I would recommend anterior disc excision and fusion, and second stage posterior fusion and corrective instrumentation (Moe *et al.* 1978).

Scoliosis

I never promised you a rose garden (Green 1964).

The prevalence of structural scoliosis in cerebral palsy differs between those who are ambulatory (spastic hemiplegia, ataxia and diplegia), and those who are not (total body involved). Several studies suggest that scoliosis is more prevalent in both groups of persons with cerebral palsy than in those with idiopathic scoliosis (Robson 1968, Balmer and MacEwen 1970, Samilson and Bechard 1973, Rosenthal *et al.* 1974, Madigan and Wallace 1981). Most studies are based upon the particular clinic population studied in a definite time-period. Consequently a true incidence cannot be stated with certainty. For example one clinic in St Louis, Missouri, reported a 5 per cent incidence of scoliosis in the years 1950 to 1959, which dropped to 3 per cent from 1970 to 1979 (Behrooz and Akbarnia 1984). Routine radiographic examinations were not performed on all patients seen in their clinics. However, it may be that in the ambulatory cerebral palsy patient the probable incidence is three times more than in the 'normal' child and adolescent population (6.0 per 100 versus 2.0 per 100). The incidence of scoliosis in 315 patients with cerebral palsy age 18 months to 21 years in my clinic from 1957 to 1975 was 6.5 per cent. In the total body involved patient the prevalence of structural scoliosis varies in the reports from 25 per cent (Samilson and Bechard 1973, Moe *et al.* 1978) to 64 per cent (Madigan and Wallace 1981). Severely involved institutionalized patients appear to have a much greater incidence and severity of scoliosis. All studies give incidence data based upon curvatures greater than 10°.

The only significance and value of the above data is to make the physician aware that scoliosis in cerebral palsy is common, and children should be regularly examined for signs of spinal curvature. When clinical evidence is found, a radiographic examination confirms and measures it so that progression can be ascertained and possibly arrested. I say 'possibly', because I am not at all certain that orthotic treatment in the total body involved is effective in preventing a progressive curvature.

The data on prevalence are also interesting. Although cerebral palsy has been with us for ages, scoliosis was thought to be almost non-existent 20 years ago (James 1967, Keats 1970). The rather sudden awareness of the problem as a serious structural change which compromises the care and function of the total body involved patient is probably related to an awareness of these patients as persons worthy of our consideration for treatment and, equally important, the emergence of effective surgical treatment due to the development of spinal instrumentation (Harrington 1962).

Etiological factors, characteristics, prognosis
The mechanism that triggers the onset of spinal curvature in cerebral palsy has not been specifically defined, but there may be similar alterations of CNS postural control circuits in the ambulatory and non-ambulatory cases. In the non-ambulatory patients, the superimposed asymmetrical spinal muscle contractions may be additive to the primary neurological mechanism and account for the greater frequency and severity of spinal curvatures in the non-ambulatory cases.

In the ambulatory patients with cerebral palsy, the development of the curve during growth, the curve pattern and prognosis for progression appear to be no different from in idiopathic scoliosis. In one study of 315 children with cerebral palsy (Bleck 1975), the incidence of scoliosis in the rare purely ataxic type was three times higher than in those who had spastic diplegia or hemiplegia. The curve patterns in ataxic cerebral palsy were identical to those found in idiopathic scoliosis (right thoracic curves) and in cases of Friedreich's ataxia, which has an 80 to 100 per cent incidence of scoliosis (Farmer 1964, Cady and Bobechko 1984). Sensory defects may be responsible according to Liszka (1961) and MacEwen (1968), who sectioned the dorsal spinal roots in experimental animals. Suzuki *et al.* (1964) found electroencephalographic abnormalities and enlargements of the third ventricle in patients with scoliosis. Further implicating the central nervous system's rôle in the mystery of idiopathic scoliosis was Martin's (1965) experiment of producing scoliosis in dogs with lesions of the caudate nucleus and reversing the spinal curvatures when the opposite caudate nucleus was destroyed.

The non-ambulatory total body involved patient develops scoliosis which is not appreciably different in pattern from those due to poliomyelitis, myelomeningocele and muscular dystrophy. Asymmetrical spasticity of the spinal musculature plays an important rôle. Abnormalities of the muscle fibers characteristic of neurogenic atrophy in total body involved scoliosis cases and the differences from normal in the distribution of fiber types were noted in the thoracis spinalis muscle biopsies in cases of idiopathic scoliosis when compared with biopsies of normal non-scoliotic subjects (Bleck *et al.* 1976). The puzzle of etiology remains because the pathological changes in the muscle were found on both sides of the curves (Bleck *et al.* 1976). Experimentally, muscle contracture has been shown in rabbits to produce scoliosis (Langenskiold 1971). But in human scoliosis we do not know whether the pathological changes in the muscles are primary or secondary.

Samilson and Bechard (1973) thought that the mechanism of the spinal curvature in total body involved patients (39 per cent of their cases were bed-confined and 92 per cent had spastic quadriplegia or tension athetosis) was a persistence of the infantile incurvatum reflex (Galant's reflex). To elicit the reflex, the skin alongside the vertebral column is stroked; the trunk bends into a concavity on the stimulated side (Beintema 1968). We tested for this reflex in 16 of our total body involved patients who had scoliosis, and could not find it in 15. One 16-month-old infant, with a long c-curve of the spine, had the reflex (Bleck 1975).

One constant observation in the total body involved patient is the absence of truncal equilibrium reactions. How these postural mechanisms affect spinal stability and might be a factor in the etiology of all scoliosis has yet to be determined. Research efforts directed along these lines have been reported in the literature (Yamada *et al.* 1969, Sahlstrand *et al.* 1978, Sahlstrand and Lidstrom 1980, Gregoric *et al.* 1981, Driscoll *et al.* 1984, Adler *et al.* 1986). Whether there are differences in the degree of equilibrium reactions in cerebral palsy and the correlation with the development of scoliosis must await objective methods of measurement of balance in patients who cannot stand without support.

Increased ligamentous laxity can probably be discounted as an etiological factor in idiopathic scoliosis and in those who have scoliosis (Bleck *et al.* 1981, Mattson *et al.* 1983).

In a search for a biochemical explanation of scoliosis development, the

443

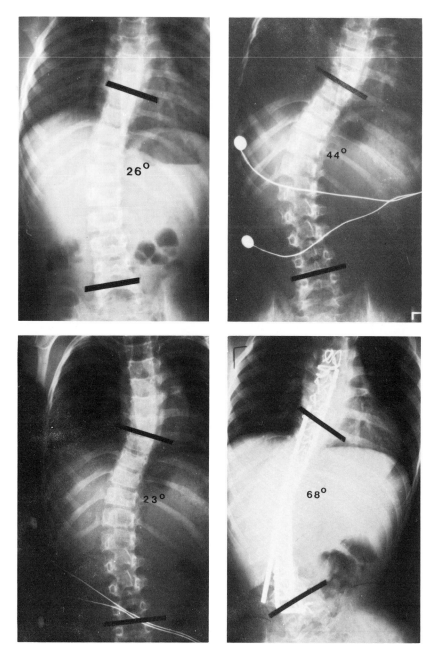

Fig. 9.39. *Top left:* anterior-posterior radiograph of spine. Curve appears similar to idiopathic scoliosis in this patient with cerebral palsy and ataxia. *Top right:* curve progressed despite two years of wear with a plastic thoracolumbar spinal orthosis (TLSO). Lateral electrical spinal stimulation tried. *Bottom left:* with lateral electrical spinal stimulator on, the curve decreased significantly. However, progression occurred. *Bottom right:* one year postoperative segmental spinal instrumentation without fusion; curve progressed and rods broke. We no longer use this method (Rinsky *et al.* 1985).

proteoglycan content of the intervertebral discs has been analyzed and found to be negative (Oegema *et al.* 1983). In this study there were no differences between cerebral palsy and idiopathic cases of scoliosis. Any changes from normal were thought to be secondary to the curvature.

Using proton NMR of human muscle extracts in idiopathic and cerebral palsy scoliosis, Arus *et al.* (1984) reported slight decreases in creatine and lactic acid in the muscle of idiopathic scoliosis and a significant decrease in cerebral palsy. These biochemical changes may indicate that the muscle is more involved and responsible for the spinal curvature in cerebral palsy.

We have no evidence that abnormalities of enchondral ossification are at work as a primary cause of idiopathic scoliosis. The studies of Enneking and Harrington (1969) showed more cartilage derangement and retarded enchondral growth on the convex side of the curves. No increased osteoplastic or osteoblastic activity could be discerned. In idiopathic scoliosis, therefore, extra-osseus causes seem to be the etiology; similar conclusions might be drawn in cerebral palsy. As in idiopathic scoliosis, the curvatures arise from a formerly straight spine and begin with a small curvature which progresses to become a severe and more rigid curve due to the secondary structural changes, first in the vertebral discs and then the vertebrae and their facet joints (Fig. 9.39).

Because hip dislocation and subluxation with pelvic obliquity often coexists with scoliosis, it has been assumed that correction of the hip problem will prevent the pelvic obliquity and the scoliosis. Muscle-release operations below the iliac crest have not prevented or altered the scoliosis. James (1956) made this observation long ago in his paper on paralytic scoliosis. Lonstein and Beck (1986) presented their data in which they could find no association between hip dislocation, pelvic obliquity and scoliosis in cerebral palsy. Scoliosis develops regardless of the hip and pelvic positions.

This review of some of the possible mechanisms of scoliosis, and the lack of a definite etiological factor to explain why some patients develop curvatures and others do not, indicates why the prevention and conservative management of scoliosis in general (and specifically in cerebral palsy) is empirical and not very effective.

Characteristics

In the total body involved patient the majority of the curves are thoracolumbar and lumbar. Very often the pelvis is part of the curve and accounts for the pelvic obliquity (Samilson and Bechard 1973). In ambulatory patients the curve pattern is usually a double major curve, with little pelvic obliquity; in some the thoracic curve predominates, with a poorly compensated lumbar curve below it (Lonstein and Beck 1986).

Because these curves begin at a younger age in the total body involved patient (in contrast to the onset in idiopathic scoliosis), and possibly because of the constant spinal muscle spasticity and contracture even at rest and recumbent, these curves become more rigid at an earlier age. This lack of flexibility in scoliosis associated with cerebral palsy is in contrast to the later-onset curvatures of idiopathic origin. Severe rotation and wedging of the vertebral bodies as well as distortion of the articular facets is usual.

The prognosis for progression of the curvature in the total body involved patient is bad, despite early diagnosis and conservative treatment. The spine curves with growth, with the most rapid growth occurring at the onset of puberty. The trunk increases its velocity of growth at the skeletal age of 11 years in boys, and 10 years in girls (Tupman 1962). The onset of puberty can be determined by observations of breast and genital development. Tanner stage 2 heralds the onset of puberty (Tanner 1962).

Numerous studies of scoliosis progression in both idiopathic and paralytic types, and the correlation with the velocity of trunk growth, have been published by Duval-Beaupère and her colleagues (Duval-Beaupère and Grossiord 1967*a*, *b*; Duval-Beaupère *et al.* 1970; Duval-Beaupère 1970, 1971; Duval-Beaupère and Combes 1971). These French publications have been summarized in English by Terver *et al.* (1980).

Spinal growth ceases for all practical purposes when the iliac apophyses are fully ossified and fusion with the body of the ilium occurs (Risser sign 5) (Risser and Ferguson 1936, Zaoussis and James 1958). If the curvature is less than 50° when skeletal maturation occurs, then progression due to growth usually does not occur.

Untreated scoliosis in 217 institutionalized patients with cerebral palsy were followed for five years by Madigan and Wallace (1986). One-third had progressive curvatures, and 76 per cent of these patients were skeletally mature. The most severely involved (presumably total body) had the greatest progression and the most severe curvatures. When pelvic obliquity was found in a radiograph of the pelvis, 96 per cent had scoliosis. Although the predictive factors have been published only for idiopathic scoliosis, the data might apply to cerebral palsy so that parents (and in these modern times, health care administrators) can be forewarned and informed (Lonstein and Carlson 1984). This information fortifies the advice on the need for regular follow-up examinations. The three consistent predictive factors were the chronological age, magnitude of the curve and the Risser sign of iliac crest apophyseal ossification. The nomogram for determining progression factors was based upon the formula: Cobb angle $- 3 \times$ the Risser sign $\div$ the chronological age. For example, if a child age 10 years has a Cobb angle of 30° and a Risser sign of zero, the nomogram shows a 100 per cent incidence of progression without treatment (this valuable nomogram can be found in the original paper by Lonstein and Carlson 1984, page 1070, Fig. 12).

Nachemson (1968) was the first to document the poor prognosis for patients who had untreated scoliosis in a 38-year follow-up study. Weinstein *et al.* (1981) in a long follow-up study of idiopathic scoliosis patients found that almost all curves over 50° progressed throughout life. The rate of progression in idiopathic curvatures can be generally stated to be 1° per year throughout life. All patients had some restriction of pulmonary function, but it was not significant or life-threatening until the thoracic curves were between 100° and 120°. Horstmann and Boyer (1984) found the greatest progression of scoliosis in quadriplegic persons with cerebral palsy after skeletal maturity and particularly in curves over 60°.

Orthotic management

In the ambulatory patient with cerebral palsy and a spinal curvature that does not involve the sacrum and pelvis, orthoses of various types used in idiopathic scoliosis are probably just as effective in cerebral palsy. The over-all rate of stopping the progression of curves in this group of patients is likely to be between 17 and 30 per cent. I have found the Milwaukee brace unsuitable in practically all patients with cerebral palsy, mainly due to their dysequilibrium which makes the wearing of this brace most difficult.

Bunnell and MacEwen (1977) reported success with plastic body jackets (TLSO) in arresting the progression of scoliosis in 48 patients with cerebral palsy, most of whom had involvement of all four limbs (N= 42). The average age of diagnosis of scoliosis was nine years. The follow-up ranged from nine to 60 months, for an average of 26.4 months. As these authors admitted, the follow-up was too short to reach a firm conclusion on the efficacy of the orthosis used. If the mean age of application of the orthosis was nine years, then the mean age at follow-up was only 11 years—almost exactly the time when spinal growth accelerates and curvatures increase dramatically.

Experienced orthopaedists use an orthosis in an attempt to 'hold' the curves in the total body involved child, and plan to stabilize the spine surgically when the child is old enough to have a spine fusion (usually after 10 years of age) at the beginning of the adolescent growth spurt. We know full well that orthoses do not prevent progression in these children but only delay definitive treatment (Moe *et al.* 1978, Winter 1986). The reason for delay, if possible, is that spinal fusion stops spinal growth.

In the total body involved patient the plastic thoracolumbar spinal orthosis (TLSO) can help hold some (but not all!) spinal curvatures. Zimbler *et al.* (1985) had little success in preventing progression of scoliosis in cerebral palsy when the curvatures were over 40° and the children were over age 10 years.

Winter (1986) has had more success in attempting to slow the progression of curvatures in the non-ambulatory patient with a polypropylene molded sitting orthosis. We have also used a 'sitting orthosis' but prefer a molded foam-padded fabric upholstered seat. Hard plastic seats are unsuitable for sitting six to eight hours at a time.

Electrical stimulation of spinal muscles with implantable stimulators has been used for the management of scoliosis in cerebral palsy by Bobechko for the past 12 years (Bobechko and Herbert 1986). They used their devices in curvatures under 40° and had excellent results: 32 per cent had more than 5° of correction; 40 per cent were unchanged; 17 per cent progressed a bit but not enough to merit surgery; 11 per cent failed and spinal fusion was necessary.

We have had no experience with this method of treatment in the scoliosis of total body involved patients. I have found no reports of the commonly used lateral electrical spinal stimulation for idiopathic scoliosis in cerebral palsy. Before using the Bobechko device, more details about the kind of patient and the age of follow-up would be essential. Curiously, Cady and Bobechko (1984) stated that there was no indication for electrical stimulation in scoliosis associated with

Years	Surgical management
1946–1956*	Posterior fusion and body cast (CP—almost none)
1957–1961*	Posterior fusion and halo cast
1959–1964*	Posterior fusion, button wire traction and halo cast
1961–1967*	Posterior fusion, Harrington instrumentation and cast (Harrington 1962)
1963	Author encouraged by Harrington instrumentation and began use for paralytic scoliosis (Bleck 1975)
1970–1972	Halo-pelvic hoop traction, posterior fusion, no cast, postoperative halo-pelvic hoop (DeWald and Ray 1970)
1967–1975*	Preoperative. Halo-femoral traction, posterior fusion and Harrington instrumentation and cast
1972–1976	Anterior fusion, Dwyer instrumentation, cast or plastic orthosis (Dwyer 1969)
1977–1979	Anterior fusion, Dwyer instrumentation, posterior fusion, Harrington instrumentation, plastic orthosis
1979–1980	Anterior fusion, Stagnara halo sitting traction, posterior fusion and Luque instrumentation, no cast or orthosis (Stagnara 1971, Luque and Cardoso 1977)
1980–1986	Anterior fusion (vertebrectomy if necessary), bed rest, posterior fusion and Luque instrumentation and no cast or orthosis
1987–	Modifications of Cotrel-Dubousset instrumentation for pelvic fixation? (Dubousset *et al.* 1986)

Pseudoarthrosis rates 1946–1977 = 20–40%
1977–1986 = >5%
*Historical data from Rancho Los Amigos Hospital, Bonnett *et al.* (1972).

Friedreich's ataxia, apparently because of the rapid and inevitable progression of spinal curvature in this condition. Surgical treatment was advised for all cases.

Surgical management

Prior to the introduction of internal fixation and instrumentation to correct scoliosis, there was little interest in attempting surgery with spine fusion in cerebral palsy. Spinal instrumentation has advanced rapidly in the past 25 years since Harrington first published his paper (Harrington 1962).

The principles and methods of stabilizing the spine with posterior element arthrodesis in scoliosis were established by Hibbs (1924), and progressively elaborated on by Cobb (1952), Risser and Nordquist (1958), Moe (1958) and Goldstein (1959). Prior to the innovation of effective instrumentation in the early 1960s, a variety of plaster body-jackets were used for correction preoperatively and postoperatively to hold the correction while posterior fusion occurred. Failure of fusion ('pseudoarthrosis' was the euphemism) at one or more levels was discouragingly common, and as high as 68 per cent (Ponseti and Friedman 1950). Goldstein's series, however, had only 12.9 per cent failure of fusion and when he added autogenous iliac bone grafts to the fusion site in 25 patients, only one had 'pseudoarthrosis' (Goldstein 1959). 'Pseudoarthrosis' was so common that some centers advised exploration of every spinal fusion six months postoperatively for a 'second look'. It is no wonder, then, that orthopaedic surgeons had little interest in attempting surgical correction and stabilization of scoliosis in cerebral palsy. I had no interest until 1963, when the Harrington instrumentation seemed to be the answer. Since that time a rapid and sometimes bewildering array of instrumen-

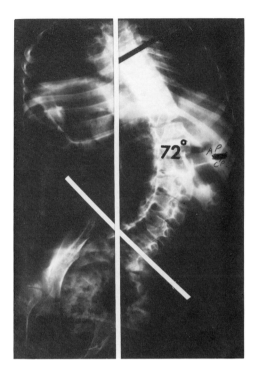

Fig. 9.40. Anterior-posterior radiograph of spine, total body involved, subluxation of left hip, pelvic obliquity due to the scoliosis. Pelvic obliquity is required to align the occiput over the sacrum.

tations and methods have been developed. An avalanche of literature has poured forth, which might make one suspect that there are as many papers and orthopaedic surgeon authors as patients. But it all has been to the good.

A summary of the evolution of the surgical management of paralytic scoliosis is presented in Table 9.III.

Indications

In cerebral palsy, surgical treatment is indicated in progressive scoliosis despite adequate orthotic use and in curvatures too severe for stabilizing with an orthosis. In the total body involved, orthotics are mainly attempts to prevent some progression until the child is old enough for spinal fusion, after 10 years. The usual thoracolumbar or lumbar curve in these patients extends to include the pelvis with resultant pelvic obliquity (Fig. 9.40).

If the curve measures over 40°, and certainly over 50°, orthoses are not likely to be effective. Unfortunately, however, most parents and other paramedical advisors want to 'wait and see' rather than put the child through the trauma of extensive surgery. This sort of emotionally driven policy in the total body involved child delays surgery until the curve is very severe (over 70°) and the patient's sitting becomes impossible and very uncomfortable. When the curves approach 90° to 100°, respiratory function is further compromised and operations become more hazardous. I have had to reject surgery in some of these patients because the risks are too great.

449

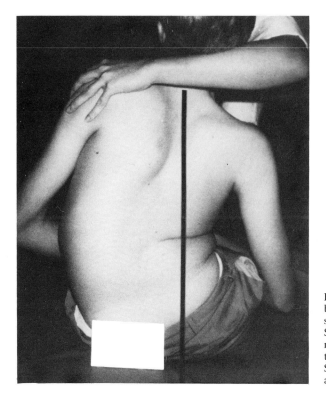

Fig. 9.41. Photograph of total body involved patient with severe scoliosis and pelvic obliquity. Spine decompensated. Lower-rib margins approximate the pelvis on the high side of the obliquity. Sitting uncomfortable and untenable.

The decision for surgery weighs the risks against the gains. Very rigid curves will require both anterior disc excision (and sometimes vertebral body excision) as well as second stage posterior instrumentation and fusion. Surgery of this magnitude may be fatal if the decision has been delayed too long, if the curve is very severe (*e.g.* 120° or more), if the adolescent's nutritional state is poor, and (most importantly) if respiratory and cardiac function severely compromised. If the patient has had a history of recurrent pneumonia and/or respiratory arrests, surgery will not be a prudent course. These patients cannot co-operate in preoperative pulmonary function studies. Blood gas determination might possibly help. The major postoperative complication I have seen is carbon dioxide retention: in this case artificial respiration may be needed for weeks or months after surgery.

In discussing risks of surgery for scoliosis, the numerical scoring system devised by Nachemson is helpful and understandable, even though we have no objective data to arrive at the score. People understand numbers, and our own 'gestalt' based upon our knowledge, assessment and experience can be expressed thus: 'If the removal of a wart is 1 point and a heart transplant is 100 points, then an ordinary Harrington instrumentation and spine fusion is 73'. In cases of paralytic scoliosis the risk can be 90 (Nachemson 1980).

Deciding on surgery, based upon the function of the mentally retarded total body involved patient, remains difficult even with the Rinsky test of assessment.

Can s/he reach for a cookie, put the cookie in the mouth or say 'cookie'? Each of these three tests reveals some function (Rinsky 1981). However, there are children and adolescents who have no oral communication or ability to feed themselves and yet are at home with loving parents who care for them much easier in a wheelchair with a seat insert and straps. When the scoliosis becomes severe and rigid, sitting becomes impossible. Then the disabled person retrogresses to bed nursing.

The major complaint of the non-ambulatory patient with a severe and progressive scoliosis is marked discomfort when sitting due to the pelvic obliquity and the lower ribs constantly pressed into the pelvic brim (Fig. 9.41). Neither seat alterations nor lateral pressure pads afford relief. The thoracic suspension body-jacket has not been satisfactory, because it will not correct passively these rigid curves and it obviously constricts respiration in a patient who already has restrictive lung disease.

Philosophical deliberations and cost-benefits might be focused on the 'person behind the handicap', the family which cares for the person and the costs of advancing the institutional placement as continuous nursing care becomes necessary. In California, 10 years of care in a State Hospital will cost at least $500,000. 10 children placed in institutions before it is necessary (*e.g.* before ageing parents can no longer care for them) will take away another $5,000,000 that might be more profitably spent in research leading to prevention of the brain damage or making treatment of the existing condition more effective. As prophesied by McLuhan (1964), our media age seems to focus on the immediate when we need a longer and broader view. Physicians often ask why we should operate on these children's spines. For them, this bit of rumination is offered.

Spinal growth does cease with spinal fusion (Johnson and Southwick 1960, Moe *et al.* 1964, Letts and Bobechko 1974). The amount of spinal growth is small and the amount of correction obtained will often make up for the slight loss in height. One can calculate that each vertebra grows in height 0.07cm per year, and if 12 vertebrae are fused at age 12 years, the loss of height at skeletal maturity at 16 years wil be 3.36cm (four years $\times$ 0.07cm $\times$ 12 vertebrae) (Moe *et al.* 1978).

Spinal flexibility must be assessed preoperatively. Anterior-posterior (or posterior-anterior) radiographs are made with the patient supine (or prone) and bending laterally to the left and right. Large radiographic cassettes are necessary so that the maximum amount of the spine is on the film. Active bending films are not usually possible in the total body involved patient, so passive bending is necessary.

Radiographs in paralytic scoliosis have been made with the patient in cervical and pelvic traction on a Risser-type table (Miller and Green 1976). I have found this difficult, and since we do not depend exclusively on traction to correct the curvatures, I no longer use this method of assessment.

I much prefer the prone-lying posterior-anterior radiograph of the spine made when the examiner's hand pushes against the apical region of the curve with the other hand providing the countervailing pressure on the opposite side of the pelvis. Examiners should wear lead gloves and an apron, to avoid excessive radiation. Exposure to radiation can be eliminated with a specially designed mechanical pushing device for the radiographic table (Hosada 1982) (Fig. 9.42). We have

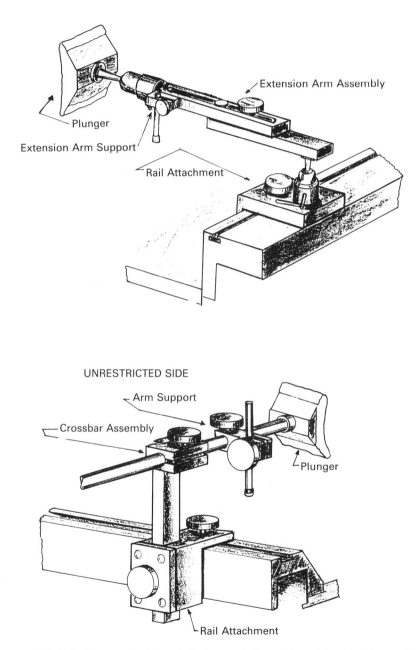

RESTRICTED SIDE

Extension Arm Assembly

Plunger

Extension Arm Support

Rail Attachment

UNRESTRICTED SIDE

Arm Support

Crossbar Assembly

Plunger

Rail Attachment

Fig. 9.42. *Top:* mechanical push device attached to radiographic table. The restricted side rests firmly against the pelvis on the side of the concavity of the spinal curvature. *Bottom:* unrestricted side of the push device attaches on the opposite side of the radiographic table. The arm is adjusted to produce maximum pressure against the apex of the convexity of the curvature (from Hosada 1982).

452

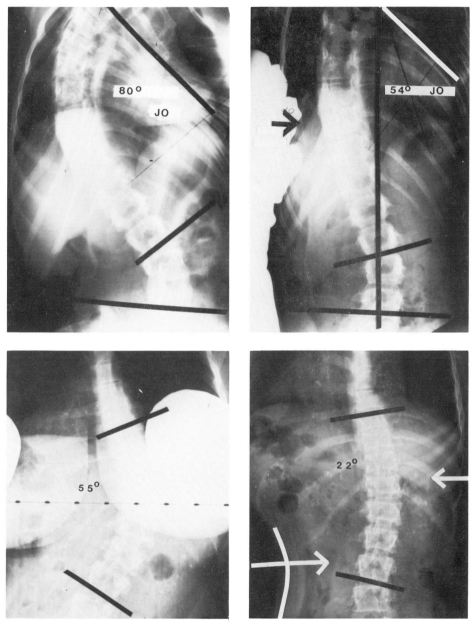

Fig. 9.43. *Top left:* anterior-posterior radiograph of spine. Scoliosis in cerebral palsy, athetosis, total body involved. *Top right:* posterior-anterior radiograph of spine with patient prone and manual compression against the apex of the curve with resistance on the lateral aspect of the opposite pelvis. The examiner must wear a lead apron and gloves. This maneuver gives a good indication of the degree of flexibility of the curve and replicates what one observes during surgery. *Bottom left:* thoracolumbar curve, mentally retarded, deaf, ataxia, age 22 years, female. Constant back pain. *Bottom right:* posterior-anterior radiograph made with mechanical 'push' device in place (see Fig. 9.42). Reduction of the curve is sufficient to indicate only posterior fusion and instrumentation.

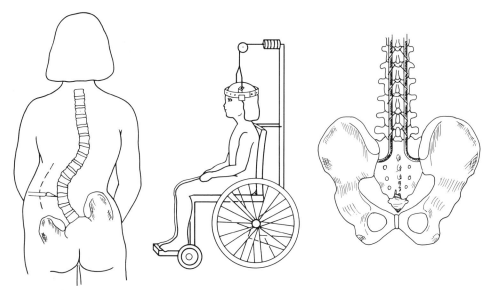

Fig. 9.44. Schematic drawing of our scheme for management of rigid paralytic scoliosis. *Left:* anterior intervertebral disc excision and fusion. *Center:* halo wheelchair traction for 14 days (we have often eliminated this step in recent years). *Right:* segmental spinal instrumentation.

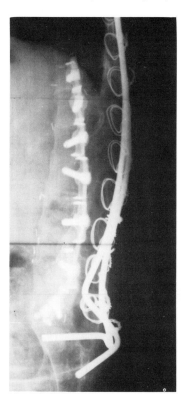

Fig. 9.45. Lateral radiograph of spine. Patient two years postoperative anterior fusion and Dwyer instrumentation, followed by second-stage segmental spinal instrumentation (Luque). Anterior fusion is very solid but the Dwyer instrumentation eliminated the lordosis. Note vertical sacrum.

found that these prone push films give as much information on flexibility of the curve as the bending films. Only one exposure is necessary (Kleinman *et al.* 1982).

I prefer the push films because they accurately simulate what we see and do at the time of posterior spinal instrumentation and fusion (Fig. 9.43).

Preoperative traction
With the invention of the halo for cervical traction, an efficient method of spinal distraction evolved and was combined with femoral traction (Nickel *et al.* 1968). We never used preoperative traction in our patients with the halo-femoral method (Bonnett *et al.* 1972). The femoral traction was practically always precluded in our patients with cerebral palsy because of the usual coexistence of hip subluxation or dislocation. We did use halo traction with the patient seated in the wheelchair after myotomy of the spinal muscles or after anterior-disc excision (Stagnara 1971). We stopped this regimen when we found that anterior-disc excision, vertebral body excision in some very rigid spines and anterior fusion was more efficient mobilization (Fig. 9.44). Pelvic traction with cervical traction (Cotrel 1975) was never tried because it was found to be insufficient mobilization for rigid idiopathic curves. It works best on curves that are flexible and do not require it!

Postoperative continuous traction with a halo-pelvic hoop apparatus was also abandoned because of improved instrumentation (DeWald and Ray 1970, O'Brien *et al.* 1971). By 1977, O'Brien's approbation of this method had diminished. The risks of bowel perforation, halo pin and pelvic pin tract infection and other complications dampened our enthusiasm for this method. Furthermore, by the time we thought about applying it to cerebral palsy, anterior spine fusion and instrumentation had appeared.

Anterior spinal fusion and instrumentation
Anterior spine fusion was pioneered by Hodgson (1968). Anterior instrumentation and fusion was the innovation of Dwyer (Dwyer *et al.* 1969, Dwyer 1973). In North America, Hall (1972) further developed the anterior thoraco-abdominal approach to the spine. The Dwyer method was used for correction of lumbar scoliosis in cerebral palsy with good early results and rapid return of function because no plaster jackets were necessary (Bonnett *et al.* 1973). By 1977 enthusiasm had cooled, because of the unacceptably high failure of fusion rate—29 per cent in neuromuscular scoliosis (Hall *et al.* 1977). Hsu *et al.* (1982), in their study of the results of Dwyer instrumentation, concluded that it might be used in idiopathic lumbar or thoracolumbar curves that had excessive lordosis. In 1972 I used the Dwyer instrumentation in two patients with cerebral palsy and severe rigid curves, but soon realised that merely excising discs was useless. Vertebral body excision would be required to mobilize some of these spines (Leatherman 1969, Heinig 1984).

I have used the Dwyer instrumentation in a severely athetoid young adult who had a progressive scoliosis in combination with the posterior instrumentation and fusion. However, in the past six years we have not used the Dwyer instrumentation in the paralytic scolioses. The major reason was that this method of anterior

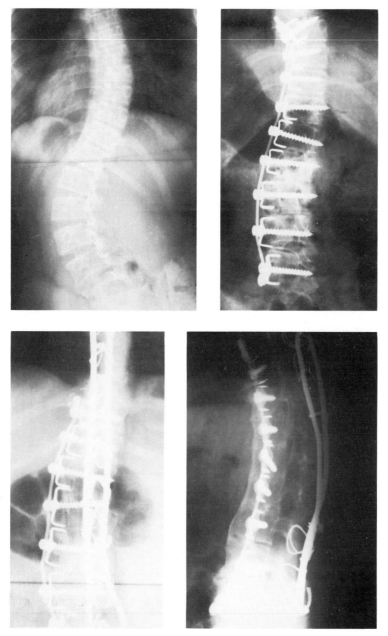

Fig. 9.46. Anterior-posterior radiographs of spine, patient MM. *Top left:* age 13 years, cerebral palsy, ambulatory, ataxia. *Top right:* postoperative Dwyer instrumentation and anterior fusion. *Bottom left:* eight years postoperative, age 21, lower Dwyer cable has broken between the fourth and fifth lumbar vertebrae. Failure of fusion at L4-L5 level and back pain. *Bottom right:* segmental spinal instrumentation and posterior fusion resulted in solid arthrodesis and relief of back pain. The lumbar lordosis is reversed due to the anterior instrumentation and fusion. This is why we have given up the Dwyer instrumentation for most cases.

fixation practically eliminated the lumbar lordosis which we found so essential for sitting with the weight properly distributed on the posterior thighs rather than on the coccygeal region (Fig. 9.45). Another important factor was the rigidity of the anterior fixation which precluded further correction with rods posteriorly at the second-stage procedure (Fig. 9.46).

In their report on the combined Dwyer instrumentation in paralytic scoliosis, O'Brien *et al.* (1971) made a significant contribution when they demonstrated that if the fifth lumbar vertebra was made level with the fourth lumbar vertebra, the pelvic obliquity might be corrected due to the strong iliolumbar ligaments which connect the fifth lumbar vertebrae to the ilium.

Zielke (1982) devised a more rigid type of anterior fixation with staples, screws and a rod. Its major advantage seems to be the ability to derotate the spine and to correct the lateral curvature. The device is very efficient for relatively short-segment correction of thoracolumbar curves. Zielke claims that his instrumentation has made the Dwyer obsolete because it is so effective in correcting rotation. We have used it only occasionally, and never in the scoliosis of the total body involved patient.

Posterior instrumentation has been modified many times since its introduction by Harrington (1962). Modifications have included square-ended rods, which could be bent to conform to the kyphosis and lordosis, and many types and shapes of distal and proximal distraction hooks, sacral fixation hooks and self-adjusting hooks (Akeson and Bobechko 1986). The principle of the Harrington instrumentation was distraction on the concave side of the curve and compression on the convex side. Many surgeons seemed to think that the compression rod was ineffective, and eliminated it. Faith in the compression rod was restored by the addition of lateral traction rods, placed horizontally between the compression and distraction rods.

Harrington instrumentation soon found its way into scoliosis in the total body involved patient. MacEwen (1969) was one of the pioneers. By 1972 he found that the use of the Harrington instrumentation was not a 'rose garden' as many had hoped (MacEwen 1972). I too had my troubles (Bleck 1975). Perhaps it is fortunate that the complications occur early in the postoperative course, and the late results concerning maintenance of correction and assurance of fusion can be ascertained in two to three years (spine fusions take about a year to mature). By 1972 it appeared obvious that paralytic scoliosis was best treated with the combined anterior and posterior staged arthrodeses (O'Brien and Yau 1972, Bonnett *et al.* 1977) (Fig. 9.47). This approach has continued, but with new types of instrumentation.

Lonstein and Akbarnia (1983), in a long-term follow-up of 107 patients with scoliosis associated with cerebral palsy or mental retardation, concluded that in those with pelvic obliquity it was always necessary to do the anterior and posterior approaches, and fusion to the sacrum was essential.

Luque (Cardoso *et al.* 1976, Luque and Cardoso 1977) introduced an entirely new principle of spinal fixation with the use of interlaminar wires fixed at each spinal segment to a semirigid rod on both sides of the curve. No postoperative plaster or orthotic immobilization was necessary with this method, which made it

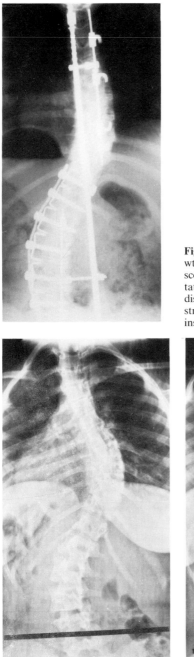

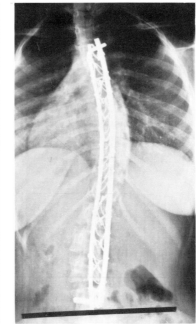

Fig. 9.47. Anterior-posterior radiograph of spine in patient wtih cerebral palsy, ataxia, mental retardation, progressive scoliosis. Postoperative anterior fusion with Dwyer instrumentation and second-stage Harrington instrumentation with distraction and compression rods and Cotrel lateral traction struts. Early mobilization. Fusion very solid. The apogee of instrumentation: no longer used by us.

Fig. 9.48. Anterior-posterior radiographs of the spine. *Left:* right thoracic, left lumbar curve, progressive. Pelvic obliquity 3°; no need to fuse into the sacrum. *Right:* postoperative posterior fusion and Luque segmental spinal instrumentation. Pelvic obliquity not significant. Both curves corrected and spine remains compensated.

Type of surgery	N
Harrington and posterior fusion	3
Luque and posterior fusion	3
Luque and Harrington combination	2
Subtotal	8
Dwyer	3
Dwyer and Harrington	12
Dwyer and Luque (1 with vertebrectomy)	5
Subtotal	20
Anterior fusion and Harrington	2
Anterior fusion and Luque (1 with vertebrectomy)	3
Subtotal	5
TOTAL	33

Complications: operative and immediate postoperative (39%)		Complications: late (24%)	
Atelectasis	2	Luque rod removed (fracture L5 lamina)	1
Pneumonia	1		
Pleural effusion	4		
Carbon dioxide retention	2	Died 2 months postoperative of pulmonary embolism	1
(10 days on respirator)			
Urinary tract infection	1	Protrusion of upper end Luque rod (kyphosis)	1
Chylothorax	1	Broken Luque rod, failure of fusion L4–L5 (ambulatory spastic diplegia)	1
Cardiac arrest during surgery; full recovery	1	Lower Harrington rod distracted from alar hook	1
Upper Harrington hook loose	1	Pressure sores left iliac crest and greater trochanter (5 years postoperative)	
		Frayed Dwyer cable, proximal screw cut out	
		Frayed Dwyer cable, L4–L5 failure of of anterior fusion (5 years postoperative)	1

Note: there were no neurological complications in this group.

very appealing for use in the total body involved child (Fig. 9.48).

The method rapidly spread throughout the globe. Many reports have appeared on its efficacy in neuromuscular scoliosis and in cerebral palsy (Allen and Ferguson 1981, 1982; Brown *et al.* 1982; Metz and Zielke 1982; Stanitski *et al.* 1982; Ferguson and Allen 1983; Allen 1983; Cardoso 1984; Thompson *et al.* 1985; Kalen *et al.* 1985).

Our results and complications in neuromuscular scoliosis in general, and cerebral palsy in particular, are not much different from others. Of 28 patients, 15 were non-ambulatory. The mean age of surgery was 16.7 years (range 10 to 31 years). The average curve was 69° (range 35° to 110°). In those who had the

combined anterior fusion and posterior fusion with segmental spinal instrumentation, the mean correction was 70 per cent. The operations were long (average seven
hours) and blood loss considerable (average 5500ml). These are not procedures to
be used recklessly. Early and late complications in our cerebral palsy patients, who
had several types of scoliosis surgery as we evolved the techniques from 1977 to
1982, are listed in Table 9.IV. This list only serves to forewarn the surgeon, patient
and family. This is not the kind of case that can be admitted to the hospital in the
morning, whisked through the operation in the afternoon and sent home five days
later.

One of the two patients who had broken rods was a 22-year-old woman who
had spastic diplegia and double major curves of 60°. Her low back pain was
intractable for two years, and she walked with a pelvic femoral fixation. Despite a
plastic orthosis, the pelvic fixation of the rods (Galveston technique, see Allen and
Ferguson 1981) could not withstand the stress. One year later, on removal of the
rods, the entire spine was solidly fused except at the fifth lumbar-first sacral level.
We had not performed anterior discectomies and fusion. The other patient had
scoliosis due to traumatic paraplegia. He felt so fine that shortly after discharge
from hospital he resumed his exercises on a horizontal bar. His rod broke.

The principle of segmental spinal fixation was added to the Harrington
distraction rod. Many surgeons use this combination ('Harri-Luke', 'Lukington',
'Luque-Harrington').

A recent modification has been the unit Luque rod which has a closed loop at
the top (Moseley *et al.* 1986). These Canadians devised this system to prevent
'translation' of the rods in neuromuscular scoliosis; most of their cases had scoliosis
due to muscular dystrophy. In their technique of fusion to the sacrum they also
used the Galveston technique of sacral fixation. In six months all showed a
'windshield-wiper' effect of the rods in the ilium, undoubtedly due to pelvic
motion. In curves with severe rotation and limited flexibility even after anterior
disc excision, I have found the unit rod difficult to use. But perhaps this is due to
the 'learning curve'.

McCarthy and McCullough (1986) invented a locking collar for the proximal
ends of the Luque rods, to prevent migration and rotation. The device was effective
in their hands. Locking the two rods together uses the same principle as the unit
rod. Leong (1985) commented on the problem of loss of correction of double major
curves due to rotation of the Luque rods. I have had similar problems. The locking
collar should be a solution.

The results of segmental spinal instrumentation in neuromuscular scoliosis
have generally been very good, despite the complications which are inherent in the
type of high-risk patient for whom both the anterior and posterior combined
procedures are indicated. The preceding historical review is presented in order to
give a perspective to the scholarly surgeon, and to prevent the kind of mistakes
made in the past.

Drummond (1984) modified segmental spinal fixation by passing the wires
through the spinous processes over a button at each level, and fixing them to a
Harrington rod on the convexity and a Luque rod on the concavity. The method

was used successfully in 34 patients with cerebral palsy. Their main curves were 82° (range 38° to 146°). The average correction was 50.5 per cent, and an average loss of just 5° of correction was recorded in a mean follow-up of 22 months (Sponseller *et al.* 1986).

The latest improvement is the Cotrel-Dubousset instrumentation from France (Dubousset *et al.* 1986, Johnson *et al.* 1986). The basis is a return to the distraction-compression principle of Harrington and hooks, but with a twist—the rod is rough and derotation of the vertebra can be achieved as well as lateral correction. It appears to be ideal for idiopathic right thoracic and thoracolumbar curves.

Surgery in young children (below age nine years) who have progressive scoliosis despite orthotics requires some method of internal fixation without spine fusion. Short fusions for congenital scoliosis are different and effective (Winter and Moe 1982). The Luque segmental spinal instrumentation without fusion failed to prevent progression of spinal curves in these young children (three of the nine had cerebral palsy) and, in some, rods broke as growth progressed (Rinsky *et al.* 1985). Eberle *et al.* (1986) had the same experience in attempting to prevent progressive curves without fusion and segmental spinal instrumentation. Like us, he advised against using the system except possibly in collapsing spines of flaccid paralysis.

The implantation of the Harrington rod over the muscles spanning the curve and distracting the rod every six months has been resumed for our patients (Moe *et al.* 1984). Ascani (1985), from Italy, has a clever modification of the distracting rod principle with two hooks on either side of the distal and proximal ends. With this system he can distract the spine through a small incision to twist the interior of the rod and distract the rod between the hooks at regular intervals. Takahashi (1986), from Japan, described to me a similar instrument to Ascani's for sequential correction of scoliosis without spinal fusion. 'Le monde est petit'.

Spinal muscle myotomy apparently is not effective. If it were, we would see many reports of successful prevention of progressive scoliosis in cerebral palsy. I have found only one report of a 21-year-old Japanese male who had severe athetosis and scoliosis with pelvic obliquity. After 'soft-tissue releases' and a transfer of the ipsilateral tensor fasciae latae to the rib cage, the scoliosis and pelvic obliquity improved 'remarkably' (Terazawa *et al.* 1980). It may be that if this young man had pure athetosis and constant alternating movements, he did not have a structural but a positional or postural type of scoliosis.

The principles of surgery in paralytic scoliosis have remained the same regardless of instrumentation:

1. Spinal fusion is essential; the instruments and devices are only temporary 'sutures' to maintain the correction while new bone formation creates a strong fusion mass.

2. The site for arthrodesis of the spine should be as far lateral as the transverse processes.

3. The facet joints should be excised—although Allen (1979) doubted that this step was essential, given the rigid internal fixation used. I have had an opportunity to explore the posterior elements of the spine 11 years after a solid anterior spinal fusion. I found most of the spinal facet joints still open and with a thin layer of

461

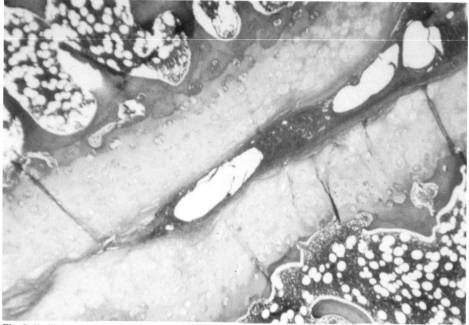

Fig. 9.49. Photomicrograph of intervertebral facets of patient MM (Fig. 9.46). Facets removed in area of solid anterior fusion eight years postoperatively. Articular cartilage still present and with viable cells. Some areas have fibrous tissue between the joint surfaces.

articular cartilage; in some areas fibrous tissue spanned the joint (Fig. 9.49).

4. Additional bone graft should be added (Goldstein 1969). In these very severe and long curvatures we use the patient's own iliac bone for grafts, and supplement this with freeze-dried allograft bone. Allografts appear to assist building the fusion mass (McCarthy *et al.* 1985) (Fig. 9.50).

Some orthopaedic surgeons routinely do rib resections on the convex side (Rinsky 1984, Hoppenfeld and Gross 1986), and these can be used for supplemental grafts.

5. The consensus is that in paralytic scoliosis of cerebral palsy and total body involved, the best results are with both anterior and posterior spine fusion (Fig. 9.50).

6. When pelvic obliquity is present (as it is in practically all these cases) the fusion should extend from the sacrum to the uppermost thoracic vertebrae (first to the third thoracic) (Fig. 9.51).

7. The pelvic obliquity should be corrected as much as possible. The goal is a level pelvis. If there are contractures below the iliac crest (hip adduction or abduction) these should be corrected first.

8. The correction should always aim for compensation of the spine—the occiput remains directly over the sacrum (Fig. 9.52).

9. Correction should not be forced beyond the limits of passive mobility of the spine. To force correction of kyphosis and scoliosis under general anesthesia with

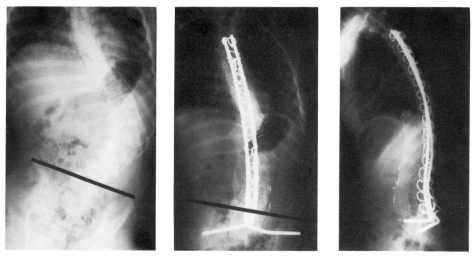

Fig. 9.50. Anterior-posterior radiographs of the spine, patient LS. *Above left:* age 14 years, progressive thoracolumbar scoliosis, cerebral palsy, total body involved, loss of sitting balance. *Above right:* three years postoperative anterior spine fusion followed in two weeks with posterior fusion and Luque segmental spinal instrumentation with Galveston method of pelvic fixation. Note the all-important lateral fusion mass in the lumbar spine. *Left:* three years postoperative, demonstrates the solid anterior body fusions and the preservation of lumbar lordosis of approximately 40°.

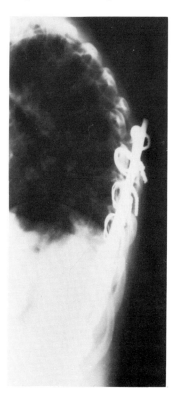

Fig. 9.51. Lateral radiograph of spine, one year postoperative posterior spinal fusion and segmental spinal instrumentation in a 17-year-old female with decompensated thoracolumbar scoliosis. The proximal ends of the rods protruded and broke through the skin due to the increasing postoperative kyphosis. Lesson: fuse the spine posteriorly as high as the second or third thoracic level particularly in thoracic kyphosis with scoliosis.

463

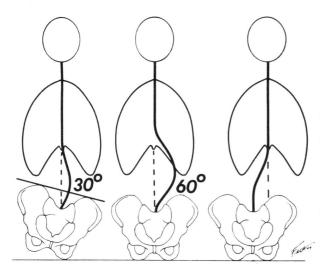

Fig. 9.52. Importance of obtaining alignment of the head and trunk over the center of the sacrum. *Left:* minimal curve but pelvic obliquity. Not satisfactory. *Center:* larger curve but well-balanced trunk and head over sacrum. *Right:* small curve, pelvis level, trunk vertical but shifted out of balance to the right. Not satisfactory. Even though *center* has the larger curve, the mechanics are better than in the diagrams *left* or *right*. (Reprinted by permission from Moe *et al.* 1978.)

powerful instruments invites neurological problems due to stretch of the spinal cord. The amount of correction on the lateral bending film (or prone-lying push film) plus 10° is the safe zone (Luque 1982).

In the total body involved patient, inadvertent paraplegia as a complication of treatment would result in loss of bladder and bowel control which is intact in almost all total body involved patients. Loss of protective skin sensation would further compromise function and care.

10. During the correction, spinal-cord monitoring using cortical evoked potentials, while not perfect, is helpful and is done at most centers (Bunch *et al.* 1983, Brown *et al.* 1984). We also do the Stagnara wake-up test in these patients, even though they have no voluntary control of their feet and lower limbs (Vauzelle *et al.* 1973). Stimulation of the plantar aspect of the feet with a small tooth forceps is sufficient stimulus to cause withdrawal of the foot and limb. This ensures continuity of the anterior columns of the spinal cord. Ginsberg *et al.* (1985) reported a case of paraplegia after surgery during which the somatosensory evoked potentials were preserved. Very recently a study has shown a 32 per cent failure of accuracy in spinal-cord monitoring in scoliosis surgery (Szalay *et al.* 1986). The problem is inability to monitor the anterior columns of the spinal cord.

Dysfunction of the spinal cord is likely to be due to interruption of the blood supply; this can occur with distraction. In the anterior discectomy and fusion, paraplegia is extremely rare; we have heard of this in one case. We can only speculate on the cause. One caution worth emphasizing is *not to attempt electrocoagulation of unseen bleeding vessels* in the intervertebral foramina on the anterior approach or anterior to the transverse processes in the posterior dissection. The blood supply of the spinal cord is known to be irregular, although we do know its major artery arises from one of the intercostal arteries or an upper lumbar vessel near the intervertebral foramen on the left, varying in origin from the sixth to the third lumbar vertebra (Keim and Hilal 1971). The objective of surgery

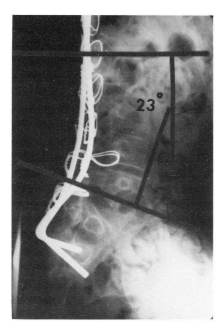

Fig. 9.53. Lateral radiograph of spine postoperative posterior fusion and segmental spinal instrumentation. Rods bent to conform to necessary lumbar lordosis. When sitting, 20° to 30° is probably sufficient to cause weight distribution to the posterior thighs rather than to the caudal end of the sacrum and coccyx.

is to provide a compensated spinal curve with a level pelvis, not a perfectly straight spine for all to admire in the radiology conference.

The speed at which surgery is performed is not the primary criterion of technical excellence. A slow meticulous operation with no neurological complications and an eventual solid arthrodesis is preferred.

11. In the total body involved patient, the goal is a comfortable sitting posture—so lumbar lordosis must be preserved. Rods have to be bent to accommodate the lordosis which should be between 40° and 60° when standing (measured by the Cobb method from the first to the fifth lumbar vertebra on the lateral radiograph). In a patient who sits and cannot walk, a lumbar lordosis between 20° and 30° seems adequate (Fig. 9.53).

Lumbar lordosis ensures that the bodyweight when sitting will be on the posterior thighs, which can accept 100mm of mercury per square inch before skin ischemia occurs. This is in contrast to the coccygeal area which can tolerate about 15mm of mercury per square inch; coccygeal weight-bearing will be the result of eliminating the lordosis of the spine (Motloch 1978).

12. Postoperatively, these patients need molded seat inserts to support the trunk and compensate for the deficient equilibrium reactions.

Our surgical management of the spinal curvature in the total body involved patient has evolved since 1979. It includes:

1. Preparation for autologous blood transfusions one month in advance, in which the one unit per week is drawn from the patient and stored to be used in the operating room.

2. For patients who usually have poor respiratory exchange, chest physical and

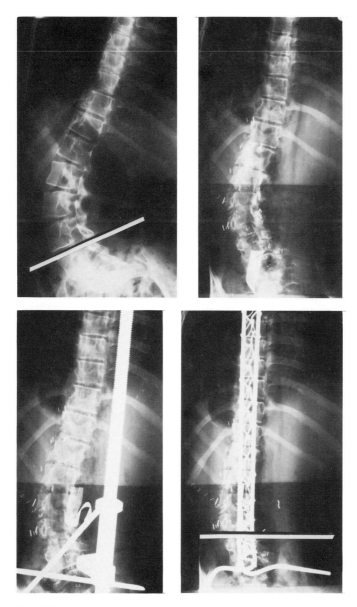

Fig. 9.54. Anterior-posterior radiographs of the spine, patient JL, female. *Top left:* age 16, total body involved, non-ambulatory, progressive scoliosis, sitting balance compromised. *Top right:* postoperative anterior-disc excision, partial vertebrectomy third lumbar vertebra, interbody fusion, approach thoracoabdominal on right removing 10th rib. *Bottom left:* intraoperative radiograph, second stage, posterior fusion, Harrington outrigger used to level pelvis. *Bottom right:* correction obtained with outrigger captured by segmental spinal instrumentation. Galveston pelvic fixation. In cases of pelvic obliquity fusion should always include the sacrum. The pure Galveston technique of pelvic fixation with the L-rods is to insert them from the region of the posterior iliac spine area obliquely through the pelvis through its thickest portion. The distal end of the rod ends approximately 2.5cm superior to the greater sciatic notch.

respiratory therapy two to three times on the first preoperative day is the least one can do for prevention of pulmonary complications.

3. Anterior thoracolumbar approach for anterior-disc excision, removal of the cartilagenous end-plates to subchondral bone, and excision of vertebral bodies when the apical vertebrae remain fixed and immovable (Heinig 1984). When vertebrae are excised, the anterior longitudinal ligament is preserved. Heinig preserves the cortex and scoops out the cancellous bone to create an 'eggshell'. The shell is crushed and the vertebral fragments replaced in the sleeve of the ligaments, like making a sausage (Fig. 9.54).

Vertebral body excision in scoliosis was done in the past, but very rarely (Compère 1932, VonLackum and Smith 1933, Wiles 1951). Although anesthesia techniques and blood-replacement advances (e.g. 'cell saver' in which blood is suctioned from the wound, washed in a machine to remove the plasma, and the cells resuspended in solution to be administered) have made vertebral body excision safer and more feasible, it is still a formidable technique. Extreme caution and care is obviously necessary. It is uncertain whether continuous cold saline lavage of the exposed dura mater and/or the administration of intravenous corticosteroids protect the spinal cord. However, I have done this in the past. Naloxone hydrocholoride (Narcan), an opiate antagonist, has protected the spinal cord from the effects of blunt trauma experimentally in animals, but the efficacy of the clinical application has yet to be shown (Young 1985).

4. The patients is kept in bed for two weeks following the first stage. No sitting is permitted. The physical therapist ensures maintainance of the range of motion of the lower limbs, and the respiratory therapist assists in obtaining maximum respiratory exchange. During these two weeks the blood hemoglobin is maintained with oral iron and blood transfusion, if necessary, in order to prepare for the second stage of surgery.

5. Posterior fusion of the spine and segmental spinal instrumentation (Luque) with the Galveston technique for pelvic fixation (Allen 1983, Allen and Ferguson 1984) (Fig. 9.55).

6. Resumption of sitting five to six days postoperatively, and the fabrication of a molded upholstered seat insert.

No plaster or plastic jackets or orthoses have been necessary unless the surgeon feels insecure about the fixation. In only two of 55 cases of paralytic scoliosis have we used anterior and posterior plastic shell-type thoracolumbar orthoses for six months postoperatively.

Neurological complications are the biggest danger in all scoliosis surgery. Of 7885 cases collected from 1965 to 1971 by the Scoliosis Research Society, acute spinal-cord lesions occurred in 87. 74 involved the spinal cord (41 complete paralyses and 33 incomplete). Complete recovery occurred in 22 of these, there was partial recovery in 28 and none in 24. Not all were associated with Harrington instrumentation; six patients became paraplegic with skeletal traction only (MacEwen *et al.* 1975).

Segmental spinal instrumentation has been no exception. Wilber *et al.* (1984) reported the occurrence of neurological complications in 137 patients who had

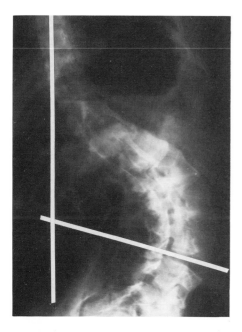

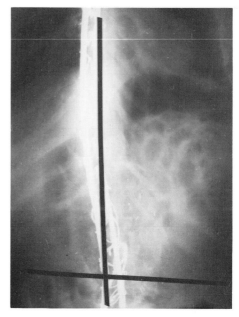

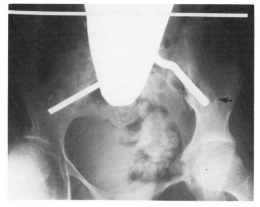

Fig. 9.55. Anterior-posterior radiographs of spine and pelvis, patient SM. *Above left:* age 21 years, total body involved, severe rigid scoliosis and pelvic obliquity. *Above right:* postoperative. First stage was anterior-disc excision and vertebrectomy of apical vertebrae which were replaced in the periosteal and ligamentous tube. Second stage, posterior fusion with segmental spinal instrumentation from third thoracic to sacral levels. *Left:* postoperative pelvic fixation. Pelvis level. Hips located. Sitting balance restored. Arrow indicates 'windshield-wiper' effect of rod in right side of pelvis due to some pelvic motion while consolidation of the spine fusion occurs.

segmental spinal instrumentation: in 49 with Harrington rods and 20 with Luque rods, neurological complications occurred in 17 per cent; 4 per cent had a major cord injury. In the 68 cases with only Harrington instrumentation and no segmental wiring, only one Brown-Sequard syndrome was reported. The minor sensory changes with segmental wiring had an incidence of 13 per cent and were transient.

Allen and Ferguson (1985) reviewed 507 cases of segmental spinal instrumentation with Luque rods, performed by 20 surgeons. The neurological complications were: two partial spinal-cord syndromes (0.4 per cent), 13 cases of truncal and limb hyperesthesia (2.6 per cent), and two other nerve injuries (0.4 per cent); one of these was a femoral neuropathy from the protruding pelvic rod, and recovery occurred later. Another 'nerve lesion' was in a patient with partial paralysis due to

468

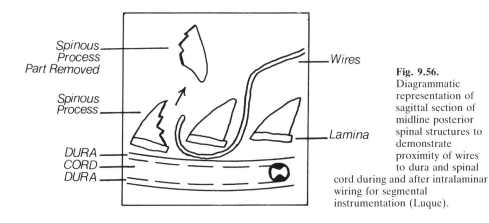

Spinous Process Part Removed

Spinous Process

Wires

DURA

CORD

DURA

Lamina

Fig. 9.56. Diagrammatic representation of sagittal section of midline posterior spinal structures to demonstrate proximity of wires to dura and spinal cord during and after intralaminar wiring for segmental instrumentation (Luque).

poliomyelitis preoperatively in one limb which was thought to be weaker after the surgery. Recovery was deemed to occur to the preoperative status in five months postoperative, and no sensory changes were ever found. The two spinal-cord lesions were both Brown-Sequard syndromes. One recovered competely and the other regained 90 per cent of her function. In this study no evidence was found to substantiate the canard of the need for a 'learning curve'.

The hyperesthesias after segmental spinal instrumentation in my patients were characterized by extreme skin tenderness over the anterior trunk and thighs. The cause remains obscure. Fortunately, all patients completely recovered from this distressing phenomenon within two weeks (our cases were part of the 1985 Allen and Ferguson study). Five of the 20 surgeons reported this complication. Biemond (1964) studied an autopsy of a patient who had this syndrome and found in the cervical cord a lesion of the posterior horns with perivascular bleeding and edema. A similar condition was described in association with cervical-spine trauma by Biemond (1964) and Braakman and Penning (1971). It was thought to be a result of trauma to the posterior spinal cord, but all patients recovered.

The animal experiments in which sublaminar wires were used and the spinal canal examined, revealing subdural hemorrhage and displacement of the posterior tracts and compression of the anterior tracts of the spinal cord, seem to confirm some of the neurological complications seen clinically (Liepones *et al.* 1984) (Fig. 9.56). How large these wires were in relationship to the spinal canal and lamina would need a more detailed study than reported in the abstract.

Nevertheless, the surgeon needs to have observed the technique before doing it, and exercise extreme caution and care when attempting to pass wires under the lamina (Yngve *et al.* 1986). Small-boned children perhaps should have 18-gauge wires, with the standard 16-gauge being reserved for those with larger skeletal structures. Epidural bleeding can possibly be diminished by keeping the wire tip tightly against the undersurface of the lamina when passing it through, and by gently packing the epidural fat area in the interspace with cellulose foam pads (Gelfoam) soaked in thrombin. When entering the epidural region between the spinous processes, the fat and vessels can be swept away with a fine Penfield probe;

469

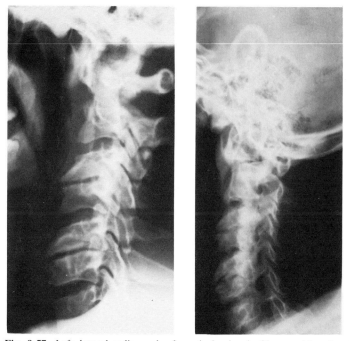

Fig. 9.57. *Left:* lateral radiograph of cervical spine in 31-year-old male with athetosis and constant rotation of head and neck to the left. Had gradual onset of weakness of left shoulder abduction. Extensive degenerative changes in intervertebral discs and in vertebral bodies. *Right:* oblique view cervical spine in same patient, marked narrowing of intervertebral foramina to almost complete occlusion. This explained the neuropathy which caused the progressive muscle weakness in the upper limb.

small up-biting rongeurs (Spurling or Cloward type) that are carefully inserted to rest tightly against the ligamentum flavum would be another precaution. Removing the ligamentum flavum in the thoracic and upper-lumbar region cannot be with the same bold technique used for excision of the herniated intervertebral disc in the lower-lumbar canal. If bleeding does occur, electrocoagulation and hemostats should on no account be used.

It is uncertain whether the administration of intravenous corticosteroids upon discovery of the hyperesthesia syndrome is effective in reducing its duration. I have the impression that doing so in decreasing doses over a five-day period reduces the very distressing symptoms to seven to 10 days rather than two to six weeks.

All of this discussion is not to suggest a return to the 'gold standard' of Harrington instrumentation in scoliosis and pelvic obliquity in the total body involved child. Some sort of segmental spinal instrumentation still remains the best method of management, when combined with the anterior discectomy and fusion as the first stage. Not all is solved, and we will await further developments in the technology while hoping for improvements in the biological approach to prevent cerebral palsy and the total body involved child, who needs our concern, care and help in the meantime.

Cervical spondylosis and myelopathies

In severe athetosis (of the tension type or mixed with spasticity), constant movement of the neck seems to play havoc with the cervical vertebrae and the intervertebral discs, eventually leading to foraminal occlusion or compression of the spinal cord. I have recently seen a 34-year-old female with severe athetosis who suddenly became quadriplegic at the fifth cervical level. She had evidence of subluxation of the fifth on the sixth cervical vertebrae, and a computerized axial tomogram combined with nitrizamide radiopaque dye in the canal showed atrophy of the spinal cord.

Another patient, a 31-year-old man, had severe athetosis and constant head-turning to the left. He had the slow onset of flaccid paralysis of his shoulder girdle musculature supplied by the fifth and sixth nerve roots. The radiographs of his cervical spine showed extensive degenerative changes and almost complete bony occlusions of the intervertebral foramina (Fig. 9.57).

McCluer (1982) reported four athetoid patients (ages 28, 41, 46 and 60 years) who had cervical spondylosis and a myelopathy. Two had an almost complete quadriplegia at the fifth cervical spinal-cord level. Three of these four patients had surgical decompressions of the cervical spinal cord with poor results. Angelini *et al.* (1982) had one case of cervical myelopathy in a child with torsion dystonia.

Whether such disasters can be prevented is moot. Even if one monitored the cervical spine anatomy regularly in these athetoid patients who have consistent head-turning, what could one do about it in the absence of neurological signs? Athetosis has become less prevalent as a motor defect in cerebral palsy: partly due to better obstetrics in preventing perinatal hypoxia, and because of the prevention of hemolytic anemia of the newborn and jaundice with early exchange transfusions and immunization against the Rh factor in the Rh-negative mother during pregnancy.

REFERENCES

Adler, N., Bleck, E. E., Rinsky, L. A., Young, W. (1986) 'Balance reactions and eye-hand coordination in idiopathic scoliosis.' *Journal of Orthopaedic Research,* **4,** 102–107.
Akeson, J., Bobechko, W. P. (1986) 'Treatment of scoliosis by instrumentation with double hook and posterior fusion.' *Orthopaedic Transactions,* **10,** 35.
Allen, B. L. Jr. (1979) *Personal communication.*
—— (1983) 'Spinal instrumentation, Part II. Segmental spinal instrumentation with L-rods.' *In: Instruction Course Lectures, American Academy of Orthopaedic Surgeons, Vol. 32.* St. Louis: C. V. Mosby.
—— Ferguson, R. L. (1981) 'The Galveston technique for L-rod instrumentation of the scoliotic spine.' *Spine,* **7,** 276–284.
—— —— (1982) 'L-rod instrumentation for scoliosis in cerebral palsy.' *Journal of Pediatric Orthopedics,* **2,** 87–96.
—— —— (1984) 'Basic considerations in pelvic fixation cases.' *In:* Luque, E. R. (Ed.) *Segmental Spinal Instrumentation.* Thorofare, New Jersey: Slack. pp. 185–220.
—— —— (1985) 'The Galveston technique of L-rod instrumentation—a second generation survey.' *Paper No. 13, read at Annual Meeting of the Pediatric Orthopaedic Society of North America, Boston.*
Alonso, J. E., Lovell, W. W., Lovejoy, J. F. (1986) 'The Altdorf hip clamp.' *Journal of Pediatric Orthopedics,* **6,** 339–402.

471

Angelini, L., Broggi, G., Nardocci, N., Savoiardo, M. (1982) 'Subacute cervical myelopathy in a child with cerebral palsy. Secondary to torsion dystonia?' *Child's Brain*, **9**, 354–357.

Arus, C., Barany, M., Westler, W. M., Markley, J. L. (1984) 'Proton nuclear magnetic resonance of human muscle extracts.' *Clinical Physiology and Biochemistry*, **2**, 49–55.

Ascani, E. (1985) *Personal communication.*

Bailey, T. E., Hall, J. E. (1985) 'Chiari medial displacement osteotomy.' *Journal of Pediatric Orthopedics*, **5**, 635–641.

Baker, L. D., Dodelin, R., Bassett, F. H. (1962) 'Pathologic changes in the hip in cerebral palsy: incidence, pathogenesis, and treatment.' *Journal of Bone and Joint Surgery*, **44A**, 1331–1342.

Balmer, G. A., MacEwen, G. D. (1970) 'The incidence of scoliosis in cerebral palsy.' *Journal of Bone and Joint Surgery*, **52B**, 134–136.

Banks, H. H., Green, W. T. (1960) 'Adductor myotomy and obturator neurectomy for correction of adduction of the hip in cerebral palsy.' *Journal of Bone and Joint Surgery*, **42A**, 111–126.

Barry, R. J., Staheli, L. T. (1986) 'Management of neuromuscular hip dysplasia by pericapsular osteotomy.' *Orthopaedic Transactions*, **10**, 149.

Beals, R. K. (1969) 'Developmental changes in the femur and acetabulum in spastic paraplegia and diplegia.' *Developmental Medicine and Child Neurology*, **11**, 303–313.

Behrooz, A., Akbania, M. D. (1984) 'Spinal deformity in patients with cerebral palsy.' *Orthopaedic Transactions*, **8**, 116.

Beintema, D. J. (1968) *A Neurological Study of Newborn Infants. Clinics in Developmental Medicine, No. 28.* London: S.I.M.P. with Heinemann.

Benson, M. K. D., Evans, D. C. J. (1976) 'The pelvic osteotomy of Chiari: an anatomical study of the hazards and misleading radiographic appearances.' *Journal of Bone and Joint Surgery*, **58B**, 164–168.

Biemond, A. (1964) 'Contusio cervicalis posterior.' *Nederlands Tijdschrift voor Geneeskunde*, **108**, 1333–1335.

Bleck, E. E. (1975) 'Deformities of the spine and pelvis in cerebral palsy.' *In:* Samilson, R. L. (Ed.) *Orthopaedic Aspects of Cerebral Palsy. Clinics in Developmental Medicine, Nos. 52/53.* London: S.I.M.P. with Heinemann; Philadelphia: J. B. Lippincott.

—— (1979) *Orthopaedic Management in Cerebral Palsy.* Philadelphia: W. B. Saunders.

—— (1980) 'The hip in cerebral palsy.' *Orthopaedic Clinics of North America*, **11**, 79–104.

—— Holstein, A. (1963) 'Iliopsoas tenotomy for spastic hip flexion deformities in cerebral palsy.' *Paper presented at Annual Meeting American Academy of Orthopaedic Surgeons, Chicago.*

—— Koehler, J. P., Dillingham, M., Trimble, S. (1976) 'Histochemical studies of thoracis spinalis and sacrospinalis muscles in scoliosis.' *American Academy of Neurology (Program Abstract).*

—— Terver, S., Wheeler, R., Csongradi, J., Rinsky, L. A. (1981) 'Joint laxity in children: statistical correlations with scoliosis, congenital dislocation of the hip and talipes equinovarus.' *Orthopaedic Transactions*, **5**, 5–6.

Bobath, K. (1966) *The Motor Deficit in Patients with Cerebral Palsy. Clinics in Developmental Medicine No. 23.* London: S.I.M.P. with Heinemann Medical; Philadelphia: J. B. Lippincott.

Bobechko, W. P., Herbert, M. A. (1986) 'Totally implantable stimulators for treatment of scoliosis in children with CP.' *Orthopaedic Transactions*, **10**, 156.

Bonnett, C., Perry, J., Brown, J. C., Greenberg, B. J. (1972) 'Halo-femoral distraction and posterior spine fusion for paralytic scoliosis.' *Journal of Bone and Joint Surgery*, **54A**, 202. (*Abstract*).

—— Brown, J. C., Brooks, H. L. (1973) 'Anterior spine fusion with Dwyer instrumentation for lumbar scoliosis in cerebral palsy.' *Journal of Bone and Joint Surgery*, **55A**, 425. (*Abstract*).

—— —— Perry, J., Nickel, V., Walinski, T., Brooks, H. L., Hoffer, M., Stiles, C., Brooks, R. (1975) 'The evolution of treatment of paralytic scoliosis at Rancho Los Amigos Hospital.' *Journal of Bone and Joint Surgery*, **57A**, 206–215.

—— —— Grow, T. (1976) 'Thoracolumbar scoliosis in cerebral palsy. Results of surgical treatment.' *Journal of Bone and Joint Surgery*, **58A**, 326–328.

Bowen, J. R., MacEwen, G. D., Mathews, P. A. (1981) 'Treatment of extension contracture of the hip in cerebral palsy.' *Developmental Medicine and Child Neurology*, **23**, 23–29.

Braakman, R., Penning, L. (1971) *Injuries of the Cervical Spine.* Amsterdam: Excerpta Medica. pp. 82–83.

Brown, J. S., Swank, S., Specht, L. (1982) 'Combined anterior and posterior spine fusion in cerebral palsy.' *Spine*, **7**, 570–573.

Brown, R. H., Nash, C. L. Jr., Berilla, J. A., Amaddio, M. D. (1984) 'Cortical evoked potential monitoring. A system for intraoperative monitoring of spinal cord function.' *Spine*, **9**, 256–261.

Bunch, W. H., Scarff, T. B., Trimble, J. (1983) 'Spinal cord monitoring.' *Journal of Bone and Joint*

Surgery, **65,** 707–710.

Bunnell, W. P. (1985) 'Varus derotational osteotomy of the hip in cerebral palsy.' *Orthopaedic Transactions,* **9,** 88.

—— MacEwen, G. D. (1977) 'Non-operative treatment of scoliosis in cerebral palsy: preliminary report on the use of a plastic jacket.' *Developmental Medicine and Child Neurology,* **19,** 45–49.

Bureau of Education for the Handicapped (1976) *Conference on Communication Aids for the Non-Vocal Severely Physically Handicapped Person, Alexandria, Virginia.*

Cady, R. B., Bobechko, W. P. (1984) 'Incidence, natural history and treatment of scoliosis in Friedreich's ataxia.' *Journal of Pediatric Orthopedics,* **4,** 673–676.

Canale, S. T., Hammond, N. L., Cotler, J. M., Sneddlen, H. E. (1975) 'Pelvic displacement osteotomy for chronic hip dislocation in myelodysplasia.' *Journal of Bone and Joint Surgery,* **57A,** 177–183.

Cardoso, A. (1984) 'Paralytic scoliosis.' *In:* Luque, E. R. (Ed.) *Segmental Spinal Instrumentation.* Thorofare, N. J.: Slack. pp. 119–146.

—— Tajonas, F. A., Luque, E. R. (1976) 'Osteotomias de columna, neuvos conceptos.' *Annals of Orthopaedic Trauma,* **12,** 105–113.

Castle, M. E., Schneider, C. (1978) 'Proximal femoral resection-interposition arthroplasty.' *Journal of Bone and Joint Surgery,* **60A,** 1051–1054.

Chiari, K. (1955) 'Ergebnisse mit der Beckenosteotomie als Pfannendachplastik.' *Zeitschrift für Orthopädie und ihre Grenzgebiete,* **87,** 14–26.

—— (1974) 'Medial displacement osteotomy of the pelvis.' *Clinical Orthopaedics and Related Research,* **98,** 55–71.

Cobb, J. R. (1952) 'Technique, after-treatment, and results of spine fusion in scoliosis.' *Instructional Course Lectures, Vol. 9.* Ann Arbor: J. W. Edwards. pp. 65–70.

Coleman, S. S. (1978) *Congenital Dysplasia and Dislocation of the Hip.* St. Louis: C. V. Mosby.

—— (1983) 'Reconstructive procedures in congenital dislocation of the hip.' *In:* McKibbin, B. (Ed.) *Recent Advances in Orthopaedics, No. 4.* Edinburgh: Churchill Livingstone. pp. 23–44.

Colton, C. L. (1972) 'Chiari osteotomy for acetabular dysplasia in young adults.' *Journal of Bone and Joint Surgery,* **54B,** 578–589.

Compere, E. L. (1932) 'Excision of hemivertebrae for correction of congenital scoliosis. Report of two cases.' *Journal of Bone and Joint Surgery,* **14,** 555–562.

Copeliovitch, Y., Mirovsky, N., Halperin, D., Hendel, D. (1983) 'Extension deformity of the hips with anterior subluxation of the head of the femur in cerebral palsy.' *Orthopaedic Transactions,* **7,** 557.

Cotrel, Y. (1975) 'Traction in the treatment of vertebral deformity.' *Journal of Bone and Joint Surgery,* **57B,** 260. *(Abstract).*

Crenshaw, A. H. (1963) *Campbell's Operative Orthopaedics.* St Louis: C. V. Mosby.

Cristofaro, R., Koffman, M., Woodward, R., Baxter, S. (1977) 'Treatment of the totally involved cerebral palsy problem sitter.' *Paper read at the Annual Meeting of the American Academy for Cerebral Palsy and Developmental Medicine, Atlanta.*

—— Taddonio, R. F., Gelb, R. (1985) 'The effect of correction of spinal deformity and pelvic obliquity on hip stability in neuromuscular disease.' *Orthopaedic Transactions,* **9,** 88.

D'Astous, J. L., Baxter, M. E. (1986) 'Proximal femoral resection-interposition arthroplasty-salvage hip surgery for the severely disabled child with cerebral palsy.' *Paper read at the Annual Meeting Pediatric Orthopedic Society of North America, Boston.*

Davis, J. B. (1954) 'The muscle-pedicle bone graft in hip fusion.' *Journal of Bone and Joint Surgery,* **33A,** 790–799.

DeWald, R. L., Ray, R. D. (1970) 'Skeletal traction for the treatment of scoliosis.' *Journal of Bone and Joint Surgery,* **52A,** 233–238.

Driscoll, D. M., Newton, R. A., Lamb, R. L., Nogi, J. (1984) 'A study of postural equilibrium in idiopathic scoliosis.' *Journal of Pediatric Orthopedics,* **4,** 677–681.

Drummond, D. S. (1984) 'The Wisconsin system: a technique of interspinous segmental spinal instrumentation.' *Contemporary Orthopaedics,* **8,** 29–37.

—— Rogala, E. J., Cruess, R., Moreau, J. (1979) 'The paralytic hip and pelvic obliquity in cerebral palsy and myelomeningocele.' *American Academy of Orthopaedic Surgeons Instructional Course Lectures,* **28,** 7–36.

Dubousset, J. (1985) 'Scolioses paralytiques et bassin oblique.' *In:* Dimeglio, A., Auriach, A., Simon, L. (Eds.) *L'Enfant Paralysé.* Paris: Masson. pp. 90–97.

—— Graf, H., Miladi, L., Cotrel, Y. (1986) 'Spinal and thoracic derotation with CD instrumentation.' *Orthopaedic Transactions,* **10,** 36.

Duval-Beaupère, G. (1970) 'Les repères de maturation dans la surveillance des scolioses.' *Revue de Chirurgie Orthopédique et Réparatrice de L'Appareil Locomoteur,* **56,** 59–76.

—— (1971) 'Pathogenic relationship between scoliosis and growth.' *In:* Zorab, P. A. (Ed.) *Scoliosis and Growth.* London: Churchill Livingstone.

—— Grossiord, A. (1967*a*) 'Les caractères évolutifs des scolioses polymyéliques; 207 cas de type respiratoire.' *Presse Médicale*, **75**, 2375–2380.

—— —— (1967*b*) 'Apport des scolioses polymyétiliques a l'étude des scolioses idiopathiques.' *Acta Orthopedica Belgica*, **33**, 575–586.

—— Dubousset, J., Queneau, P., Grossiord, A. (1970) 'Pour une théorie unique de l'évolution des scolioses.' *Presse Médicale*, **78**, 1141–1146.

—— Combes, J. (1971) 'Segments supérieur et inférieur au cours de la croissance physiologique des filles.' *Archives Françaises de Pédiatrie*, **28**, 1057–1070.

Dwyer, A. F., Newton, C., Sherwood, A. A. (1969) 'An anterior approach in scoliosis: a preliminary report.' *Clinical Orthopaedics and Related Research*, **62**, 192–202.

—— (1973) 'Experience of anterior correction of scoliosis.' *Clinical Orthopaedics and Related Research*, **93**, 191–206.

Eberle, D. F., Al-Saati, F., Al-Saudairy, M. (1986) 'Complications following segmental spinal instrumentation without fusion in management of paralytic scoliosis.' *Orthopaedic Transactions*, **10**, 17.

Eilert, R. E., MacEwen, G. D. (1977) 'Varus derotational osteotomy of the femur in cerebral palsy.' *Clinical Orthopaedics and Related Research*, **125**, 168–172.

Enneking, W. F., Harrington, P. (1969) 'Pathological changes in scoliosis.' *Journal of Bone and Joint Surgery*, **51A**, 165–184.

Eyre-Brook, A. L., Jones, D. A., Harris, F. C. (1978) 'Pemberton's iliac acetabuloplasty for congenital dislocation or subluxation of the hip.' *Journal of Bone and Joint Surgery*, **60B**, 18–24.

Farmer, T. W. (1964) *Pediatric Neurology.* New York: Hoeber.

Ferguson, A. B. (1973) 'Primary open reduction of congenital dislocation of the hip using a median adductor approach.' *Journal of Bone and Joint Surgery*, **55A**, 671–689.

—— (1975) *Orthopaedic Surgery in Infancy and Childhood.* Baltimore: Williams & Wilkins.

—— Allen, B. L. Jr. (1983) 'Staged correction of neuromuscular scoliosis.' *Journal of Pediatric Orthopedics*, **3**, 555–562.

Fettweis, E. (1979) 'Addukotrenspasmus, Praluxationen und Luxationen und den Huftgelenken bei spastisch gelähmten Kindern und Jugendlichen, klinische Beobachtungen zur Ätiologie, Pathogenese, Therapie und Rehabilitation. Part I.' *Zeitschrift für Orthopädie*, **117**, 39–49.

Fulford, G. E., Cairns, T. P., Sloan, Y. (1982) 'Sitting problems of children with cerebral palsy.' *Developmental Medicine and Child Neurology*, **24**, 48–53.

Gandy, D. J., Meyer, L. C. (1983) 'Long-term study of the dislocating hip in cerebral palsy.' *Orthopaedic Transactions*, **7**, 387.

Ginsberg, H. H., Shetter, A. G., Raudzens, P. A. (1985) 'Postoperative paraplegia with preserved intraoperative somatosensory evoked potentials.' *Journal of Neurosurgery*, **63**, 296–300.

Goldstein, L. A. (1959) 'Results in the treatment of scoliosis with turnbuckle plaster cast correction and fusion.' *Journal of Bone and Joint Surgery*, **41A**, 321–335.

—— (1969) 'Treatment of idiopathic scoliosis by Harrington instrumentation and fusion with fresh autogenous iliac bone grafts.' *Journal of Bone and Joint Surgery*, **51A**, 209–222.

Green, H. (1964) *I Never Promised You a Rose Garden.* New York: Holt, Rinehart, Winston.

Greene, W. (1985) 'Cary plate fixation for varus derotation femoral osteotomy in cerebral palsy.' *Paper read at Annual Meeting of American Academy for Cerebral Palsy and Developmental Medicine, Seattle.*

Gregorič, M., Pečak, F., Trontelj, J. V., Dimitrijevic, M. R. (1981) 'Postural control in scoliosis.' *Acta Orthopaedica Scandinavica*, **52**, 59–63.

Griffith, B., Donavan, M. M., Stephenson, C. T., Franklin, T. (1982) 'The adductor transfer and iliopsoas recession in the cerebral palsy hip.' *Orthopaedic Transactions*, **6**, 94–95.

Grogan, T. J., Krom, W., Oppenheim, W. L. (1986) 'The Chiari osteotomy for hip containment in cerebral palsy.' *Orthopaedic Transactions*, **10**, 143.

Gross, M. S., Ibrahim, K., Wehner, J., Dvonch, V. (1984) 'Combined surgical procedure for treatment of hip dislocation in cerebral palsy.' *Orthopaedic Transactions*, **8**, 113.

Guillot, M., Terver, S., Betrand, A., Vanneuville, G. (1977) 'Radiographie, electromyographie et approche functionnelle du muscle psoas-iliaque.' *Acta Anatomica*, **99**, 274. (*Abstract.*)

Gurd, A. R. (1984) 'Surgical correction of myodesis of the hip in C.P.' *Orthopaedic Transactions*, **8**, 112.

Hall, J. E. (1972) 'The anterior approach to spinal deformities.' *Orthopedic Clinics of North America*, **3**, 81–93.

474

—— (1981) *Personal communication.*

—— Gray, J., Allen, M. (1977) 'Dwyer instrumentation and spinal fusion: a follow-up study.' *Journal of Bone and Joint Surgery,* **59B,** 117. (*Abstract.*)

Harrington, P. (1962) 'Treatment of scoliosis. Correction and internal fixation by spinal instrumentation.' *Journal of Bone and Joint Surgery,* **44A,** 591–610.

Harris, N. H., Lloyd-Robert, G. C., Gallien, R. (1975) 'Acetabular development in congenital dislocation of the hip.' *Journal of Bone and Joint Surgery,* **57B,** 46–52.

Heinig, J. (1984) 'Eggshell procedure' *In:* Luque, E. R. (Ed.) *Segmental Spinal Instrumentation.* Thorofare, N.J.: Slack. pp. 221–234.

Herold, H. H., Daniel, D. (1979) 'Reduction of neglected congenital dislocation of the hip in children over the age of six years.' *Journal of Bone and Joint Surgery,* **61B,** 1–6.

Hibbs, R. A. (1924) 'A report of fifty-nine cases of scoliosis treated by the fusion operation.' *Journal of Bone and Joint Surgery,* **6,** 3–37.

Hirose, G., Kadoya, S. (1984) 'Cervical spondylotic radiculo-myelopathy in patients with athetoid-dystonic cerebral palsy: clinical evaluation and surgical treatment.' *Journal of Neurology, Neurosurgery, Psychiatry,* **47,** 775–780.

Hiroshima, K., Ono, K. (1979) 'Correlation between muscle shortening and derangement of hip joint in spastic cerebral palsy.' *Clinical Orthopaedics and Related Research,* **144,** 186–193.

Hodgson, A. R. (1968) 'Correction of fixed spinal curves.' *Journal of Bone and Joint Surgery,* **47A,** 1222–1227.

Hoffer, M. M. (1986) 'Management of the hip in cerebral palsy.' *Journal of Bone and Joint Surgery,* **68A,** 629–631.

—— Abraham, E., Nickel, V. (1972) 'Salvage surgery at the hip to improve sitting posture of mentally retarded, severely disabled children with cerebral palsy.' *Developmental Medicine and Child Neurology,* **14,** 51–55.

—— Bullock, M. (1981) 'The functional and social significance of orthopaedic rehabilitation of mentally retarded patients with cerebral palsy.' *Orthopedic Clinics of North America,* **12,** 185–191.

Hoffman, D. V., Simmons, E. H., Barrington, T. W. (1974) 'The results of the Chiari osteotomy.' *Clinical Orthopaedics and Related Research,* **98,** 162–170.

Holte, R., Siekman, A. (1983) *Fundamentals of Postural Seating. Special Bulletin of Rehabilitation Engineering Center.* Palo Alto, California: Children's Hospital at Stanford.

Hoppenfeld, S., Gross, A. M. (1986) 'Posterior rib resection in scoliosis surgery.' *Orthopaedic Transactions,* **10,** 27.

Horstmann, H. M. (1986) 'Skeletal maturation in cerebral palsy.' *Orthopaedic Transactions,* **10,** 152.

—— Boyer, B. (1984) 'Progression of scoliosis in cerebral palsy patients after skeletal maturity.' *Orthopaedic Transactions,* **8,** 116.

—— Rosabal, D. G. (1984) 'Varus derotation osteotomy.' *Orthopaedic Transactions,* **9,** 192.

Hosada, G. (1982) 'Push-film device.' *Special Project: Rehabilitation Engineering Intern.* Palo Alto, California: Children's Hospital at Stanford.

Houkom, J. A., Roach, J. W., Wenger, D. R., Speck, G., Herring, J. A., Norris, R. N. (1986) 'Treatment of acquired hip subluxation in cerebral palsy.' *Journal of Pediatric Orthopedics,* **6,** 285–290.

Howard, D. B., McKibbin, B., Williams, L. A., Mackie, I. (1985) 'Factors affecting the incidence of hip dislocation in cerebral palsy.' *Journal of Bone and Joint Surgery,* **67B,** 530–532.

Hsu, L. C. S., Zucherman, J., Tang, S. C., Leong, J. C. Y. (1982) 'Dwyer instrumentation in the treatment of adolescent idiopathic scoliosis.' *Journal of Bone and Joint Surgery,* **64B,** 536–541.

Ibrahim, K., Gross, M., Wehner, J. (1986) 'Combined procedure helps relieve pain in cerebral palsy patients.' *Orthopedics Today,* Sept. 4.

James, J. I. P. (1956) 'Paralytic scoliosis.' *Journal of Bone and Joint Surgery,* **38B,** 660–685.

—— (1967) *Scoliosis.* Edinburgh: E. & S. Livingstone. p. 145.

Johnson, J. T. H., Southwick, W. O. (1960) 'Bone growth after spine fusion.' *Journal of Bone and Joint Surgery,* **42A,** 1396–1412.

Johnson, J. R., Wingo, C. F., Holt, R. T., Leatherman, K. D. (1986) 'A preliminary report of 36 patients treated with the Cotrel-Dubousset procedure.' *Orthopaedic Transactions,* **10,** 36.

Jones, E. T. (1986) 'Adductor tendonotomy in cerebral palsy.' *Orthopaedic Transactions,* **10,** 142.

Kalen, V. (1985) *Personal communication.*

—— Gamble, J. G. (1984) 'Resection arthroplasty of the hip in paralytic dislocations.' *Developmental Medicine and Child Neurology,* **26,** 341–346.

—— Bleck, E. E. (1985) 'Prevention of spastic paralytic dislocation of the hip.' *Developmental Medicine and Child Neurology,* **27,** 17–24.

475

—— —— Rinsky, L. A. (1985) 'Preliminary results of Luque instrumentation in neuromuscular scoliosis.' *Orthopaedic Transactions*, **9**, 94–95.

Keats, S. (1970) *Operative Orthopaedics in Cerebral Palsy*. Springfield, Ill.: C. C. Thomas. p. 225.

—— Morgese, A. N. (1967) 'A simple anteromedial approach to the lesser trochanter of the femur for the release of the iliopsoas tendon.' *Journal of Bone and Joint Surgery*, **49A**, 632–636.

Keim, H. A., Hilal, S. K. (1971) 'Spinal angiography in scoliosis patients.' *Journal of Bone and Joint Surgery*, **53A**, 904–912.

Kleinman, R. G., Csongradi, J. J., Rinsky, L. A., Bleck, E. E. (1982) 'The radiographic assessment of spinal flexibility in scoliosis.' *Clinical Orthopaedics and Related Research*, **162**, 47–53.

Klisic, P. C., Jankovic, L. (1976) 'Combined procedure of open reduction and shortening of the femur in treatment of congenital dislocation of the hip in older children.' *Clinical Orthopaedics and Related Research*, **119**, 60–69.

Koffman, M. (1981) 'Proximal femoral resection or total joint replacement in severe disabled cerebral palsy spastic patients.' *Orthopedic Clinics of North America*, **12**, 91–100.

Langenskiold, A. (1971) 'Growth disturbance of muscle: a possible factor in the pathogenesis of scoliosis.' *In:* Zorab, P. A. (Ed.) *Scoliosis and Growth*. London: Churchill Livingstone. p. 85.

Larsen, L. (1971) *Lecture, Orthopaedic Grand Rounds, Stanford University School of Medicine, Stanford, California*.

Lau, J. H. K., Parker, J. C., Hsu, L. C. S., Leong, J. C. Y. (1986) 'Paralytic hip instability in poliomyelitis.' *Journal of Bone and Joint Surgery*, **68B**, 528–533.

Leatherman, K. C. (1969) 'Resection of vertebral bodies.' *Journal of Bone and Joint Surgery*, **51A**, 206. (*Abstract*.)

Le Foll, D. (1980) 'Contribution à l'étude de la luxation de la hanche chez l'infirme moteur d'origine cérébrale.' *Thèse pour le Doctorat en Médecine, Académie de Paris, Université René Descartes, Faculté de Médecine Chochin Port, France*.

—— Dubesset, J., Queneau, P. (1981) 'Les défauts de centrage de la tête fémorale chez l'infirme moteur d'origine cérébrale.' *Revue de Chirurgie Orthopédique*, **67**, 121–131.

Letts, R. M., Bobechko, W. P. (1974) 'Fusion of the scoliotic spine in young children.' *Clinical Orthopaedics and Related Research*, **101**, 136–145.

—— Shapiro, L., Mulder, K., Klasen, O. (1984) 'The windblown hip syndrome in total body cerebral palsy.' *Journal of Pediatric Orthopedics*, **4**, 55–62.

Liepones, J. V., Bunch, W. H., Lonser, R. E., Daley, R. L., Gogan, W. J. (1984) 'Spinal cord injury during segmental sublaminar spinal instrumentation: an animal model.' *Orthopaedic Transactions*, **8**, 173.

Liszka, O. (1961) 'Spinal cord mechanisms leading to scoliosis in animal experiments.' *Acta Medica Polonia*, **2**, 45–63.

Lonstein, J. E., Akbarnia, A. (1983) 'Operative treatment of spinal deformities in patients with cerebral palsy or mental retardation. An analysis of one hundred and seven cases.' *Journal of Bone and Joint Surgery*, **65A**, 43–55.

—— Carlson, J. M. (1984) 'The prediction of curve progression in untreated idiopathic scoliosis during growth.' *Journal of Bone and Joint Surgery*, **66A**, 1061–1071.

—— Beck, K. (1986) 'Hip dislocation and subluxation in cerebral palsy.' *Journal of Pediatric Orthopedics*, **6**, 521–526.

Luque, E. R. (1982) 'Segmental spinal instrumentation for correction of scoliosis.' *Clinical Orthopaedics and Related Research*, **163**, 192–198.

—— Cardoso, A. (1977) 'Segmental correction of scoliosis with rigid fixation. Preliminary report.' *Orthopaedic Transactions*, **1**, 136–137.

McCarthy, R. E., Peek, R. D., Morrissy, R. T. (1985) 'Allograft bone in spinal fusions for scoliosis.' *Orthopaedic Transactions*, **9**, 438.

McCluer, S. (1982) 'Cervical spondylosis with myelopathy as a complication of cerebral palsy.' *Paraplegia*, **20**, 308–312.

MacEwen, G. D. (1968) 'Experimental scoliosis.' *In:* Zorab, P. A. (Ed.) *Proceedings of a Second Symposium on Scoliosis: Causation*. Edinburgh: Churchill Livingstone. p.18.

—— (1969) 'The incidence and treatment of scoliosis in cerebral palsy.' *Paper Presented at Annual Meeting of American Academy for Cerebral Palsy, Miami Beach, Florida*.

—— (1972) 'Operative treatment of scoliosis in cerebral palsy.' *Reconstructive Surgery and Traumatology*, **13**, 58–67.

—— Bunnell, W. P., Sriram, M. (1975) 'Acute neurological complications in the treatment of scoliosis. A report of the Scoliosis Research Society.' *Journal of Bone and Joint Surgery*, **57A**, 404–408.

McIvor, W. C., Samilson, R. L. (1966) 'Fractures in patients with cerebral palsy.' *Journal of Bone and*

476

Joint Surgery, **48A,** 858–866.

McLuhan, M. (1964) *Understanding the Media: Extension of Man.* New York: McGraw.

McNaughton, S. (1975) 'Visual symbols: a system of communication for the nonverbal physically handicapped child.' *Regional Course, American Academy for Cerebral Palsy, Palo Alto, California.*

Madigan, R. R., Wallace, S. L. (1981) 'Scoliosis in the institutionalized cerebral palsy population.' *Spine,* **6,** 583–590.

—— —— (1986) 'Scoliosis in cerebral palsy: short term follow-up and prognosis in untreated institutionalized patients.' *Orthopaedic Transactions,* **10,** 17.

Malefijt, M. C., Dew, W., Hoogland, T., Nielsen, H. K. L. (1982) 'Chiari osteotomy in the treatment of congenital dislocation and subluxation of the hip.' *Journal of Bone and Joint Surgery,* **64A,** 996–1004.

Martin, J. P. (1965) 'Curvature of the spine in post-encephalitic Parkinsonism.' *Journal of Neurology, Neurosurgery and Psychiatry,* **28,** 395–400.

Mattson, G., Haderspeck-Grib, K., Schultz, A., Nachemson, A. (1983) 'Joint flexibilities in structurally normal girls and girls with idiopathic scoliosis.' *Journal of Orthopaedic Research,* **1,** 57–62.

Metz, P., Zielke, K. (1982) 'Erste Ergebnisse der Operation nach Luque. Voräufiger Bericht über 12 Fälle.' *Zeitschrift für Orthopädie,* **120,** 337–338.

Miller, G. R., Green, W. B. (1976) 'Preoperative predictability of Harrington rod correction for scoliosis: stretch x-ray technique.' *Scientific Exhibit, Annual Meeting American Academy of Orthopaedic Surgeons, New Orleans.*

Miranda, S. (1979) 'Outcomes of spastic diplegia.' *Unpublished study. Palo Alto, California: Children's Hospital at Stanford.*

Mitchell, G. P. (1974) 'Chiari medial displacement osteotomy.' *Clinical Orthopaedics and Related Research,* **98,** 146–150.

Moe, J. H. (1958) 'A critical analysis of methods of fusion for scoliosis. An evaluation in two hundred and sixty-six patients.' *Journal of Bone and Joint Surgery,* **40A,** 529–554.

—— Sundberg, A. B., Gustilo, R. (1964) 'A clinical study of spine fusion in the growing child.' *Journal of Bone and Joint Surgery,* **46B,** 784–785. *(Abstract.)*

—— Winter, R. B., Bradford, D. S., Lonstein, J. E. (1978) *Scoliosis and Other Spinal Deformities.* Philadelphia: W. B. Saunders.

Molloy, M. K. (1986) 'The unstable paralytic hip: treatment by combined pelvic and femoral osteotomy and transiliac psoas transfer.' *Journal of Pediatric Orthopedics,* **6,** 533–538.

Morigana, H. (1973) 'An electromyographic study on the function of the psoas major muscle.' *Journal of the Japanese Orthopaedic Association,* **47,** 351–365.

Moseley, C., Mosca, V., Lawton, L., Koreska, J. (1986) 'Improved stability in segmental instrumentation in neuromuscular scoliosis.' *Orthopaedic Transactions,* **10,** 5.

Motloch, W. (1978) 'Analysis of medical costs associated with healing of pressure sores in adolescent paraplegics.' *Thesis for Bachelor of Science Degree in Business Administration, University of San Francisco.*

Mowery, C. A., Houkom, J. A., Roach, J. W., Sutherland, D. H. (1986) 'A simple method of hip arthrodesis.' *Journal of Pediatric Orthopedics,* **6,** 7–10.

Murbarat, J. J., Mortensen, W., Katz, W. (1986) 'Combined pelvic (Dega) and femoral osteotomies in the treatment of paralytic hip dislocation.' *Developmental Medicine and Child Neurology* (Suppl. 53), **28,** 33–34. *(Abstract.)*

Murray, W. R., Lucas, D. B., Inman, V. T. (1964) 'Femoral head and neck resection.' *Journal of Bone and Joint Surgery,* **46A,** 1184–1197.

Nachemson, A. (1968) 'A long-term follow-up study of non-treated scoliosis.' *Acta Orthopaedica Scandinavica,* **39,** 466–476.

—— (1980) *Lectures, International Pediatric Orthopaedic Seminar, Chicago.*

Nickel, V. L., Perry, J., Garrett, A., Heppenstall, M. (1968) 'The halo, a spinal skeletal traction fixation device.' *Journal of Bone and Joint Surgery,* **50A,** 1400–1409.

O'Brien, J. P. (1977) 'The management of severe spinal deformities with the halo-pelvic apparatus; pitfalls and guidelines in its use.' *Journal of Bone and Joint Surgery,* **59B,** 117–118. *(Abstract.)*

—— Yau, A. C. M. C., Smith, T., Hodgson, A. R. (1971) 'Halo-pelvic traction.' *Journal of Bone and Joint Surgery,* **53B,** 217–229.

—— (1972) 'Anterior and posterior correction and fusion for paralytic scoliosis.' *Clinical Orthopaedics and Related Research,* **86,** 151–153.

O'Brien, J. J., Sirkin, R. B. (1977) 'The natural history of the dislocated hip in cerebral palsy.' *Paper presented at the Annual Meeting of the American Academy for Cerebral Palsy and Developmental Medicine, Atlanta.*

477

Oegema, T. R., Bradford, D. S., Cooper, K. M., Hunter, R. E. (1983) 'Comparison of the biochemistry of proteoglycans isolated from normal, idiopathic scoliotic and cerebral palsy spines.' *Spine,* **8,** 378–384.

Onimus, M., Vergnat, L. (1980) 'La médialisation du cotyle et les déplacements parasites dans l'ostéotomie pelvienne de Chiari.' *Revue de Chirurgie Orthopédique,* **66,** 299–309.

Parsch, V. K. (1985) 'Hanche et infirmité motrice cérébrale.' *In:* Dimeglio, A., Auriach, A., Simon, L. (Eds.) *L'Enfant Paralysé.* Paris: Masson.

Paul, I. T., Holte, R. N., VonKampen, E. (1980) 'Factors influencing design of modular inserts for disabled children.' *Proceedings of International Conference on Rehabilitation Engineering,* 161–162.

Pemberton, P. A. (1965) 'Pericapsular osteotomy of the ilium for treatment of congenital subluxation and dislocation of the hip.' *Journal of Bone and Joint Surgery,* **47A,** 65–86.

Peterson, L. T. (1950) 'Tenotomy in the treatment of spastic paraplegia with special reference to tenotomy of the iliopsoas.' *Journal of Bone and Joint Surgery,* **32A,** 875–885.

Phelps, W. M. (1959) 'Prevention of acquired dislocation of the hip in cerebral palsy.' *Journal of Bone and Joint Surgery,* **41A,** 440–448.

Ponseti, I. V., Friedman, B. (1950) 'Changes in the scoliotic spine after fusion.' *Journal of Bone and Joint Surgery,* **32A,** 381–395.

Pous, J. G. (1985) 'Cartilagenous iliac crest transfer to stabilize neurologic hip.' *Orthopaedic Transactions,* **9,** 192.

Propst-Proctor, S. L., Bleck, E. E. (1983) 'Radiographic determination of lordosis and kyphosis in normal and scoliotic children.' *Journal of Pediatric Orthopedics,* **3,** 344–346.

—— Rinsky, L. A., Bleck, E. E. (1983) 'The cisterna chyli in orthopaedic surgery.' *Spine,* **7,** 787–792.

Rab, G. T. (1978) 'Biomechanical aspects of Salter osteotomy.' *Clinical Orthopaedics and Related Research,* **132,** 82–87.

—— (1981*a*) 'Containment of the hip: a theoretical comparison of osteotomies.' *Clinical Orthopaedics and Related Research,* **154,** 191–196.

—— (1981*b*) 'Preoperative roentgenographic evaluation for osteotomies about the hip in children.' *Journal of Bone and Joint Surgery,* **63A,** 305–309.

Raih, T. J., Comfort, T. H., Beck, K. O., Vanden Brink, K. D. (1985) 'Proximal femoral resections in severe cerebral palsy.' *Orthopaedic Transactions,* **9,** 492.

Rang, M. (1986) *Course on Cerebral Palsy, Scottish Rite Children's Hospital, Atlanta, Georgia.*

—— Douglas, G., Bennet, G. D., Koreska, J. (1981) 'Seating for children with cerebral palsy.' *Journal of Pediatric Orthopedics,* **1,** 279–287.

—— Silver, R., de la Garza, J. (1986) 'Cerebral palsy.' *In:* Lovell, W. W., Winter, R. B. (Eds.) *Pediatric Orthopaedics, 2nd Edn.* Philadelphia: J. B. Lippincott.

Reimers, J. (1980) 'The stability of the hip in children. A radiological study of the results of muscle surgery in cerebral palsy.' *Acta Orthopaedica Scandinavica (Supplement),* **184,** 1–97.

—— Poulsen, S. (1984) 'Adductor transfer versus tenotomy for stability of the hip in spastic cerebral palsy.' *Journal of Pediatric Orthopedics,* **4,** 52–54.

Ring, N. O., Nelhman, L., Pearson, D. A. (1978) 'Molded supportive seating for the disabled.' *Prosthetics and Orthotics International,* **2,** 30–34.

Rinsky, L. A. (1981) *Personal communication.*

—— (1984) *Personal communication.*

—— Gamble, J. G., Bleck, E. E. (1985) 'Segmental instrumentation without fusion in children with progressive scoliosis.' *Journal of Pediatric Orthopedics,* **5,** 687–690.

Risser, J. C., Ferguson, A. B. (1936) 'Scoliosis: its prognosis.' *Journal of Bone and Joint Surgery,* **18,** 667–670.

—— Nordquist, D. M. (1958) 'A follow-up study of the treatment of scoliosis.' *Journal of Bone and Joint Surgery,* **40A,** 555–569.

Robson, P. (1968) 'The prevalence of scoliosis in adolescents and young adults with cerebral palsy.' *Developmental Medicine and Child Neurology,* **10,** 447–452.

Root, L. (1977*a*) 'The totally involved cerebral palsy patient.' *Instructional Course Lectures, Annual Meeting American Academy of Orthopaedic Surgeons, Las Vegas.*

—— (1977*b*) 'Total hip replacement in cerebral palsy.' *Paper Presented at the Annual Meeting of the American Academy for Cerebral Palsy and Developmental Medicine, Atlanta.*

—— (1982) 'Total hip replacement in young people with neurological disease.' *Developmental Medicine and Child Neurology,* **24,** 186–188. *(Annotation.)*

—— Broumann, S. N. (1985) 'Combined pelvic osteotomy with open reduction and femoral shortening for dislocated hips.' *Orthopaedic Transactions,* **9,** 942–943.

—— Goss, J. R., Mendes, J. (1986) 'The treatment of the painful hip in cerebral palsy by total hip replacement or hip arthrodesis.' *Journal of Bone and Joint Surgery,* **68A,** 590–598.

Rosenthal, D. K., Levine, D. D., McCarver, C. L. (1974) 'The occurrence of scoliosis in cerebral palsy.' *Developmental Medicine and Child Neurology,* **16,** 664–667.

Sahlstrand, T., Ortengren, R., Nachemson, A. (1978) 'Postural equilibrium in adolescent scoliosis.' *Acta Orthopaedica Scandinavica,* **49,** 354–365.

—— Lidström, J. (1980) 'Equilibrium factors as predictors of the prognosis in adolescent scoliosis.' *Clinical Orthopaedics and Related Research,* **152,** 232–236.

Salter, R. B. (1961) 'Innominate osteotomy in the treatment of congenital dislocation and subluxation of the hip.' *Journal of Bone and Joint Surgery,* **43B,** 518–539.

—— (1966) 'Role of innominate osteotomy in the treatment of congenital dislocation and subluxation of the hip in the older child.' *Journal of Bone and Joint Surgery,* **48A,** 1413–1439.

Salvati, E. A., Wilson, P. D. (1974) 'Treatment of irreducible hip subluxation by Chiari's iliac osteotomy.' *Clinical Orthopaedics and Related Research,* **98,** 151–161.

Samilson, R. L. (1970) *Personal communication.*

—— (1981) 'Orthopedic surgery of the hips and spine in retarded cerebral palsy patients.' *Orthopedic Clinics of North America,* **12,** 83–90.

Tsou, P., Aamoth, G., Green, W. M. (1972) 'Dislocation and subluxation of the hip in cerebral palsy.' *Journal of Bone and Joint Surgery,* **54A,** 863–873.

—— Bechard, R. (1973) 'Scoliosis in cerebral palsy.' *In:* Ahstrom, J. P. (Ed.) *Current Practice in Orthopaedic Surgery.* St. Louis: C. V. Mosby. p. 183.

Schultz, R. S., Chamberlain, S. E., Stevens, P. M. (1984) 'Radiographic comparison of adductor procedures in cerebral palsied hips.' *Journal of Pediatric Orthopedics,* **4,** 741–744.

Sharrard, W. J. W., Allen, J. M. H., Heaney, S. H., Prendiville, G. R. G. (1975) 'Surgical prophylaxis of subluxation and dislocation of the hip in cerebral palsy.' *Journal of Bone and Joint Surgery,* **57B,** 160–166.

—— Burke, J. (1982) 'Iliopsoas transfer in the management of established dislocation and refractory progressive subluxation of the hip in cerebral palsy.' *International Orthopaedics,* **6,** 149–154.

Sherk, H. H., Pasquariello, P. D., Doherty, J. (1983) 'Hip dislocation in cerebral palsy: selection for treatment.' *Developmental Medicine and Child Neurology,* **25,** 738–746.

Smith, W. S., Ireton, R. J., Coleman, C. R. (1958) 'Sequelae of experimental dislocation of a weight-bearing ball-and-socket joint in a young growing animal.' *Journal of Bone and Joint Surgery,* **40A,** 1121–1127.

Somerville, E. W. (1959) 'Paralytic dislocation of the hip.' *Journal of Bone and Joint Surgery,* **41B,** 279–288.

Sponseller, P. D., McBeath, A. A., Perpich, M. (1984) 'Hip arthrodesis in young patients. A long-term follow-up study.' *Journal of Bone and Joint Surgery,* **66A,** 853–859.

—— Whiffen, J. R., Drummond, D. S. (1986) 'Interspinous process segmental spinal instrumentation for scoliosis in cerebral palsy.' *Journal of Pediatric Orthopedics,* **6,** 559–563.

Stagnara, P. (1971) 'Traction cranienne par le 'Halo' de Rancho los Amigos.' *Revue de Chirurgie Orthopédique,* **57,** 287–300.

Staheli, L. T. (1981) 'Slotted acetabular augmentation.' *Journal of Pediatric Orthopaedics,* **1,** 321–327.

Stanitski, C. L., Micheli, L. J., Hall, J. E., Rosenthal, R. M. (1982) 'Surgical correction of spinal deformity in cerebral palsy.' *Spine,* **7,** 563–569.

Steeger, D., Wunderlich, T. (1982) 'Zur Problematik der Korrekturosteotmie am Hüftgelenk spastisch behinderter Kinder.' *Zeitschrift für Orthopädie,* **120,** 221–225.

Steel, H. H. (1977) 'Triple osteotomy of the innominate bone.' *Clinical Orthopaedics and Related Research,* **122,** 116–127.

Stephenson, C. T., Donavan, M. M. (1971) 'Transfer of hip adductor origins to the ischium in spastic cerebral palsy.' *Developmental Medicine and Child Neurology,* **13,** 247. *(Abstract.)*

Sutherland, D. H., Greenfield, R. (1977) 'Double innominate osteotomy.' *Journal of Bone and Joint Surgery,* **59A,** 1082–1091.

Suzuki, J., Inoue, S., Tsuji, K., Mitsuhasi, M. (1964) 'Studies on brain changes in scoliosis.' *Journal of the Chiba Medical Society,* **40,** 165.

Szalay, E. A., Roach, J. W. Houkom, J. A., Wenger, D. R., Herring, J. A. (1986*a*) 'Extension-abduction contracture of the spastic hip.' *Journal of Pediatric Orthopedics,* **6,** 1–6.

—— Carollo, J. J., Roach, J. W. (1986*b*) 'Sensitivity of spinal cord monitoring to intraoperative events.' *Journal of Pediatric Orthopedics,* **6,** 437–441.

Tanner, J. M. (1962) *Growth at Adolescence. 2nd Edn.* Oxford: Blackwell.

Tachdjian, M. O., Minear, W. L. (1956) 'Hip dislocation in cerebral palsy.' *Journal of Bone and Joint Surgery,* **38A,** 1358–1364.

479

Terazawa, K., Nasu, M., Takata, H., Watanabe, T., Hayshi, T. (1980) 'A case of severe scoliosis associated with cerebral palsy showing remarkable improvement following soft tissue release around the hip and axilla and transfer of the m.tensor fasciae latae to the ribs.' *International Orthopaedics*, **4**, 115–120.

Terver, S. (1981) *Personal communication.*

—— Kleinman, R., Bleck, E. E. (1980) 'Growth landmarks and the evolution of scoliosis: a review of pertinent studies on their usefulness.' *Developmental Medicine and Child Neurology*, **22**, 675–684.

Thompson, G. H., Wilber, R. G., Shaffer, P. V., Scoles, A., Kalamchi, A., Nash, C. L. F. Jr. (1985) 'Segmental spinal instrumentation in neuromuscular spinal deformities.' *Orthopaedic Transactions*, **9**, 485.

Trefler, E., Tooms, R. E., Hobson, D. A. (1978) 'Seating for cerebral palsied children.' *Interclinic Information Bulletin*, **17**, 1–8.

Tupman, G. S. (1962) 'A study of bone growth in normal children and its relationship to skeletal maturation.' *Journal of Bone and Joint Surgery*, **44B**, 42–67.

Tylowski, C. M., Rosenthal, R. K., Simon, S. R. (1980) 'Proximal femoral osteotomy in cerebral palsy.' *Clinical Orthopaedics and Related Research*, **151**, 183–192.

Uehara, A. (1986) *Personal communication.*

Uematsu, A., Bailey, H. C., Winter, W. G., Brouwer, T. D. (1977) 'Results of posterior iliopsoas transfer for hip instability caused by cerebral palsy.' *Clinical Orthopaedics and Related Research*, **126**, 183–189.

Vanderbrink, K. D., Beck, K. O., Comfort, T. H. (1984) 'Management of the hip in severe cerebral palsy.' *Orthopaedic Transactions*, **8**, 454.

Vauzelle, C., Stagnara, P., Jouvinroux, P. (1973) 'Functional monitoring of spinal cord activity during spinal surgery.' *Journal of Bone and Joint Surgery*, **55A**, 441. (*Abstract.*)

Vidal, M. (1982) *L'Infirme Moteur Cérébrale Spastique. Troubles Moteurs et Orthopédiques.* Paris: Masson.

Von Lackum, W. H., Smith, A.deF. (1933) 'Removal of vertebral bodies in the treatment of scoliosis.' *Surgery, Gynecology and Obstetrics*, **57**, 250–256.

Weinert, C., Ireland, M. L. (1985) 'Abduction osteotomy for the severely contracted hip in spastic quadriplegia—a new technique with rigid fixation using the compression hip screw system.' *Orthopaedic Transactions*, **9**, 101.

Weinstein, S. L., Zavala, D. C., Ponseti, I. V. (1981) 'Idiopathic scoliosis. Long term follow-up and prognosis in untreated patients.' *Journal of Bone and Joint Surgery*, **63A**, 702–711.

Wheeler, J. E., Weinstein, S. L. (1984) 'Adductor tenotomy–obturator neurectomy.' *Journal of Pediatric Orthopedics*, **4**, 48–51.

Wiberg, G. (1939) 'Studies on dysplastic acetabula and congenital subluxation of the hip joint with special reference to the complication of osteoarthritis.' *Acta Chirurgica Scaninavica*, **83**, Suppl. 58.

Wilber, R. G., Thompson, G. H., Shaffer, J. W., Brown, R. H., Nash, C. L. (1984) 'Postoperative neurological deficits in segmental spinal instrumentation.' *Journal of Bone and Joint Surgery*, **66A**, 1178–1187.

Wiles, P. (1951) 'Resection of dorsal vertebrae in congenital scoliosis.' *Journal of Bone and Joint Surgery*, **33A**, 151–154.

Winter, R. B. (1986) 'The spine in cerebral palsy.' *Lecture notes from Pediatric Orthopaedic Seminar, Fitzsimmons Army Hospital, Denver.*

—— Moe, J. H. (1982) 'The results of spine arthrodesis for congenital spinal deformity in patients younger than five years.' *Journal of Bone and Joint Surgery*, **64A**, 419–432.

Yamada, K., Ikata, T., Yamamoto, H., Nakagawra, Y., Tanaka, H., Tesuka, H. (1969) 'Equilibrium function in scoliosis and active corrective plaster jacket for the treatment.' *Yokushima Journal of Experimental Medicine*, **16**, 1–7.

Yngve, D. A., Burke, S. W., Price, C. A., Riddick, M. F. (1986) 'Technique. Sublaminar wiring.' *Journal of Pediatric Orthopedics*, **6**, 605–608.

Young, C. (1954) *Personal communication.*

Young, W. (1985) *Personal communication.*

Zaoussis, A. L., James, J. I. P. (1958) 'The iliac apophysis and the evolution of curves in scoliosis.' *Journal of Bone and Joint Surgery*, **40B**, 442–453.

Zielke, K. (1982) 'Ventrale Derotationspondylodese. Behandlungsergebnisse bei idiopathischen Lumbalskoliosen.' *Zeitschrift für Orthopädie*, **120**, 320–329.

Zimbler, S., Craig, C., Harris, J., Sohn, R., Rosenberg, G. (1985) 'Orthotic management of severe scoliosis in spastic neuromuscular disease—results of treatment.' *Orthopaedic Transactions*, **9**, 78.

Zuckerman, J. D., Staheli, L. T., McLaughlin, J. F. (1984) 'Augmentation for progressive hip subluxation in cerebral palsy.' *Journal of Pediatric Orthopedics*, **4**, 436–442.

APPENDIX

ABOUT X-RAYS IN CHILDREN*

Introduction

As parents and patients, we know you are interested in knowing the dangers associated with an x-ray examination. Today, we are more aware of potential health hazards to which we are exposed. Just how potentially harmful is the radiation to which we are exposed in an x-ray examination? And how does this exposure compare to that radiation which we encounter in merely living on this planet?

Natural everyday radiation

The average person in the United States receives about 200 *milliroentgens* of radiation per year. Half of this is derived from 'natural' background radiation. 'Natural' radiation includes such sources as cosmic rays and radioactivity in rocks and building materials. The living organisms of this planet have been exposed continuously to these sources since life began. There is no practical way to avoid such exposure.

Risk and benefits of x-rays

What are the risks of radiation exposure? It must be emphasized that we are dealing with statistical probabilities; quantitative assessment of *risk* cannot readily be applied to a given individual and a particular x-ray examination. An x-ray examination of the chest gives an exposure equivalent to a whole body dose of about 10 milliroentgens. This is equivalent to the cosmic ray exposure (i) from traveling across this country four times by jet airplane, or (ii) from living in Denver, Colorado, for two months[1]. The risk of cancer from any of the common x-ray examinations done here at Children's Hospital is less than one chance in 50,000[2]. For children, our calculations suggests a maximum leukemia risk of one in 750,000 from age 0 to 9 years. Because the benefit from proper diagnosis is usually much larger, no law limits the radiation dose to a patient for their own medically prescribed x-rays. However for sake of comparison, a member of the public may legally be exposed to 500 milliroentgens per year as a by-product of others' use of radiation.

*Reprinted by permission of the authors: S. L. Propst-Proctor MD (Fellow, Pediatric Orthopaedic and Rehabilitation Services), Roland Finston PhD (Director, Health Physics Office), Johnny Payne (Chief Technologist, Department of Radiology), Colleen Murphy Wynne RN (Head Nurse, Orthopaedic Service), Eugene E. Bleck MD (Professor, Orthopaedic and Surgery), Children's Hospital at Stanford and Department of Surgery, Orthopaedic Division, Stanford University School of Medicine.

Table 1A: Extremities

Patient age	1 year	5 years	15 years
Foot (AP[1] & Lat[2])	8*	13	27
Ankle (3-way)	10	20	34
Tibia (AP & Lat)	12	19	38
Knee (AP & Lat)	45	78	363
(Notch)	24	52	213
(Patellar)	6	14	21
Femur (AP & Lat)	25	45	191
Hand (AP & Lat)	9	15	21
Wrist (AP & Lat)	14	23	32
Forearm (AP & Lat)	14	18	32
Humerus: (AP & Lat)	14	20	40
Shoulder: (AP & oblique)	68	190	410

Table 1B: Spine and pelvis

Patient age	1 year	5 years	15 years
Pelvis (AP[1])	30*	52	136
(Lat[2])	26	47	164
Cervical spine			
(AP & Lat)	60	120	222
(Obliques)	58	122	222
Thoracic spine			
(AP & Lat)	180	270	541
Lumbar spine			
(AP & Lat)	124	410	954
Lumbar spot	133	380	870
Scoliosis (AP)	26	54	106

Table 1C: Other X-rays

Patient age	1 year	5 years	15 years
Bone age	9*	15	21
Scanograms of lower extremities	59	122	411
Entire lower extremities	27	69	381
Femoral anteversion	110	182	942
Skull			
(AP[1] & Lat[2])	417	565	1141
(Towne's view)	208	243	605
Abdomen			
(AP)	30	47	135
(Upright)	34	61	177
Chest			
(PA[3] & Lat)	11	12	26

* Milliroentgen
[1] anterior-posterior
[2] lateral
[3] posterior-anterior

Why are x-rays necessary?

There is always a risk, albeit small, associated with any radiation exposure. The risk must be weighed against the benefit that can be obtained by taking the x-ray picture. It is necessary for the Orthopaedic Surgeon to visualize bone and joints and this can only be done by utilizing x-rays. To detect progression of a scoliotic curve of the spine, healing of a broken bone, presence of a tumor or infection, or abnormality of limb from birth, the doctor must order x-rays.

Protection

One way of protecting parts of the body that are at most risk is to shield or cover that area. For *shielding*, a lead or lead-equivalent barrier is placed between the x-ray beam and a part of the body. The gonads (ovaries in females and testes in males) are routinely shielded so long as this shield does not interfere with obtaining the diagnostic information. Breasts of female patients, whenever possible, are shielded during the taking of spine films.

Definitions

A REM is a *unit of measurement of dose equivalent* that takes into consideration the biological effectiveness of the radiation. It is a means of comparing various sources of radiation exposure to one another.

A RAD is the *unit of absorbed dose*. One rad is the dose when any ionizing radiation deposits 100ergs per gram in any material. One rad is usually equivalent to one roentgen in soft tissue. One rad from X-RAYS is also equal to one rem.

A ROENTGEN is the *unit of exposure* in which the amount of x-ray or gamma radiation will produce 1 esu of charge per cc of air under standard conditions. A MILLIROTENTGEN is one thousandth of a roentgen.

X-RAYS, like gamma rays, are part of the electromagnetic energy spectrum which also includes radio waves, visible light, and ultra-violet light. x-rays have high energies and short wavelengths and readily penetrate matter.

Radiation doses

The following figures represent the total radiation doses for a single set of x-rays. *Skin and bone marrow* doses have been measured for x-ray studies commonly obtained for patients of the Pediatric Orthopaedic Service at Children's Hospital at Stanford.

Skin exposure (Tables 1A, 1B and 1C)

Skin exposures are measured using dosimeters that can be applied directly on the skin where the beam enters the body. The unit of measurement is the *milliroentgen*.

Active bone marrow dose (Tables 2A, 2B and 2C)

Active bone marrow doses are calculated from data obtained by skin monitors because directly measuring the dose received by the internal organs or bone marrow, would require invasive monitoring devices[3,4,5]. The values for active bone marrow doses are considerably smaller than the entrance skin exposures, as only a fraction of the marrow is within the direct beam of radiation in any single x-ray.

The dose to the bone marrow is chosen as a measurement because bone marrow tissue is widely distributed and thus is representative of the overall dose/risk of each x-ray examination. The lifetime risk of leukemia (a bone marrow cancer) for children from birth to 9 years is 4/100,000,000 for each millirad of bone marrow dose. For children from the age of 10 to 19, the risk is 2/100,000,000[5]. Active bone marrow doses are measured in *millirads*.

Table 2A: Extremities

Patient age	1 year	5 years	15 years
Foot (AP[1] & Lat[2])	*	*	*
Ankle (3-way)	*	*	*
Tibia (AP & Lat)	*	*	*
Knee (AP & Lat)	*	2+	*
(Notch)	*	1	*
(Patellar)	*	*	*
Femur (AP & Lat)	2	4	2
Hand (AP & Lat)	*	*	*
Wrist (AP & Lat)	*	*	*
Forearm (AP & Lat)	*	*	*
Humerus (AP & Lat)	*	*	*
Shoulder (AP & oblique)	6	10	4

Table 2B: Spine and pelvis

Patient age	1 year	5 years	15 years
Pelvis			
(AP)	3+	4	6
(Lat)	2	2	10
Cervical spine			
(AP[1] & Lat[2])	2	4	3
(Obliques)	1	2	2
Thoracic spine			
(AP & Lat)	24	33	17
Lumbar spine			
(AP & Lat)	17	25	39
Scoliosis			
(AP)	3	6	12

+ Millirads
[1]anterior-posterior
[2]lateral
* No measurable dose

484

Table 2C: Other X-rays

Patient age	1 year	5 years	15 years
Bone age	*	*	*
Scanograms of lower extremities	4+	5	3
Entire lower extremities (AP)	2	7	2
Femoral anteversion	8	14	7
Skull			
(AP[1] & Lat[2])	16	20	32
(Towne's view)	8	10	20
Abdomen			
(AP)	3	4	7
(Upright)	3	5	5
Chest			
(PA[3] & Lat)	2	2	2

+ Millirads
[1]anterior-posterior
[2]lateral
[3]posterior-anterior
* No measurable dose

REFERENCES

1. *Natural Background Radiation in the United States.* Washington, D.C.: National Council on Radiation
   Protection and Measurements, NCRP No. 45, 1975.
2. Laws, P. W., Rosenstein, M. (1978) 'A somatic dose index for diagnostic radiology.' *Health Physics*, **35**, 629–642.
3. Rosenstein, M., Beck, T. J., Warner G. G. (1979) *Handbook of Selected Organ Doses for Projections Common in Pediatric Radiology,* Rockville, MD.: U.S. Dept. of Health, Education, and Welfare, Publication (FDA) 79–8079.
4. Rosenstein, M. (1976) *Handbook of Selected Organ Doses for Projections Common in Diagnostic Radiology,* Rockville, MD.: U.S. Dept. of Health, Education and Welfare, Publication (FDA) 76–8031.
5. National Academy of Science, The Effects of Populations of Exposure to Low Levels of Ionizing Radiation, Washington, D.C., Committee on the Biological Effects of Ionizing Radiations, 1980.

485

INDEX

486

490

493

Triradiate cartilage, growth arrest of 423
Truncal sway 33
Two-point discrimination test (Moberg's) 47

U

Ulna, posterior bowing 134
Upper limb
 assessment 41–7
 structural changes 134
Upper limb surgery 214–40
 hand *see* Hand

V

Valium (diazepam) 197 (table), 197
Varus derotation subtrochanteric osteotomy 422
Vastus intermedius muscle 296
Vastus lateralis muscle 296
Vastus medialis muscle 296
Vein of Galen, tearing of 126–7
Vestibular reflexes 112
Vestibular stimulation
 cerebral palsy 164
 Down's syndrome 164
Vestibular system 112–13
 neuronitis 112
 weightlessness effect 113
Vestibulo-ocular system 112
Videotape recording 72
Visual cortex, spines on apical dendrites 114–15
Visual defect 41
Visual-motor tests 67–8
Voice, synthetic 185
Vojta method of physical therapy 151, 155–6, 158, 165–6

Volar capsulodesis 237
V-type osteotomies, Swanson's 266

W

Walkers 172–3
 steerable 186
 weight-relieving 173, 174 (fig.)
Walking 33–40, 142–3, 146
 ability 143
 age of 122–3
 mental retardation effect 124
 motor quotient 123–4
 prognosis tests 121–2
 severity index 124
 see also Gait
Walking aids 172–4
Weight-bearing radiograph of child's foot 264 (fig.)
Wheelchair 186–8
 cost 189
 electric 187 (fig.), 188
 simple materials 147 (fig.)
'Windblown' ('windswept') posture 395, 396 (fig.)
Winter sports 169
Wrist arthrodesis 235–6
Wrist-flexion deformities 233
 tendon lengthening 233–5
 postoperative care of tendon lengthenings/ transfers 235

X

X-ray examination in childhood 481–5
 active bone marrow dose 484